Shawn M. Talbott, PhD

A Guide to Understanding
Dietary Supplements

Pre-publication
REVIEWS,
COMMENTARIES,
EVALUATIONS . . .

D0226287

"Finally, the truth about dietary supplements! No hype, no innuendos, no falsehoods, no slander—just the facts!

Dr. Talbott's book cuts through common fallacies, inaccuracies, and ignorance to deliver the most accurate and even-handed review on all aspects of dietary supplements available. I have frequently been asked if there is a book that explains all about dietary supplements and how to use them. Until this book, I was not satisfied with anything out there. This book is it!

The book describes how dietary supplements are regulated and how the dietary supplement industry really operates. This is the reality consumers are not getting from the media, their doctors, the government, or even the industry itself. It provides just the right balance between delivering enough facts to cover all the important points about dietary supplements without bogging down in minutiae. You will understand dietary supplements after reading this book!

A Guide to Understanding Dietary Supplements is a valuable resource. It will stand as the definitive comprehensive review on dietary supplements for many years."

Luke R. Bucci, PhD
Vice President, Research,
Weider Nutrition International,
Salt Lake City, UT

"*A Guide to Understanding Dietary Supplements* provides a contemporary perspective on the value of dietary supplements. Most chapters begin with a discussion of healthful lifestyle behaviors that may elicit the most benefits for a specific performance or health condition, followed by a discussion of dietary supplements that may also be helpful. The book explains the complexities of the Dietary Supplement Health and Education Act, and provides a detailed view of the process for developing and marketing a new dietary supplement along with the different types of research that may be used to support product claims.

The book focuses on more than 130 different individual dietary supplements, including vitamins, minerals, amino acids, herbals, and other constituents, which are evaluated in regard to their effect on fourteen performance or health conditions. Dr. Talbott presents both the pros and cons of using each specific supplement. Of particular value to the reader is the Master Supplement Chart, highlighting which supplements may be used for specific performance or health conditions. This book may be helpful to dietitians, nutrition educators, and other health professionals, and consumers with a science background."

Melvin H. Williams, PhD, FACSM
Eminent Scholar Emeritus,
Department of Exercise Science,
Old Dominion University,
Norfolk, VA

❧

"This book is one of the most thorough, informative, up-to-date, and objective reviews of dietary supplements that is available. I was quite impressed by the author's objectivity and clarity of writing in an arena that can be very confusing. Talbott is relatively unbiased in his evaluation of the Dietary Supplement Act, the process of substantiation of claims, and his evaluation of the claims of the various supplements. His approach is science-based and objective.

The audience interested in the efficacy of dietary supplements is quite diverse, ranging from the evangelist to the scientist, so it is no wonder that one book might not be expected to please all. This book may come close, due to the author's objectivity and willingness to consider and discuss both traditional claims and folklore as well as published scientific evidence, both with animal models and human clinical trials.

Talbott's overview of the dietary supplement industry and the Dietary Supplement Health Education Act is particularly helpful in gaining an understanding of this topic. This is a very complex topic because it is a mixture of politics, economics, and science, which tends to polarize different groups of people depending upon their particular interests. Talbott's background as a nutritionist and nationally known scientist, and his experience in both education and industry, gives him a unique perspective in addressing this topic.

A particularly useful aspect of the book is its organization into chapters based upon the particular application of the dietary supplement. I believe this text will find useful application in college-level nutrition instruction and will be a valuable reference text for dietitians, pharmacists, pharmacologists, physiologists, physicians, and other health care professionals."

E. W. Askew, PhD
Professor and Director,
Division of Foods and Nutrition,
University of Utah, Salt Lake City

The Haworth Press®
New York • London • Oxford

A Guide to Understanding Dietary Supplements

THE HAWORTH PRESS
Nutrition, Exercise, Sports, and Health
Robert E. C. Wildman, PhD, RD, LD
Senior Editor

The Nutritionist: Food, Nutrition, and Optimal Health by Robert Wildman

A Guide to Understanding Dietary Supplements by Shawn M. Talbott

Fragments: Coping with Attention Deficit Disorder by Amy Stein

A Guide to Understanding Dietary Supplements

Shawn M. Talbott, PhD

The Haworth Press®
New York • London • Oxford

The Haworth Press, Inc., 10 Alice Street, Binghamton, NY 13904-1580.

PUBLISHER'S NOTE
The development, preparation, and publication of this work has been undertaken with great care. However, the publisher, employees, editors, and agents of The Haworth Press are not responsible for any errors contained herein or for consequences that may ensue from use of materials or information contained in this work. The opinions expressed by the author(s) are not necessarily those of The Haworth Press, Inc.

Pencil drawings copyright © Elizabeth Russell.

Cover design by Marylouise E. Doyle.

Library of Congress Cataloging-in-Publication Data

Talbott, Shawn M.
    A guide to understanding dietary supplements / Shawn M. Talbott.
        p. cm.
    Includes bibliographical references and index.
    ISBN 0-7890-1455-6 (hard : alk. paper)—ISBN 0-7890-1456-4 (soft : alk. paper)
    1. Dietary supplements. 2. Dietary supplements industry. I. Title.

RM258.5 .T354 2002
615.1—dc21

2002068770

CONTENTS

Chapter 6. Supplements for Boosting Energy Levels   181

Chapter 7. Supplements for Bone Health   217

ABOUT THE AUTHOR

Dr. Shawn Talbott received his master's degree in exercise physiology from the University of Massachusetts in Amherst and his PhD in nutritional biochemistry from Rutgers University in New Jersey, where his research focused on sports nutrition, human performance, bone metabolism, and weight loss issues. He has received several competitive research awards and has published more than 100 articles on nutrition, health, and fitness. An accomplished athlete, Dr. Talbott has competed at the national and international levels in rowing, cycling, and triathlons.

Dr. Talbott has held positions in product development, strategic marketing, and consulting in the food, wellness, and dietary supplement industries, and serves as an advisor to numerous nutrition journals/magazines, health-oriented Web sites, and athletic organizations. He is currently Adjunct Assistant Professor in the Department of Nutrition at the University of Utah in Salt Lake City, and holds the position of Senior Scientist in New Product Development and Nutrition Research at Pharmanex.

Foreword

To supplement or not to supplement . . . that is the question. This restatement of Hamlet's moral and philosophical dilemma continues to perplex thousands, perhaps even millions of individuals trying to determine whether or not nutritional supplementation is right for them.

Now, with the publication of *A Guide to Understanding Dietary Supplements,* Dr. Shawn Talbott has provided an important contribution and useful information to help people make an informed decision concerning nutritional supplements and health.

By any criteria, supplements are a big business. Over half of the adult population in the United States consumes a least one dietary supplement on a regular basis. The marketplace for supplements exceeds 16 billion dollars each year in the United States alone (more than is spent on all of primary care medicine) and is growing at a rate of greater than 10 percent per year. Like it or not, supplements are here to stay. The American public has clearly voted with its feet.

Why have nutritional supplements become so popular? Probably for many reasons. As Dr. Talbott points out in this book, 80 percent of Americans feel that they do not receive adequate levels of vitamins and minerals in their diets. To a large degree they are probably correct. Less than 1 percent of adults in the United States population consume the recommended five servings of fruits and vegetables on a daily basis.

At their best, nutritional supplements can contribute to a positive lifestyle and good health. When consumed in conjunction with regular exercise, proper nutrition, and attention to weight management, supplements may further enhance disease prevention and risk factor reduction. There has been an explosion of well-conducted research trials in the past decade linking various nutritional practices, including the consumption of some supplements and improved health outcomes. Furthermore, as the population in the United States and other industrialized countries continues to grow older, the desire to take proactive steps to improve lifestyle and lower the risk of chronic disease has become even stronger.

But are all of those individuals who feel they are improving their health by taking supplements actually correct? Are some supplements better than others? Are some supplements potentially dangerous? Sorting through the vast field of supplements containing literally thousands of products is a daunting task even for the most committed and curious consumer. The best hope for achieving positive outcomes by adding supplements to the diet can only come if consumers (and health care professionals) become more educated in the whole area of supplementation.

For all of these reasons, this book is a welcome addition to the educational process concerning supplements. The book is authoritative and exhaustive. It is loaded with worthwhile information presented in a user-friendly and non-biased manner. The author is well qualified to write on this topic by virtue of his doctorate in nutritional biochemistry, as well as his years of practical experience in both the food and supplement industries.

Dr. Talbott's book comes at a very important time when many individuals are trying to determine whether or not taking supplements is the right choice for them. It also comes at a time when important new science is being discovered on a daily basis in the areas of nutritional supplementation and good health. I believe this book will serve as a valuable guide both to consumers and health care professionals and will clear up much confusion about which supplements are beneficial, which are possibly beneficial and which are either of questionable value or even dangerous. To his credit, Dr. Talbott does not attempt to answer the question of whether or not to supplement. What he does do, however, is provide an excellent framework for each consumer to make an informed decision.

James M. Rippe, MD
Founder and Director, Rippe Lifestyle Institute
Rippe Health Assessment
at Florida Hospital Celebration Health

Foreword

The dietary supplement industry is a multibillion-dollar business, marketing products designed mainly to enhance health and performance. Advertisements and supplement labels make claims such as *rapid weight loss, higher energy levels,* or *improved heart health,* and such claims entice 40 percent of Americans or more to use dietary supplements on a regular basis. In the 1990s information about the research base supporting dietary supplement claims was not readily accessible to health professionals and consumers, but that is changing in this new millennium with the publication of scientific books evaluating the efficacy and safety of dietary supplements.

A Guide to Understanding Dietary Supplements by Shawn M. Talbott, PhD, provides a contemporary, balanced perspective on the value of dietary supplements. Dr. Talbott clearly notes that a dietary supplement, as defined, is simply a product used to *supplement* the diet, not *replace* it. Indeed, most chapters begin with a discussion of healthful lifestyle behaviors, particularly nutritional and exercise behaviors, that may elicit the most benefits for a specific performance or health condition, which is followed by a discussion of dietary supplements that also may be helpful.

Dr. Talbott explains the complexities of the Dietary Supplement Health and Education Act (DSHEA) and provides a detailed overview of the process for developing and marketing a new dietary supplement, along with the different types of research that may be used to support product claims for performance and health and for safety. Overall, these introductory chapters provide the reader with an understanding of why the public is often confused regarding the use of dietary supplements. The heart of the book focuses on more than 130 different individual dietary supplements, including vitamins, minerals, amino acids, herbals, and other constituents, which are evaluated in regard to their effect on fourteen performance or health conditions, such as weight control, sports performance, brain function, heart health, immune function, and bone and joint health. Each individual supplement is defined chemically, and then discussed in terms of product claims, theory underlying its use, scientific support for its efficacy and safety, appropriate dosage, and its overall value. Of particular value to the reader is a Dietary Supplement Master Chart, highlighting which supplements may be used for specific performance or health conditions.

Based on the totality of available scientific evidence, which is substantial for some supplements but rather limited for others, Dr. Talbott presents both the pros and cons of using each specific supplement. In other words, does it work and is it safe? Dietary supplements are not *magic bullets,* but neither are they necessarily *modern snake oil* as some dietary supplements, if used judiciously, may be helpful as a means to enhance performance or health in certain individuals.

Dietitians and other health professionals who provide advice on dietary supplements will find this book an excellent addition to their library.

Melvin H. Williams, PhD, FACSM
Eminent Scholar Emeritus
Department of Exercise Science
Old Dominion University
Norfolk, VA

Preface

Widespread Use of Supplements

At no other time in our history has the public interest in self-care and the use of "natural" health remedies been so widespread. According to several public health surveys, as much as 50 to 60 percent of the American adult population consumes a dietary supplement on a regular basis. The reasons for the widespread use of supplements are addressed in other parts of this book, but it is abundantly clear that using dietary supplements to promote health and reduce disease is here to stay.

Widespread Confusion

Unfortunately, right along with the enthusiastic public acceptance of dietary supplements has also come a great deal of confusion. The dizzying array of product claims, marketing pitches, and late-night testimonials is understandably bewildering to consumers, health professionals, and even nutritionists and dieticians. In many cases, a substantial percentage of potential supplement users (people who might have benefited from a judicious use of supplements) have instead become so confused that they've decided to forgo supplement usage at all.

This is unfortunate because, for many people, the regular use of certain nutritional supplements can be a cost-effective strategy for both promoting short-term health and reducing longer-term disease risks. A large and growing body of scientific evidence exists to show a clear health benefit of certain dietary supplements, such as calcium and vitamin D for bone health, folic acid for preventing neural tube defects, and B-complex vitamins for reducing the risk of heart disease. However, the relationship between other dietary supplements and purported health benefits is less clear, such as the equivocal evidence for the effects of vitamin E and fiber in preventing heart disease and colon cancer, respectively. Likewise, the scientific evidence is conflicting on the potential role of antioxidant nutrients such as vitamin C, selenium, and beta-carotene in the prevention of certain cancers and in slowing the very process of aging itself.

Reasons for the Confusion

The vast majority of American consumers, as much as 80 percent of the population, feel that they do not consume adequate levels of vitamins and minerals in their diets. National nutrition surveys tend to support this perception, with U.S. Department of Agriculture (USDA) statistics indicating that less than 1 percent of U.S. adults regularly consume five or more servings of fruits and vegetables daily and more than 70 percent of the population fails to achieve even RDA levels for many vitamins and minerals. National and regional surveys clearly indicate that millions of American consumers are using dietary supplements on a regular basis. When queried regarding their reasons for selecting a particular supplement, however, responses tend to gravitate toward the more general benefits, such as "for more energy" or "as nutritional insurance," rather than for specific health concerns.

Over the past three decades, there has been an explosion in the amount of scientific evidence linking nutrition and health. Unfortunately, the sheer amount of nutrition information and the conflicting health messages that are generated in response to each new study serve only to compound the confusion faced by consumers. In 1994, the Dietary Supplement Health and Education Act (DSHEA) established a framework for the U.S. regulation of dietary supplements. Depending on your perspective, DSHEA is either good because it enables the delivery of information to consumers that enables them to make their own decisions about supplements, or it is bad because it permits manufacturers and marketers to make unsubstantiated claims for particular ingredients based on their "structure" or "function" in the body (e.g., glucosamine for joints or amino acids for muscle building). The reality is that DSHEA is neither good nor bad and consumers need to have at least a superficial understanding of the law in order to fully appreciate and evaluate the claims made for various supplements. For example, the types of structure/function claims permitted by DSHEA require little to no actual research—and a good biochemistry text is the only tool needed for generating many claims.

Finally, the popular press has perpetuated a common public misconception that the dietary supplement industry is unregulated. The truth of the matter is that although the Food and Drug Administration (FDA) does not expressly *approve* the introduction of specific supplements, numerous regulations are in place that require FDA notification of new products, require product claims to be "clear and not misleading," and require companies to have adequate evidence of safety and efficacy for all products and ingredients. The trick, of course, is that the FDA has neither the resources nor the public mandate to aggressively police the claims language used to promote the hundreds of thousands of supplement products on the market.

Does the Product Actually Work?

At this point in the evolution of dietary supplements, for better or worse, a simple structure/function claim is often enough evidence for enthusiastic "early adopters" to take the plunge and start using a new supplement—even though many aspects of safety and efficacy may not be fully addressed. As consumers become more highly educated, however, and learn to ask the right questions (about ingredients, dosages, and mechanisms), they will also become more skeptical (of product claims) and more demanding (for actual clinical evidence from *human* studies), which will force supplement companies to conduct more research to *prove* the value of their products to potential customers.

Only a handful of supplement companies take the initiative (and spend the money) to go beyond the basic structure/function claims and support their product or ingredient claims with solid research, including both safety and toxicity studies (in animals) and well-designed clinical trials (randomized, double-blind, placebo-controlled studies conducted in an appropriate population of human subjects). Anything less is clearly of questionable value from a scientific perspective and (hopefully) will soon be of little value from a marketing and business perspective as well.

Achieving the right balance between the business and marketing objectives of a supplement company and the scientific and regulatory considerations of a health professional or government agency is always a difficult task. On one hand, government regulations are quite flexible in their allowance of claims that can be made for dietary supplements, so most companies are reluctant to commit large financial investments for research that can be "poached" by competitors. On the other hand, consumers are beginning to demand high-quality, well-controlled scientific evidence of a product's safety and efficacy before they will make a purchase. The very idea of science as a compelling marketing tool has become quite popular within the past few years—and it is likely to become a much more important consideration as consumers become further educated about supplements and the supplements themselves become more sophisticated in their mechanism and mode of action.

Clearing Up the Confusion

Within the past couple of years, several media outlets, public universities, and private companies have started to address the growing public confusion surrounding dietary supplements. Unfortunately, much of the dietary supplement coverage in the popular press has only added to the confusion by raising hypothetical questions about the dangers of dietary supplements. It is clear from the scientific and medical literature, however, that the vast majority of dietary supplements, when used as directed, have an outstanding safety profile.

Private health education companies such as SupplementWatch (www.supplementwatch.com) and The Natural Pharmacist (www.tnp.com) have done a tremendous job of bringing the scientific evidence (or lack thereof) for various supplements from the research journals to the public. Both companies accomplish their mission of educating and guiding lay consumers through the pros and cons of using dietary supplements—and both do so with no financial ties to the supplement industry. Through the educational efforts of these and other organizations, consumers are achieving a higher degree of what I refer to as open-minded skepticism about which supplements may provide benefits, which ones seem to be ineffective, and which others may be downright dangerous.

From even a casual glance at the current state of the dietary supplement landscape, it is abundantly clear that we need *far* more research and scientific substantiation of product and ingredient claims. The answer to the obvious question of how much research for dietary supplements is enough, however, may well ultimately come from consumers and marketers, rather than from scientists. As reliably as the sun comes up each morning, scientists and health professionals will insist on more research for a particular supplement—a critically important position that will undoubtedly help to refine our understanding of the mechanisms by which supplements work (or don't). Unfortunately, more research is not necessarily the most prudent approach when viewed in light of the market pressures under which supplement companies operate. From one viewpoint, "enough" research could be defined as that amount needed to convince a skeptical consumer to become a regular user.

For some of the most popular nutritional supplements (e.g., calcium/vitamin D for bone health), the evidence for benefits is so clearly established for certain populations that they should automatically be included in the diet. For many other supplements, including most herbal supplements, the existing data are tantalizing enough to put some scientists and most self-care enthusiasts into the "might help" frame of mind—which means that many consumers will try the supplement before all the data are in. The final category where a handful of supplements reside is "might hurt"—and primarily includes hormone precursors, glandular extracts, central nervous system stimulants, and others with direct toxic effects on the liver, kidneys, or other body systems. Unfortunately, this last category of supplements will continue to be available until educated consumers begin to assert their open-minded skepticism and demand that supplement manufacturers demonstrate that their products satisfy scientific standards for safety and efficacy. I hope that this book can be a part of that effort.

Final Thoughts

The whole idea behind this book, *A Guide to Understanding Dietary Supplements,* is to provide a critical look at the dietary supplement industry and the scientific evidence for (or against) the hundreds of supplement ingredients currently on the market—and to do so from a consumer's perspective by providing education and guidance in deciding whether to try a given supplement.

Despite the large number of supplements outlined in the following chapters, this guide barely scratches the surface of the thousands of products presently available in the marketplace. As much as possible, I have attempted to distill the most directly relevant information about each supplement in an effort to clarify the primary (substantiated) benefit for a particular ingredient. In many cases, supplements may have overlapping indications, such as vitamin E, which has benefits for the heart, brain, eyes, and skin—so although this book covers specific supplements in specific chapters, it is important to note that many "multifunction" supplements exist (see Dietary Supplement Master Chart for the extent of each overlap).

One final note needs to be made about the clear limitations of any book dealing with health, disease, and self-care issues—that being the obvious fact that no two people are alike and that each person has specific health needs that must be addressed on an individual basis in consultation with his or her own health care provider. In no way should the information presented in this book be construed as medical advice or as an alternative to professional medical care. Instead, this book is meant as a first step in exposing the reader to the pros and cons of using dietary supplements as well as an attempt to raise the public awareness of the level of scientific substantiation behind these products—and the need for more research.

Acknowledgments

No book is an effort of one. I would like to acknowledge with deep gratitude the tremendous assistance of my students and colleagues in providing invaluable feedback on the development of this book. Special thanks to Wayne Askew, PhD, for first understanding that students could benefit from a course devoted to a critical evaluation of dietary supplements, to Robert Wildman, PhD, for convincing me to write the text in support of those classes, and to Carsten Smidt, PhD, for his unwavering encouragement to challenge the claims made for dietary supplements and to subject those claims to the harsh light of scientific evidence. Sincere appreciation is also extended to Dove Bunkin, MS, for her many hours of research into specific herbal remedies and her incorporation of that information into the text, as well as to Elizabeth Russell for her contribution of artwork to enhance the ideas presented in this book.

Chapter 1

Overview of the Dietary Supplement Industry and the Dietary Supplement Health and Education Act

INTRODUCTION

According to the Food and Drug Administration's (FDA) Office of Special Nutritionals, more than half of the U.S. adult population uses some form of dietary supplement. The growth of the dietary supplement market has been phenomenal—with annual sales increasing from about $8 billion in 1996 to over $14 billion in 1999 and an expected $18 billion to $20 billion by the end of 2001 (*Nutrition Business Journal,* June 2000).

It is quite interesting to note, however, that even as dietary supplements rack up billions in sales, consumer confusion about supplement claims, effectiveness, and safety is at an all-time high. Much of the growth in dietary supplements comes in the wake of the 1994 Dietary Supplement Health and Education Act (DSHEA), which established the first legal definition of dietary supplements and set up a new framework for FDA regulation of supplements. In passing DSHEA, Congress emphasized that consumers believe dietary supplements can provide "significant health benefits" and that they want "unobstructed access" to products and information to determine whether supplements may help them (or not).

It is important to note that although supplement manufacturers are required by law to notify the FDA about the supplements that they intend to market (premarket notification), the FDA's premarket review of dietary supplements is less than that of other regulated products such as drugs and food additives. A key difference between drugs and supplements is that prior to any marketing, drugs are required to undergo a series of preclinical and clinical studies to determine effectiveness, safety, possible interactions with other substances, and appropriate dosages. The FDA must review the data from the drug trials and authorize a drug's use before it can be introduced to the market. The FDA does not authorize or test dietary supplements—making it crucial for consumers to educate themselves about the safety and potential effectiveness of dietary supplements that they may consider using.

WHAT ARE DIETARY SUPPLEMENTS?

The term "dietary supplement" is legally defined by DSHEA as "any product (other than tobacco) intended to supplement the diet that contains one or more of the following ingredients: a vitamin, mineral, herb or other botanical, an amino acid; a concentrate, metabolite, constituent, extract or combination of any of these ingredients" (P.L. 103417, 108 Stat. 4325). As you can see, the definition of what constitutes a dietary supplement is quite broad, and thousands of ingredients can legally be marketed as supplements. The Center for Food Safety and Applied Nutrition (CFSAN) oversees the FDA's activities related to dietary supplement products, and supplements are a high-priority area for CFSAN.

We'll deal with the specifics of DSHEA in another section, but it is important to note that the fact that a particular product is legally available for sale does not say anything about its effectiveness or safety. It is also important to understand, before we get into topics such as claims substantiation and critical evaluation of supplements (Chapter 3), that dietary supplements are hugely popular among large groups of the American (and worldwide) public. It is quite instructive to ask why, within the space of five to ten years, dietary supplements have become so popular.

WHY ARE DIETARY SUPPLEMENTS SO POPULAR?

There is no denying that dietary supplements are popular with the American public. From 1994 to 1999, the nutritional supplement industry has grown by 10 percent or more each year. This phenomenal level of growth is expected to continue for the foreseeable future—much of it driven by societal trends such as the aging of the worldwide population and the growing interest among consumers who want to take charge of their own health and well-being through natural remedies and self-care.

A Nutritional Approach to Health

The public appetite for health and nutrition news has created a demand for both medical journals and mass media to devote significant coverage to the positive (and negative) effects of nutritional supplements. Early reports focused on the correlation between certain nutrients and a reduced risk of certain diseases, but more contemporary reports have begun to show the direct relationship between dietary supplements and support of key physiological and biochemical processes in the body. Because of the public interest in dietary supplements and the wide array of both balanced and biased health reporting, public acceptance and the popularity of supplements for optimal health and performance are at an all-time high—but so is the confusion about what works, what doesn't, and how to decide what to take.

We're Not Getting Any Younger

It's old news that the largest demographic group in the history of the United States, the "baby boomers," is reaching middle age. Within the next ten to fifteen years, nearly 80 million more individuals will join this group, concerned with preserving their health and fitness and directly increasing the demand for dietary supplements and self-care strategies. The trend toward maintaining good health, rather than simply dealing with the effects of ill-health, is largely driven by the understanding among most people that it's a heck of a lot better to stay healthy than to recover from the effects of an unhealthy lifestyle (not to mention less expensive). The collective health consciousness that began nearly twenty years ago is gaining momentum, and along with exercise, it embraces nutritional supplements.

Scientific Understanding of the Nutrient-Disease Relationship Is Evolving

Increased scientific research into the relationship between nutrients and health has been the impetus for the majority of recent news stories concerning dietary supplements. As science progresses, we learn more about how diet is inextricably linked to overall health and well-being. Through the combined efforts of corporate, academic, and governmental bodies, research into the role of dietary supplements in maintaining health and preventing disease has experienced dramatic growth. On the corporate front, the most trusted and reputable manufacturers in the supplement, pharmaceutical, and food industries are devoting millions of dollars each year to funding research efforts to elucidate the health and wellness benefits of various ingredients. On the governmental front, Congress has established both the Office of Alternative Medicine (OAM) and the Office of Dietary Supplements (ODS) within the National Institutes of Health (NIH).

Favorable Regulatory Environment

In 1994 Congress enacted the Dietary Supplement Health and Education Act, which established regulatory guidelines for the manufacture, marketing, and distribution of dietary supplements. Through DSHEA, responsible nutrition companies are provided a regulatory environment within which they can satisfy the public demand for safe and effective nutritional products. Within the guidelines of DSHEA, companies are encouraged to self-regulate on many fronts, but the FDA ultimately has the last say when it comes to overall supervision.

Mass-Merchandiser Availability of Supplements

No longer are nutritional supplements confined to health food stores. Increasingly, supplements are sold in the more traditional outlets for other consumer products. In addition to traditional health food outlets such as General Nutrition Centers (GNC), vitamins, minerals, herbs, and other categories of dietary supplements can be found in most mass merchandiser outlets, including discount department stores such as Wal-Mart and Kmart, large grocery chains such as Kroger and Fred Meyer, and in pharmacy chains such as Walgreens and CVS—not to mention the hundreds of supplements that are sold exclusively on the Internet. Through these traditional consumer product channels, millions of shoppers are exposed to dietary supplements as they become more mainstream products.

DSHEA

A large part of the explosion in dietary supplements is due to the passage of House Bill S. 784—otherwise known as the Dietary Supplement Health and Education Act. President Bill Clinton signed the legislation into law (PL 103-417) on October 25, 1994. The ultimate passage of DSHEA followed several years of intense lobbying from both grassroots consumer organizations (concerned about government regulation of supplements) and representatives from the dietary supplement industry. Against the bill were representatives from the Food and Drug Administration and various groups desiring tighter regulation of dietary supplements as well as FDA oversight of supplements as drugs. In the end, Congress ruled in favor of relaxed regulations and restrictions on the manufacturing and marketing of dietary supplements—yet the debate continues to this day.

In general, proponents of less regulation feel that DSHEA strikes a balance between consumer access to supplements and the role of government to protect consumer safety. Opponents of DSHEA claim that the law blocks the FDA from fulfilling its role of protecting the American public. On balance, DSHEA gives great leeway to manufacturers and retailers of dietary supplements in what they can say about their products—but it also requires some evidence that the products are both safe and effective. Without going into an exhaustive account of the details of DSHEA, the following highlights will suffice to explain the current legislative framework for dietary supplements.

Section 3 of DSHEA

Section 3 gives the legal definition of a dietary supplement and also provides that a supplement must be in "dosage forms such as capsules, tablets, liquids, powders, or soft gels and may not be represented as a conventional food or as a sole item of a meal or of the diet" (so a soup or margarine or other food item could not be represented as a dietary supplement). In addition, dietary supplements must be labeled as supplements.

Section 4 of DSHEA

Section 4 describes issues relating to the safety of dietary supplements. The key concept from this section is that the burden of proof for showing that a particular supplement is unsafe falls on the FDA, *not* the supplement manufacturer. This provision is both good and bad. First the good—in the days before DSHEA, all the FDA needed to remove a supplement from the shelves and restrict its sale was an affidavit from an FDA scientist or consultant (quite a low standard of evidence). Now the bad—under the current DSHEA regulations, a supplement ingredient may only be deemed unsafe if:

- it presents a significant or unreasonable risk of illness or injury under the conditions of use recommended or suggested on the label or labeling;
- it is unsafe under the Food, Drug, and Cosmetic Act's standard for food;
- the Secretary of Health and Human Services declares that a supplement poses an imminent hazard to public health or safety; or
- the supplement is a new product for which there is inadequate information to provide a reasonable assurance that the ingredient does not present a significant or unreasonable risk of illness or injury.

These provisions clearly place the burden of proof for safety squarely on the shoulders of the FDA. In other words, supplement manufacturers have no obligation to prove that a particular ingredient is safe before introducing it to the market, whereas the FDA must prove that an ingredient is *not* safe before restricting its sale or removing it from the market.

An example of the burden of proof for safety concerns falling on the FDA is illustrated by the mid-1997 case concerning the FDA's proposed limitation on the amount of ephedrine alkaloids in dietary supplements and the proposal to require warnings about side effects (nervousness, dizziness, elevated blood pressure, heart palpitations, heart attack, stroke, seizures, and death). The proposal was initiated by the FDA's review of Adverse Event Reports and public comments, but was challenged by supplement industry groups as well as the General Accounting Office as a scientifically unsound position. In another case, also in 1997, the FDA identified contamination of the herbal ingredient plantain with the harmful herb *Digitalis lanata* after receiving a report of a complete heart block in a young woman. The FDA traced all uses of the contaminated ingredient and asked manufacturers and retailers to withdraw these products from the market.

Another important consideration within this section of DSHEA is that safety standards for particular ingredients are qualified by the phrase "under recommended use." This means that any challenge to the safety of a particular ingredient would have to prove the safety risk associated with the levels of intake or use suggested on the label, and dosages in excess of the suggested amount cannot be challenged. To use a contemporary example, the popular weight loss and energy herb ma huang (ephedra) is typically recommended at dosages in the range of 10 to 30 milligrams (mg) per dose (not more than 100 mg per day). At higher doses, the stimulant effects of this herb would almost certainly be considered a safety concern for many people (particularly individuals with hypertension and heart disease)—but at suggested use levels, the mild stimulatory effects on the central nervous system are unlikely to pose significant risk for healthy individuals.

In most cases, ethical manufacturers will voluntarily provide specific dosage recommendations along with appropriate cautions and warnings on supplement labels. Allowing manufacturers to include such warnings on supplement labels is a change from the past, when the FDA viewed such warnings as an indication that the product was a drug.

If you feel that you have experienced a problem or illness caused by a dietary supplement, the FDA can be contacted by mail or phone to report general complaints or concerns. In addition, either you or your health care provider can also report any adverse experiences by calling the FDA's MedWatch hotline at 1-800-FDA-1088 or by using the Web site <http://www.fda. gov/medwatch> (the MedWatch program collects reported problems possibly caused by FDA-regulated products such as drugs, medical devices, medical foods, and dietary supplements).

Section 5 of DSHEA

Section 5 addresses the ability of supplement manufacturers and retailers to use third-party publications to promote their products. Before DSHEA was passed, the FDA considered the use of any third-party literature about a product to be labeling it as an unapproved drug. The current regulation, however, expressly allows "articles, chapters in books, and other publications, if reprinted in their entirety" to be used to promote the sale of dietary supplements. Literature used in this capacity must meet the following criteria:

- It may not be false or misleading.
- It may not promote a particular manufacturer or brand of dietary supplement.
- It must be displayed or presented with other literature to present a balanced view of the available scientific information on the supplement.
- It must be physically separate from the supplement if displayed in an establishment.
- It must not have appended to it any information by sticker or other method.

Section 6 of DSHEA

Section 6 outlines the use of claims for products—also known as "statements of nutritional support" and "structure/function" claims. Prior to DSHEA, the FDA only allowed claims of nutritional support for vitamins and minerals with an established Recommended Dietary Allowance (RDA)—meaning that herbs, amino acids, and other supplements were unable to carry specific claims. Under the new DSHEA regulations, supplements are allowed to carry claim statements that fall into one of the following four general categories:

- A claim of benefit relating to a classical nutrient deficiency disease which also discloses the prevalence of that disease in the United States
- A claim that describes the role of a nutrient or dietary ingredient which is intended to affect the structure or function of the body

- A claim that characterizes the documented mechanism by which a nutrient or dietary ingredient acts to maintain a bodily structure or function
- A claim that describes general well-being from consuming a nutrient or dietary ingredient

None of the claims of nutritional support need to have specific clearance or approval from the FDA, but the manufacturer is obligated to have some substantiation that the statements made are "truthful and not misleading" and must further notify the FDA within thirty days following the first use of the claim in the market. Although the FDA does not provide approval of structure/function claims, the agency does provide guidance in this area by notifying supplement manufacturers who they feel have stepped over the line by using claims reserved for drugs. The FDA will typically notify a manufacturer of any problems with specific claims via a "courtesy letter" that outlines how a claim violates one of the four criteria. There are also a number of "approved health claims" that are permitted by the FDA for use on dietary supplements (explained more fully in Chapter 3).

Dietary supplements that make a statement of nutritional support must also display the following disclaimer: "This statement has not been approved by the Food and Drug Administration. This product is not intended to diagnose, treat, cure or prevent a disease."

In January 2000, the FDA published a final ruling that defined the types of structure/function statements that could be made concerning the effect of a dietary supplement on the structure or function of the body. This ruling attempted to distinguish prohibited "disease" claims from permitted "structure/function" claims by precluding both *express* disease claims such as "prevents osteoporosis" and *implied* disease claims such as "prevents bone fragility in postmenopausal women" without prior FDA review. It is important to note that a product need not actually state a claim for it to be implied. For example, an implied disease claim can be made through the name of a product (such as "CholestaCure") as well as through the use of pictures or symbols. Health maintenance claims are allowed (such as "maintains a healthy circulatory system"), as well as claims for minor symptoms associated with life stages (such as "hot flashes" and "symptoms of PMS"). The FDA believes that this recent clarification on appropriate structure/function claims will ultimately provide consumers with better information that will help them select appropriate dietary supplement products.

It is important to note that the FDA does not regulate advertisements for dietary supplements. Instead, the Federal Trade Commission (FTC) handles advertising for dietary supplements and most other products sold to consumers, but the FDA does work very closely with FTC officials in this area.

The FDA also does not routinely analyze the content of dietary supplements. Due to very limited resources, the FDA tends to focus first on public health emergencies and on specific products that may be linked to serious safety concerns, injury, or illness. A secondary focus is on products thought to be fraudulent or in direct violation of the law. Although routine monitoring of products pulled from store shelves is certainly within the limits of FDA authority, this does not tend to be a top priority.

Section 7 of DSHEA

Section 7 is meant to ensure that supplement labels are accurate and that they provide consumers with pertinent information about the product. Under DSHEA, dietary supplement labels must include:

- the name of each ingredient in the product,
- the quantity of each ingredient (if the product is a proprietary blend or formula, the total weight of all ingredients in the blend),
- the identity of any part of the plant from which the botanical ingredient is derived, and
- the term "dietary supplement."

Section 8 of DSHEA

Section 8 distinguishes between new dietary ingredients and those that were already on the market in the United States prior to October 15, 1994, when DSHEA was passed. "New" ingredients fall into a special class of substances and are subject to a special safety standard (see Section 4). The DSHEA regulations prohibit the introduction of new dietary ingredients into supplements unless the ingredient meets one of the following criteria:

- The supplement contains only ingredients that have been present in the food supply as a food in a form which has not been chemically altered.
- There is a history of use or other evidence supporting the ingredient's safety when used under the conditions recommended or as suggested in the labeling. (In this case, the manufacturer must provide the FDA with some evidence, such as published articles, that the ingredient is safe, and they must do so within seventy-five days prior to introducing the ingredient to the market).

The practical application of this regulation is that ingredients marketed as supplements prior to October 15, 1994, have been "grandfathered" so that they cannot be removed from the market unless the FDA legally proves that a legitimate public safety concern exists. Again, the burden of proving safety (or lack thereof) is on the FDA because manufacturers are only obligated to provide "some" evidence of safety to the FDA and are not responsible for *proving* that a new ingredient is indeed safe. Although one would hope that all supplement manufacturers would exercise the highest ethical and scientific standards to develop strong safety evidence before introducing a new product, such is not always the case.

Other Sections of DSHEA

Other sections broadly call for the establishment of good manufacturing practices (GMPs), a Commission on Dietary Supplement Labels, and an Office of Dietary Supplements Research within the National Institutes of Health. It is also important to note that Congress, in enacting DSHEA, also set forth several findings relating to dietary supplements, which include the following:

- The importance of nutrition and the benefits of dietary supplements in health promotion and disease prevention have been documented increasingly in scientific studies.
- There is a link between ingestion of certain nutrients or dietary supplements and the prevention of chronic diseases such as cancer, heart disease, and osteoporosis.
- Preventive health measures, including education, good nutrition, and appropriate use of safe nutritional supplements will limit the incidence of chronic diseases and reduce long-term health care expenditures.
- Consumers should be empowered to make choices about preventive health care programs based on data from scientific studies of health benefits related to particular dietary supplements.
- There is a growing need for emphasis on the dissemination of information linking nutrition and long-term good health.
- National surveys have revealed that almost 50 percent of the 272,690,818 (U.S. Census Bureau, July 1, 1999) Americans regularly consume dietary supplements of vitamins, minerals, or herbs as a means of improving their nutrition.
- Legislative action that protects the right of access of consumers to safe dietary supplements is necessary in order to promote wellness.

- Dietary supplements are safe within a broad range of intake, and safety problems with supplements are relatively rare.
- Although the federal government should take swift action against products that are unsafe or adulterated, the federal government should not impose unreasonable regulatory barriers limiting or slowing the flow of safe products and accurate information to consumers.
- A rational federal framework must be established to supersede the current ad hoc, patchwork regulatory policy on dietary supplements.

WORKS CONSULTED

Burdock GA. Dietary supplements and lessons to be learned from GRAS. Regul Toxicol Pharmacol. 2000 Feb;31(1):68-76.

Chang J. Scientific evaluation of traditional Chinese medicine under DSHEA: A conundrum. Dietary Supplement Health and Education Act. J Altern Complement Med. 1999 Apr;5(2):181-9.

Israelsen LD. Phytomedicines: The greening of modern medicine. J Altern Complement Med. 1995 Fall;1(3):245-8.

Nesheim MC. What is the research base for the use of dietary supplements? Public Health Nutr. 1999 Mar;2(1):35-8.

Nutrition Business Journal, June 2000:1-6.

Radimer KL, Subar AF, Thompson FE. Nonvitamin, nonmineral dietary supplements: Issues and findings from NHANES III. J Am Diet Assoc. 2000 Apr; 100(4):447-54.

SOURCES FOR ADDITIONAL INFORMATION ON DIETARY SUPPLEMENTS

Food and Drug Administration (FDA)
Office of Consumer Affairs, HFE-88
Rockville, MD 20857
1-800-FDA-4010
<www.cfsan.fda.gov>

Federal Trade Commission
Public Reference Branch, Room 130
Washington, DC 20580

SupplementWatch, Inc.
648 E. Rocky Knoll
Draper, UT 84020
(801) 572-1905
<www.supplementwatch.com>

Consumer Labs, LLC
1 North Broadway, Suite 410
White Plains, NY 10601
(201) 261-5616

Chapter 2

The Product Development Process
for Dietary Supplements

INTRODUCTION

Where do new products come from and how do they get to the shelf? One place that they rarely come from is a "Eureka!" moment of breakthrough in the lab of a lone scientist. In almost any successful company, effective product development is a process that proceeds through many steps from the idea to the finished market-ready product. In general terms, product development can be defined as:

> A process of defining the features and benefits of a product/service, coordinating technical and market research and development, developing product and process specifications, and building/testing prototypes.

Now that you have read and memorized a traditional definition of what product development is supposed to be—please forget it. Blot it from your mind. Pretend that you never saw it. The new rule in product development, particularly within the dietary supplement industry, is "fast and lean"—anything else and you are behind the curve and involved in a continual game of catch-up.

One of the primary drivers of the changes in the new product development (NPD) process is that it is simply becoming more difficult to develop breakthrough products. In addition, consumers are less loyal to specific brands, and they are increasingly aware of the variety of options available to them. Within the supplement industry, brand awareness is virtually nonexistent, so in many ways the traditional new product design and marketing approaches are poorly suited to developing successful products.

The purpose of this chapter is to expose you to the multidisciplinary process commonly referred to as "product development." As you will learn in the next several pages, the development of new dietary supplement products is an ever-changing process, almost unwieldy at times, that needs to be constantly adjusted, tweaked, and customized for specific projects, timelines, and objectives. The development of new dietary supplement products often falls somewhere between the processes followed by pharmaceutical companies and those of consumer products companies (such as food and beverage processors). As such, there is no "right" or "wrong" way to approach the new product development process for supplements—but the following pages present some scenarios that have been used effectively in the past and that may prove valuable for current and future projects.

DRUG DEVELOPMENT AS A MODEL
FOR DIETARY SUPPLEMENTS

A number of dietary supplement companies are fond of comparing their product development process to pharmaceutical standards. Just to put this comparison into the proper perspective, consider that, on average, it takes about twelve years for a new drug to proceed from the lab bench to the pharmacy shelves, while a new dietary supplement frequently takes less than twelve months to travel from idea to market. In terms of selectivity, only about one in a thousand compounds that enter preclinical drug testing even make it to human testing—and only one out of five experimental drugs tested in people is ever approved as a new drug.

Despite all the progress made by dietary supplement manufacturers in recent years in terms of extraction techniques, safety evaluation, and clinical efficacy testing, there is clearly a wide gap between the research on supplements versus that on pharmaceuticals—and there always will be. Part of the economics of the drug discovery and development process is that on average, it costs over $350 million to bring a single new medicine from the lab to the market—substantially more than the total valuation of many supplement companies. Research-based pharmaceutical companies invest more than $13 billion annually in research and development activities—that's almost as much as the entire annual sales for all of the U.S.-based dietary supplement market!

As a point of reference, the new drug development process proceeds through a highly regulated series of steps that includes the following:

- *Preclinical testing* typically involves two to four years of laboratory and animal studies to show the biological activity of the compound against the targeted disease and initial safety considerations.
- *Investigational new drug application (IND)* is filed with the FDA to begin human testing of the drug. The IND outlines previous experi-

mental results, how, where, and when the studies will be conducted, the chemical structure of the compound, how it is thought to work, any toxic effects found in animal studies, and how the compound is manufactured. The IND becomes effective if the FDA does not disapprove it within thirty days. The IND also must be reviewed and approved by the institutional review board where the studies will be conducted, and progress reports on clinical trials must be submitted at least annually to the FDA.

- *Phase I clinical trials* take about a year and typically involve fewer than 100 normal, healthy volunteers to test a drug's safety profile, dosage range, duration of action, and pharmacokinetics (how the drug is absorbed, distributed, metabolized, and excreted).
- *Phase II clinical trials* take about two years and involve controlled studies of approximately 100 to 300 volunteer patients (people with the disease) to assess the drug's effectiveness.
- *Phase III clinical trials* take about three years and may involve several thousand patients in multiple locations to monitor efficacy and adverse reactions.
- *New drug application (NDA)* is filed with the FDA following completion of all three clinical trial phases and analysis of the data (assuming the studies show safety and effectiveness). The FDA typically takes one to two years to review an NDA (although the process is supposed to take only six months).
- *Approval.* If the FDA approves the NDA, the new drug becomes available for physicians to prescribe, and the company continues to submit periodic reports about any cases of adverse reactions to the FDA. For some new drugs, the FDA may require additional studies (Phase IV) to evaluate long-term effects.

CONSUMER PRODUCT DEVELOPMENT AS A MODEL FOR DIETARY SUPPLEMENTS

Even a casual look at the dietary supplement market reveals a market saturated with variety—it's capitalism run amok! Not only do consumers want more choices, they also have rising expectations about what a given product should do, how fast it should work, and how much it should cost—and these expectations are only likely to increase. The result is that most supplement companies are forced to think of the present rather than the future. In a market that can completely reinvent itself in the space of a few months to a year, there is little room or patience for a traditional five-year business plan or three-year marketing model. The solution for fast-moving supplement companies is to consider how the business is designed today so that it can handle whatever comes down the pike in the future.

In terms of what supplement consumers are looking for, it is almost certainly not a traditional mass-market supplement designed for every Tom, Dick, and Harry. Instead, supplement consumers are looking for products specifically designed for them—they need to be customized, tailored, and targeted to their specific needs and wants. In today's increasingly "customized" world, if consumers don't get the specific product that they are looking for from you, then they'll get it from your competitors. Addressing the move toward customization is a trend in dietary supplement product development and marketing known as "niche marketing"—narrow market segments are identified and products are developed to fulfill the needs of people in that niche.

Part of identifying niche categories and developing new products to fill those niches is developing a coordinated system that can help you efficiently get from idea to product. You'll need to identify the niche, figure out who are the consumers that fall into that niche (enthusiastic early adopters), and coordinate all efforts to develop the product and communicate its benefits. Marketing people need to learn how to think in technical terms, and technical people need to be aware of marketing objectives. Market-driven engineering uses market feedback to guide product refinements in the same way that technology-driven marketing helps guide alterations in product direction.

The most successful products will go through an evolutionary process in which some products, often the early ones, will fail. Often it may take three, four, or five iterations to create that blockbuster supplement—and those first few attempts are learning exercises. Thus, it is important for the people who are developing those products to do at least a portion of their learning from firsthand consumer feedback, so the company can respond rapidly to customer needs. The practical bottom line for development of new dietary supplement products is "Get it to market first" (or at least *fast*)—and start work on the second generation the day you go to market with the first. Consumer feedback is used to spur and guide the refinement process—you're not just addressing consumer needs, wants, and concerns, you're also enhancing the product. This is a never-ending process!

The traditional NPD process calls for multiple departments to work through a century-old "pass-off" model—product development moves in a linear fashion, with engineering passing the project to manufacturing, then to marketing and sales, then to distribution, and finally down to the customers. While it is quite logical to have a systematic approach and framework established to guide the NPD process, a system that becomes too rigid and divisionalized is less likely to generate the successful products that the company needs.

All companies use a variety of approaches to develop new products. While no single process is suited for all companies, there are common elements among effective processes. Effective management of the new product development process requires a road map to provide directions to the final destination—new commercial products. In many dietary supplement companies, however, new product initiatives fail at the astonishing rate of 50 to 75 percent—meaning that only about one-quarter to one-half of the new supplement products that reach the market in a given year will survive into the next year (if they even make it that long). The reasons for new product failures among supplement companies are many—but many can be traced to a failure to set a clear direction ahead of the actual product development initiatives.

NEW PRODUCT DEVELOPMENT APPROACHES

Depending on the company, various approaches to coming up with ideas for new products may dominate. The traditional conceptual approach to the NPD process is "consumer-driven"—an idea for a new product generates a solution to a consumer problem (e.g., an energy-boosting supplement for tired consumers). Within the supplement industry, intense competitive pressures often cause NPD to be "competition-driven"—the market is analyzed in terms of competitive niches and potential product ideas that may fit each niche. Because lead time to market is often a critical success factor, NPD projects driven by competitive pressures often end up as "me-too" products with little innovation—but with the significant benefit of being able to quickly enter a rapidly growing niche (e.g., energy bars for active consumers). Although it less frequently drives product development in the dietary supplement industry, "technology-driven" product development is becoming more common as strong science becomes a marketing advantage. In this scenario, a new type of technology serves as the impetus for a new product that may not have been possible previously (e.g., time-released herbal supplements that have a longer-lasting effect).

With enough financial, marketing, and research resources backing it, virtually *any* process will suffice to churn out new products. Unfortunately, most companies, including all dietary supplement companies, are limited by both human and financial resources, so the NPD process needs to be streamlined and tailored to a company's specific needs. Part of the streamlining process—allocating precious resources to a given project—can be accomplished by approaching the NPD process in two distinct stages: direction/goal setting and product development.

Direction Setting

Well before the NPD teams get down to the actual development of specific products, the long-term objectives and overall business strategy of the company have to be defined in specific terms and used to guide the subsequent NPD process. The following steps are often part of the direction-setting phase:

- Develop a strategy for defining new product goals, strategic roles that new products will fill, and screening criteria to be applied to new categories and concepts.
- Identify categories that may warrant further attention for new products.
- Screen categories against business directions and select the most attractive ones.

Depending on the company, this direction-setting phase may take anywhere from a few weeks to a few months—but the time that it saves in reducing confusion at later stages of the NPD process is well worth the initial effort. The direction established during this first phase should result in two very valuable pieces of information: (1) a new product strategy, and (2) a prioritized ranking of attractive categories. You now have a compass to guide actual NPD activities (the "real" development process) for the next year or so.

Product Development

With the new product direction established, the NPD team can get down to what many in the industry see as the real work—the generation of ideas that will become new dietary supplements on the shelf. Again, the NPD process is much more than a few idea people sitting around and coming up with breakthrough concepts for new products. If it were just a bunch of big thinkers, then the dietary supplement industry wouldn't be the dynamic and growing industry that it is today—and there would be little need for this book! The following outline provides several steps that many, although not all, successful companies utilize in their NPD process to develop specific product concepts that satisfy the strategic goals identified during the direction-setting phase. Keep in mind that the entire NPD process should be viewed as an iterative process—meaning that each step builds on previous steps—and even feeds back or "recycles" into earlier steps.

Problem Identification

Before idea generation begins, exploratory market and consumer research is an important component of the NPD process. This first stage of the process looks at the market, competing products, health and lifestyle trends, competitive environment, and needs and wants of specific consumer segments (men/women/athletes/etc.) to identify problems and opportunities that exist. This type of exploratory research is common to virtually all supplement companies, as it provides a basis for developing creative solutions for specific consumer problems, needs, or desires.

Idea Generation

Even within the average supplement company, there is rarely a lack of ideas—but coordinating those ideas within the previously defined categories (direction setting) is often the more daunting challenge. A variety of problem-solving and creative approaches (brainstorming sessions) are used to generate new ideas. Initial ideas may come from virtually any angle, but some common areas from which new product ideas may come include:

- Consumer problems and needs
- Lifestyle and behavior trends
- Category developments
- Competitor analysis
- Foreign products successes or failures
- Internal company strengths
- Technical developments
- Many others

Concept Development

Turning an idea into a true concept requires the idea to take some substance in the form of the benefits that a consumer might expect to obtain from using the product. Development of an effective concept will also address issues related to price, packaging, and product description and positioning for ideas that pass initial screenings. It is obvious that some amount of prior knowledge of the category, ingredients, or health-disease relationship needs to be in place for effective development and evaluation of proposed concepts. Thus, at least a minimal amount of analysis of the market and of competitive factors should have been made prior to this point. Additional considerations that are unique to dietary supplement NPD can be considered subsections of the concept development phase, including:

- *Toxicity/safety:* Are there any known or suspected side effects associated with the ingredients under consideration? (See additional safety and quality control considerations below.)
- *Ingredient stability/compatibility:* Are the proposed ingredients stable over a prolonged period of time? Will they retain their full range of activity for the entire shelf life? Is each of the ingredients in the blend compatible with all the others?
- *Ingredients/product efficacy:* Do the proposed ingredients retain their desired effects with this dosage and delivery format? Will additional studies be required?
- *Raw material sourcing/quality/specifications:* Are the proposed ingredients readily available from reputable sources in sufficient amounts and at different times of year?
- *Ingredient processing/extraction/standardization:* Does the product/ingredient blend need to be subjected to special processing methods? Can the production process be standardized to ensure consistent quality and efficacy in each batch?
- *Development of marketing claims:* What can or will be said about this new product to explain its benefits and differentiate it from competitors?
- *Legal claims substantiation:* Can the proposed marketing claims be legally substantiated with available scientific evidence (FTC considerations)? Are more studies required prior to launch or can it be launched with the available evidence?

Business Analysis

For each concept, a rough assessment of market and competitive factors is compiled. This may include an examination of the dynamics of the category and the competition, consumer buying patterns, and fit with internal strengths and weaknesses. Rough financial projections may need to be compiled for a "go/no go" decision before proceeding to the next phase.

Prototype Development

Nothing frustrates manufacturing experts more than being handed a project that simply will not work outside of the "ivory tower" of the laboratory. Development of a prototype product is an important phase of the NPD process because it will test the performance of the formulation against real-world factors such as manufacturing limitations, cost, stability, and a myriad of other factors. It is at this stage that a concept is subjected to the harsh light of reality—will it really work as a product? The overall objectives of this stage of the NPD process are to produce prototypes in a form suitable for consumer testing and to learn what problems are likely to be encountered during the scale-up and commercialization phases. It is vital that product development experts (the idea people) remain involved throughout the prototype development phase and don't simply hand off the project to the technical people. It is highly likely that prototype development will reveal opportunities to alter the product formulation to make the end product better, easier to manufacture, or less expensive to produce.

Market Testing

Assuming that the product can be made and that the prototype stands up to initial expectations, market testing, when possible, can be useful for judging consumer purchase intent in the open market. Market testing allows the company to objectively evaluate whether this "great" new product concept is really a winner with potential consumers. Unfortunately, the rapid pace of the supplement industry and the pressure to be first to market with new products precludes most supplement manufacturers from conducting extensive market testing. This is changing, however, as larger multinational corporations enter the profitable category for dietary supplements and functional foods. Recent examples are major test marketing efforts by Nestlé (LC-1 probiotic), Mead Johnson (Viactiv calcium chews), McNeil (Aflexa glucosamine), and Whitehall-Robins (Flexagen glucosamine).

Scale-Up

Whether or not market testing is possible, the scale-up stage is where the final go/no go decision must be made. This stage tests the volume of plant production, evaluates product quality at these volumes, and determines any additional equipment and manufacturing needs for producing the product in commercial volumes.

Commercialization/Marketing

In many instances, the ultimate success or failure of the new product may be determined by the efforts in this stage of the process, where the product is finally introduced to the market (trade and consumers). Examples abound of "excellent" dietary supplement products that were unsuccessful because of flaws in execution during their introduction to the market (the commercialization phase). The critical success factors that operate at this phase are many, but timing, communication, and flawless execution are the cornerstones of a successful launch. It is important to educate and motivate the sales force about the benefits of the new product—just as they will do to excite consumers and entice them to make a purchase. Far from being left as a last-minute consideration, initial plans for marketing the new product (target consumer, claims development, product positioning, competitive advantages) need to be considered way back during idea generation and concept development.

Postlaunch Analysis

Quite often, many supplement companies overlook postlaunch analysis—despite the fact that analysis of the new product's performance can be quite useful information for guiding future NPD development. In most cases, product sales over a period of six to twelve months following launch are compared to the original sales and profit projections to help gauge success or failure of the new product, as well as opportunities for future NPD efforts.

Safety

Within the traditional consumer products approach to developing dietary supplements, certain aspects of the pharmaceutical model need to be incorporated (safety and efficacy testing) along with requirements that are unique to dietary supplements (development and legal approval of claims). The legal framework for dietary supplements established by DSHEA was outlined in Chapter 1. Although the legal process of evaluating and approving specific product claims is an integral part of the NPD process (concept development), it will be covered in more detail in Chapter 3.

Because safety considerations should hold a prominent place in any NPD process for dietary supplements, it is good news that a 1999 white paper from the Nutraceutical Institute (a partnership between Rutgers University and Saint Joseph's University) reported that supplement manufacturers held up safety as their number one product development priority—ahead of both commercial interests and consumer education.

As described in Chapter 1, the dietary supplement industry has no legal responsibility to prove the safety of a given product—instead it is incumbent upon the FDA to demonstrate that a supplement is unsafe ("innocent until proven guilty") prior to removing it from the market. Nevertheless, certain basic safety considerations must be adequately addressed prior to introducing a new supplement product into the general marketplace, including:

- *Literature review:* Should seek information on the structure, mode of action, target tissues, metabolites, and records/reports/accounts of traditional use.
- *Test systems:* Employing a combination of gene and oral toxicity tests is recommended. The preliminary screening may include the traditional LD50 (lethal dose for 50 percent of the animals) testing—a single dose of the substance is fed to rodents followed by a fourteen-day observation period. The LD50 typically requires at least three doses, which can be determined from the literature or from preliminary studies, and is useful for bracketing the safety limits for the supplement, predicting its toxicity, and estimating the doses needed for subsequent tests.
- *Subchronic safety:* Short-term repeated dose testing calls for continued administration of the ingredient over a twenty-eight-day period, during which time the animals are observed for behavioral abnormalities (or death). They are examined for tissue toxicity (liver, kidney, brain, etc.) at the conclusion of the study. Like single-dose LD50 testing, subchronic studies also require at least three dosage levels in addition to a zero-dose "negative" control group. Doses are selected to establish a lowest observed adverse effect level (LOAEL) and a no observed adverse effect level (NOAEL).
- *Chronic safety:* Long-term repeated dosing is recommended for supplements that may be consumed regularly over a long period of time. Like the subchronic testing, at least three dosage levels and a zero-dose control group are recommended.
- *Specialized toxicity:* Additional studies may be recommended to evaluate reproductive toxicity, developmental toxicity, neurotoxicity, and immunotoxicity.

In addition to evaluating safety considerations, supplement companies also have an ethical obligation to ensure that certain basic quality control systems are in place (often referred to collectively as "GMPs," good manufacturing practices), including the following:

- Standardized production procedures (including extraction/processing steps)
- Specifications developed for both raw materials and finished product

- Valid test methods to certify the purity of the finished product (including chemical analysis and microbiological assays to screen for contaminants such as pesticides, herbicides, fertilizers, and potentially harmful microorganisms)
- A reporting system to track each batch of raw material and finished product
- Determination of stability and storage characteristics
- A documentation system to record each of the checkpoints in the system

ADAPTING THE NPD PROCESS

There is certainly no shortage of factors that can delay or derail the NPD process—and some techniques for guiding the process may work better for one company versus another. By establishing a functional framework to guide the NPD process, however, many of the problems commonly associated with new product development can be avoided. The first step, in any company, is to identify three or four categories that represent the most attractive opportunities for the company. Despite the fact that many supplements companies want to be everything to every consumer, this is simply not possible. By narrowing down the choices to a handful of specific categories, the company is able to focus its strengths and resources to become the leader in certain categories. New product ideas can then be prioritized to focus on concepts that fit within these predefined high-potential categories.

Depending on the specific company and its unique short- and long-term goals, potential categories may be identified by a variety of approaches such as market considerations (size or growth rate) or internal strengths (existing brand equity, processing expertise, or distribution strength). In considering internal company strengths, however, it is also important to realize that the best way to sell a product is not to sell something that you can make; it's to sell something somebody needs. Regardless of the approach used to determine appropriate high-potential categories for NPD efforts, however, a variety of questions can be used to help refine both the potential of the category and the range of product candidates that may fit within each category:

- What are the current product entries in the category?
- What is the overall size of this category in units or dollars?
- What differentiates successful products in this category from less successful ones?

- Who are the existing competitors in the category? What are their strengths/weaknesses?
- Who is the consumer of products in this category?
- What benefit is this consumer deriving from products in this category?
- What new product trends are occurring with this category?
- How long will it take my company to enter this category?
- Will entry into this category pose any risk to my company (dilution of existing brand equity, significant capital, or advertising expenditures)?
- Are raw material sources readily available and stable?
- Is there an effective distribution network for products in this category?
- Is this category fully developed? Is it a passing fad? Is it seasonal?
- Will consumers understand new products in this category or will they require education?
- Can products in this category be sold to my existing customers?

ENCOURAGING CREATIVITY

Now that you have some concept of the system and process of NPD, let us consider for a moment the most important aspect of new product development—the people. Creative people will not be unduly or unnecessarily harnessed—and if they feel that they are, they will leave. So how to best manage creativity within a commercial environment?

Are the best new product developers the creative "right-brain" people or the logical "left-brain" technicians? *Yes!* The best NPD professionals are those individuals who can harness their creative energies within a logical process or framework. The most effective product developers (and companies) are successful because they understand that having a systematic and orderly NPD process in place can help guide the creative process without suppressing the creativity that is needed to spark new product ideas. The process, as outlined throughout this chapter, is a sequential step-by-step process that feeds back onto itself and provides enough flexibility to be tailored to particular new product ideas or divergent company cultures.

As mentioned previously, there is seldom a lack of new ideas within a given supplement company, but the execution of those ideas by way of assessment, screening, prioritization, and development varies substantially from one company to the next. Obviously, companies that are most effective at encouraging creativity, harnessing the best ideas, and shepherding them through the development process toward commercialization are the companies that emerge as the most successful.

Within the NPD community, there is a widespread misconception that creativity and new product idea generation is an abstract free-for-all that cannot and should not be managed for fear that creativity will be squelched in its tracks. Subscribers to this point of view tend to forget that creativity does not occur in a vacuum, but instead occurs most reliably when stimulated by a constant flow of information, feedback, conjecture, emotions, and free association (an old saying among creativity experts is that "ambiguity is essential for innovation"). Ideas for new products in and of themselves are less valuable to a company than practical ideas generated within a systematic framework—because that framework can help bring those ideas to the market to solve a consumer problem, address a health need, or extend benefits into a new demographic.

Managing creativity in NPD is nothing if not challenging. In many companies, NPD is considered to be one group while marketing is another, operations another, quality assurance yet another, and so on. Within the typical framework, artificial walls are established between the various divisions whereby NPD comes up with the idea/concept, operations makes it, marketing creates the story, and the business model and so on. The problem, of course, is that the NPD process is much more effective as a multidisciplinary endeavor that requires, and indeed thrives upon, input and feedback from each division at almost every step of the process. In many ways, the NPD manager must develop a wider range of skills than managers of clearly defined departments such as finance, legal, and others, simply due to the multidisciplinary nature of guiding a new product from idea to launch.

SUMMARY

Managing the NPD process can be enhanced by grounding the development steps within a direction-setting framework. Such a sequential, step-by-step process can still retain a high degree of flexibility that permits "free-flowing" creativity to be harnessed within an orderly and efficient framework. Once the NPD process is established within a particular company, it is beneficial to leave it alone for awhile to allow the multidisciplinary teams to become accustomed to the process.

Chapter 3

Critical Evaluation of Dietary Supplements

INTRODUCTION

Since the passage of DSHEA in 1994, the sheer number of different dietary supplement products introduced to the market is mind-boggling. It is no exaggeration to estimate that *several hundred thousand* unique dietary supplement products are currently on the market. With such a large number of products to choose from, and with a variety of claims being made for each product, it is no wonder that consumers are confused when it comes to selecting specific supplements.

Recall from Chapter 1 that dietary supplements can contain one or more ingredients such as vitamins, minerals, herbs, botanicals, or amino acids and that although the FDA requires substantiation and notification for all claims, there is no specific approval process for supplements. As such, the various claims of nutritional support made for many supplements are often vague and confusing to consumers. This chapter provides an outline for evaluating the claims made by and for various dietary supplements on the market.

In general, the process of critically evaluating dietary supplements should proceed through at least three steps (and potentially many more) including (at least) history of use, claims substantiation, and scientific support—each of which is outlined more fully in the following sections.

HISTORY OF USE AND SAFETY

In the majority of cases, especially when it comes to herbal supplements, there is often a story about how the supplement in question has been used for "centuries" as a treatment for specific conditions in "ancient" cultures. The very reason that many supplements are even on the market has to do with the fact that they were used as natural medicines before the advent of modern pharmaceuticals.

With the growing number of consumers relying on dietary supplements as part of their self-care and health maintenance regimens, issues of safety, efficacy, and quality are of paramount importance. A significant challenge for manufacturers of dietary supplements, particularly for botanical extracts, is the complexity of the formulations, which may have multiple active (and inactive) ingredients (as opposed to a single-ingredient formulation, which is the norm for most pharmaceutical preparations). Because herbs and other plants are highly complex organisms with thousands of organic compounds, the therapeutic benefits associated with a particular phytomedicine may be due to one or many active compounds. Ensuring a consistent level of therapeutic efficacy while still maintaining the safety and "essence" of the whole herb is a significant challenge for modern formulators of dietary supplements. Even early practitioners of herbal medicine, the shamans of ancient times, used extraction methods to concentrate the active components of medicinal herbs (pressed juices, tea infusions, alcoholic tinctures, etc.). Today, modern supplement extraction techniques are also aimed at concentrating the active compounds (whether known or suspected) from a plant while also trying to standardize the formulation so that it consistently provides a quantifiable amount of active (or marker) compounds from batch to batch.

Standardized Extracts

Because herbal preparations can vary widely in total content of both active and inactive ingredients, a popular approach to delivering dietary supplements with consistent effects is to try to produce products with standard levels of particular compounds or classes of chemicals. In the modern pharmaceutical industry, it is generally quite easy for manufacturers to list the milligrams of a particular compound in the formula because it may only contain one ingredient (such as aspirin, which is a single chemical called acetylsalicylic acid). Because one aspirin tablet is the same as the next, consumers can select their product based on milligrams of acetylsalicylic acid and price. The same is not true of herbs and other dietary supplements, in which thousands of active and inactive compounds may contribute to the overall effect of the supplement. Adding to the confusion is the fact that the absolute levels and relative proportion of those compounds can vary widely from one crop to the next due to conditions of growing, harvesting, storage, and processing methods.

The bottom line is that because of the great potential for variation, there really is no perfect way to differentiate one dietary supplement product from another—but the standardization process can help. Because standardization can produce an herbal extract according to a defined process and with a reproducible content of either active or marker compounds, it can generally be expected that if that extract shows benefits in clinical testing, then other extracts that are produced by the same standards should also have the same benefits. For example, if we know that a particular leaf extract, such as ginkgo biloba, has benefits for a particular condition, such as Alzheimer's disease, it is reasonable to expect that ginkgo leaf extract produced under the same conditions as those shown to be effective in clinical studies should also be effective. Now, let's assume that the ginkgo is grown under fixed conditions, harvested during midsummer, extracted for twelve hours in a mixture of 30 percent alcohol and hot water, and dried to contain a certain percentage and total amount of a specific class of chemicals, and you can begin to gain an appreciation for the complexity of producing an extract with equivalent efficacy. A ginkgo supplement that is produced by a different process may or may not have equal effectiveness, even if it is standardized to the same percentage of active compounds, because different manufacturing processes could result in different levels of other active or inactive ingredients.

Active versus Marker Compounds

It is both the strength and weakness of herbal medicine and dietary supplementation that because of the complexity of the active and inactive constituents, we simply do not know whether a certain extract works unless it is put through a series of clinical studies. Unfortunately, many supplement manufacturers routinely "borrow" studies done on herbal formulations that are different from the ones that they sell—and make the very large assumption that all extracts standardized for a given class of compounds are identical. In many ways, standardization brings a certain amount of undeserved credibility to some supplement products because, although it certainly increases reproducibility, it does not necessarily indicate effectiveness.

If the therapeutic effect of a given plant can be linked directly to a precise chemical constituent (or group of compounds), then an extract of the plant can be standardized to contain a specified amount of the given active compound(s). In the majority of cases, however, the activity of botanicals is due to a group of related compounds, rather than to a single chemical entity—so herbal extracts are frequently standardized to contain a total content of active compounds within a particular class of compounds. For example, the activity of red yeast rice (*Monascus purpureus* Went), a popular dietary supplement for lowering serum cholesterol levels, is due to a class of about a dozen compounds known as monacolins, which have an effect on inhibiting a liver enzyme that is needed for cholesterol synthesis (HMG-CoA reductase). Standardized versions of red yeast rice typically contain a certain percentage of total monacolins (about 0.4 percent) and may also be standardized for unsaturated fatty acid content (about 0.8 percent). In this case, because it is known that the monacolins inhibit HMG-CoA reductase activity in the liver, they are thought to provide the primary effect on reducing cholesterol synthesis and lowering serum cholesterol levels in the body.

Very often, however, the precise compounds responsible for the therapeutic effect of a given botanical are either not known or are difficult or impractical to measure. In these cases, an extract may be standardized based on its content of another compound (a marker compound) that can be more easily quantified on a repeated basis. This approach assumes that when the extract is properly standardized to a marker compound, then the other active constituents, whatever they might be, will also be present in sufficient quantities. The obvious limitation of standardizing extracts based on marker compounds is that variations in extraction or processing methods may influence marker and active constituents to varying degrees. In most cases, however, both clinical and laboratory evidence has supported the practical use of marker compounds to help ensure consistent efficacy of products. An example of using markers to ensure efficacy is the popular herbal antidepressant St. John's wort *(Hypericum perforatum)*, which is typically standardized to contain 0.3 percent hypericin—despite the fact that hypericin is almost certainly not the compound responsible for the antidepressant effects of the herb. Nonetheless, because clinical studies have demonstrated that extracts standardized to 0.3 percent hypericin are effective and because hypericin is relatively easy to measure, even though hypericin is not the active compound, it is a good marker that can be used to ensure consistent efficacy in end products.

Standardized versus Concentrated Extracts

Instead of being standardized to a specific level or concentration of active or marker compounds, concentrated extracts are simply expressed in terms of a ratio of the concentration to the crude (unconcentrated) herb. For example, a ginseng extract may be expressed as a 10:1 root extract—meaning that ten parts of the unconcentrated crude ginseng root are needed to produce one part of the concentrated extract. The primary limitation of concentrated versus standardized extracts is that natural variability in crude botanicals (due to variations in climate, geography, harvesting methods, etc.) can result in an extract with highly variable amounts of active constituents (or even none at all).

CLAIMS SUBSTANTIATION

With such a wide variety of dietary supplements available in the marketplace, manufacturers and marketers are under pressure to differentiate their products from the rest—and bold claims are part of doing so. For example, benefit claims for different brands of echinacea extract may range from the cautious "supports healthy immune function" all the way up to the bold "prevents colds and infections." In another example, competing brands of glucosamine may differ in their claims language from the conservative "maintains healthy joints" to the more aggressive "rebuilds joint cartilage" and even to the barely legal "reduces the pain and stiffness of arthritis."

In each example, the claims are within the same ballpark, but nuances in the wording are what distinguish one product from another on the shelf. The question that a consumer must ask himself or herself is whether the available scientific evidence can substantiate a particular claim. The answer will be provided by a thorough examination of the scientific literature—although this is typically neither very realistic for most consumers nor convenient when one is confronted with dozens of product choices at the local health food store. So what is a consumer to do?

As with any decision that will ultimately influence your health, it is certainly in your best interest to educate yourself as much as possible about the particular self-care remedy that you are considering. Taking the example of glucosamine, it is clear that all of the claims for various products have something to do with joints. It is unclear, however, where to draw the line in terms of claims. If you were able to scan the scientific literature on glucosamine supplementation, you would find that the majority of clinical studies in humans show efficacy in reducing the pain and stiffness associated with osteoarthritis, while a handful of animal and test-tube studies suggest a stimulation of cartilage tissue growth, and virtually no studies support a maintenance of existing joint health. This may seem a bit counterintuitive—that the most aggressive product claims have the strongest scientific support, while the more conservative claims actually mislead the consumer into thinking that a particular effect exists when little or no objective evidence exists to support such a claim.

SCIENTIFIC SUPPORT

Has the Product Been Studied?

Because it is often quite difficult to gain access to and effectively evaluate the existing scientific literature on a particular dietary supplement, perhaps the best way for consumers to know whether particular products are effective is to use a brand that has been subjected to well-designed clinical studies. The ideal situation is to know the specific product or extract that was used in a particular study and then to select that one.

It is important to understand that all research is not created equal, and some types of studies are considered "stronger" than others. In general, the most reliable type of research is a randomized, double blind, placebo-controlled study, sometimes called a randomized clinical trial or RCT. In addition, it is always best if the study was conducted in a group of volunteers that closely resembles the group to which the product is targeted (such as a group of athletes for a muscle-building supplement). Certainly, other types of scientific research can be quite valuable in learning how a supplement works or if it is safe, but the RCT is generally considered the gold standard of study design.

Randomized, Double-Blind, Placebo-Controlled Trials

In this type of study, volunteers are recruited and randomly assigned to receive either the real supplement or an inactive fake (placebo) that resembles the supplement under study. Because neither the volunteers nor the principal researchers know which people are receiving the supplement or the placebo, the study is referred to as "double-blind." The double-blind design helps to avoid a common psychological effect of many treatments called the placebo effect—in which about 30 percent of people will feel an effect of the treatment even when they have been assigned to the placebo group. Having a placebo group as part of the study design allows the researchers to attribute any changes found in the supplement group to an effect of the supplement and not to chance.

Single-Blind, Unblinded, or Open-Label Studies

A number of research study designs are used when it is not possible or practical to use a double-blind or placebo-controlled design. For example, sometimes it may be important for a physician or researcher to know which subjects are taking a particular treatment—so the patients can be kept blind to the treatment that they are receiving, while the researcher remains aware of each subject's treatment to monitor for side effects. This type of design, called a single-blind study, controls for the placebo effect among the subjects, but is still subject to possible bias from the researcher. Another popular study design, called open-label, means that everyone involved with the study, volunteers and researchers, knows who receives the supplement (because there is no placebo group). Although open-label studies can be quite effective in identifying potential safety issues (assuming they are large enough), they cannot tell us the effectiveness of a particular supplement. The major drawback with an open-label study is that, because there is no control group, it is impossible to say whether any benefits observed in the treatment group are in fact due to the supplement or to another reason.

Observational or Epidemiological Studies

Observational studies follow large groups or entire populations of people for several years to determine which diet and lifestyle factors might be associated with specific diseases, better overall health, and longer life. In many cases, observational studies are the only way to learn how lifestyle factors lead to (or prevent) diseases that occur over long periods of time (such as cancer and heart disease). Not only are these types of studies impractical for most dietary supplement companies, their results can be difficult to understand. For example, let's say that an observational study of rural Chinese farmers found that drinking several cups of green tea each day is associated with reduced cancer rates. Great news to be sure, but it may not necessarily be the green tea that is responsible for the overall effect (although it may help). It is important to keep in mind that this population of people also gets a lot more exercise and consumes a lot less fat and sugar as well as a lot more fruits and vegetables than the average American—so it may be that overall lifestyle habits play a more important role than green tea per se. The bottom line with observational studies is that because of the difficulty in deciphering which factors are the most important, more research is almost always needed before conclusive recommendations can be made. For these reasons, observational studies are typically used by scientists to raise questions and guide the development of RCTs.

Laboratory (Animal) and Test-Tube (In Vitro) Studies

Test-tube studies, also called in vitro studies (which means "in glass" in Greek), can be used very effectively to help scientists determine the hows and whys of a particular supplement's mechanism of action. The downside, of course, is that because test-tube conditions are so far removed from conditions within the human body, these types of studies can rarely be used to support consumption of a particular supplement. Unfortunately, there are numerous examples of how test-tube data is improperly used to support supplement use. For example, there are hundreds of reports detailing how various plant extracts can "stimulate" the activity of immune cells in test tubes. These studies are often used to support the concept of consuming the plant extract as a way to strengthen the immune system—a somewhat logical, but inaccurate conclusion. Test-tube studies used as support for dietary supplementation fail to account for the fact that anything consumed orally must first be digested and absorbed through the gastrointestinal tract, transported in the bloodstream, delivered to the tissues, and *still* manage to remain effective when diluted by body fluids. In a similar manner, data collected from animal studies can be very helpful in determining initial efficacy, dosing, safety, and toxicity issues, but animals often process nutrients differently, so clinical studies in humans are needed to confirm any findings drawn from studies in animals.

As you can clearly see, a number of study designs can be used to claim scientific support for a particular supplement—but the strongest and most reliable type of evidence comes from the randomized, double-blind, placebo-controlled human trials. When confronted with making a purchase decision (which product to buy), consumers should look first to those products which have been used in RCTs (see Table 3.1 for some examples).

TABLE 3.1. Products That Have Been Tested by RCT

Herb	Use (dose)	Products
Black cohosh *(Cimicifuga racemosa)*	Menopause/hot flashes (40 mg twice daily)	Remifemin (Enzymatic Therapy) Remifemin (Schaper & Brummer)
Ginkgo *(Ginkgo biloba)*	Senile dementia/ Alzheimer's disease (120-240 mg daily)	Ginkgold (Nature's Way) Ginkoba (Pharmaton) Quanterra (Warner-Lambert) Ginkai (Lichtwer) Tebonin/Egb761 (Schwabe) Kaveri/LI-1370 (Lichtwer)
Horse chestnut *(Aesculus hippocastanum)*	Chronic venous insufficiency/varicose veins (250 mg twice daily)	Venostat (Pharmaton) Venostasin (Klinge Pharma)
Saw palmetto *(Serenoa repens)*	Benign prostatic hyperplasia/enlarged prostate (160 mg twice daily)	ProstActive (Nature's Way) Quanterra (Warner-Lambert) Prostagutt (Schwabe) Permixon (Pierre Fabre)
St. John's wort *(Hypericum perforatum)*	Mild-moderate depression (900 mg daily)	Kira (Lichtwer) Quanterra (Warner-Lambert) Movana (Pharmaton) Perika (Nature's Way) Jarsin/LI-160 (Lichtwer) Neuroplant (Schwabe)

Does the Product Actually Work?

A glaring problem in the dietary supplement industry is the overwhelming lack of research on specific products. In most cases, supplements come to market with a substantial history of use, a logical mechanism of action, and a small amount of substantiation for any benefits that are claimed. As stated previously, the best approach to selecting a particular dietary supplement is to use the specific extract or product that has been used in clinical studies. When this is not possible, consumers are forced into the imperfect scenario of educating themselves about the history, mechanism, and substantiation issues. This scenario is flawed because it is not uncommon for a supplement to meet each of these criteria and yet still fail to stand up to the rigors of a well-designed clinical study.

An example of a dietary supplement with a long history of use, a logical mechanism of action, and a certain level of claims substantiation is the popular diet supplement hydroxycitric acid (HCA). HCA is the active ingredient extracted from the rind of a little pumpkin-like fruit, *Garcinia cambogia,* that grows in India and Southeast Asia. Dietary supplements and a wide variety of weight loss formulas contain *Garcinia* extract (standardized for HCA levels) as a way to inhibit fat production and suppress appetite.

The theory behind why HCA *should* work for promoting weight loss is relatively sound—HCA can inhibit an enzyme in cells, citrate lyase, which is needed for the conversion of carbohydrates into fat. In the cell, carbohydrates are broken down into citrate compounds, which are then converted (by citrate lyase) into acetyl coenzyme A (acetyl CoA)—the metabolic building block for fat synthesis. By blocking the conversion of citrate into acetyl CoA, HCA can suppress fat synthesis (at least in test-tube studies). It is important to note, however, that the citrate lyase enzyme is only significantly active under conditions of carbohydrate overconsumption. In other words, unless you're eating a lot of carbohydrate-type foods (bagels, pasta, potatoes), and overloading your carbohydrate storage capacity (muscle and liver glycogen stores), there is no significant conversion of carbohydrates into fatty acids.

Unfortunately, the scientific support for HCA as an effective weight loss supplement is not nearly as clear-cut as its theory. Animal studies have certainly shown that HCA decreases weight gain in rodents—primarily by suppressing appetite and reducing food intake. At least one rat study has also shown a loss of body weight and reduced fat mass due to an 11 percent increase in daily energy expenditure. HCA also appears to be effective in both lean and obese rats, where it can reduce food intake, body weight, body fat accumulation, fat cell size, and serum triglycerides.

Studies of HCA supplementation in humans, however, have been equivocal. In some studies, 1,000 to 2,400 mg of HCA per day led to a doubling or tripling of weight loss compared to placebo groups. In 1998, however, the *Journal of the American Medical Association* (JAMA, 280(18)) published a study showing no effect of *Garcinia cambogia* on weight loss in overweight men and women. In the study, a commercially available product (1,500 mg HCA per day for twelve weeks) did not augment weight loss compared to the placebo group. The JAMA study has been criticized by pro-HCA camps on a number of criteria including the restrictive nature of the diet (low energy—1,210 kilocalories [kcal] per day), the high fiber content (which decreases absorption of HCA), and the failure to assess HCA absorption (to see if it actually got into the cells where it becomes active). In defense of the study, however, the authors assert that they wanted to test the compound under conditions in which people might normally try to lose weight (thus the low-calorie diet). They also noted that the possibility for HCA to be effective in blocking fat synthesis may be more evident when people fall off their diets or relapse and start consuming lots of high-carbohydrate foods.

The debate on the efficacy of HCA and other dietary supplements will undoubtedly continue to rage for years to come. The point, however, is that despite a long history of use (as a weight loss tea in India), a logical theory and mechanism of action (citrate lyase inhibition), and a degree of claims substantiation (lots of skinny lab rats), the end result is that the supplement may not work when subjected to use under real-world conditions.

THIRD-PARTY SCREENING
OF DIETARY SUPPLEMENTS

If anything should be crystal-clear to the reader at this point, it is that the world of dietary supplements is quite confusing—even for the well-educated consumer. Between the thousands of products and the millions of claims being made, consumers and health practitioners alike are confused and frustrated. Because there are no established testing protocols or approval procedures for dietary supplements, variations in product consistency, dosage size, and levels of standardization remain a huge issue for many manufacturers.

To fill this void, a number of independent companies have initiated screening, testing, and review programs as a way to provide consumers with some guidance in selecting and using (or avoiding) various dietary supplements. Among those taking the lead in educating consumers right now are Consumer Labs and Supplement Watch, but established media outlets such as *Consumer Reports, The Los Angeles Times, The Boston Globe,* and *The*

Washington Post as well as university researchers around the world have been raising the issue of supplement quality for several years now.

ConsumerLab.com

ConsumerLab.com conducts independent laboratory analysis of supplement products to see whether or not they match up to their label claims. The names of products that pass the lab testing are posted on their Web site (www.consumerlab.com), and manufacturers of those products can license the ConsumerLab.com seal of approval for their labels. It is unclear whether or not offering to sell a seal of approval to supplement manufacturers would create any conflict of interest or pressure to "pass" more products to generate more sales. It will be interesting to see how commercial products fair in ConsumerLab.com's testing process. Because of the many technical difficulties associated with analytical testing of herbal products, however, not all types of supplements can be easily tested (see Complexity of Testing). For example, differences between analytical methods may give widely different results, and the presence of certain compounds in a given extract may interfere with the accuracy of measuring levels of another compound.

SupplementWatch

SupplementWatch takes a different approach to reviewing dietary supplements—by not accepting advertising or financial support from supplement manufacturers. Instead, SupplementWatch licenses its product reviews to supplement retailers as an educational tool to help consumers select products with proven safety and efficacy. SupplementWatch conducts reviews of specific dietary supplement products and recommends brands that score 80 percent or higher in their 100-point rating system covering areas such as claims, theory/scientific support, safety, and value. The product ratings are targeted to consumers, who can access the information for free at the SupplementWatch Web site (www.supplementwatch.com), as well as to retailers, who can use the information to help them decide which products to stock on their shelves and to help them educate customers about which products to try.

The U.S. Pharmacopoeia (USP)

Many dietary supplements have started to use the USP designation on their labels to show consumers that the products meet the USP standards for purity, potency, disintegration, and dissolution. The USP is a nongovernmental, voluntary organization established in 1820 to help set quality standards for drug quality. Since the early 1900s, the USP has been recognized as the organization that establishes standards for product strength, quality, and purity—and the standards established by USP for drug products are legally enforceable by the FDA. To better understand exactly what the USP standards are evaluating, and what these standards mean for selecting specific supplement products, the following brief explanations are provided:

- *Disintegration* indicates how fast a tablet or capsule breaks into small pieces so the nutrients can dissolve. If a tablet or capsule does not break down completely within a certain amount of time, it may not dissolve and may pass through the body without being absorbed.
- *Dissolution* is a measurement of how fast a supplement dissolves. If the tablet or capsule does not dissolve (following dissolution of the tablet/capsule) its ingredients cannot be absorbed.
- *Strength* is the amount of a specific vitamin, mineral, or herbal in each tablet or capsule. To meet USP product quality standards, the amount present must be within a limited range of the amount declared on the label.
- *Purity* assures that the product is within a range for acceptable impurities (from contamination or degradation).
- *Expiration date* must be listed on the label indicating the date beyond which the supplement may no longer meet USP standards of purity, strength, and/or quality.

Complexity of Testing

One of the current debates raging within the dietary supplement industry is the need for and benefit of analytical laboratory testing. On the surface, the need for chemical analysis may be obvious—to ensure that products contain precisely what their labels claim. The problem, however, is that analytical testing procedures are quite different and much more complex than methods used to test for drug purity. Pharmaceutical preparations are typically manufactured with a single active ingredient (or at least a defined few), while most botanical supplements are a complex mixture of hundreds of chemical structures. Exactly which active ingredients deliver the health benefit is often unknown, as is the contribution of various inactive compounds to the overall effect of the supplement. The confusion is compounded by the fact that the analytical methodology (the actual tests) is itself very complex—and different methods can be used to test for the same ingredient (often with quite different results). In some cases, not even the manufacturer of the supplement has a good handle on the precise analytical method that may be most appropriate for testing for a particular range of compounds (and finding out may take several months to a year of lab work). In addition, because different manufacturers use different formulas and procedures for creating supplements in the same category (e.g., joint supplements), the same type of supplement, but with a different formula, may also call for a different test method (making it even harder to compare different brands of supplements head to head). Some of the questions that need to be answered prior to analytical testing of specific brands of dietary supplements include:

- Which of the active components should be analyzed for?
- What test methods accurately measure the existence of those ingredients?
- How much of these components should be present? In what ratios?
- Will the presence of one component interfere with the measurement of another?
- Can a test detect products that have been "doctored" with synthetic compounds?
- Even if a given product actually provides 100 percent of its label claim, what does this say about the safety and efficacy of the product when used as directed?

PUTTING DIETARY SUPPLEMENT CLAIMS INTO THE PROPER PERSPECTIVE

There is little doubt that some structure/function claims made for dietary supplement products stray quite close to the line in terms of touting specific health benefits. Chapter 1 outlined the *legality* of such claims, but just because a particular claim is legal says nothing about its scientific validity or its overall merit in educating or confusing consumers.

Supplement manufacturers and marketers use a variety of nutrient-content claims, disease claims, and nutrition support claims (which include structure/function claims) to sell their products. Remember from Chapter 1 that *nutrient content claims* describe the level of a nutrient in a food or dietary supplement (e.g., "High in calcium" for a 200 mg calcium tablet or "Excellent source of vitamin C" for supplements with at least 12 mg, 20 percent of the DV, of ascorbic acid). *Nutrition support claims* can describe a link between a nutrient and the deficiency disease that can result if the nutrient is lacking in the diet (e.g., vitamin C prevents scurvy), but the label must also indicate the prevalence of the disease in the United States. Nutrition support claims also cover the most popular of supplement claims—the structure/function claims that are used to refer to the effect of the supplement on the body's structure, function, or overall well-being (e.g., calcium builds strong bones, antioxidants maintain cell integrity, fiber maintains bowel regularity). *Disease claims* show a link between a food/nutrient and a disease—and the FDA only allows certain claims based on a review of the scientific evidence (Table 3.2). Currently, dietary supplements are permitted to carry disease claims for the following:

- Folic acid and decreased risk of neural tube defects
- Calcium and a lower risk of osteoporosis
- Psyllium seed husk and heart disease
- Soy protein and heart disease
- Omega-3 fatty acids and heart disease
- B vitamins (folic acid, B_6, and B_{12}) and heart disease

How to Spot Fraudulent Products

Both the FDA and FTC monitor dietary supplement claims—the FDA for safety and unauthorized drug/disease claims and the FTC for false advertising. Some common clues that can be used to spot fraudulent claims:

- Claims that the product is a "secret cure" or is part of "breakthrough" research
- Undefined or vague claims for a product's ability to "detoxify" or "purify" the body
- Claims that the product can cure a wide range of unrelated diseases
- Claims that a product is "backed by scientific studies"—but no list of references is provided
- Claims that the supplement has no side effects yet offers powerful effects
- Accusations that medical professionals and drug companies are suppressing information about effective alternative treatments

FDA GUIDANCE ON SCIENTIFIC REVIEW OF HEALTH CLAIMS

When evaluating *health* claims for dietary supplements (different than nutrition support claims), the scientific review process that the FDA uses to evaluate whether or not certain claims are warranted is quite comprehen-

TABLE 3.2. Authorized Health Claims That Can Be Made for Foods and/or Dietary Supplements

Nutrient/disease relationship	Sample claim	Requirements
Calcium and osteoporosis	Regular exercise and a healthy diet with enough calcium helps teen and young adult white and Asian women maintain good bone health and may reduce their high risk of osteoporosis later in life.	Food or supplement must be high in calcium and must not contain more phosphorus than calcium. Claims for products with more than 400 mg of calcium per day must state that a daily intake over 2,000 mg offers no added known benefit to bone health.
Sodium and hypertension	Diets low in sodium may reduce the risk of high blood pressure, a disease associated with many factors.	Foods must meet criteria for "low sodium."
Dietary fat and cancer	Development of cancer depends on many factors. A diet low in total fat may reduce the risk of some cancers.	Foods must meet criteria for "low fat" and fish and meats must meet criteria for "extra lean."
Dietary saturated fat and cholesterol and risk of coronary heart disease	While many factors affect heart disease, diets low in saturated fat and cholesterol may reduce the risk of this disease.	Foods must meet criteria for "low saturated fat," "low cholesterol," and "low fat." Fish and meats must meet criteria for "extra lean."
Fiber-containing grain products, fruits and vegetables, and cancer	Low-fat diets rich in fiber-containing grain products, fruits, and vegetables may reduce the risk of some types of cancer, a disease associated with many factors.	Foods must meet criteria for "low fat" and, without fortification, be a "good source" of dietary fiber.
Fruits, vegetables, and grain products that contain fiber, particularly soluble fiber, and risk of coronary heart disease	Diets low in saturated fat and cholesterol and rich in fruits, vegetables, and grain products that contain some types of dietary fiber, particularly soluble fiber, may reduce the risk of heart disease, a disease associated with many factors.	Foods must meet criteria for "low saturated fat," "low fat," and "low cholesterol." They must contain, without fortification, at least 0.6 g of soluble fiber per reference amount, and the soluble fiber content must be listed.
Fruits and vegetables and cancer	Low-fat diets rich in fruits and vegetables may reduce the risk of some types of cancer, a disease associated with many factors.	Foods must meet criteria for "low fat" and, without fortification, be a "good source" of fiber, vitamin A, or vitamin C.

TABLE 3.2 *(continued)*

Nutrient/disease relationship	Sample claim	Requirements
Folate and neural tube birth defects	Healthful diets with adequate folate may reduce a woman's risk of having a child with a brain or spinal cord birth defect.	Foods must meet or exceed criteria for "good source" of folate—that is, at least 40 mcg of folic acid per serving (at least 10 percent of the Daily Value).
		A serving of food cannot contain more than 100 percent of the DV for vitamin A and vitamin D because of their potential risk to fetuses.
Dietary sugar alcohol and dental caries (cavities)	Frequent between-meal consumption of foods high in sugars and starches promotes tooth decay. The sugar alcohols in this food do not promote tooth decay. Shortened claim (small packages): "Does not promote tooth decay."	Foods must meet the criteria for "sugar free." The sugar alcohol must be xylitol, sorbitol, mannitol, maltitol, isomalt, lactitol, hydrogenated starch hydrolysates, hydrogenated glucose syrups, erythritol, or a combination of these.
Dietary soluble fiber, such as that found in whole oats and psyllium seed husk, and coronary heart disease	Diets low in saturated fat and cholesterol that include 3 g of soluble fiber from whole oats per day may reduce the risk of heart disease. One serving of this whole-oats product provides ____ g of this soluble fiber.	Foods must meet criteria for "low saturated fat," "low cholesterol," and "low fat." Foods that contain whole oats must contain at least 0.75 g of soluble fiber per serving. Foods that contain psyllium seed husk must contain at least 1.7 g of soluble fiber per serving.
Soy protein and heart disease	Diets low in saturated fat and cholesterol that include 25 g of soy protein a day may reduce the risk of heart disease. One serving of (name of food) provides ____ g of soy protein.	In order to qualify for this health claim, a food must contain at least 6.25 g of soy protein per serving (one-fourth of the effective level of 25 g per day).
Omega-3 fatty acids and heart disease	The scientific evidence about whether omega-3 fatty acids may reduce the risk of coronary heart disease (CHD) is suggestive, but not conclusive. Studies in the general population have looked at diets containing fish, and it is not known whether diets or	Must include a qualifying statement about the importance of low saturated-fat diets in reducing heart disease risk—such as "It is known that diets low in saturated fat and cholesterol may reduce the risk of heart disease."

Nutrient/disease relationship	Sample claim	Requirements
	omega-3 fatty acids in fish may have a possible effect on reduced risk of CHD. It is not known what effects omega-3 fatty acids may or may not have on risk of CHD in the general population.	
B vitamins and heart disease	The scientific evidence about whether folic acid, vitamin B_6, and vitamin B_{12} may reduce the risk of heart and other vascular diseases is suggestive, but not conclusive. Studies in the general population have generally found that these vitamins lower homocysteine, an amino acid found in the blood. It is not known whether elevated levels of homocysteine may cause vascular disease or whether homocysteine levels are caused by other factors. Studies that will directly evaluate whether reducing homocysteine may also reduce the risk of vascular disease are not yet complete.	Must include a qualifying statement about the importance of low saturated-fat diets in reducing heart disease risk—such as "It is known that diets low in saturated fat and cholesterol may reduce the risk of heart disease."

sive. The standard of scientific validity for a health claim includes two components: (1) that the totality of the publicly available evidence supports the substance/disease relationship that is the subject of the claim, and (2) that there is "significant scientific agreement" among qualified experts that the relationship is valid.

Because of the limitations of the various research methods used to study the relationship between nutrients and disease, it is not possible to specify the exact type or number of studies needed to support a health claim. An additional limitation is the dependence on data derived from studies that were not specifically designed or conducted for the purpose of supporting a health claim. In reviewing a health claim petition, the FDA identifies specific studies to review. In general, interventional studies provide the strongest evidence for a beneficial nutrient/disease effect, but the overall quality and relevance of each individual study is considered in assessing its contribution to the weight of the evidence for the proposed nutrient/disease relationship. The evaluation of study design, protocol, measurement, and statistical issues for individual studies serves as the starting point from which the FDA determines the overall strengths and weaknesses of the data and assesses the weight of the evidence. Criteria that are considered by the FDA in assessing the quality of individual studies of substance/disease relationships include the following:

- Adequacy and clarity of the design.
- Were the questions to be answered by the study clearly described at the outset?
- Was the methodology used in the study clearly described and appropriate for answering the questions posed by the study?
- Was the duration of the study intervention or follow-up period sufficient to detect an effect on the outcome of interest?
- Were potential confounding factors identified, assessed, and/or controlled?
- Was subject attrition (subjects leaving the study before the study is completed) assessed, explained, and reasonable?
- Population studied.
- Was the sample size large enough to provide sufficient statistical power to detect a significant effect? (If the study is underpowered, it may be impossible to conclude that the absence of an effect is not due to chance.)
- Was the study population representative (for factors such as age, gender distribution, race, socioeconomic status, geographic location, family history, health status, and motivation) of the population to which the health claim will be targeted?
- Were criteria for inclusion and exclusion of study subjects clearly stated and appropriate?
- Were recruitment procedures that minimized selection bias used?
- For controlled interventions, were subjects randomized? If matching was employed to assign the subjects to control and treatment groups, were appropriate demographic characteristics and other variables used for the matching? Was randomization successful in producing similar control and intervention groups?
- Were analytical methodology and quality control procedures to assess dietary intake adequate?
- Was the dietary intervention or exposure well defined and appropriately measured?

- For intervention studies, was an appropriate level of intake (i.e., the level hypothesized to be effective) for the food substance of interest planned, monitored, and achieved?
- Were the background diets to which the test substance was added, or the control and interventional diets, adequately described, measured, and suitable?
- Was a lead-in period employed for dietary interventions? (Because changes in the diet may induce compensatory metabolic changes, the effect of an intervention should be measured after stabilization has occurred, i.e., a lead-in period.)
- In studies with crossover designs, was there an appropriate washout period (period during which subjects do not receive an intervention) between dietary treatments? (Lack of a sufficient washout period between interventions may lead to confusion as to which intervention produced the health outcome.)
- Were the form and setting of the intervention representative of the real world?
- Were other possible concurrent changes in diet or health-related behavior (weight loss, exercise, alcohol intake, smoking cessation) during the study that could account for the outcome identified, assessed, and/or controlled?
- Were the disease outcomes well defined and appropriately measured? If biomarkers (intermediate or surrogate endpoint markers) were measured, has their relevance to disease outcomes been validated?
- Were efforts made to detect harmful as well as beneficial effects? (For example, increasing the consumption of some food substances may increase the risk of a chronic disease, and extracting or concentrating some food substances may render them injurious to health.)
- Were appropriate statistical analyses applied to the data?
- Was statistical significance interpreted appropriately? (For example, differences that are not statistically significant should be described as not demonstrating a difference rather than as showing a trend.)

Some individuals and organizations have proposed various scoring methods for grading studies (e.g., "A/1" for the largest, longest, and most well-controlled studies, down to "F/5" for studies with significant flaws in experimental design). Although both codes (I, II, III, A, B, C) and quantitative scores may be appropriate for rating *individual* studies, they do not adequately describe the evidence as a whole. For example, these methods do not capture the number of studies or consistency of findings. *At present, a universally applicable system for evaluation of the evidence as a whole is not available*. In addition to the study design, many other factors contribute to the strength of the evidence, including:

- the *number of studies* in support of the association,
- the *consistency* of results across different settings and types of populations,
- whether *conflicting* results exist and whether they necessarily disprove an association (because elements of the study design may account for the lack of an effect in negative studies), and
- the *magnitude of the effect* (larger is better, and strong statistical significance with narrow confidence intervals is even better).

In general, the ultimate question that must be answered is whether the evidence in support of the nutrient/disease relationship outweighs the evidence against it and whether the available body of evidence is sufficient to permit the conclusion that a change in the dietary intake of that nutrient will result in a change in the disease endpoint (e.g., that consuming more calcium equals a reduced risk of osteoporosis).

Significant scientific agreement cannot be reached without a strong, relevant, and consistent body of evidence on which experts in the field may base a conclusion that a nutrient/disease relationship exists. It is important to appreciate the fact that there is considerable potential for incorrect conclusions if only preliminary evidence (emerging science) is available for review. Perhaps the best example of this situation is illustrated by the body of evidence for the association between beta-carotene and cancer risk. At the time of the FDA's health claim review, no results from relevant clinical trials had been reported—but several human epidemiological studies were available, and several laboratory studies had proposed mechanistic theories on how beta-carotene might reduce cancer risk.

While there was strong evidence that a high intake of fruits and vegetables rich in carotenoids was associated with a reduced risk of cancer, it was unclear whether the active components of fruits and vegetables were beta-carotene, other carotenoids, fiber, or some other compounds yet to be identified. Animal studies, however, strongly suggested a positive effect of beta-carotene in lowering the frequency and severity of experimental cancer.

The FDA review concluded that existing evidence was inconclusive and that significant scientific agreement did not yet exist; the animal studies could not be applied directly to humans because the type and amount of carcinogen exposure in the experimental conditions were not similar to human exposure. Subsequently, the FDA's decision to deny the health claim was further supported when a randomized, controlled trial in Finland found that not only did beta-carotene *not* prevent the development of lung cancer in high-risk Finnish men with a history of smoking, but it actually caused a significant *increase* in the rate of lung cancer among the beta-carotene supplemented group (an unexpected outcome based on the preliminary evidence).

In determining whether there is significant scientific agreement, the FDA also takes into account the viewpoints of qualified experts outside the agency, if evaluations by such experts have been conducted and are publicly available. For example, the FDA will take into account:

- review publications that critically summarize data and information in the scientific literature;
- documentation of the opinion of an expert panel that is specifically convened for this purpose by a credible, independent body; and
- the opinion or recommendation of a federal government scientific body such as the National Institutes of Health (NIH) or the Centers for Disease Control and Prevention; or the National Academy of Sciences; or an independent, expert body such as the Committee on Nutrition of the American Academy of Pediatrics, the American Heart Association, American Cancer Society, or task forces or other groups assembled by the NIH.

ADVERTISING AND CLAIMS SUBSTANTIATION FOR DIETARY SUPPLEMENTS

The Federal Trade Commission and the Food and Drug Administration work together but have divided responsibilities with regard to dietary supplement regulation. As applied to dietary supplements, the FDA has primary responsibility for claims on product labeling, including packaging, inserts, and other promotional materials distributed at the point of sale. The FTC has primary responsibility for claims in advertising (including print and broadcast ads, infomercials, catalogs, and direct marketing materials, including marketing on the Internet). Because of their shared jurisdiction, the two agencies work closely to ensure that their enforcement efforts are consistent to the fullest extent possible.

The FTC's truth-in-advertising law can be boiled down to two common-sense propositions: (1) advertising must be truthful and not misleading; and (2) before disseminating an ad, advertisers must have adequate substantiation for all objective product claims. A deceptive ad is one that contains a misrepresentation or omission that is likely to mislead consumers acting reasonably under the circumstances, to their detriment. The FTC's substantiation standard typically means "competent and reliable scientific evidence"—but it also covers all claims, whether *express* or *implied*, that the ad conveys to consumers.

Identifying Express and Implied Claims

The first step in evaluating the truthfulness and accuracy of advertising is to identify all express and implied claims that an ad conveys to consumers. Advertisers must make sure that whatever they say expressly in an ad is accurate. Often, however, an ad conveys other claims beyond those expressly stated. Under FTC law, an advertiser is equally responsible for the accuracy of claims suggested or implied by the ad. Advertisers cannot suggest claims that they could not make directly.

> *Example:* An advertisement for your product claims that "university studies prove" that a mineral supplement can improve athletic performance. You, as the advertiser, are responsible for having the studies to document the advertised benefit. Furthermore, the ad strongly implies to consumers that those studies, because they were conducted at a university, are scientifically sound.

> *Example:* An ad for an herbal supplement makes the claim that the product "boosts the immune system to help maintain a healthy nose and throat during the winter season." The ad features the product name Flu-Gone and includes images of people sneezing and coughing. The various elements of the ad—the product name, the depictions of cold and flu sufferers, and the reference to nose and throat health during the winter season—likely convey to consumers that the product helps prevent colds. Therefore, the advertiser must be able to substantiate that claim. Even without the product name and images, the reference to nose and throat health during the winter season may still convey a cold prevention claim.

Disclosure of Qualifying Information/Clear and Prominent Disclosure

Advertisements are required to disclose information if it is "material in light of representations made or suggested by the ad, or material considering how consumers would customarily use the product" (Federal Trade Commission, "Dietary Supplements: An Advertising Guide for Industry"). This standard means that because certain information is not disclosed, con-

sumers may be misled into thinking that a particular product works differently than if they had been provided all relevant information. Likewise,
when the disclosure of qualifying information is necessary to prevent an ad
from being deceptive, that information should be presented clearly and
prominently so that it is actually noticed and understood by consumers. A
fine-print disclosure at the bottom of a print ad, a disclaimer buried in a
body of text, a brief video superscript in a television ad, or a disclaimer that
is easily missed on an Internet Web site are not likely to be adequate.

> *Example:* An ad for a weight loss supplement cites a placebo-
> controlled, double-blind clinical study as demonstrating that the prod-
> uct resulted in an average weight loss of fifteen pounds over an eight-
> week period. The weight loss for the test group is, in fact, significantly
> greater than for the control subjects. However, both the control and
> test subjects engaged in regular exercise and followed a calorie-
> restricted diet as part of the study regimen. The advertisement should
> make clear that users of the supplement must follow the same diet and
> exercise regimen to achieve the claimed weight loss results.

> *Example:* The same weight loss supplement is advertised with the
> headline "FAST & EASY WEIGHT LOSS" along with dramatic be-
> fore and after pictures and ad copy that describes how the product
> helps users lose weight easily. A fine-print disclosure at the bottom of
> the ad indicating that in addition to taking the supplement, users must
> also follow a "low-calorie diet and regular exercise program" would
> not be sufficiently prominent to qualify the headline and the overall
> impression that the product alone will cause weight loss.

The Amount and Type of Evidence

A guiding principle for determining the amount and type of evidence that
will be sufficient is the amount that "experts in the relevant area of study
would generally consider to be adequate." As a general rule, well-controlled
human clinical studies are the most reliable form of evidence. Results obtained in animal and in vitro studies will also be examined, particularly
where they are widely considered to be acceptable substitutes for human research or where human research is not possible. Although there is no requirement that any specific *number* of studies support a dietary supplement
claim, the replication of research results in an independently conducted
study adds to the weight of the evidence. In most situations, the quality of
studies will be more important than quantity. When a clinical trial is not possible (e.g., in the case of a relationship between a nutrient and a condition

that may take decades to develop), epidemiological evidence may be an acceptable substitute for clinical data, especially when supported by other evidence, such as research explaining the biological mechanism underlying the claimed effect. Anecdotal evidence about the individual experience of consumers is clearly not sufficient to substantiate claims about the effects of a supplement. Even if those experiences are genuine, they may be attributable to a placebo effect or other factors unrelated to the supplement. Individual experiences are not a substitute for scientific research.

> *Example:* A supplement is advertised for its benefits in "maintaining good vision into old age." In addition to a long-term, large-scale epidemiological study showing a strong association between lifelong high consumption of the principal ingredient in the supplement and better vision in those over the age of sixty, scientific experts in the area have discovered a plausible biological mechanism that might explain the effect. Because a clinical intervention trial would be very difficult and costly to conduct, such a claim would be permitted.

The Quality of the Evidence

In addition to the amount and type of evidence, the FTC examines the validity of each piece of evidence. While there is no set protocol for how to conduct research that will be acceptable under the FTC substantiation doctrine, there are several well-accepted scientific principles that can be used to assess the validity of test results (placebo-controlled, blinding of subjects/researchers, longer duration, etc.).

> *Example:* A supplement is advertised to help reduce appetite in people trying to lose weight. There are three studies supporting the effect and no contrary evidence. One study consists of subjects tested over a one-week period, with no control group. The second study is well-controlled, of longer duration, but shows only a slight effect that is not statistically significant. The third study administers the compound through injection and shows a significant appetite-suppressant effect, but there is some question whether the compound would be absorbed into the bloodstream if administered orally. Because the studies all have significant limitations, it would be difficult to draft even a carefully qualified claim that would adequately convey to consumers the limited nature of the evidence. The advertiser should not base a claim on these studies.

The Totality of the Evidence

Studies cannot be evaluated in isolation. The surrounding context of the scientific evidence is just as important as the internal validity of individual studies. Advertisers should consider all relevant research relating to the claimed benefit of their supplement and should not focus only on research that supports the effect, while discounting research that does not. Wide variation in outcomes of studies and inconsistent or conflicting results will raise serious questions about the adequacy of substantiation. Where there are inconsistencies in the evidence, it is important to examine whether there is a plausible explanation for those inconsistencies. In some instances, for example, the differences in results are attributable to differences in dosage, the form of administration (e.g., oral or intravenous), the population tested, or other aspects of study methodology.

> *Example:* A supplement is advertised to "help increase metabolism and reduce body fat," and the product is supported by two controlled, double-blind studies showing a modest but statistically significant loss of fat at the end of a six-week period. However, there is an equally well-controlled, blinded twelve-week study showing no statistically significant difference between test and control groups consuming the same product. Assuming other aspects of methodology are similar, the studies taken together suggest that, if the product has any effect on body fat, it would be very small. Given the totality of the evidence on the subject, the claim is likely to be unsubstantiated.

The Relevance of the Evidence to the Specific Claim

A common problem in substantiation of advertising claims occurs when an advertiser has valid studies, but the studies do not support the claim made in the ad. Claims that do not match the science, no matter how sound that science is, are likely to be considered unsubstantiated by the FTC. Advertising should not exaggerate the extent, nature, or permanence of the effects achieved in a study and should not suggest greater scientific certainty than actually exists. Although emerging science can sometimes be the basis for a carefully qualified claim, advertisers must make consumers aware of any significant limitations or inconsistencies in the scientific literature.

> *Example:* An ad for a supplement claims that a particular nutrient helps maintain healthy cholesterol levels. A substantial body of epidemiological evidence suggests that foods high in that nutrient are as-

sociated with lower cholesterol levels. There is no science, however, demonstrating a relationship between the specific nutrient and cholesterol, although it would be feasible to conduct such a study. If there is a basis for believing that the health effect may be attributable to other components of the food, or to a combination of various components, a claim about the cholesterol maintenance benefits of the supplement product is likely not substantiated by this evidence.

Example: An energy-boosting supplement is advertised to "help increase alertness safely and naturally." The product contains two herbs known to have a central nervous system stimulant effect and the manufacturer has compiled reliable scientific research that each of the herbs, individually, is safe and causes no significant side effects in the recommended dose. This evidence may be inadequate to substantiate an unqualified safety claim if there is any reason to suspect that the combination of multiple ingredients might result in interactions that would alter the effect or safety of the individual ingredients.

Claims Based on Consumer Experiences or Expert Endorsements

An overall principle suggested by the FTC is that advertisers should not make claims through either consumer or expert endorsements that would be deceptive or could not be substantiated if made directly. It is not enough that a testimonial represents the honest opinion of the endorser. Under FTC law, advertisers must also have appropriate scientific evidence to back up the underlying claim. Ads that include consumer testimonials about the efficacy or safety of a supplement still need to be backed up by adequate substantiation that the testimonial experience is representative of what consumers will generally achieve when using the product. When a supplement is advertised by an "expert" endorser, the advertiser or manufacturer should make sure that the endorser has appropriate qualifications to be represented as an expert and has conducted testing of the product that would be generally recognized in the field as sufficient to support the endorsement. In addition, whenever an expert or consumer endorser is used, the advertiser should disclose any material connection between the endorser and the advertiser of the product (such as a financial interest).

Example: An ad for a weight loss supplement features before and after pictures of a woman along with her quote stating, "I lost thirty pounds in thirty days while using Fat-Burners." An asterisk next to the quotation references a disclaimer in fine print at the bottom of the ad that reads, "Results may vary." The experience of the woman is accurately represented, but the research on the effectiveness of the supplement showed an average weight loss of only eight pounds in thirty days. Therefore, the disclosure does not adequately convey to consumers that they would likely see much less dramatic results. The placement and size of the disclaimer is also insufficiently prominent to qualify the claim effectively.

Example: An infomercial for a dietary supplement features an expert referred to as a "doctor" and a "leading clinician in joint health" discussing the effect of a supplement product on the maintenance of healthy joints. The expert is not licensed to practice medicine but has a graduate degree and is a trained physical therapist, running a sports clinic. The expert has not conducted any review of the scientific literature on the active component of the supplement. In return for appearing in the infomercial, she is given a paid position as an officer in the company. The ad is likely to be deceptive for several reasons. First, her qualifications as an expert have been overstated, and she has not conducted sufficient examination of the product to support the endorsement. In addition, her connection to the company is one that consumers might not expect and may affect the weight and credibility of her endorsement. Even if she is adequately qualified and has conducted an adequate review of the product, her position as an officer of the company should be clearly disclosed.

"Traditional Use" Claims

Claims based on historical or traditional use should be confirmed by well-controlled scientific studies or should be presented in such a way that consumers understand that the sole basis for the claim is a history of use of the product for a particular purpose. A number of supplements, particularly botanical products, have a long history of use as traditional medicines to treat certain conditions or symptoms. Several European countries have a separate regulatory approach to these traditional medicines, allowing manufacturers to make certain limited claims about their traditional use for treating certain health conditions. It is important for advertisers to be sure that they can document the extent and manner of historical use and that they be careful not to overstate such use.

Example: A supplement is marketed in the same formulation used for centuries in China as a tonic for improving mental function. The manufacturer prepares the product in a manner consistent with Chinese preparation methods. The ad claims, "Traditional Chinese Medicine—Used for Thousands of Years to Bring Mental Clarity and Improve Memory." The ad also contains language that clearly conveys that the efficacy of the product has not been confirmed by research, and that traditional use does not establish that the product will achieve the claimed results. The ad is likely to adequately convey the limited nature of support for the claim.

Example: A supplement is marketed as a capsule containing a concentrated extract of a botanical product that has been used in its raw form in China to brew teas for increasing energy. The advertisement clearly conveys that the energy benefit is based on traditional use and has not been confirmed by scientific research. The ad may still be deceptive, however, because the concentrated extract is not consistent with the traditional use of the botanical in raw form and may produce a significantly different effect.

Use of the DSHEA Disclaimer in Advertising

Under section 6 of DSHEA, a two-part disclaimer must accompany all statements of nutritional support for dietary supplements on the product label: that the statement has not been evaluated by FDA and that the product is not intended to "diagnose, treat, cure or prevent any disease."

Example: You market a joint flexibility supplement using a product name and packaging that is similar in color and design to a nonprescription drug used to treat joint pain associated with arthritis. The advertising for this product may lead consumers to believe that the supplement is, in fact, an approved drug, or may give consumers more general expectations that the product has been subjected to similar government review for safety and efficacy.

Example: You advertise a dietary supplement with various structure/function claims and a statement that the product "Complies with FDA notification procedures of the Dietary Supplement Health and Education Act." This statement may suggest to consumers that FDA has authorized the claims made in the ad or that it has reviewed the support for the claims and found the product to be effective. Because there is no review and authorization process for such claims under DSHEA, this would be deceptive.

Third-Party Literature

As outlined in Chapter 1, section 5 of DSHEA permits the use of third-party literature, within specific guidelines, to help educate consumers about dietary supplements. From an advertising and sales perspective, however, advertising that refers to specific third-party literature to promote your product is typically not permitted.

> *Example:* You refer to a book, *The Alzheimer's Miracle Cure,* whether it mentions your supplement specifically by name or not, in advertising for your brain health supplement. Even if the book does not endorse or otherwise mention your supplement brand, by referring to the book in advertising materials (e.g., "as mentioned in *The Alzheimer's Miracle Cure*"), as the advertiser, you would be responsible for substantiating any claims about the product that are conveyed by your references to the book, whereas the book itself, as noncommercial speech, would not be subject to the FTC's jurisdiction over advertising.

What Needs to Be in Your "Substantiation File"

- *Notification letter:* A copy of the notification letter should be included.
- *Identification of dietary supplement ingredients:* The identity and quantity of the dietary supplement ingredient that is the subject of the statement of nutritional support should be included. If possible, the active component and mechanism of action should also be indicated.
- *Evidence to substantiate statements of nutritional support:* Such evidence should include copies of key references to experimental or clinical data and/or findings of authoritative bodies and other evidence. References should include relevant information, positive or negative. Research or monographs from appropriate foreign sources may be cited, along with evidence that specific uses or claims are approved in other countries. An interpretive synopsis by individuals or groups qualified by training and experience to evaluate the evidence should accompany the literature citations and should assess clearly the evidence supporting the statement. Evidence for efficacy should include the dosage at which effects are observed. Where historical use is cited as the evidence for a statement, the composition of the product should correspond with the material for which such claims of historical use may be made. The complexity of a product may affect the substantiation required.

- *Evidence to substantiate safety:* The file should indicate the basis of the manufacturer's conclusion that the product can reasonably be expected to be safe at intended levels of use.
- *Good manufacturing practices:* Assurance that GMPs were followed in the manufacture of the product should be indicated.
- *Qualifications of reviewers:* The qualifications of those who reviewed the evidence should be included. Substantiation should be assembled by an individual or group qualified by training and experience to assess the evidence, and the file should list the qualifications of those who reviewed the data on safety and efficacy. If an external advisory body was consulted, it should be identified.

Chapter 4

Supplements for Weight Loss

INTRODUCTION

Weight loss products are the Holy Grail for the supplement industry. Aside from multivitamins, weight loss is the largest (no fat jokes!) category in terms of sales—racking up several billion dollars in 1999 alone. Around the world, the prevalence of overweight and obesity has been steadily increasing over the past fifty years, and studies in developed countries (e.g., the United States, Canada, and Great Britain) suggest that this trend will continue at an alarming rate. Overweight is defined as having a body mass index (BMI) of over 27.0 kg/m^2, and obese is defined as a BMI greater than 30 kg/m^2 (or about 30 percent above ideal body weight).

Over the past two decades or so (1976-1994), the prevalence of obesity in the American population increased from 12.8 percent to 22.5 percent. Further, in 1999, over half (61 percent) of U.S. adults were classified as overweight or obese (according to the National Health and Nutrition Examination Surveys, or NHANES). The increase in the number of overweight and obese adults is a major health concern because obesity contributes to an increased risk of heart disease, hypertension, diabetes, and some cancers, and is now considered one of the primary risk factors for cardiovascular disease (along with smoking, high cholesterol, hypertension, and sedentary lifestyle).

EXERCISE VERSUS DIET

It is obvious that as we age, we have a tendency to gain weight, particularly fat weight. It is unclear, however, if this age-related weight gain is an unavoidable condition. Regular exercise is often promoted as a tool for preventing weight gain—and there is good evidence that people who are more active have a reduced risk of gaining weight. In one study, a large group of men were followed over two years. At the beginning of this period, the most active men and those that watched fewer hours of television were less likely to be overweight (it seems that *Who Wants to Be a Millionaire* contributes directly to obesity). After two years, those who were most active and watched fewer hours of television gained less weight (moral of the story— kill your television). Data from several national surveys (in both the United States and other countries) clearly show that people who maintain higher levels of physical activity are less likely to gain weight, or at least gain less weight than their inactive counterparts.

However, whether exercise is a good tool for promoting weight loss is somewhat controversial. A recent review of studies related to the effect of physical activity in the treatment of adulthood overweight and obesity concluded that adding exercise to a reduction in caloric intake only leads to modest additional weight loss (5 to 7 lb), but that regular participation in exercise is strongly associated with *maintenance* of weight loss. Thus, although exercise may not be the best approach for initial weight loss, it is an important factor in prevention of weight regain.

So, with most of the available evidence suggesting that physical activity plays a more important role in reducing age-related weight gain than in actually promoting weight loss, the obvious question is, "Why is exercise not more effective in promoting weight loss?" The answer is because of the difficulty in promoting a substantial negative energy balance with exercise alone. Negative energy balance is a state in which one expends more energy (calories) than one consumes. To achieve a state of negative energy balance, one must consume fewer calories, expend more energy, or both. This seems like a pretty simple task, but the reality is that most adult Americans do not have a good understanding of the energy value of different foods or exercises. Most people tend to underestimate the caloric value of the food consumed and overestimate the caloric value of exercise. Consider some of the values in Table 4.1.

STEP FAR AWAY FROM THE CHEESECAKE

A caloric deficit of approximately 3,500 calories (kcal) is needed to lose 1 pound (lb) of body fat. If your goal is to lose 1 to 2 lb per week (a reasonable goal for most overweight individuals), this would require a caloric deficit of 500-1,000 kcal *each day!* For most people, this would mean 30 to 60 minutes of intense exercise daily. Unfortunately, most American adults are extremely sedentary—with about one-third getting *no* physical activity and most people becoming less and less active as they age (exactly the opposite way that the trend should be heading).

More striking is the fact that the benefits of exercise can easily be offset with inappropriate food choices. It is easy to see that the amount of energy

TABLE 4.1. Calories Burned by Exercise Compared to Those Supplied by Food

Energy (calories)	Exercise for 30 minutes*	Dietary equivalent
100	Walking, leisurely pace	¾ cup of ice cream
150	Walking, brisk pace	6 Oreo cookies
200	Stationary cycling, easy	3 tablespoons of peanut butter
240	Lap swimming, leisurely	20 potato chips or French fries
240	Aerobic exercise class	1 slice of pizza
300	Lap swimming, vigorous	12 Hershey Kisses
300	Stationary cycling, vigorous	1 fried chicken leg
300	Running, slow pace	1 Burger King cheeseburger
500	Running, fast pace	1 Taco Bell bean burrito with cheese

*For a person who weighs more than 175 lb, the estimated energy expenditure is slightly higher, and slightly lower for those who weigh less than 175 lb.

expended during 30 minutes of walking can easily be offset with a handful of potato chips, a slice of pizza, or six to eight Oreos! This should not scare one into avoiding these foods at all costs, but it should be recognized that all of us need to consider our "calorie budgets" very carefully.

So, how much physical activity is needed to (1) prevent weight gain and (2) promote substantial weight loss? This is not an easy question to answer, especially considering that exercise will have different effects on appetite and food intake in different people. However, most people will find that their food intake and hunger will not increase much when they begin exercising. In one study, women who had lost weight were followed over the subsequent twelve months. The threshold level of physical activity required to prevent weight regain (less than 10 lb) corresponded to approximately *80 minutes of brisk walking per day.* People enrolled in the National Weight Control Registry (NWCR) report a similar level of walking (the NWCR is a large database of individuals who have maintained a 30 lb weight loss for at least one year). In addition, recent data from Japan suggest that accumulating 12,000 to 16,000 steps per day reduces the risk of weight gain. Thus, using a pedometer to track your daily step totals may provide feedback as to whether you are reaching an activity level high enough to help manage your weight.

It is essential to remember that it is *total* daily energy expenditure that is important. If you increase your daily amount of exercise, but become more inactive during other parts of the day, the impact of exercise on body weight will be minimized. Perhaps the best strategy is to increase the amount of daily *planned* physical activity (e.g., add a 15 to 30 minute walk at lunch or in the evening), but to also increase your amount of *unplanned* physical activity (e.g., take the stairs instead of the elevator, avoid escalators, park your car a few blocks from work).

SUPPLEMENTS THAT MAY HELP

Although exercise can play an important role in helping you prevent further weight gain (or regain), diet will represent the primary way to shed unwanted pounds. Although it might sound easy on paper—to simply put less food in your mouth—the reality is that reducing calorie intake is a huge problem for most of us. Some of the supplements outlined in this chapter may be helpful in suppressing appetite and controlling food cravings, while others may provide a mild increase in caloric expenditure or benefits in related metabolic pathways (see Table 4.2). *None* of the ingredients should be viewed as anything remotely close to a magic bullet to help "melt away" fat (marketing hype notwithstanding)—but some of them may be modestly effective as an addition to a reduced-calorie diet and a program of moderate exercise (they are supplements after all).

Chromium is one of the most popular dietary supplements marketed for weight loss—so popular, in fact, that a number of companies have been slapped with FTC penalties for making "fat-burner" types of claims for chromium-based products. Even though chromium is no magic fat-melting bullet, it does play a vital role in carbohydrate metabolism. As a dietary supplement, chromium may be helpful in controlling blood sugar (by enhancing insulin action) and by doing so may help some people reduce appetite and food cravings. Vanadium is another mineral that has effects in promoting the actions of insulin and therefore may also be beneficial in controlling blood sugar.

Conjugated linoleic acid, or CLA, is a mixture of different forms (isomers) of the essential fatty acid linoleic acid. CLA is found in the diet primarily in beef and dairy products—but as most of us eat less of these foods when we are attempting weight loss, our daily intake of CLA is fairly low. Several studies, both animal and human, have shown CLA supplements (about 3 grams [g] per day) to promote an increase in lean body mass (muscle), while causing a decrease in body fat percentage (although weight frequently does not change). One study in particular gave subjects 3 g of CLA for ninety days and found a 20 percent reduction in body fat and a 5 percent increase in lean muscle.

TABLE 4.2. Dietary Supplements Promoted for Weight Loss and Weight Maintenance

Ingredient	Dose (per day)	Action
5-Hydroxytryptophan	300-900 mg	Mood balance/appetite control
Banaba leaf	32-48 mg	Blood sugar/appetite control
Bladderwrack	N/A	Thermogenic
Carnitine	2-6 g	Fat oxidation
Chitosan	2-6 g	Fat binding
Chromium	200-1,000 mcg	Blood sugar/appetite control
Citrus aurantium (synephrine)	4-20 mg	Thermogenic/appetite suppressant
Conjugated linoleic acid (CLA)	3-5 g	Thermogenic
Fiber	20-40 g	Fat binding
Garcinia cambogia (hydroxycitric acid)	750-1,500 mg	Thermogenic/appetite suppressant
Glucomannan	1-4 g	Fat binding
Green tea	125-500 mg	Thermogenic
Guarana (caffeine)	100-500 mg	Thermogenic/appetite suppressant
Gymnema sylvestre	200-400 mg	Blood sugar/appetite control
Ma huang/*Sida cordifolia* (ephedra)	12-24 mg	Thermogenic/appetite suppressant
Pyruvate	5-20 g	Thermogenic
Quercetin	100-1,000 mg	Thermogenic
St. John's wort	450-900 mg	Mood balance/appetite control
Vanadium	10-100 mcg	Blood sugar/appetite control
White willow (salicin)	100-120 mg	Thermogenic

Banaba leaf and *Gymnema sylvestre* are popular supplement ingredients in products targeting blood sugar control and diabetes. Both herbs are quite effective in reducing elevated blood sugar levels—a hallmark of diabetes and a key factor for many people in controlling appetite. Banaba appears to lower blood sugar levels by increasing the uptake of glucose into cells, while gymnema seems to control blood sugar by slowing the absorption of sugar from the intestinal tract. Because blood sugar fluctuations can be closely related to hunger, energy levels, and food cravings in many people, adequate control of blood sugar levels throughout the day may be quite effective in promoting weight loss and maintenance.

Fiber and chitosan are often used in weight loss supplements for their "fat-binding" properties, which may help reduce the intestinal absorption of a small amount of fat.

Garcinia cambogia, a plant native to India, contains a relatively high concentration of hydroxy citric acid (HCA). Some small-animal studies suggest that HCA may promote weight maintenance by reducing appetite and the conversion of carbohydrates into fat (by inhibiting the action of an enzyme, citrate lyase).

Green tea has become an extremely popular dietary supplement for weight loss following the publication of a study in the *American Journal of Clinical Nutrition.* The study, which fed green tea extract (containing 50 mg of caffeine and 90 mg of EGCG, one of the catechins naturally found in green tea) three times per day, found a significant 4 percent increase in energy expenditure throughout the day as well as an increase in the amount of fat burning. This has led a number of companies to add green tea to their products and tout the "thermogenic" and "fat oxidation" effects of green tea. Although the study did not measure weight loss over time, it was able to show that the benefits of green tea were not due entirely to the caffeine content (because they also looked at pure caffeine, which was not as effective in increasing caloric expenditure or fat metabolism).

Guarana is a South American herb that is found in a number of weight loss products as a natural source of caffeine. Just like the caffeine in your morning cup of coffee, guarana is effective in suppressing appetite and causing a slight elevation in energy expenditure (as a stimulant).

Ma huang, also known as ephedra, is the granddaddy of weight loss herbs—primarily due to the success of Metabolife and related products. Ephedra is, like caffeine, a central nervous system stimulant—so it can suppress appetite and cause a slight increase in energy expenditure. Unfortunately, a number of adverse side effects are common in many (but not all) people—such as headaches, insomnia, elevated blood pressure, irritability, and heart palpitations. The weight loss effects of ephedra are generally enhanced by combination with caffeine and aspirin, the popular "ECA stack"—but the side effects are also more common and more pronounced.

Pyruvate, a three-carbon sugar molecule, has been promoted as a weight loss aid following the publication of two clinical studies in which pyruvate supplements enhanced the amount of weight and fat lost by subjects consuming a low-calorie diet. The mechanism behind this effect may cause a slight increase in metabolic rate and the number of calories burned each day while consuming the supplement.

St. John's wort and 5-HTP are two supplements used primarily for their effects in elevating serotonin levels, relieving mild depression, and promoting emotional well-being. Because low serotonin levels have also been theorized to contribute to hunger and overeating, some supplements include St. John's wort or 5-HTP as a way to balance serotonin levels and control appetite. After the "fen-phen" debacle a few years ago, a number of national weight loss centers began prescribing Prozac as a weight loss aid. Because Prozac is a selective serotonin reuptake inhibitor (SSRI), it keeps serotonin levels elevated by blocking serotonin from being taken back up into brain cells. St. John's wort may work in a similar way (reducing reuptake), while 5-HTP appears to increase the synthesis of serotonin.

Quercetin and white willow bark are common minor ingredients in several weight loss formulations. Both ingredients have anti-inflammatory properties because they inhibit prostaglandins. A side effect of blocking prostaglandin activity is an inhibition of norepinephrine breakdown—so the ultimate effect of quercetin and white willow supplements is to have more norepinephrine around. Norepinephrine is known to interact with a special kind of receptor found on fat cells (the beta-3 receptor) to stimulate the breakdown of fat. See where this is going? Both quercetin and white willow appear to increase norepinephrine levels, which may stimulate fat metabolism, which may lead to enhanced weight loss. That's a lot of maybes, and neither ingredient is thought to be effective on its own.

SUMMARY

As you can undoubtedly see from the information in this chapter, lasting weight loss comes from close attention to diet, exercise for prevention of weight gain, and (possibly) dietary supplements to provide an added measure of support to your diet and exercise efforts. Remember—there are no magic bullet supplements (or drugs) that will "melt fat" or result in weight loss without changes in diet and exercise (it's not exactly an exciting story, but it's the truth). Supplements are, after all, meant to be used as *supplements* to a healthy lifestyle—not as stand-alone miracles, as they are often touted.

CONJUGATED LINOLEIC ACID (CLA)

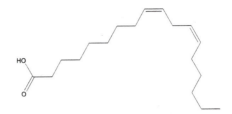

Linoleic Acid

What Is It?

Linoleic acid (LA) is one of the two essential fatty acids (the other is linolenic acid). Linoleic acid is an omega-6 fatty acid, meaning that it is unsaturated, with a double bond occurring at the sixth carbon atom. *Conjugated* linoleic acid (CLA) is an isomer of LA, which refers to a slight rearrangement of the molecular structure (conjugation), resulting in a fatty acid with altered chemical functions. The rearrangement in this case is a conjugated double bond occurring at carbons 10 and 12 or at carbons 9 and 11. Linoleic acid is found in the diet in vegetable oils, whereas the conjugated variety, CLA, is found primarily in meat and dairy products. The form of CLA found most commonly in dietary supplements is manufactured from vegetable oils such as sunflower oil.

Claims

- Builds muscle
- Burns fat
- Increases thermogenesis (calorie expenditure)
- Fights cancer
- Suppresses catabolic hormones
- Antioxidant

Theory

The antitumor/anticancer properties attributed to CLA may be due to an antioxidant effect or to an undefined interaction between CLA and various carcinogens. CLA is also thought to increase the production of prostaglandins, which are derived from fatty acid molecules and have been linked to an elevated synthesis of growth hormone. In athletes, increased growth hormone levels are viewed as beneficial to promote enhanced muscle growth and strength. Some prostaglandins may also increase blood circulation to the muscles and adipose tissue—an effect that has been suggested to improve muscle function and fat mobilization.

Scientific Support

The majority of research on the dietary intake of CLA has been conducted in animals. Several studies have indicated an antitumor effect of CLA in normal doses—close to what an average person might consume daily from food (1 to 4 g)—assuming a typical intake of meat and dairy products. Studies in rats and mice have shown that animals fed CLA-supplemented diets display reduced food intake, lower body weight, and a drastic reduction in tumors. Weight loss studies in rodents have also shown a beneficial effect of CLA feeding—with supplemented rats gaining less body fat, but more lean body mass, compared to control animals. In livestock studies (cattle, pigs, chickens), supplemental CLA has been shown to promote growth and prevent muscle wasting, whereas body fat accumulation may be suppressed due to an increase in energy expenditure. In rabbits with high cholesterol, CLA feeding reduces low-density lipoprotein (LDL) and triglycerides.

Of the small amount of human clinical data, for example, an abstract presented at a strength and conditioning conference showed no differences between two groups of weight lifters on measures of body weight, fat mass, or fat-free mass following a month of CLA supplementation. Another small study followed ten subjects consuming 3 to 4 g of CLA each day for three months and compared them to ten subjects consuming a placebo. Results showed no difference in weight loss between CLA and placebo, but those taking CLA dropped somewhat more body fat. In one study of seventeen healthy women, CLA supplements (3 g per day) or a sunflower oil placebo for sixty-four days, resulted in no change in body weight, fat-free mass, fat mass, or percentage of body fat. Likewise, CLA had no significant effect on energy expenditure, fat oxidation, or respiratory exchange ratio at rest or during exercise.

Safety

No side effects are reported with CLA supplementation—but caution is advised as the majority of the work has been done in animals.

Value

More research is needed to prove out the claims of weight loss and weight maintenance in humans.

Dosage

Typical dosage recommendations are 3 to 5 g per day. Most people ingest less than 1 g per day from meat and dairy foods.

WORKS CONSULTED

Cook ME, Miller CC, Park Y, Pariza M. Immune modulation by altered nutrient metabolism: Nutritional control of immune-induced growth depression. Poult Sci. 1993 Jul;72(7):1301-5.

Stangl GI. Conjugated linoleic acids exhibit a strong fat-to-lean partitioning effect, reduce serum VLDL lipids and redistribute tissue lipids in food-restricted rats. J Nutr. 2000 May;130(5):1140-6.

Yang M, Pariza MW, Cook ME. Dietary conjugated linoleic acid protects against end stage disease of systemic lupus erythematosus in the NZB/W F1 mouse. Immunopharmacol Immunotoxicol. 2000 Aug;22(3):433-49.

Zambell KL, Keim NL, Van Loan MD, Gale B, Benito P, Kelley DS, Nelson GJ. Conjugated linoleic acid supplementation in humans: Effects on body composition and energy expenditure. Lipids. 2000 Jul;35(7):777-82.

HYDROXYCITRIC ACID (HCA)

What Is It?

Hydroxycitric acid is the active ingredient extracted from the rind of a little pumpkin-like fruit, *Garcinia cambogia,* from India and Southeast Asia. Dietary supplements and a wide variety of weight loss formulas contain garcinia extract to inhibit fat production and suppress appetite. A number of products include extracts (about 50 percent HCA) under the brand names Citrin (Sabinsa) and CitriMax (InterHealth). A new one called Regulator is a 98 percent pure potassium HCA from a small Irish supplement company.

Claims

- Promotes weight loss
- Suppresses appetite
- Reduces blood lipids
- Increases fat oxidation/mobilization
- Promotes glycogen synthesis
- Increases energy levels

Theory

HCA can inhibit an enzyme in cells, citrate lyase, which is needed for the conversion of carbohydrates into fat. In the cell, carbohydrates are broken down into citrate compounds, which are then converted (by citrate lyase) into another compound, acetyl coenzyme A (acetyl CoA)—the metabolic building block for fat synthesis. By blocking the conversion of citrate into acetyl CoA, HCA can suppress fat synthesis. Acetyl CoA is further converted into malonyl CoA, a compound that may block the actions of carnitine acyltransferase in shuttling fatty acids into the mitochondria to be burned (and cause HCA to promote fat burning).

It is important to note, however, that the citrate lyase enzyme is only significantly active under conditions of carbohydrate overconsumption. If you're chowing down on low-fat, high-carb foods at every meal, then your glycogen stores will be overflowing and your citrate lyase enzymes are going to be working overtime converting those excess carbs to fat.

Now that you've blocked the fat production, you have to do something with those excess carbs. They can't be stored as glycogen because those stores in liver and muscle are already full, so it is thought that the body disposes of them by increasing carbohydrate oxidation (burning them). As a result of these fully loaded glycogen stores, some researchers have suggested that a side effect of HCA supplementation may be a suppression of appetite—which would reduce food intake and promote weight loss.

Scientific Support

Animal studies have shown that hydroxycitrate decreases weight gain—primarily by suppressing appetite and reducing food intake. At least one rat study has also shown a loss of body weight and reduced fat mass due to an 11 percent increase in daily energy expenditure. HCA appears to be effective in both lean and obese rats, where it can reduce food intake, body weight, body fat accumulation, fat cell size, and serum triglycerides.

Studies of HCA supplementation in humans have been equivocal. In some studies, 1,000 to 2,400 mg of HCA per day led to a doubling or tripling of weight loss compared to placebo groups. In 1999, however, JAMA published a study showing no effect of *Garcinia cambogia* on weight loss in overweight men and women. In the study, a commercially available product (Thermogenic Ultra Lean from Great American Nutrition, Salt Lake City, Utah), providing 1,500 mg of HCA per day did not augment weight loss compared to the placebo group in the twelve-week study.

The authors of the JAMA study concluded that their results do not support a role for *Garcinia cambogia* in facilitating weight loss beyond the effects observed with a low-calorie, high-fiber diet. Evidence from animal studies and human trials of high carbohydrate diets, however, suggest otherwise—and support the use of HCA for inhibiting fat synthesis and reducing body weight. Additionally, in individuals consuming a normal diet, HCA may provide some measure of appetite suppression, which may curtail food cravings and help to support weight maintenance. For example, one small study indicated that subjects taking HCA were better able to adhere to a weight loss diet than subjects taking a placebo. An unpublished study from the makers of the Regulator brand of HCA showed an effect on suppressing appetite and reducing body weight (4 to 12 lb greater than placebo). The study looked at fifty subjects who consumed 1.5 to 6 g of the HCA supplement daily for one month.

Another study used a double-blind, placebo-controlled, randomized, crossover study design to investigate whether three days of HCA supplementation (3 g per day) had any influence on metabolic parameters with or without moderately intense exercise (40 to 60 percent VO2max [maximal oxygen consumption]). The study examined ten sedentary men across four lab visits (consuming a 30 to 35 percent fat diet) and found no significant differences for measures of fat/carbohydrate oxidation (respiratory quotient) or other aspects of metabolism.

Safety

No serious adverse side effects are associated with intake of *Garcinia cambogia* or hydroxycitric acid supplements, aside from some minor gastrointestinal distress induced by high doses.

Value

For weight loss, regular intake of *Garcinia cambogia* and HCA is supported by animal studies (and high-carbohydrate diets), where it reduces food intake and body fat accumulation. Some data from human trials support the effectiveness of HCA for weight control in humans, but here the data is not particularly strong, and much more research is needed to confirm the degree of weight loss that can be expected from regular HCA supplementation.

Given the apparent safety profile of garcinia/HCA supplements and the clear difficulty associated with maintaining a reduced body weight following weight loss, HCA may be most effective as an aid to preventing weight regain rather than as an approach to stimulating significant fat loss (which is best achieved by lifestyle modifications in diet, behavior, and exercise patterns). Those individuals who have succeeded in losing body weight and fat mass (not an easy task) may be better able to adhere to their new diet and maintain their new lower body weight more effectively with the help of HCA dietary supplements.

Dosage

Typical doses associated with suppression of appetite and reductions in body weight are 750 to 1,500 mg of *Garcinia cambogia* (standardized for at least 50 percent HCA) taken in two to three divided doses about 30 to 60 minutes before eating. Because of the variation in hydroxycitric acid content between various brands of *Garcinia cambogia* extract, it is recommended to choose a brand that is standardized to a high level of HCA.

WORKS CONSULTED

Badmaev V, Majeed M, Conte AA. Garcinia cambogia for weight loss. JAMA. 1999 Jul 21;282(3):233-4; discussion 235.

Firenzuoli F, Gori L. Garcinia cambogia for weight loss. JAMA. 1999 Jul 21; 282(3):234; discussion 235.

Heymsfield SB, Allison DB, Vasselli JR, Pietrobelli A, Greenfield D, Nunez C. Garcinia cambogia (hydroxycitric acid) as a potential antiobesity agent: A randomized controlled trial. JAMA. 1998 Nov 11;280(18):1596-600.

Kriketos AD, Thompson HR, Greene H, Hill JO. (–)-Hydroxycitric acid does not affect energy expenditure and substrate oxidation in adult males in a postabsorptive state. Int J Obes Relat Metab Disord. 1999 Aug;23(8):867-73.

McCarty MF. Inhibition of citrate lyase may aid aerobic endurance. Med Hypotheses. 1995 Sep;45(3):247-54.

McCarty MF. Utility of metformin as an adjunct to hydroxycitrate/carnitine for reducing body fat in diabetics. Med Hypotheses. 1998 Nov;51(5):399-403.

Schaller JL. Garcinia cambogia for weight loss. JAMA. 1999 Jul 21;282(3):234; discussion 235.

CHITOSAN

What Is It?

Chitosan is a dietary fiber derived from chitin. Chitin is an amino-polysaccharide (combination of sugar and protein) that comes from the shells of shellfish. Chitin used to be nothing more than a waste product of the shellfish industry, but a bit of chemical treatment and voila! a new fiber is born. Chitosan is typically found in dietary supplements for reducing cholesterol levels and promoting weight loss.

Claims

- Reduces fat absorption
- Lowers cholesterol levels
- Promotes weight loss

Theory

Because chitosan is a positively charged compound, it is able to attract and bind to fatty acids (which carry a negative charge). As such, chitosan can absorb up to four to six times its weight in fat (including cholesterol) and prevent that fat from being absorbed into the body. This means that for every gram of chitosan that you consume as a supplement, you'll prevent the absorption of about 4 to 6 g of fat (a very rough approximation). If you're consuming 3 to 5 g of chitosan each day, you could be blocking anywhere from 100 to 300 fat calories from ever being absorbed. The only catch is that the chitosan has to be in your digestive system at the same time as the fat—so typical recommendations are to consume it along with fatty meals (like pizza with extra cheese).

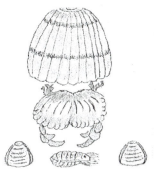

Scientific Support

The majority of research on chitosan has been done in animals, where it has been shown to effectively bind to fats in the digestive tract and prevent their absorption. In one study, high doses of chitosan reduced fat absorption by almost half (but these animals were on a very high fat diet and they probably experienced severe diarrhea from all the fat in their stools). The main beneficial effect of chitosan supplements appears to be a mild to moderate reduction in serum levels of LDL cholesterol (the bad kind).

When evaluated as a weight loss supplement, however, results for chitosan's effectiveness have not been consistent. In one Italian study, the combination of chitosan supplements and a thirty-day low-calorie diet (1,000 calories per day) showed chitosan to be effective in promoting weight loss (16 lb) compared to a placebo (7 lb) in obese subjects. More recent studies of overweight volunteers, however, gave 1,000 to 2,400 mg of chitosan per day over the course of one month but found no significant effect of chitosan in promoting weight loss. In one study, thirty-four overweight volunteers were assigned to receive either 2 g of chitosan or placebo for one month (randomized, placebo-controlled, double-blind design) while maintaining their normal diet. After four weeks of treatment, there were no significant changes in body weight, body mass index, or serum levels of cholesterol, triglycerides, or nutrients (vitamins A, D, and E, and beta-carotene). In the more recent studies, participants were allowed to "eat normally" and were instructed to not change their diets. It may be that chitosan is more effective in promoting weight loss when used in conjunction with a reduced-calorie and reduced-fat diet—some researchers have suggested that even though chitosan may block fat absorption quite well, people still end up consuming more calories from other sources throughout the day.

Safety

Unfortunately, the fact that chitosan prevents fat absorption also means that it can cause gas, bloating, and diarrhea (due to fermentation of the fat in the large intestine). The possibility also exists for chitosan, at high intakes, to interfere with absorption of fat-soluble vitamins (A, D, E, and K) and the carotenoids (such as beta-carotene, lycopene, lutein, and zeaxanthin)—similar to the way the "fake fat" Olestra can reduce absorption of these nutrients.

Value

As a supplement to promote a mild reduction in fat absorption and serum levels of LDL cholesterol, chitosan appears to be effective. As a weight loss agent, however, chitosan only appears to offer benefits when used in conjunction with a low-fat, reduced-calorie diet. Thus, chitosan supplements should not be expected to deliver significant weight loss effects unless significant dietary alterations are followed.

Dosage

Typical recommendations for chitosan supplements are 2 to 6 g per day, usually consumed in divided doses of about 1 g with each meal.

WORKS CONSULTED

Deuchi K, Kanauchi O, Imasato Y, Kobayashi E. Effect of the viscosity or deacetylation degree of chitosan on fecal fat excreted from rats fed on a high-fat diet. Biosci Biotechnol Biochem. 1995 May;59(5):781-5.

Deuchi K, Kanauchi O, Shizukuishi M, Kobayashi E. Continuous and massive intake of chitosan affects mineral and fat-soluble vitamin status in rats fed on a high-fat diet. Biosci Biotechnol Biochem. 1995 Jul;59(7):1211-6.

Egger G, Cameron-Smith D, Stanton R. The effectiveness of popular, non-prescription weight loss supplements. Med J Aust. 1999 Dec 6-20;171(11-12):604-8.

Han LK, Kimura Y, Okuda H. Reduction in fat storage during chitin-chitosan treatment in mice fed a high-fat diet. Int J Obes Relat Metab Disord. 1999 Feb;23(2):174-9.

Kanauchi O, Deuchi K, Imasato Y, Shizukuishi M, Kobayashi E. Mechanism for the inhibition of fat digestion by chitosan and for the synergistic effect of ascorbate. Biosci Biotechnol Biochem. 1995 May;59(5):786-90.

Okunevich IV, Kliueva NN, Solov'eva MA, Triufanov VF, Ryzhenkov VE. The hypolipidemic activity of natural substances. Eksp Klin Farmakol. 1992 Sep-Oct;55(5):44-7.

Ormrod DJ, Holmes CC, Miller TE. Dietary chitosan inhibits hypercholesterolaemia and atherogenesis in the apolipoprotein E-deficient mouse model of atherosclerosis. Atherosclerosis. 1998 Jun;138(2):329-34.

Pittler MH, Abbot NC, Harkness EF, Ernst E. Randomized, double-blind trial of chitosan for body weight reduction. Eur J Clin Nutr. 1999 May;53(5):379-81.

Razdan A, Pettersson D. Effect of chitin and chitosan on nutrient digestibility and plasma lipid concentrations in broiler chickens. Br J Nutr. 1994 Aug;72(2):277-88.

Razdan A, Pettersson D. Hypolipidaemic, gastrointestinal and related responses of broiler chickens to chitosans of different viscosity. Br J Nutr. 1996 Sep;76(3):387-97.

Sugano M, Fujikawa T, Hiratsuji Y, Nakashima K, Fukuda N, Hasegawa Y. A novel use of chitosan as a hypocholesterolemic agent in rats. Am J Clin Nutr. 1980 Apr;33(4):787-93.

Vachoud L, Zydowicz N, Domard A. Physicochemical behaviour of chitin gels. Carbohydr Res. 2000 Jun 30;326(4):295-304.

Wuolijoki E, Hirvela T, Ylitalo P. Decrease in serum LDL cholesterol with microcrystalline chitosan. Methods Find Exp Clin Pharmacol. 1999 Jun;21(5):357-61.

GLUCOMANNAN/KONJAC

What Is It?

Glucomannan is a polysaccharide (long chains of simple sugars, primarily mannose and glucose) that is classified as a soluble fiber. Because glucomannan can absorb up to 200 times its weight in water, it has been used as a dietary supplement to promote weight loss (via increasing feelings of fullness). Glucomannan is derived from several plants, but the primary source is an Asian plant called konjac.

Claims

- Lowers cholesterol and triglyceride levels
- Reduces fat absorption
- Promotes blood sugar control
- Promotes feeling of fullness (satiety)
- Promotes weight loss

Theory

Like many soluble fibers, glucomannan can bind with a variety of substances in the digestive tract to slow digestion, relieve constipation, and reduce the absorption of fat and carbohydrates. As such, glucomannan is often used in products intended to reduce blood cholesterol and triglyceride levels as well as blood sugar. Because it can absorb a great deal of water and promote a feeling of fullness, glucomannan is frequently used in supplements intended to promote weight loss.

Scientific Support

A handful of clinical studies confirm that glucomannan lowers cholesterol (total and LDL). In childhood obesity, glucomannan has been shown to decrease cholesterol and triglyceride levels significantly. In one study, two groups of twenty-five severely obese patients underwent very low calorie diet therapy for three months (with or without a 4 g per day glucomannan supplement). The results showed that the glucomannan group had a significant loss of body weight and fat mass compared to the group receiving diet therapy alone. The glucomannan group also had a more pronounced change in lipid status and carbohydrate tolerance. In another study, twenty obese subjects were given 1 g of glucomannan with 8 oz of water one hour prior to each meal for two months (versus a placebo). Subjects were instructed not to change their eating or exercise patterns. Results showed a significant weight loss (5.5 lb) as well as a drop in serum levels of total and LDL cholesterol (15 to 20 mg/dl) in the glucomannan group, but no significant change in the placebo group.

In terms of gastrointestinal benefits, seven to ten days of glucomannan consumption has been shown to increase the growth of beneficial bacteria in the gut *(Bifidobacterium)* and relieve constipation (3 to 4 g per day in divided doses) without causing excessive diarrhea or flatulence.

In animal studies, glucomannan has been shown to help control blood sugar levels—possibly by slowing the absorption of glucose into the bloodstream.

Safety

Like other soluble fibers, glucomannan has the potential to bind with and reduce the absorption of certain nutrients—so a daily multivitamin supplement may be advisable for individuals consuming high doses of glucomannan on a regular basis. In high doses, glucomannan may lead to diarrhea, bloating, and flatulence, but cutting back the dose relieves these unpleasant side effects.

Value

As a weight loss aid, glucomannan is sometimes combined with other fibers, such as chitosan, to increase the fat-binding effects and feelings of fullness—both of which may be effective in promoting weight loss and weight maintenance as well as for controlling mildly elevated cholesterol and blood sugar levels.

Dosage

Typical dosage recommendations for glucomannan are 1 g consumed with at least 8 oz of water approximately one hour prior to a meal (can be repeated 3 to 4 times per day at each meal). If combined with other fibers, follow the directions on the specific product, because different fiber products may have different dosage/use recommendations.

WORKS CONSULTED

Arvill A, Bodin L. Effect of short-term ingestion of konjac glucomannan on serum cholesterol in healthy men. Am J Clin Nutr. 1995 Mar;61(3):585-9.

Cairella M, Marchini G. Evaluation of the action of glucomannan on metabolic parameters and on the sensation of satiation in overweight and obese patients. Clin Ter. 1995 Apr;146(4):269-74.

Doi K. Effect of konjac fibre (glucomannan) on glucose and lipids. Eur J Clin Nutr. 1995 Oct;49 (Suppl 3):S190-7.

Hou YH, Zhang LS, Zhou HM, Wang RS, Zhang YZ. Influences of refined konjac meal on the levels of tissue lipids and the absorption of four minerals in rats. Biomed Environ Sci. 1990 Sep;3(3):306-14.

Hozumi T, Yoshida M, Ishida Y, Mimoto H, Sawa J, Doi K, Kazumi T. Long-term effects of dietary fiber supplementation on serum glucose and lipoprotein levels in diabetic rats fed a high cholesterol diet. Endocr J. 1995 Apr;42(2):187-92.

Livieri C, Novazi F, Lorini R. The use of highly purified glucomannan-based fibers in childhood obesity. Pediatr Med Chir. 1992 Mar-Apr;14(2):195-8.

Signorelli P, Croce P, Dede A. A clinical study of the use of a combination of glucomannan with lactulose in the constipation of pregnancy. Minerva Ginecol. 1996 Dec;48(12):577-82.

Vido L, Facchin P, Antonello I, Gobber D, Rigon F. Childhood obesity treatment: Double blinded trial on dietary fibres (glucomannan) versus placebo. Padiatr Padol. 1993;28(5):133-6.

Vita PM, Restelli A, Caspani P, Klinger R. Chronic use of glucomannan in the dietary treatment of severe obesity. Minerva Med. 1992 Mar;83(3):135-9.

Vuksan V, Jenkins DJ, Spadafora P, Sievenpiper JL, Owen R, Vidgen E, Brighenti F, Josse R, Leiter LA, Bruce-Thompson C. Konjac-mannan (glucomannan) improves glycemia and other associated risk factors for coronary heart disease in type 2 diabetes. A randomized controlled metabolic trial. Diabetes Care. 1999 Jun;22(6):913-9.

Walsh DE, Yaghoubian V, Behforooz A. Effect of glucomannan on obese patients: A clinical study. Int J Obes. 1984;8(4):289-93.

Yoshida M, Sawa J, Hozumi T, Mimoto H, Ishida Y, Kazumi T, Doi K, Baba S. Effects of long-term high-fiber diet on macrovascular changes and lipid and glucose levels in STZ-induced diabetic SD rats. Diabetes Res Clin Pract. 1991 Sep;13(3):147-52.

MA HUANG/EPHEDRA

What Is It?

Ma huang is a Chinese herb that is also referred to as Chinese ephedra and herbal ephedrine. The active compounds, ephedra or ephedrine alka- loids, are also found in other herbals such as Mormon tea and *Sida cordifolia* (about forty species of plants contain versions of ephedra). Ma huang, and its various herbal cousins, function as sympathomimetics, meaning that they mimic some of the effects of the body's own sympathetic (stimulant) hormones such as epinephrine and norepinephrine (either by increasing the levels of these hormones or by reducing their breakdown). Ephedrine is a nonselective sympathomimetic, which means that it acts as a general stimu- lant on many parts of the body simultaneously (lungs, heart, blood vessels, adrenal glands, etc.). It is most often used as a central nervous system stimu- lant (for alertness or energy), as a decongestant (for asthma or as a breathing aid), and as an appetite suppressant in a wide variety of weight loss and thermogenic-type products.

Claims

- Increases alertness
- Speeds up metabolism
- Aids weight loss
- Enhances athletic performance
- Mental sharpness

Theory

Because ephedrine acts as a general sympathetic nervous system stimulant, it can give users a boost or pickup similar to what you might feel after a cup or two of strong coffee. By mimicking the effects of epinephrine, ephedra can increase the out- put of blood from the heart, enhance mus- cle contractility, raise blood sugar levels, and open bronchial pathways for easier breathing. In many cases, ephedra can re- sult in a temporary suppression of appetite, which may help efforts aimed at dietary re- striction and weight loss.

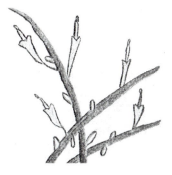

Scientific Support

The research findings concerning the effects of ma huang and other ephedra-containing products is equivocal—some studies show absolutely no beneficial effect, while a handful of others show a modest increase in metabolic rate, suppression of appetite, and enhanced weight loss when compared to a placebo. A possible reason for the inconsistent findings is the variable levels of the active alkaloids responsible for the stimulatory effects associated with ma huang and other ephedra-containing products. As with many naturally derived compounds, levels of the active chemicals can vary significantly from product to product and from batch to batch—a *major* problem in light of the potential adverse side effects associated with ephedra-containing products (see Safety).

Because ephedrine is a stimulant, it is logical that either a single dose or chronic repeated use would elevate metabolic rate somewhat (meaning that you would burn more calories at rest and during exercise). One study showed that overweight men and women who were dieting were better able to maintain their resting metabolic rate (which typically falls during a weight loss program) when they consumed 150 mg of ephedrine per day (although no additional weight loss was noted). The combination of ephedrine (20 to 40 mg) and caffeine (200 to 400 mg), sometimes combined with theophylline from tea (50 mg) or salicylates from white willow (100 mg), has been found to work better than either agent alone in producing a slight increase in resting metabolism and appears to be about as effective as prescription weight loss medications such as dexfenfluramine. In another study, ephedrine (30 mg) combined with caffeine (100 mg) and aspirin (300 mg) increased energy expenditure following a meal in obese women. This combination, known to many consumers as the ECA stack (for ephedrine/caffeine/aspirin), has become one of the most popular weight loss supplements on the market.

Safety

Ephedrine can be converted into the street drug methamphetamine (meth or speed), and sales of ephedrine and pseudoephedrine have been restricted in sixteen states. Ephedrine is considered a banned substance by the International Olympic Committee (IOC), the United States Olympic Committee (USOC), and the National Collegiate Athletic Association (NCAA). The FDA has received nearly 1,000 reports of adverse events from consumers using any of over 100 supplements containing ephedrine alkaloids. Complaints have ranged from nervous system and cardiovascular system effects such as elevated blood pressure, heart palpitations, insomnia, irritability, and headaches to serious adverse effects such as seizures, stroke, heart attack, and even death (about fifteen to twenty thus far). Most of these adverse events occurred in otherwise healthy young to middle-aged adults using the products for weight control or increased energy. In response to the relatively large number of adverse reports (compared to other dietary supplements), the FDA proposed to limit the amount of ephedra alkaloids that could be consumed per dose (8 mg) and per day (24 mg). Quite recently, however, the General Accounting Office (GAO) has determined that the majority of these reports cannot be substantiated or linked directly to any ephedra-containing product, nor did the FDA have adequate scientific evidence that any restrictions on ephedra dosing or daily intake were needed. To put the overall safety question into proper perspective, ephedrine alkaloids are *not* for everyone—but 1,000 adverse reports out of several hundred million doses over the last couple of years hardly qualifies as the public health menace that many media stories have suggested.

Virtually all dietary supplements that contain ephedra alkaloids also carry a strong warning on their labels which reads:

> Women who are pregnant or nursing should avoid using ephedra-containing products. Keep out of reach of children. Avoid using ephedrine-containing products if you have high blood pressure, heart or thyroid disease, diabetes, difficulty in urination due to prostate enlargement, or if taking monoamine oxidase (MAO) inhibitors or any other prescription drug. Reduce or discontinue use if nervousness, tremor, irritability, rapid heartbeat, sleeplessness, loss of appetite, or nausea occur.

If you have a complaint of your own to lodge, you can report any adverse effects at the FDA's MedWatch Web site: <http://www.fda.gov/ medwatch>.

Value

Ephedra-containing dietary supplements and herbal stimulant/weight loss teas are likely to appeal to individuals seeking an energy boost. Extreme caution should be used, however, by people with high blood pressure or existing heart disease. Because ephedrine is commonly found in many weight loss and thermogenic products, overweight individuals, who may be at higher risk for hypertension and heart disease, should be especially aware of possible adverse side effects.

Dosage

Because ephedrine is similar in structure to amphetamines and can increase heart rate and blood pressure in susceptible individuals, the FDA has recommended that ephedrine consumption should be limited to less than 24 mg per day and that dietary supplements contain no more than 8 mg of ephedrine or related alkaloids per serving (recently, the FDA has indicated that they may be backing away from this recommendation, but it still stands in the public record for now). It is very important, should you decide to use ephedra-containing products, to understand that a variety of ephedrine-like compounds (alkaloids) are present in ma huang and related herbs, including ephedrine, norephedrine, pseudoephedrine, methylephedrine, and norpseudoephedrine—and products should be standardized to a *total alkaloid content*. For example, a product that states it has 356 mg of ma huang or related herb per serving and is standardized to 6 percent ephedra alkaloids would have 21.36 mg of ephedra alkaloids per serving ($356 \times 0.06 = 21.36$)—make sure that the standardization is to total alkaloids rather than simply to ephedrine.

In the few studies that have been conducted on ephedra-containing products for weight loss, the total amount of ephedrine ingested per day has ranged between 60 to 75 mg (usually in three divided doses of 20 to 25 mg per dose).

These dosage recommendations should be considered in light of a recent study from the University of Arkansas that analyzed the content of ephedra alkaloids in twenty dietary supplements. The study showed that the alkaloid content varied considerably among products—from *zero* to 18.5 mg per dose, and significant lot-to-lot variations in alkaloid content were observed for at least four products (meaning that even if you selected the same brand each time, you would be getting a different level of ephedra). For one product, the alkaloid content varied by as much as 1,000 percent between lots. Perhaps the most disturbing finding of the study was that fully half of the products showed discrepancies of more than 20 percent between the label claim for ephedra alkaloids and the actual alkaloids measured in the study.

WORKS CONSULTED

Astrup A, Breum L, Toubro S. Pharmacological and clinical studies of ephedrine and other thermogenic agonists. Obes Res. 1995;3(Suppl 4):537S-40S.

Astrup A, Breum L, Toubro S, Hein P, Quaade F. The effect and safety of an ephedrine/caffeine compound compared to ephedrine, caffeine and placebo in obese subjects on an energy restricted diet. A double blind trial. Int J Obes Relat Metab Disord. 1992;16(4):269-77.

Breum L, Pederson JK, Ahlstrom F, Frimodt-Moller J. Comparison of an ephedrine/caffeine combination and dexfenfluramine in the treatment of obesity. A double-blind multi-centre trial in general practice. Int J Obes Relat Metab Disord. 1994;18(2):99-103.

Bruno A, Nolte KB, Chapin J. Stroke associated with ephedrine use. Neurology, 1993;43(7):1313-6.

Capwell RR, Ephedrine-induced mania from an herbal diet supplement [letter]. Am J Psychiatry. 1995;152(4):647.

Daly PA, Krieger DR, Dulloo AG, Young JB, Landsberg L. Ephedrine, caffeine and aspirin: Safety and efficacy for treatment of human obesity. Int J Obes Relat Metab Disord. 1993;17(Suppl 1):S73-8.

Flurer CL, Lin LA, Satzger RD, Wolnik KA. Determination of ephedrine compounds in nutritional supplements by cyclodextrin-modified capillary electrophoresis. J Chromatogr B Biomed Appl. 1995 Jul 7;669(1):133-9.

Gurley BJ, Gardner SF, Hubbard MA. Content versus label claims in ephedra-containing dietary supplements. Am J Health Syst Pharm. 2000 May 15;57(10): 963-9.

Gurley BJ, Gardner SF, White LM, Wang PL. Ephedrine pharmacokinetics after the ingestion of nutritional supplements containing Ephedra sinica (ma huang). Ther Drug Monit. 1998 Aug;20(4):439-45.

Gurley BJ, Wang P, Gardner SF. Ephedrine-type alkaloid content of nutritional supplements containing Ephedra sinica (Ma-huang) as determined by high performance liquid chromatography. J Pharm Sci. 1998 Dec;87(12):1547-53.

Josefson D. Herbal stimulant causes US deaths [news]. Br Med J. 1996;312(7043): 1378-9.

Ros JJ, Pelders MG, De Smet PA. A case of positive doping associated with a botanical food supplement. Pharm World Sci. 1999 Feb;21(1):44-6.

Roxanas MG, Spalding J. Ephedrine abuse psychosis. Med J Aust. 1977;2(19): 639-40.

Toubro S, Astrup AV, Breum L, Quaade F. The acute and chronic effects of ephedrine/caffeine mixtures on energy expenditure and glucose metabolism in humans. Int J Obes Relat Metab Disord. 1993a;17(Suppl 3):S73-7; discussion S82.

Toubro S, Astrup AV, Breum L, Quaade F. Safety and efficacy of long-term treatment with ephedrine, caffeine and an ephedrine/caffeine mixture. Int J Obes Relat Metab Disord. 1993b;17(Suppl 1):S69-72.

Van Mieghem W, Stevens E, Cosemans J. Ephedrine-induced cardiopathy. Br Med J. 1978;1(6116):816.

White LM, Gardner SF, Gurley BJ, Marx MA, Wang PL, Estes M. Pharmacokinetics and cardiovascular effects of ma-huang (Ephedra sinica) in normotensive adults. J Clin Pharmacol. 1997 Feb;37(2):116-22.

GUARANA

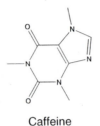

Caffeine

What Is It?

Guarana *(Paullinia cupana)* comes from the seeds of a South American shrub, most of which originates in Brazil. Traditional uses of guarana by natives of the Amazon rain forest include adding crushed seeds to foods and beverages for increasing alertness and reducing fatigue. As a dietary supplement, it's no wonder that guarana is an effective energy booster—it contains about twice the caffeine found in coffee beans (about 3 to 4 percent caffeine in guarana seeds compared to 1 to 2 percent for coffee beans). Concentrated guarana extracts, however, can contain as much as 40 to 50 percent caffeine, with popular supplements delivering 50 to 200 mg of caffeine per day (about the same amount found in one to two cups of strong coffee). As with any caffeine-containing substance, too much can lead to nervousness, tension, and headaches.

Claims

- Increases energy levels/reduces fatigue
- Enhances physical and mental performance
- Promotes weight loss
- Suppresses appetite

Theory

The theory behind how guarana works is relatively straightforward. The major active constituents are caffeine (sometimes called "guaranine" to make you think it's different in some way) and similar alkaloids such as theobromine and theophylline (which are also found in coffee and tea). Each of these compounds has well-known effects as nervous system stimulants. As such, they may also have some effect on increasing metabolic rate, suppressing appetite, and enhancing both physical and mental performance.

Scientific Support

The seeds of guarana are known to be rich in xanthines (caffeine) and have been widely used as a tonic in many South American countries, particularly Brazil. In studies that have determined the total xanthine content of guarana powder, caffeine content typically averages 30 to 50 percent (depending on the extract). Related compounds such as theobromine and theophylline are found at levels of 1 to 3 percent and, like caffeine, can be detected in the urine for up to nine days following guarana intake.

Most of the scientific evidence on caffeine as a general stimulant and an aid to exercise performance shows convincingly that caffeine is effective. Consuming 3 to 6 mg of caffeine per kilogram (2.2 lb) of body weight (about 350 mg for an average sized man or 250 mg for a woman) approximately one hour before exercise improves endurance performance without raising urinary caffeine levels above the IOC's doping threshold. To reach that level, you'd need to take in about 800 mg of caffeine, which is about the amount found in eight cups of coffee or eighteen cans of Coke.

As a weight loss aid, however, although caffeine may suppress appetite somewhat at high levels, on its own it does not seem to be a very effective supplement for increasing calorie expenditure (thermogenesis). When combined with other stimulant-type supplements such as ma huang (ephedra), however, it appears that caffeine can extend the duration of action of ephedra in suppressing appetite and increasing caloric expenditure (although it may also increase the risk of adverse side effects associated with ephedra and caffeine).

There are several natural forms of each compound in the ECA stack; ephedra (as ma huang and *Sida cordifolia*), caffeine (as guarana, maté, and kola nut), and aspirin (as white willow bark). The ECA combination appears to be more effective in promoting weight loss than any of the individual ingredients on their own. For example, about 150 mg of ephedrine per day can increase metabolic rate by 3 to 5 percent over a twenty-four-hour period, whereas a lower dose of ephedrine (60 mg per day) increases daily caloric expenditure by nearly 8 percent when combined with caffeine (200 to 400 mg per day) and aspirin (80 to 160 mg per day of salicin).

Safety

The toxicity of guarana has been assessed in cellular and animal studies. In most cases, there is no significant danger, aside from the side effects of high caffeine intake, associated with guarana consumption. At least one study, however, found water extracts of guarana to cause genetic damage in cell cultures—although it is unclear whether this suggests any health risk for humans consuming guarana extract as a dietary supplement. As with any caffeine-containing food, guarana extracts can lead to insomnia, nervousness, anxiety, headaches, high blood pressure, and heart palpitations. Guarana is not recommended for women who are pregnant or lactating.

Value

Guarana is certainly an effective stimulant that can help increase the general state of arousal and enhance mental and physical performance. For an athlete or exerciser who needs a little boost before athletic competition or exercise, a moderate amount of guarana (caffeine) may be helpful. For individuals attempting to lose weight, however, guarana and caffeine do not appear to be especially effective as stand-alone weight loss aids, but in combination with other thermogenic and nervous system stimulants (the ECA stack), the caffeine may extend the activity and potency of certain supplement ingredients.

Dosage

Caffeine intake of 180 to 450 mg a day (about the amount in two to four cups of brewed coffee or 500 to 1000 mg of guarana extract) has been associated with mild stimulant properties and enhanced physical and mental performance. Higher levels of intake are not associated with additional increases in performance, but may result in adverse side effects such as tension, irritability, and nausea.

WORKS CONSULTED

Bempong DK, Houghton PJ. Dissolution and absorption of caffeine from guarana. J Pharm Pharmacol. 1992 Sep;44(9):769-71.

Benoni H, Dallakian P, Taraz K. Studies on the essential oil from guarana. Z Lebensm Unters Forsch. 1996 Jul;203(1):95-8.

Bydlowski SP, D'Amico EA, Chamone DA. An aqueous extract of guarana (Paullinia cupana) decreases platelet thromboxane synthesis. Braz J Med Biol Res. 1991;24(4):421-4.

Bydlowski SP, Yunker RL, Subbiah MT. A novel property of an aqueous guarana extract (Paullinia cupana): Inhibition of platelet aggregation in vitro and in vivo. Braz J Med Biol Res. 1988;21(3):535-8.

Carlson M, Thompson RD. Liquid chromatographic determination of methylxanthines and catechins in herbal preparations containing guarana. J AOAC Int. 1998 Jul-Aug;81(4):691-701.

da Fonseca CA, Leal J, Costa SS, Leitao AC. Genotoxic and mutagenic effects of guarana (Paullinia cupana) in prokaryotic organisms. Mutat Res. 1994 May;321(3):165-73.

Donadio V, Bonsi P, Zele I, Monari L, Liguori R, Vetrugno R, Albani F, Montagna P. Myoglobinuria after ingestion of extracts of guarana, ginkgo biloba and kava. Neurolog Sci. 2000 Apr;21(2):124.

Espinola EB, Dias RF, Mattei R, Carlini EA. Pharmacological activity of Guarana (Paullinia cupana Mart.) in laboratory animals. J Ethnopharmacol. 1997 Feb;55(3):223-9.

Galduroz JC, Carlini EA. Acute effects of the Paulinia cupana, "Guarana" on the cognition of normal volunteers. Rev Paul Med. 1994 Jul-Sep;112(3):607-11.

Galduroz JC, Carlini EA. The effects of long-term administration of guarana on the cognition of normal, elderly volunteers. Rev Paul Med. 1996 Jan-Feb;114(1):1073-8.

Katzung W. Guarana—a natural product with high caffeine content. Med Monatsschr Pharm. 1993 Nov;16(11):330-3.

Mattei R, Dias RF, Espinola EB, Carlini EA, Barros SB. Guarana (Paullinia cupana): Toxic behavioral effects in laboratory animals and antioxidants activity in vitro. J Ethnopharmacol. 1998 Mar;60(2):111-6.

Miura T, Tatara M, Nakamura K, Suzuki I. Effect of guarana on exercise in normal and epinephrine-induced glycogenolytic mice. Biol Pharm Bull. 1998 Jun;21(6):646-8.

Rommelspacher H. Guarana. Dtsch Med Wochenschr. 1995 Mar 17;120(11):384.

Salvadori MC, Rieser EM, Ribeiro Neto LM, Nascimento ES. Determination of xanthines by high-performance liquid chromatography and thin-layer chromatography in horse urine after ingestion of Guarana powder. Analyst. 1994 Dec;119(12):2701-3.

Santa Maria A, Lopez A, Diaz MM, Munoz-Mingarro D, Pozuelo JM. Evaluation of the toxicity of guarana with in vitro bioassays. Ecotoxicol Environ Saf. 1998 Mar;39(3):164-7.

Schafer AT. Microscopic examination of Guarana powder—Paullinia cupana Kunth. Arch Kriminol. 1999 Jul-Aug;204(1-2):23-7.

SYNEPHRINE/ZHI SHI

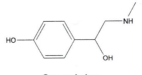

Synephrine

What Is It?

Synephrine is the main active compound found in the fruit of a plant called *Citrus aurantium*. The fruit is also known as zhi shi (in traditional Chinese medicine), and as green orange, sour orange, and bitter orange in other parts of the world. Synephrine is chemically very similar to the ephedrine and pseudoephedrine found in many over-the-counter cold/allergy medications and in a number of weight loss and energy supplements that contain ma huang.

Claims

- Increases metabolic rate
- Increases caloric expenditure
- Fat burner
- Promotes weight loss
- Increases energy levels

Theory

Because synephrine is a stimulant, similar to caffeine and ephedrine, it is thought to have similar effects in terms of providing an energy boost, suppressing appetite and increasing metabolic rate and caloric expenditure. In traditional Chinese medicine (TCM), zhi shi is used to help stimulate the Qi (energy force). Although synephrine and several other compounds found in zhi shi are structurally similar to ephedrine and are known to act as stimulants (via adrenergic activity), zhi shi does not appear to have the same negative central nervous effects as ma huang (ephedra). Through its stimulation of specific adrenergic receptors (beta-3, but not beta-1, beta-2, or alpha-1), zhi shi is theorized to stimulate fat metabolism without the negative cardiovascular side effects experienced by some people with ma huang (which stimulates *all* beta-adrenergic receptors).

Scientific Support

The effects of synephrine alone or in combination with other ingredients such as kola nut and guarana (caffeine sources) or with salicylates such as white willow (a natural form of aspirin) generally fall into the category of a mild stimulant. The extract of *Citrus aurantium,* in addition to synephrine, also contains tyramine and octopamine. Octopamine may be related in some way to appetite control, as it is thought to influence insect behavior by stopping bugs from eating citrus fruit (so if you're an insect, this may be the perfect weight loss supplement for you). Importantly, each of these related compounds (synephrine, ephedrine, and octopamine) can result in elevated blood pressure.

A recent study conducted in dogs suggests that synephrine and octopamine can increase metabolic rate in a specific type of fat tissue known as brown adipose tissue (BAT). This effect would be expected to increase fat loss in humans, except for one small detail—adult humans don't have brown adipose tissue. As it stands now, *Citrus aurantium* extract is one of the most overhyped ingredients on the weight loss scene. There are some interesting theories on how it might work to increase metabolic rate and promote weight loss, but most are couched in pseudoscientific mumbo jumbo and none are backed by any credible scientific evidence of effectiveness in humans.

Safety

Both isolated synephrine and *Citrus aurantium* extract have been shown to raise blood pressure in animal studies. Until more studies are conducted on the safety, pharmacology, and efficacy of *Citrus aurantium* as a thermogenic supplement, it should be treated as an ingredient with mild stimulant properties and should be avoided by individuals with cardiovascular concerns such as hypertension.

Value

The most likely explanation for weight loss effects attributed to *Citrus aurantium* supplements is the amphetamine-like effects of the alkaloids. Although this effect is likely to be somewhat less dramatic than effects induced by ma huang (ephedra alkaloids), users can expect variable effects including reduced appetite and heightened feelings of energy (similar to caffeine)—both of which are likely to result in weight loss.

Dosage

Because synephrine is but one small component of the *Citrus aurantium* fruit, a standardized extract is recommended. A dose of 4 to 20 mg of synephrine per day is typical in products providing 200 to 600 mg of a standardized *Citrus aurantium* extract (3 to 6 percent synephrine).

WORKS CONSULTED

Candelore MR, Deng L, Tota L, Guan XM, Amend A, Liu Y, Newbold R, Cascieri MA, Weber AE. Potent and selective human beta(3)-adrenergic receptor antagonists. J Pharmacol Exp Ther. 1999 Aug;290(2):649-55.

Carpene C, Galitzky J, Fontana E, Atgie C, Lafontan M, Berlan M. Selective activation of beta3-adrenoceptors by octopamine: Comparative studies in mammalian fat cells. Naunyn Schmiedebergs Arch Pharmacol. 1999 Apr;359(4):310-21.

Chen X, Liu LY, Deng HW, Fang YX, Ye YW. The effects of Citrus aurantium and its active ingredient N-methyltyramine on the cardiovascular receptors. Yao Hsueh Hsueh Pao. 1981 Apr;16(4):253-9.

Fontana E, Morin N, Prevot D, Carpene C. Effects of octopamine on lipolysis, glucose transport and amine oxidation in mammalian fat cells. Comp Biochem Physiol C Pharmacol Toxicol Endocrinol. 2000 Jan;125(1):33-44.

Galitzky J, Carpene C, Bousquet-Melou A, Berlan M, Lafontan M. Differential activation of beta 1-, beta 2- and beta 3-adrenoceptors by catecholamines in white and brown adipocytes. Fundam Clin Pharmacol. 1995;9(4):324-31.

Galitzky J, Carpene C, Lafontan M, Berlan M. Specific stimulation of adipose tissue adrenergic beta 3 receptors by octopamine. C R Acad Sci III. 1993; 316(5):519-23.

Hu S, Wang G. Textual studies on shangzhou zhiqiao fructus Aurantii. Chung Kuo Chung Yao Tsa Chih. 1996 Mar;21(3):137-8, 189.

Langin D, Portillo MP, Saulnier-Blache JS, Lafontan M. Coexistence of three beta-adrenoceptor subtypes in white fat cells of various mammalian species. Eur J Pharmacol. 1991 Jul 9;199(3):291-301.

Miyazawa M, Okuno Y, Fukuyama M, Nakamura S, Kosaka H. Antimutagenic activity of polymethoxyflavonoids from Citrus aurantium. J Agric Food Chem. 1999 Dec;47(12):5239-44.

Satoh Y, Tashiro S, Satoh M, Fujimoto Y, Xu JY, Ikekawa T. Studies on the bioactive constituents of Aurantii Fructus Immaturus. Yakugaku Zasshi. 1996 Mar;116(3):244-50.

Zhang ZZ, Fan CS, Huang AH. A study on the quality of fruits of Citrus aurantium L. (zhishi and Zhiqiao) produced in Jiangxi. Chung Kuo Chung Yao Tsa Chih. 1989 Sep;14(9):520-2, 573.

Zhao NK. Cultivation of Citrus aurantium. Chung Yao Tung Pao. 1984 Mar;9(2):56-7.

CARNITINE

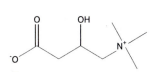

Carnitine

What Is It?

Carnitine is an amino acid that is synthesized in the liver and kidneys from lysine and methionine. The major function of carnitine is to facilitate the transport and metabolism of long-chain fatty acids into the mitochondria for beta-oxidation and energy generation. Carnitine can be also found in the diet in foods such as meat and dairy products.

Claims

- Enhances endurance
- Increases fat metabolism
- Lowers cholesterol and triglyceride levels
- Cardioprotective

Theory

Carnitine supplementation could potentially be beneficial under several conditions. First, because of carnitine's role in facilitating fatty acid transport into the mitochondria for oxidation, it is possible that elevated carnitine levels would permit a greater or faster transport of fat leading to increased fat oxidation, which may impact weight loss and/or endurance performance. A greater reliance on fat for energy may also result in a sparing of muscle glycogen and a subsequent enhancement of exercise performance. It is also theorized that supplemental carnitine could have some effect on reducing lactic acid accumulation in muscles by buffering pyruvate and, therefore, extending exercise capacity before fatigue.

Scientific Support

Studies of the role of carnitine as an ergogenic aid have been equivocal, with several suggesting a beneficial effect of supplements and others indicating no effect at all. Several early studies suggested an indirect effect of carnitine (2 to 6 g per day) on endurance performance by showing a reduction in the respiratory exchange ratio (RER), which indicates a greater reliance on fats for energy generation. Other studies have failed to indicate any glycogen-sparing effect of carnitine supplements (6 g per day). It has also been shown that with supplements, although blood carnitine levels go up, the acyl-enzyme system for fatty acid transport into the mitochondria is not augmented—suggesting that the body does a pretty good job of packing enough carnitine into the mitochondrial membrane without the help of dietary supplements.

In terms of weight loss, the very low calorie diets (less than 800 calories per day) that are used for intensive obesity treatment have been shown to result in lower levels of carnitine in the blood and tissues—possibly due to an increase in carnitine excretion. Because carnitine transports fatty acids into mitochondria for oxidation, any reduction in carnitine status in people trying to lose weight may be viewed as detrimental. A double-blind investigation tested the weight loss effects of carnitine in thirty-six moderately overweight women over two months (eighteen received 4 g of carnitine per day and eighteen received placebo). Subjects also completed 30 minutes of walking exercise (60 to 70 percent of maximum heart rate) four days per week. Results indicated no significant changes in body weight, fat mass, or the amount of fat oxidation either at rest or during exercise—suggesting that carnitine may not be particularly effective for promoting weight loss.

In support of the beneficial role of carnitine supplements, however, studies in kidney dialysis patients show that low carnitine levels in the dialysate can lead to elevated levels of blood lipids. Likewise, studies of heart disease patients have shown that carnitine supplements (2 g per day over six months) can reduce cholesterol and triglyceride levels. Perhaps the most convincing data on the benefits of carnitine as a dietary supplement come from several studies of patients with heart disease. Among individuals who had suffered a heart attack, carnitine supplements (2 to 3 g per day over four to eight weeks) resulted in a reduction in the amount of damage to the heart muscle and an increase in heart muscle viability. Among those suffering from angina (chest pain), carnitine reduces the incidence of angina and cardiac arrhythmias as well as reducing the need for antiangina and antiarrhythmic medications. In addition, carnitine (2 g per day for six months) can also increase exercise tolerance in patients with angina—meaning that they can exercise longer and at a higher level before experiencing chest pain.

These data suggest that although the ergogenic benefits of carnitine supplements are probably unfounded, or at least hard to measure, the benefits in terms of heart function and blood lipid maintenance are interesting. Under conditions in which the heart muscle is deprived of oxygen (i.e., heart attack and angina), fat breakdown and energy production are reduced. It also appears that carnitine concentrations may be somewhat reduced in cardiac cells undergoing such stress. Supplemental levels of carnitine may help replenish the lost carnitine and facilitate a return to adequate levels of fatty acid transport and energy production in the heart muscle.

Safety

Doses of 2 to 6 g per day over a period of six months have been studied with no observed adverse side effects.

Value

For weight loss, carnitine does not appear to be particularly effective for promoting weight loss or enhancing fat burning. For athletes, as an ergogenic aid, carnitine is not recommended except for vegetarians, who may not consume adequate levels of carnitine or its precursor amino acids (lysine and methionine) in their diets. For cardioprotective benefits, carnitine is recommended as a daily supplement to help maintain blood lipid profile and promote fatty acid utilization within heart muscle.

It is important to note that some supplemental forms of carnitine actually contain the physiologically inactive form of carnitine (D-carnitine) rather than the form which is active in humans (L-carnitine). Oversaturation of the tissue with the D- form could possibly displace the active form of carnitine in tissues and lead to muscle weakness.

Dosage

Doses of 2 to 6 g per day are typically recommended for cardiovascular, sports performance, and weight loss benefits—although the effectiveness of any dose of carnitine for sports or weight loss effects are not impressive. As a "heart health" nutrient, approximately 2 g per day of carnitine may provide some benefits in terms of promoting general heart function.

WORKS CONSULTED

Bogden JD, Baker H, Frank O, Perez G, Kemp F, Bruening K, Louria D. Micronutrient status and human immunodeficiency virus (HIV) infection. Ann N Y Acad Sci. 1990;587:189-95.

Davis AT, Davis PG, Phinney SD. Plasma and urinary carnitine of obese subjects on very-low-calorie diets. J Am Coll Nutr. 1990 Jun;9(3):261-4.

Janssens GP, Buyse J, Seynaeve M, Decuypere E, De Wilde R. The reduction of heat production in exercising pigeons after L-carnitine supplementation. Poult Sci. 1998 Apr;77(4):578-84.

Kelley DE, Goodpaster B, Wing RR, Simoneau JA. Skeletal muscle fatty acid metabolism in association with insulin resistance, obesity, and weight loss. Am J Physiol. 1999 Dec;277(6 Pt 1):E1130-41.

Lolic MM, Fiskum G, Rosenthal RE. Neuroprotective effects of acetyl-L-carnitine after stroke in rats. Ann Emerg Med. 1997 Jun;29(6):758-65.

McCarty MF. Optimizing exercise for fat loss. Med Hypotheses. 1995 May; 44(5):325-30.

McCarty MF. Utility of metformin as an adjunct to hydroxycitrate/carnitine for reducing body fat in diabetics. Med Hypotheses. 1998 Nov;51(5):399-403.

Pahl MV, Vaziri ND, Seo M. Intestinal absorption of carnitine in experimental azotemia. Res Commun Chem Pathol Pharmacol. 1990 Dec;70(3):337-47.

Papamandjaris AA, MacDougall DE, Jones PJ. Medium chain fatty acid metabolism and energy expenditure: Obesity treatment implications. Life Sci. 1998; 62(14):1203-15.

Simoneau JA, Veerkamp JH, Turcotte LP, Kelley DE. Markers of capacity to utilize fatty acids in human skeletal muscle: Relation to insulin resistance and obesity and effects of weight loss. FASEB J. 1999 Nov;13(14):2051-60.

Villani RG, Gannon J, Self M, Rich PA. L-Carnitine supplementation combined with aerobic training does not promote weight loss in moderately obese women. Int J Sport Nutr Exerc Metab. 2000 Jun;10(2):199-207.

Williams MH. Ergogenic and ergolytic substances. Med Sci Sports Exerc. 1992 Sep;24(9 Suppl):S344-8.

PYRUVATE

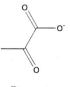

Pyruvate

What Is It?

Pyruvate is a "salt" form of pyruvic acid—a three-carbon molecule derived from the breakdown of glucose. The form of pyruvic acid found in dietary supplements is combined with various minerals such as sodium, calcium, magnesium, or potassium to improve stability. In the body, glucose (six carbons) is split into two pyruvic acid molecules (three carbons each) in the end stages of cellular glycolysis. When enough oxygen is present, pyruvic acid can be converted into acetyl CoA in the mitochondrion of the cell to produce energy. Under anaerobic conditions, however, pyruvic acid becomes lactic acid, which can build up and lead to muscle fatigue.

Claims

- Enhances weight loss and reduces weight regain
- Decreases appetite
- Elevates energy levels
- Increases endurance levels
- Increases muscle glycogen
- Reduces fatigue

Theory

Because glucose (the chief sugar used by cells for energy) is broken down into pyruvic acid, an increased level of pyruvic acid in the body is theorized to enhance a cell's ability to generate energy.

Scientific Support

In general, the scientific support for pyruvate as either a weight loss aid or a way to boost energy levels is somewhat controversial. At least a couple of human studies, however, have shown that daily consumption of 25 g of pyruvate plus 75 g of dihydroxyacetone (DHA, another three-carbon sugar derived from glucose) over one week can help improve endurance performance. For weight loss, subjects consuming pyruvate tend to lose somewhat more fat and weight (about 2 to 6 lb extra) compared to control groups given a placebo. The problem, of course, is that these interesting results have really been blown out of proportion by wildly enthusiastic marketers at a number of companies (read more under Value).

In one small study, thirteen obese women consumed a low-calorie diet for three weeks along with DHA and pyruvate. Subjects fed DHA and pyruvate showed a greater loss of weight and fat (about 2 lb) compared to placebo. Another small study (fourteen subjects) by the same researchers found again that subjects fed pyruvate showed a greater weight loss of about 2 to 3 lb compared to placebo over a period of several weeks while also consuming a low-calorie diet. A slightly larger study (thirty-four subjects) of subjects fed a low-calorie diet along with 22 to 44 g per day of pyruvate or placebo for one month again showed an enhancement of weight loss and fat loss (but no change in plasma concentrations of cholesterol, LDL, triglycerides, or HDL). A more recent study took a somewhat different approach—looking not at promotion of weight loss, but at suppression of weight regain following loss. In this study, pyruvate and DHA were fed to seventeen obese women (nine received the supplement, eight received placebo) following three weeks of weight loss via a low-calorie diet. During the supplementation phase, subjects adhered to a "weight gain" diet providing calories at levels 50 percent above energy requirements. Results indicated that weight and fat gain were significantly less in patients receiving the supplement compared to placebo (again, about 2 lb difference between groups)—suggesting that pyruvate and DHA supplements may be effective in helping to prevent weight regain following weight loss.

Safety

No significant side effects are expected with the levels of pyruvate found in most commercially available dietary supplements (which is typically quite low due to the high cost of pyruvate). In some studies, subjects consuming relatively large doses of pyruvate have reported minor gastrointestinal disturbances such as diarrhea and flatulence.

Value

Like many of the newer dietary supplement ingredients, don't expect to find pyruvate products hanging out on the discount rack—pyruvate is not cheap ($25 to $60 for a one-month supply). The main problem, however, is that the vast majority of commercial products contain only about 250 to 1,500 mg of pyruvate per serving—or about *100 times less* than the levels shown to be effective in the clinical studies just outlined. Powdered forms are available that can increase serving sizes to 5 or 6 g per serving, but we're still looking at miniscule levels when compared to the 25 to 40 g used in most studies.

Dosage

Although 1 to 5 g of pyruvate are typically recommended per day, this is more of a market consideration (people will actually pay for products with this much pyruvate). Most studies have used 20 g or more (which would be far too expensive to sell as a dietary supplement). Most commercial preparations contain 500 mg to 1 g of pyruvate with two to three servings recommended per day.

WORKS CONSULTED

Bryson JM, King SE, Burns CM, Baur LA, Swaraj S, Caterson ID. Changes in glucose and lipid metabolism following weight loss produced by a very low calorie diet in obese subjects. Int J Obes Relat Metab Disord. 1996 Apr;20(4):338-45.

Fields AL, Cheema-Dhadli S, Wolman SL, Halperin ML. Theoretical aspects of weight loss in patients with cancer. Possible importance of pyruvate dehydrogenase. Cancer. 1982 Nov 15;50(10):2183-8.

Fields AL, Falk N, Cheema-Dhadli S, Halperin ML. Accelerated loss of lean body mass in fasting rats due to activation of pyruvate dehydrogenase by dichloroacetate. Metabolism. 1987 Jul;36(7):621-4.

Stanko RT, Arch JE. Inhibition of regain in body weight and fat with addition of 3-carbon compounds to the diet with hyperenergetic refeeding after weight reduction. Int J Obes Relat Metab Disord. 1996 Oct;20(10):925-30.

Stanko RT, Reynolds HR, Hoyson R, Janosky JE, Wolf R. Pyruvate supplementation of a low-cholesterol, low-fat diet: Effects on plasma lipid concentrations and body composition in hyperlipidemic patients. Am J Clin Nutr. 1994 Feb;59(2):423-7.

Stanko RT, Tietze DL, Arch JE. Body composition, energy utilization, and nitrogen metabolism with a 4.25-MJ/d low-energy diet supplemented with pyruvate. Am J Clin Nutr. 1992 Oct;56(4):630-5.

Stanko RT, Tietze DL, Arch JE. Body composition, energy utilization, and nitrogen metabolism with a severely restricted diet supplemented with dihydroxyacetone and pyruvate. Am J Clin Nutr. 1992 Apr;55(4):771-6.

Sukala WR. Pyruvate: Beyond the marketing hype. Int J Sport Nutr. 1998 Sep;8(3):241-9.

BLADDERWRACK

What Is It?

Bladderwrack *(Fucus vesiculosus)* is a brown seaweed or algae. As a dietary supplement, bladderwrack is often used to stimulate metabolic rate and promote fat and weight loss. Like many seaweeds, bladderwrack has a relatively high concentration of iodine.

Claims

- Increases levels of thyroid hormones
- Promotes weight loss
- Increases energy levels

Theory

The primary theory explaining how a brown seaweed can help increase energy levels and stimulate weight loss is that bladderwrack contains a relatively high concentration of iodine. One of the key functions of iodine is in the thyroid gland, which requires it to produce adequate levels of thyroid hormones. Low levels of thyroid hormones are associated with reduced energy levels and weight gain—so maintaining optimal levels is a key factor in promoting stamina and healthy body weight.

Scientific Support

Although the underlying theory for using bladderwrack as a dietary supplement for increased energy and weight loss appear to be logical, it has not been evaluated by well-controlled clinical studies. A few things that we *do* know about the biological effects of bladderwrack extracts include reduction of platelet aggregation (anticoagulant), reduction of blood glucose, and even inhibition of certain enzyme activity in HIV (the virus that causes AIDS).

Safety

No long-term safety studies have been conducted on bladderwrack—but it is not recommended in high doses or for prolonged periods of time because of the high iodine content and the risk of iodine overdose. The well-respected herbal monographs from Germany's Commission E list bladder-wrack as an unapproved herbal medication.

Value

For its most frequently made claims as a dietary supplement (increased energy and weight loss), bladderwrack has not been shown to be effective. As such, its primary value is probably as a crude source of iodine (but an expensive one at that).

Dosage

There are no accepted dosage recommendations for bladderwrack. Rarely available as a stand-alone supplement, bladderwrack is typically included as part of various herbal blends targeted to weight loss, cellulite reduction, increased energy, or thyroid support.

WORKS CONSULTED

Beress A, Wassermann O, Tahhan S, Bruhn T, Beress L, Kraiselburd EN, Gonzalez LV, de Motta GE, Chavez PI. A new procedure for the isolation of anti-HIV compounds (polysaccharides and polyphenols) from the marine alga Fucus vesiculosus. J Nat Prod. 1993 Apr;56(4):478-88.

Durig J, Bruhn T, Zurborn KH, Gutensohn K, Bruhn HD, Beress L. Anticoagulant fucoidan fractions from Fucus vesiculosus induce platelet activation in vitro. Thromb Res. 1997 Mar 15;85(6):479-91.

Fujimura T, Shibuya Y, Moriwaki S, Tsukahara K, Kitahara T, Sano T, Nishizawa Y, Takema Y. Fucoidan is the active component of fucus vesiculosus that promotes contraction of fibroblast-populated collagen gels. Biol Pharm Bull. 2000 Oct;23(10):1180-4.

Lamela M, Anca J, Villar R, Otero J, Calleja JM. Hypoglycemic activity of several seaweed extracts. J Ethnopharmacol. 1989 Nov;27(1-2):35-43.

WHITE WILLOW

What Is It?

The bark of the white willow tree *(Salix alba)* is a source of salicin and other salicylates—compounds which are similar in structure to aspirin (acetyl salicylic acid). Native Americans are thought to have used ground willow bark and willow bark tea as a remedy for everything from pain relief to fevers. Today, white willow bark is often used as a natural alternative to aspirin, but perhaps the most common use in dietary supplements is as an adjunct for weight loss (as the "A" in ECA stacks).

Claims

- Pain reliever (headaches, arthritis, minor injuries)
- Fever reducer
- Anti-inflammatory
- Enhances weight loss (only in combination with other ingredients)

Theory

As a weight loss aid, white willow bark extract offers little to no benefit by itself. In combination with other dietary supplements, however, white willow is thought to extend or increase the activity of several thermogenic ingredients in elevating energy expenditure and promoting fat metabolism.

Scientific Support

The primary active compound in white willow bark is salicin. In the body, salicin can be converted into salicylic acid, which has powerful effects as an anti-inflammatory and pain reliever. Until synthetic aspirin could be produced in large quantities, white willow bark was the treatment of choice for reducing fevers, relieving headache and arthritis pain, and controlling swelling. Although synthetic aspirin is clearly a more effective pain reliever and anti-inflammatory agent than the weaker natural bark extract, white willow can also serve as a source of tannins—a combination that may be synergistic in ele-

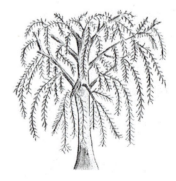

vating energy expenditure by interfering with prostaglandin production and inhibiting norepinephrine breakdown. Although this mild elevation of norepinephrine concentrations would not be expected to significantly elevate resting energy expenditure on its own, its effect appears to be enough, when used in combination with other thermogenic supplements, to help promote increased fat oxidation (examples include ma huang, synephrine, green tea, guarana, and quercetin).

Safety

Stomach ulcers and other gastrointestinal complaints (nausea and diarrhea) are common side effects from prolonged high-dose consumption of either synthetic aspirin or white willow bark extracts. Long-term use of high doses of either salicin source is not recommended, although the natural bark extract is often tolerated much better than the more powerful synthetic aspirin. Individuals with concerns about blood clotting and bleeding time should use aspirin and white willow with caution, as both have the potential to interfere with platelet aggregation and prolong bleeding time (i.e., a blood-thinning effect).

Value

If you have a pounding headache that you want to go away quickly, chances are you will experience better results with regular aspirin from your local pharmacy or grocery store (at a better price than white willow). For those looking for a gentler approach to either temporary inflammation or weight management (thermogenesis), lower-dose white willow may be an effective alternative to aspirin.

Dosage

Standardized extracts of white willow bark are available in which total salicin intake is typically 60 to 120 mg per day for relief of acute pain, fever, or inflammation. For longer-term consumption as an adjunct to weight management and thermogenesis, smaller doses are generally tolerated much better.

WORKS CONSULTED

Chrubasik S, Eisenberg E, Balan E, Weinberger T, Luzzati R, Conradt C. Treatment of low back pain exacerbations with willow bark extract: A randomized double-blind study. Am J Med. 2000 Jul;109(1):9-14.

Daly PA, Krieger DR, Dulloo AG, Young JB, Landsberg L. Ephedrine, caffeine and aspirin: Safety and efficacy for treatment of human obesity. Int J Obes Relat Metab Disord. 1993 Feb;17(Suppl 1):S73-8.

Dulloo AG, Miller DS. Aspirin as a promoter of ephedrine-induced thermogenesis: Potential use in the treatment of obesity. Am J Clin Nutr. 1987 Mar;45(3):564-9.

Dulloo AG, Miller DS. Ephedrine, caffeine and aspirin: "Over-the-counter" drugs that interact to stimulate thermogenesis in the obese. Nutrition. 1989 Jan-Feb;5(1):7-9.

Geissler CA. Effects of weight loss, ephedrine and aspirin on energy expenditure in obese women. Int J Obes Relat Metab Disord. 1993 Feb;17(Suppl 1):S45-8.

Krieger DR, Daly PA, Dulloo AG, Ransil BJ, Young JB, Landsberg L. Ephedrine, caffeine and aspirin promote weight loss in obese subjects. Trans Assoc Am Physicians. 1990;103:307-12.

Levesque H, Lafont O. Aspirin throughout the ages: A historical review. Rev Med Interne. 2000 Mar;21(Suppl 1):8s-17s.

Norton WL, Meisinger MA. An overview of nonsteroidal antiinflammatory agents. Inflammation. 1977 Mar;2(1):37-46.

Toubro S, Astrup AV, Breum L, Quaade F. Safety and efficacy of long-term treatment with ephedrine, caffeine and an ephedrine/caffeine mixture. Int J Obes Relat Metab Disord. 1993 Feb;17(Suppl 1):S69-72.

Chapter 5

Sports Supplements and Ergogenic Aids

INTRODUCTION

Sports nutrition may seem like a no-brainer for many people—eat some carbs before your workout, drink some water during exercise, and get a good night's sleep to help your body recover—Right? WRONG! What to consume before, during, and after exercise is *far* from being an easy question to answer. As we dig into the complexity of sports nutrition, we see that many variables affect what our bodies need. Is the exercise a maximal effort, a long endurance run, or a series of repetitive maximal bouts? Is our goal to sustain speed or performance, or to reduce muscle soreness and improve recovery? Have we been training using a specific drink or food prior to the exercise bout? For each athletic event, training session, and individual athlete, there will be unique nutrition needs that have to be satisfied to promote optimal performance. What follows is a breakdown of physiology, nutrient needs, and real-world recommendations to satisfy nutrient needs before, during, and after exercise.

The market for sports supplements is about $3 billion annually—that's a lot of Powerbars! The main problem with selecting a sports supplement, however, is that most people simply have no idea how to use them the right way. There are certainly some very useful products on the market—but you'll have to do more than scarf down an energy bar while watching the Olympic games on TV.

When it comes to sports nutrition, it's quite helpful to break things down into three distinct periods of time—before, during, and after exercise. Another way to categorize products is by their main mode of action—such as muscle building, endurance, or recovery. This chapter takes a look at sports nutrition products from both perspectives.

SUPPLEMENTS FOR USE WITH EXERCISE

Before Exercise

Your Body Physiology

If you've been training for a good while for a specific race, your body has gone through some adaptations that affect you both physiologically and nutritionally. With endurance training, your body now has increased mitochondria (in the trained muscles), increased myoglobin, increased vascularization, and increased oxygen transport mechanisms among a long list of physiological changes. Due to these changes, your muscle cells are capable of holding more water and more glycogen than when you were untrained. Your body now has a larger fuel tank for its endurance workout—but realize that a larger fuel tank does you no good, unless you fill it to the top with premium fuel!

What Your Body Needs

Starting forty-eight hours prior to your exercise bout, be sure to increase your intake of both water and carbohydrates. Your body is capable of holding a lot of water, which is ultimately necessary for maximum performance. Your muscle cells also crave fuel. Carbohydrates are the preferred fuel for intense activity, whether aerobic or anaerobic, so an increase in the amount of carbs that you consume prior to an intense effort will give your muscles the fuel that they need. Note: Do not increase your total calories above what you are normally used to, or you will simply gain weight (as fat).

Recommendation

Starting forty-eight hours prior to your event, minimize the amount of fat and protein in your diet. In the same ratio, substitute carbohydrates for protein and fat in each meal. Be sure not to consume any carbohydrates or supplements to which you are unaccustomed (stick to things that you've already had experience with in training), as this will only increase the risk of gastric distress. Your daily caloric intake should consist of at least 70 percent carbohydrates. You cannot drink too much water (or at least you would have to try really hard to do so). Minimize or, even better, eliminate any diuretics including caffeine.

Example: Let's say your standard dinner includes two chicken breasts with rice, salad, and a Coke. Before your big race, try substituting a cup of pasta for one chicken breast and two large glasses of water or prerace drink for the Coke (keep the salad and rice).

During Exercise (and Two Hours Prior)

Your Body Physiology

As you begin a long, low-intensity exercise bout, your heart rate increases and your body starts burning both carbohydrates and fat. As long as the intensity is low, you can expect your body to burn primarily fat as it conserves carbohydrates. When intensity increases, the body looks for a more efficient fuel to keep up with demand, and it begins burning more carbohydrates. If you exercise too long, your body will run out of stored carbohydrates (glycogen), and you'll need to supply additional carbs orally to keep your "machine" running. Without ingesting carbohydrates, at the right time and in the right amounts, you can expect a drastic decrease in performance—a nasty situation referred to as "hitting the wall" or "bonking."

What Your Body Needs

Hopefully you have taken the recommendations in the previous section and fueled your body properly with carbohydrates and water. If you did not, then you can minimize your losses with the following recommendations, but realize that it is too late to optimize your fuel stores.

Prior to exercise, your body is capable of storing, within the muscle cell, high levels of glycogen and water. Two hours prior to exercise you may want to top off those levels to assure maximum performance (at this point be sure to only use carbohydrates with a low glycemic index [LGI]. (LGI carbohydrates are carbohydrate sources that are digested and absorbed at a slow rate.) Consuming LGI carbohydrates immediately before exercise will help stabilize blood sugar, so that your body burns fat instead of glucose or glycogen. This allows your body to spare its carbohydrates so you can exercise longer before you bonk or hit the wall. Note: Antioxidants prior to exercise can also reduce muscle damage and delay the onset of muscle soreness following exhaustive exercise.

Recommendation

Two hours prior to exercise, consume about 1 to 2 g of LGI carbs per kilogram of body weight (1 kg equals 2.2 lb, so about 0.45 to 0.9 g are needed per pound of body weight). In addition, consume 8 oz of water for every 50 lb of body weight. About 30 minutes prior to exercise, again consume LGI carbs and water—but only at about 1 to 2 g of carbs and 1 oz of water per 10 lb of body weight. Some athletes like to snack on LGI foods and water for the entire two hours before the race.

Time before exercise	LGI Carbs (for a 200 lb athlete)	Fluid intake
2 h	100 to 200 g	32 oz
30 min	20 to 40 g	20 oz
During	20 to 40 g/h	16 oz/h

For the first hour of the race, be sure to consume at least 4 oz of water every 15 minutes or so. If you can stomach it, and have been training this way, you can use your carbohydrate drink (such as Cytomax, Gatorade, Perform, etc.). About an hour into the race, be sure to switch exclusively to a carbohydrate drink. At this point you are trying to spare your stored muscle glycogen by offering your body some oral carbohydrates. A combination of high glycemic and low glycemic carbohydrates (50/50 split) works best at a concentration of less than 7 percent. Concentrations higher than 7 percent can delay gastric emptying. In other words, you cannot digest the carbohydrates and water quickly enough, and it becomes a detriment. Be sure that the sports drink that you consume contains adequate levels of sodium, calcium, potassium, and chloride, which help to replace electrolyte losses and provide energy.

> *Example:* Two hours prior: Eat ½ cup dried apricots, one 8 oz glass of skim milk, and rice bran with 24 oz of water. During your race, use a carbo/fluid replacement beverage of your choice—but only if you have been using it during your training (or train with the sponsored race drink).

After Exercise

Your Body Physiology

Congratulations! You have now depleted your body of glycogen, electrolytes, and water. In order to survive, your body has a built-in defense mechanism—a high affinity for each of these nutrients. Your body also needs to repair torn muscle fibers and is seeking protein to do so. The good news is that your body is very sensitive to these nutrients for about 20 minutes following exercise and has a relatively high sensitivity for two hours after. As such, it is vitally important to feed your body's needs as soon as possible after crossing the finish line or hearing the end of game buzzer.

What Your Body Needs

Upon completion of your exercise, you can expect your body to be depleted of glycogen, sodium, chloride, potassium, creatine, glutamine, and water. As the body hungers for these nutrients, insulin sensitivity is increased, and water and glycogen resynthesis is in demand! It could take 48 to 72 hours to replenish these stores optimally (if not done properly) so do what it takes to optimize nutrients immediately after exercise. Adding protein to this mix also helps with the repair of muscle fibers and helps reduce muscle soreness.

Recommendation

Immediately following exercise, consume a drink containing high glycemic index (HGI) carbohydrates (HGI carbs rush sugar into the blood) with protein at a 4:1 ratio. This maximizes glycogen resynthesis more than carbohydrates or protein alone. Make sure that the drink contains high levels of sodium, chloride, and potassium. Added levels of specific amino acids such as creatine, glutamine, and taurine can work synergistically with the protein and glucose to improve recovery time even more.

> *Example:* Within 20 minutes after exercise, consume a small meal composed of HGI carbs and protein. A fast option might be some instant rice with a baked potato and some tuna fish (two HGI carbs plus some protein), but many athletes prefer a "recovery-focused" post-exercise beverage, many of which are formulated specifically with these recovery criteria in mind.

Other Factors

There are a number of factors to consider when choosing the specific nutrients to fuel your body and develop your before, during, and after exercise nutrition regimen:

- *How long is my race or exercise bout?* Races under an hour may not need any oral glucose or water—but this also depends on your training state.

- *Will I be doing repeated bouts or only one?* Repeated bouts of exercise throughout the day have entirely different needs than a single long bout of aerobic exercise.
- *At what intensity will I be working out?* Low intensity burns fat and conserves carbohydrates. High-intensity exercisers may be better off ingesting HGI carbohydrates immediately before exercise.
- *What is the purpose of the drink I am about to consume?* Am I trying to optimize electrolyte and fluid replacement, replace carbohydrate, or enhance recovery?
- *How well trained am I?* A better-trained athlete has more adaptations to training than a nontrained individual and may be able to race for nearly two hours without ingesting glucose.
- *Have I used any specific nutrients during my training?* Do not attempt to use something foreign to your digestive system on the day of the race. Practice all these recommendations during training to see how your body responds to each one.

FUNCTIONAL CATEGORIZATION OF SPORTS SUPPLEMENTS

Another useful way to categorize sports nutrition products, beyond the before/during/after approach outlined above, is by their primary effect or mode of action. Using this method, sports nutrition products fall primarily into three categories (with some overlap between categories):

- Muscle strength and mass
- Endurance and energy
- Recovery

Muscle Strength and Mass

Creatine

Creatine is stored primarily in skeletal muscle as creatine phosphate (CP), where its main role is to restore adenosine diphosphate (ADP) to adenosine triphosphate (ATP), which can then be used as an energy source to support muscle contractions (and possibly to help reduce lactic acid accumulation). Creatine can also cause muscle cells to swell due to an influx of fluid—the result of which is a muscle cell with an increased cell volume and cross-sectional area—both of which may stimulate protein synthesis and lead to increased muscle size and strength. There is some evidence that creatine supplements may aid muscle function in patients with muscular dystrophy and muscle-wasting conditions (such as aging).

Much speculation has associated creatine use with several adverse side effects such as muscle cramping and strained muscles—effects that are thought to be due less to creatine per se than to athletes exceeding their capabilities and trying to do more work than their muscles are ready to do. A real concern may be the possibility of dehydration (due to retained fluid inside the muscle cell)—but an increased intake of fluids easily remedies this situation.

Protein Powders

Protein powders are available from virtually every supplement manufacturer—with claims for everything from increasing muscle mass to losing (or gaining) weight. The most common sources of protein come from milk (casein and whey), egg, and soy.

Aside from their use in weight loss and muscle building applications, protein supplements are also being used in some of the newer "recovery" formulations. Because the body's protein needs increase dramatically (and disproportionately to caloric needs) during physical trauma and injury, supplemental protein added to the diet can not only enhance recovery from exercise, but may also boost immunity and help prevent injuries from repeated training (and overtraining).

Protein sources are often classed based on their biological value (BV), a term that refers to the amount of protein deposited in tissues per gram of protein absorbed. In general, the higher the BV, the more effective will be the utilization of protein in the body. Whey protein is often considered to be the protein source with the highest BV (100), but using a more precise calculation of protein "quality," other concentrated sources of protein such as egg, casein (milk), and soy now rival whey proteins. Depending on how soy protein is processed, it may also retain various levels of estrogenic compounds known as isoflavones (genistein and daidzein), and whey protein isolates may deliver a blend of immunoglobulin compounds that have been linked to increased immune function (again, depending on processing methods).

Amino Acids

Because amino acids are the building blocks of protein, most protein supplements provide a full complement of amino acids. In some cases, however, the use of higher levels of specific amino acids may provide an additional benefit. It is important to note, however, that excessive ingestion of any individual amino acid may interfere with the absorption and metabolism of other amino acids (a situation with the potential to create deficiencies of essential amino acids).

Branched-Chain Amino Acids (BCAA)

BCAAs (leucine, isoleucine, and valine) are essential amino acids, meaning the body is not able to synthesize them, and they need to be supplied in the diet. The BCAAs are believed to be important in delaying "central" fatigue, which originates in the central nervous system (as opposed to "peripheral" fatigue that results from biochemical events within the muscles). Proponents of the central fatigue hypothesis believe that BCAA supplementation can help delay the production of serotonin in the brain and result in a longer duration of exercise before fatigue sets in. BCAA supplementation may also decrease protein breakdown during strenuous exercise.

Other supplements that fall into the "muscle strength and mass" category include:

- Androstenedione
- Dehydroepiandrosterone (DHEA)
- Beta-hydroxy beta-methylbutyrate (HMB)
- *Tribulus terrestris*
- Vanadium
- Boron
- Zinc

Endurance and Energy

Ma Huang

Ma huang is one of the most popular stimulant herbs. It contains ephedra (two alkaloids, ephedrine and pseudoephedrine), which has been used in over-the-counter remedies for colds, flu, and asthma (to alleviate nasal congestion and open airways). Ephedra compounds are quite effective weight loss aids, as they stimulate metabolism and suppress appetite. They also appear to be even more effective when combined with other stimulants such as caffeine (often from guarana or kola nut) and salicylates (aspirin-like compounds often supplied as white willow bark). Some people can use ephedra-based supplements with no side effects, while other individuals experience elevated heart rate and blood pressure, as well as insomnia, anxiety, irrita-bility, heart palpitations, and other unpleasant side effects.

Many other supplement ingredients promoted as energy products overlap with popular weight loss or thermogenic products, some of which are:

- B-complex vitamins
- Bee pollen
- Blue-green algae
- Ciwuja (Siberian ginseng)
- Cordyceps
- Ginseng
- Royal jelly

Recovery

Glucosamine and Chondroitin

Glucosamine, whether used alone or in combination with chondroitin, appears to be quite effective in alleviating the pain and inflammation associ-ated with arthritis. Many sports supplements are beginning to include these ingredients in recovery formulas designed to help repair and prevent dam-age to muscles, joints, and other connective tissue structures.

Sports Drinks

Sports drinks usually contain water, electrolytes, and carbohydrates (usually a combination of glucose/dextrose, glucose polymers, and/or fruc-tose). Depending on the product, various amounts of protein, vitamins, min-erals, and ergogenic agents may also be present. The level of carbohydrate and other nutrients will determine whether a given beverage is intended for use primarily during exercise for energy and rehydration or before and after exercise for recovery.

Glycerol

Glycerol (glycerin, glycerine, glycerate) naturally occurs as part of tri-glycerides, but as a dietary supplement or component of sports drinks, glyc-erol causes cells to hold water and may help to delay dehydration during ex-ercise and promote rehydration following exercise. About 1 g of glycerin per kilogram of body weight is mixed with water or sports drink (1 g of glycerin per ounce of water) and consumed one to three hours before exercise. The downside of glycerol use can include headaches and nausea.

Other recovery nutrients include:

- Antioxidants
- B-complex vitamins
- Glutamine
- Zinc
- Beta-sitosterol

SUMMARY

Athletes and recreational exercisers alike are using sports nutrition supplements to promote improvements in muscle mass and strength, energy and endurance, and recovery after exercise (Table 5.1). Using these products the right way, in the right amounts, and in the right situations can help improve exercise performance, bolster adaptations to training, and promote optimal recovery from exercise training.

TABLE 5.1. Dietary Supplements Promoted for Sports Performance

Supplement	Dosage (per day)	Primary claim
Alpha-ketoglutarate (AKG/OKG)	10-20 g	Increases muscle mass
Androstenedione	50-200 mg	Increases testosterone
Beta-hydroxy beta-methylbutyrate (HMB)	3 g	Reduces muscle catabolism
Branched-chain amino acids (BCAA)	3-20 g	Recovery/fatigue prevention
Carnosine	1-3 g	Muscle recovery
Cordyceps sinensis	2-4 g	Increases oxygen uptake
Creatine	5-25 g	Increases muscle mass
Dehydroepiandrosterone (DHEA)	50-100 mg	Increases testosterone
Gamma-oryzanol	100-500 mg	Increases testosterone

Supplement	Dosage (per day)	Primary claim
Glycerol	70 g (for a 70-kg athlete)	Delays dehydration
Medium-chain triglycerides (MCTs)	1-2 tbsp	Improves endurance
Protein	0.8-1.6 g/kg BW	Various
Proteolytic enzymes	Varies	Reduces pain/inflammation
Ribose	3-10 g	Increases muscle energy
Sodium bicarbonate	21 g (for a 70-kg athlete)	Reduces lactic acid
Tribulus terrestris	250-1,500 mg	Increases testosterone

CREATINE

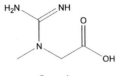

Creatine

What Is It?

Creatine is an amino acid. It is normally produced in the body from arginine, glycine, and methionine. Creatine plays a vital role in cellular energy production as creatine phosphate (phosphocreatine) in regenerating adenosine triphosphate (ATP) in skeletal muscle. Without ATP, muscle contraction is not possible. Oral administration of creatine increases muscle stores and may increase muscle strength and improve exercise performance. In the diet, creatine is found in meat and fish, although cooking destroys most of it.

Claims

- Increases energy
- Enhances muscle size and strength
- Increases power output

Theory

Most of the creatine in the diet comes from meat (an 8 oz steak might have a gram), but about half of the body's supply is manufactured in the liver and kidneys. On average, your muscles require about 2 g of creatine a day (somewhat more for muscular people, a bit less for skinny folks), but more or less depending on your activity level and degree of muscle mass.

Creatine is stored in muscle cells as phosphocreatine and is used to help generate cellular energy for muscle contractions. It also may increase the amount of water that each muscle cell holds—thus increasing the size of the muscle (and possibly its function as well). Creatine is used in the body to produce creatine phosphate or CP, which can be thought of as a storage form of quick energy. The function of CP is to regenerate the primary supply of cellular energy—which comes from ATP. ATP supplies energy for all cells in your body. Upon giving up some of its energy, ATP becomes ADP (diphosphate) and needs to be regenerated into ATP to do it all over again. CP performs this crucial ATP regeneration step by donating a phosphate group to ADP (ADP + P = ATP).

Under conditions in which rapid resynthesis of ATP is important, such as during repeated bouts of high intensity exercise, a higher muscle concentration of CP may serve as a reservoir of stored energy and therefore enhance performance. Although it has not been studied extensively, there may also be a role for creatine in maintaining muscle mass and preventing the muscle wasting that occurs as a result of old age and in chronic conditions such as AIDS and heart failure.

Scientific Support

Creatine is one of the new breed of dietary supplements—those based on sound scientific theory and backed up by well-controlled studies. At this writing, at least twenty published articles exist to support the efficacy of creatine supplements in improving performance in high-intensity, repeated-bout activities (weight lifting, sprinting, jumping). Creatine supplements do not appear to enhance physical performance, however, among subjects performing lower-intensity endurance activity such as cycling or running. Although increased muscle mass could conceivably enhance endurance performance, the weight gain from water and muscle weight may even result in a decline in performance.

The benefits of creatine are likely to be due, at least in part, to an increased ability to train harder—thus increasing strength. This might be good news to athletes who are training intensely, but it means that creatine alone (without exercise) would probably have very little effect on the muscle mass of sedentary individuals.

A significant gain in physical performance in high-intensity exercise has been shown with creatine doses of 20 to 30 g per day, but more recent research is indicating that similar performance benefits are possible with much lower doses in the range of 2 to 5 g per day (although benefits may take longer to be noticed).

Taking very large doses of creatine daily also seems to increase the strength of muscular dystrophy patients' muscles by about 10 percent. Although that may be considered a relatively small gain, it may be very important to a person who can pick up a glass of water because of it. Supplementation with 10 g of creatine per day for five days followed by 5 g per day for another week has produced increases in muscle strength in the legs, hands, and feet of patients with muscular dystrophy. Such patients usually have lower creatine levels than healthy people, so boosting muscle stores may help augment cellular energy production and support muscular contraction.

Safety

Because of its effects on muscle size and strength, creatine is often confused with anabolic steroids. Steroids, which mimic the effects of the male sex hormone testosterone, can result in a wide variety of adverse side effects such as severe acne, hair loss, testicular shrinkage, and psychological problems. Although the long-term effects of prolonged creatine use have not been examined, no obvious adverse effects have been linked to use of creatine as a dietary supplement. Side effects reported anecdotally include gastrointestinal distress, nausea, dehydration, and muscle cramping—but none of these effects have been documented in scientific studies.

Although no serious side effects have been scientifically verified in subjects using relatively brief (less than twelve weeks) creatine regimens, some athletes have reported muscle cramps, muscle tears, and dehydration. Caution is also advised for people with kidney disorders and for those at risk for dehydration (such as those who exercise in extreme heat or who are losing weight for wrestling or lightweight crew).

Value

Consumers spent well over $200 million on creatine supplements in 2000. Creatine has become one of the hottest sports supplements for one major reason—it works. Creatine appears to be effective in specific situations—high-intensity activities that require short bouts of repeated activity (e.g., weight lifting and football). Athletes in other sports may achieve a significant indirect benefit, as creatine supplements may allow more intense levels of weight training, with strength and power benefits transferring to the sport.

Dosage

The most common regimen for creatine supplementation follows a two-phase cycle with a five- to ten-day loading phase (20 to 25 g per day) followed by a variable length maintenance phase (2 to 5 g per day) to maintain muscle saturation. It is unclear, however, whether the loading phase is actually needed to achieve the same end result. Creatine absorption appears to be enhanced when the supplement is taken with a high-carbohydrate drink such as fruit juice.

WORKS CONSULTED

Aaserud R, Gramvik P, Olsen SR, Jensen J. Creatine supplementation delays onset of fatigue during repeated bouts of sprint running. Scand J Med Sci Sports. 1998 Oct;8(5 Pt 1):247-51.

Archer MC. Use of oral creatine to enhance athletic performance and its potential side effects. Clin J Sport Med. 1999 Apr;9(2):119.

Becque MD, Lochmann JD, Melrose DR. Effects of oral creatine supplementation on muscular strength and body composition. Med Sci Sports Exerc. 2000 Mar;32(3):654-8.

Benzi G. Is there a rationale for the use of creatine either as nutritional supplementation or drug administration in humans participating in a sport? Pharmacol Res. 2000 Mar;41(3):255-64.

Bermon S, Venembre P, Sachet C, Valour S, Dolisi C. Effects of creatine monohydrate ingestion in sedentary and weight-trained older adults. Acta Physiol Scand. 1998 Oct;164(2):147-55.

Casey A, Greenhaff PL. Does dietary creatine supplementation play a role in skeletal muscle metabolism and performance? Am J Clin Nutr. 2000 Aug;72(2 Suppl):607S-17S.

Culpepper RM. Creatine supplementation: safe as steak? South Med J. 1998 Sep;91(9):890-2.

Feldman EB. Creatine: A dietary supplement and ergogenic aid. Nutr Rev. 1999 Feb;57(2):45-50.

Graham AS, Hatton RC. Creatine: A review of efficacy and safety. J Am Pharm Assoc (Wash). 1999 Nov-Dec;39(6):803-10; quiz 875-7.

Guerrero-Ontiveros ML, Wallimann T. Creatine supplementation in health and disease. Effects of chronic creatine ingestion in vivo: Down-regulation of the expression of creatine transporter isoforms in skeletal muscle. Mol Cell Biochem. 1998 Jul;184(1-2):427-37.

Jacobs I. Dietary creatine monohydrate supplementation. Can J Appl Physiol. 1999 Dec;24(6):503-14.

Jones AM, Atter T, Georg KP. Oral creatine supplementation improves multiple sprint performance in elite ice-hockey players. J Sports Med Phys Fitness. 1999 Sep;39(3):189-96.

Juhn MS. Does creatine supplementation increase the risk of rhabdomyolysis? J Am Board Fam Pract. 2000 Mar-Apr;13(2):150-1.

Juhn MS, O'Kane JW, Vinci DM. Oral creatine supplementation in male collegiate athletes: A survey of dosing habits and side effects. J Am Diet Assoc. 1999 May;99(5):593-5.

Juhn MS, Tarnopolsky M. Oral creatine supplementation and athletic performance: A critical review. Clin J Sport Med. 1998 Oct;8(4):286-97.

Kamber M, Koster M, Kreis R, Walker G, Boesch C, Hoppeler H. Creatine supplementation—Part I: Performance, clinical chemistry, and muscle volume. Med Sci Sports Exerc. 1999 Dec;31(12):1763-9.

Kraemer WJ, Volek JS. Creatine supplementation. Its role in human performance. Clin Sports Med. 1999 Jul;18(3):651-66.

Kreider RB. Dietary supplements and the promotion of muscle growth with resistance exercise. Sports Med. 1999 Feb;27(2):97-110.

Kreis R, Kamber M, Koster M, Felblinger J, Slotboom J, Hoppeler H, Boesch C. Creatine supplementation—Part II: In vivo magnetic resonance spectroscopy. Med Sci Sports Exerc. 1999 Dec;31(12):1770-7.

LaBotz M, Smith BW. Creatine supplement use in an NCAA Division I athletic program. Clin J Sport Med. 1999 Jul;9(3):167-9.

Leenders NM, Lamb DR, Nelson TE. Creatine supplementation and swimming performance. Int J Sport Nutr. 1999 Sep;9(3):251-62.

Mujika I, Padilla S, Ibanez J, Izquierdo M, Gorostiaga E. Creatine supplementation and sprint performance in soccer players. Med Sci Sports Exerc. 2000 Feb;32(2):518-25.

Poortmans JR, Francaux M. Long-term oral creatine supplementation does not impair renal function in healthy athletes. Med Sci Sports Exerc. 1999 Aug;31(8):1108-10.

Rawson ES, Clarkson PM. Acute creatine supplementation in older men. Int J Sports Med. 2000 Jan;21(1):71-5.

Rico-Sanz J, Zehnder M, Buchli R, Dambach M, Boutellier U. Muscle glycogen degradation during simulation of a fatiguing soccer match in elite soccer players examined noninvasively by 13C-MRS. Med Sci Sports Exerc. 1999 Nov;31(11):1587-93.

Robinson SJ. Acute quadriceps compartment syndrome and rhabdomyolysis in a weight lifter using high-dose creatine supplementation. J Am Board Fam Pract. 2000 Mar-Apr;13(2):134-7.

Schedel JM, Terrier P, Schutz Y. The biomechanic origin of sprint performance enhancement after one-week creatine supplementation. Jpn J Physiol. 2000 Apr;50(2):273-6.

Silber ML. Scientific facts behind creatine monohydrate as sport nutrition supplement. J Sports Med Phys Fitness. 1999 Sep;39(3):179-88.

Terjung RL, Clarkson P, Eichner ER, Greenhaff PL, Hespel PJ, Israel RG, Kraemer WJ, Meyer RA, Spriet LL, Tarnopolsky MA, Wagenmakers AJ, Williams MH. American College of Sports Medicine roundtable. The physiological and health effects of oral creatine supplementation. Med Sci Sports Exerc. 2000 Mar;32(3):706-17.

Theodorou AS, Cooke CB, King RF, Hood C, Denison T, Wainwright BG, Havenetidis K. The effect of longer-term creatine supplementation on elite swimming performance after an acute creatine loading. J Sports Sci. 1999 Nov;17(11):853-9.

Vandebuerie F, Vanden Eynde B, Vandenberghe K, Hespel P. Effect of creatine loading on endurance capacity and sprint power in cyclists. Int J Sports Med. 1998 Oct;19(7):490-5.

Wyss M, Kaddurah-Daouk R. Creatine and creatinine metabolism. Physiol Rev. 2000 Jul;80(3):1107-213.

Yu PH, Deng Y. Potential cytotoxic effect of chronic administration of creatine, a nutrition supplement to augment athletic performance. Med Hypotheses. 2000 May;54(5):726-8.

RIBOSE

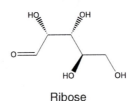

Ribose

What Is It?

Ribose is a five-carbon simple sugar (a pentose) that forms the carbohydrate portion, or backbone, of RNA and DNA molecules. When combined with adenine, ribose produces adenosine, one of the components of the energy currency of the cell—ATP (adenosine triphosphate). Ribose is used in the body in several specific ways. It can be converted into pyruvate and enter into the pathways of energy metabolism, or it can be used to manufacture nucleotides—the primary building blocks for important structures in the body such as RNA, DNA, and ATP.

Claims

- Increases energy
- Reduces fatigue
- Increases muscle strength
- Aids weight loss
- Improves cardiac function

Theory

Because ribose can serve as a precursor to adenosine (the "A" in ATP) and seems to stimulate the production of ATP, the theory behind ribose supplementation is that it may maximize ATP stores and, therefore, increase cellular energy stores for improved exercise performance and fatigue prevention.

In the cell, ATP loses its phosphate groups to generate energy. Losing one phosphate turns ATP ("tri"-phosphate) into ADP ("di") and finally into AMP ("mono"). Adenine/adenosine (no phosphates) can either be reconverted to AMP or lost from the cell. The conversion to AMP/ADP/ATP, or "salvage" of adenosine, requires a ribose-containing molecule known as 5-phosphororibosyl-1-pyrophosphate (PRPP). If this salvage does not take place, the adenosine is lost and will need to be converted from scratch—a process known as de novo synthesis, which again requires the ribose-containing PRPP.

Scientific Support

Ribose has been under study as a therapy for cardiac ischemia (reduced blood flow to the heart) for a number of years. The data from these studies clearly indicate that ribose can help improve heart function during and following periods of reduced blood flow and oxygen delivery. Under conditions of constricted blood and oxygen flow to heart and muscle tissue, ATP levels have been shown to decrease by as much as 50 percent. This finding is not unexpected, but the fact that creatine phosphate levels recover relatively quickly, while ATP levels may remain depressed for several days, suggests that adenosine levels may not be adequately maintained. In animal studies, supplemental ribose permits recovery of approximately 85 percent of normal ATP levels within twenty-four hours following restricted circulation.

In patients with coronary artery disease, supplemental ribose allows subjects to exercise significantly longer than they could before they consumed ribose and longer than subjects who consumed a placebo supplement. During intense exercise, ATP levels are reduced 10 to 20 percent, which may be attributed to the loss of adenosine and inadequate resynthesis of ATP. In some muscle fibers, complete resynthesis of ATP may require twenty-four to ninety-six hours (one to four days) to fully recover from exhaustive exercise. Supplemental ribose has the potential to increase the rate of adenosine production and ATP synthesis approximately three- to fourfold, meaning that recovery of ATP stores can be reduced from one to four days to six to twenty-four hours.

Safety

Because ribose is found in all cells of the body, it is generally recognized as a nontoxic substance. The total body stores of ribose amount to approximately 1 to 4 mg per 100 ml of blood. At supplemental doses, as much as 60 g per day have been given with no significant side effects. At such high levels, the possible occurrence of gastrointestinal distress, diarrhea, and hypoglycemia are more likely.

Value

Clearly, anyone concerned with managing diminished blood flow to the heart of muscle tissues would be interested in ribose supplementation. In particular, those who experience chest pain, shortness of breath, or leg pain during exercise may want to consider ribose as a daily dietary supplement. The casual or occasional exerciser is unlikely to benefit from ribose supplements except in the case of several back-to-back days of intense exercise. The weekend warrior will probably have enough time between exercise sessions to fully recover his or her ATP levels, so supplemental ribose is not recommended. Competitive athletes, however, who may be training once or more per day could notice benefits such as increased power output and increased time to exhaustion with regular ribose supplementation (due to enhanced ATP resynthesis following exercise-induced depletion).

Dosage

Doses of as much as 60 g per day have been used in studies of myocardial ischemia. For purposes of maintaining elevated levels of ribose in the blood, smaller doses of 3 to 10 g of ribose may be sufficient. Taking ribose in divided doses before and after exercise is thought to provide the greatest benefits in terms of ATP synthesis and prevention of exercise-induced ischemia. The combination of ribose with other energy-promoting supplements such as creatine, pyruvate, or carnitine may provide additional benefits in terms of promoting exercise performance.

WORKS CONSULTED

De Jong JW, Van der Meer P, Owen P, Opie LH. Prevention and treatment of ischemic injury with nucleosides. Bratisl Lek Listy. 1991 Mar-Apr;92(3-4): 165-73.

Dow JW, Nigdikar S, Bowditch J. Adenine nucleotide synthesis de novo in mature rat cardiac myocytes. Biochim Biophys Acta. 1985 Nov 20;847(2):223-7.

Erickson D. Sugar fix? A simple sugar may help hearts heal. Sci Am. 1990 Dec;263(6):119, 122.

Gatsura VV. Pentosephosphate cycle metabolites as energy-supplying anti-ischemic agents. Farmakol Toksikol. 1991 Jul-Aug;54(4):4-8.

Kalsi KK, Smolenski RT, Pritchard RD, Khaghani A, Seymour AM, Yacoub MH. Effects of dipyridamole and adenine/ribose on ATP concentration and adenosine production in cardiac myocytes. Adv Exp Med Biol. 1998;431:781-4.

Mahoney JR Jr, Sako EY, Seymour KM, Marquardt CA, Foker JE. A comparison of different carbohydrates as substrates for the isolated working heart. J Surg Res. 1989 Dec;47(6):530-4.

Muller C, Zimmer H, Gross M, Gresser U, Brotsack I, Wehling M, Pliml W. Effect of ribose on cardiac adenine nucleotides in a donor model for heart transplantation. Eur J Med Res. 1998 Dec 16;3(12):554-8.

Olivares J, Dubus I, Barrieux A, Samuel JL, Rappaport L, Rossi A. Pyrimidine nucleotide synthesis is preferentially supplied by exogenous cytidine in adult rat cultured cardiomyocytes. J Mol Cell Cardiol. 1992 Nov;24(11):1349-59.

Pasque MK, Wechsler AS. Metabolic intervention to affect myocardial recovery following ischemia. Ann Surg. 1984 Jul;200(1):1-12.

Pliml W, von Arnim T, Stablein A, Hofmann H, Zimmer HG, Erdmann E. Effects of ribose on exercise-induced ischemia in stable coronary artery disease. Lancet. 1992 Aug 29;340(8818):507-10.

Siess M, Delabar U, Seifart HJ. Cardiac synthesis and degradation of pyridine nucleotides and the level of energy-rich phosphates influenced by various precursors. Adv Myocardiol. 1983;4:287-308.

Smolenski RT, Kalsi KK, Zych M, Kochan Z, Yacoub MH. Adenine/ribose supply increases adenosine production and protects ATP pool in adenosine kinase-inhibited cardiac cells. J Mol Cell Cardiol. 1998 Mar;30(3):673-83.

St Cyr JA, Bianco RW, Schneider JR, Mahoney JR Jr, Tveter K, Einzig S, Foker JE. Enhanced high energy phosphate recovery with ribose infusion after global myocardial ischemia in a canine model. J Surg Res. 1989 Feb;46(2):157-62.

Tan ZT. Ruthenium red, ribose, and adenine enhance recovery of reperfused rat heart. Coron Artery Dis. 1993 Mar;4(3):305-9.

Tan ZT, Bhayana JN, Bergsland J, Wang XW, Hoover EL. Concanavalin A, ribose, and adenine resuscitate preserved rat hearts. J Cardiovasc Pharmacol. 1997 Jul;30(1):26-32.

Tan ZT, Wang XW. Verapamil, ribose and adenine enhance resynthesis of postischemic myocardial ATP. Life Sci. 1994;55(18):PL345-9.

Wagner DR, Gresser U, Zollner N. Effects of oral ribose on muscle metabolism during bicycle ergometer in AMPD-deficient patients. Ann Nutr Metab. 1991; 35(5):297-302.

Ward HB, Wang T, Einzig S, Bianco RW, Foker JE. Prevention of ATP catabolism during myocardial ischemia: A preliminary report. J Surg Res. 1983 Apr;34(4):292-7.

Zharova TV, Vinogradov AD. A competitive inhibition of the mitochondrial NADH-ubiquinone oxidoreductase (complex I) by ADP-ribose. Biochim Biophys Acta. 1997 Jul 4;1320(3):256-64.

Zimmer HG, Ibel H. Ribose accelerates the repletion of the ATP pool during recovery from reversible ischemia of the rat myocardium. J Mol Cell Cardiol. 1984 Sep;16(9):863-6.

AMINO ACIDS

Amino acids are the basic building blocks of protein and can be obtained in an almost endless variety of supplemental forms including capsules, tablets, bars, and powdered mixtures. Products are available that provide a foodlike mixture of all twenty nutritionally important amino acids, while other products focus on the specific characteristics of isolated amino acids.

Amino acids are typically categorized based on their nutritional role as essential or nonessential (see Table 5.2). The body cannot produce essential amino acids, so they must be obtained from a dietary source. Nonessential amino acids can either be manufactured directly by the body or can be obtained by conversion from another amino acid. It is important to keep in mind that "nonessential" does not mean that these amino acids are unimportant. It simply means that, under ideal circumstances, there are routes other than the diet by which they can be obtained. Several of the nonessential amino acids are considered to be "conditionally essential"—meaning

TABLE 5.2. Essential and Nonessential Amino Acids

Essential amino acids	Nonessential amino acids
Isoleucine	Arginine
Leucine	Alanine
Lysine	Asparagine
Methionine	Aspartic acid
Phenylalanine	Cysteine
Threonine	Glutamine
Tryptophan	Glutamic acid
Valine	Glycine
Histidine (conditionally essential)	Proline
	Serine
	Tyrosine

Note: There are many other amino acids, but some can be produced in the body by combining or processing other amino acids from the diet (example: lysine and methionine are combined to produce carnitine).

that under certain conditions, such as injury, disease, increased stress, or intense physical activity, the body's machinery is unable to generate adequate levels, and supplemental dietary sources are required.

The recommended dietary allowance for protein is 0.8 g per kilogram of lean body mass per day for a healthy adult. There is widespread controversy concerning the question of whether athletes should consume more protein than the average individual. There is good scientific support for the concept that a greater availability of amino acids promotes protein synthesis and reduces muscle loss that occurs during training. It is fairly well accepted now that athletes probably need closer to 1.0 to 1.8 g of protein per kilogram of body weight per day, particularly during strenuous training.

In most cases, amino acids and total protein intake are considered to be synonymous. In some cases, however, a specific amino acid may have unique characteristics that may lend beneficial effects in treating certain metabolic states. Some are as follows:

- Alanine—enlarged prostate
- Arginine—heart function, growth hormone stimulation
- Branched chain amino acids (valine, leucine, isoleucine)—sports performance
- Carnitine—heart support, sports performance, chronic fatigue, diabetes
- Creatine—sports performance
- Cysteine and N-acetylcysteine (NAC)—lung function (bronchitis), antioxidant support
- Glutamic acid—enlarged prostate
- Glutamine—immune support, gastrointestinal maintenance
- Glycine—enlarged prostate
- Ornithine and ornithine alpha-ketoglutarate (OKG)—sports performance, wound healing
- Phenylalanine—depression
- Taurine—diabetes, epilepsy, high blood pressure
- Tyrosine—alcohol withdrawal, Alzheimer's disease, depression, increased alertness

WORKS CONSULTED

Antonio J, Street C. Glutamine: A potentially useful supplement for athletes. Can J Appl Physiol. 1999 Feb;24(1):1-14.

Barnett DW, Conlee RK. The effects of a commercial dietary supplement on human performance. Am J Clin Nutr. 1984 Sep;40(3):586-90.

Buchman AL, O'Brien W, Ou CN, Rognerud C, Alvarez M, Dennis K, Ahn C. The effect of arginine or glycine supplementation on gastrointestinal function, muscle injury, serum amino acid concentrations and performance during a marathon run. Int J Sports Med. 1999 Jul;20(5):315-21.

Davis JM, Welsh RS, De Volve KL, Alderson NA. Effects of branched-chain amino acids and carbohydrate on fatigue during intermittent, high-intensity running. Int J Sports Med. 1999 Jul;20(5):309-14.

di Luigi L, Guidetti L, Pigozzi F, Baldari C, Casini A, Nordio M, Romanelli F. Acute amino acids supplementation enhances pituitary responsiveness in athletes. Med Sci Sports Exerc. 1999 Dec;31(12):1748-54.

Dohm GL. Protein nutrition for the athlete. Clin Sports Med. 1984 Jul;3(3):595-604.

Elam RP, Hardin DH, Sutton RA, Hagen L. Effects of arginine and ornithine on strength, lean body mass and urinary hydroxyproline in adult males. J Sports Med Phys Fitness. 1989 Mar;29(1):52-6.

Kingsbury KJ, Kay L, Hjelm M. Contrasting plasma free amino acid patterns in elite athletes: Association with fatigue and infection. Br J Sports Med. 1998 Mar;32(1):25-32; discussion 32-3.

Kreider RB. Dietary supplements and the promotion of muscle growth with resistance exercise. Sports Med. 1999 Feb;27(2):97-110.

Lambert MI, Hefer JA, Millar RP, Macfarlane PW. Failure of commercial oral amino acid supplements to increase serum growth hormone concentrations in male body-builders. Int J Sport Nutr. 1993 Sep;3(3):298-305.

Mero A. Leucine supplementation and intensive training. Sports Med. 1999 Jun;27(6):347-58.

van Hall G, Saris WH, Wagenmakers AJ. Effect of carbohydrate supplementation on plasma glutamine during prolonged exercise and recovery. Int J Sports Med. 1998 Feb;19(2):82-6.

Wagenmakers AJ. Amino acid supplements to improve athletic performance. Curr Opin Clin Nutr Metab Care. 1999 Nov;2(6):539-44.

Williams MH. Facts and fallacies of purported ergogenic amino acid supplements. Clin Sports Med. 1999 Jul;18(3):633-49.

Yaspelkis BB 3rd, Ivy JL. The effect of a carbohydrate—arginine supplement on postexercise carbohydrate metabolism. Int J Sport Nutr. 1999 Sep;9(3):241-50.

BRANCHED-CHAIN AMINO ACIDS (BCAAS)

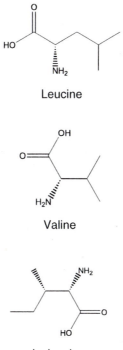

Leucine

Valine

Isoleucine

What Is It?

Branched-chain amino acids (BCAAs) are three essential amino acids: leucine, valine, and isoleucine. The recommended dietary allowance for BCAAs is about 3 g per day—an amount that should be easily obtained from protein foods. Supplements have been used at levels around 5 to 20 g per day.

Claims

- Increases endurance
- Prevents fatigue
- Improves mental performance
- Increases energy levels

Theory

The idea behind BCAA supplements relates to a phenomenon known as central fatigue, which holds that mental fatigue in the brain can adversely affect physical performance in endurance events. The central fatigue theory suggests that low blood levels of BCAA may accelerate the production of serotonin, a key neurotransmitter in the brain, and prematurely lead to fatigue. Tryptophan, an amino acid that circulates in the blood, is a precursor of serotonin, and can be more easily transported into the brain to increase serotonin levels when BCAA levels in the blood are low (because high blood levels of BCAA can block tryptophan transport into the brain). During exercise, as muscle and liver glycogen are depleted for energy, blood levels of BCAA may also decrease and fatty acid levels increase to serve as an additional energy source. The problem with extra fatty acids in the blood is that they need to attach to a carrier protein called albumin for proper transport. In doing so, the fatty acids displace tryptophan from its place on albumin and facilitate the transport of tryptophan into the brain for conversion into serotonin. Therefore, due to the combination of reduced BCAA and elevated fatty acids in the blood, more tryptophan enters the brain and more serotonin is produced, leading to central fatigue. Supplementing the diet with additional levels of BCAA is thought to block the tryptophan transport and, therefore, delay fatigue.

Scientific Support

Although the general theory of central fatigue and BCAA supplementation is sound, the research findings have not all been positive. In general, however, acute BCAA supplementation (immediately prior to or during exercise) has been shown to increase mental performance, improve cycling endurance, and reduce the time to complete a marathon. Chronic BCAA supplementation (two weeks) has also been shown effective in improving time-trial performance in trained cyclists. However, a number of studies in trained and untrained subjects have shown no effect of BCAA supplements on exercise performance or mental performance. In some cases, BCAAs have been compared to carbohydrate supplementation during exercise with similar results (both delay fatigue to similar degrees).

Safety

Supplemental intakes of BCAAs have been studied in the range of 3 to 20 g per day in tablet and liquid form with no adverse side effects. Higher intakes should be avoided due to the possibility of competitive inhibition of the absorption of other amino acids from the diet and the risk of gastrointestinal distress.

Value

For endurance athletes, particularly those competing in longer races (two-plus hours) such as marathons, triathlons, road cycling, backpacking, and orienteering, BCAA supplements may be warranted to help delay central fatigue. Participation in shorter duration events is unlikely to result in substantial changes in blood levels of BCAA, tryptophan, or fatty acids, so BCAA supplementation is probably not needed.

Dosage

Three to 20 g per day, taken before or during exercise to delay fatigue or immediately following exercise as an aid to recovery.

WORKS CONSULTED

Blomstrand E, Celsing F, Newsholme EA. Changes in plasma concentrations of aromatic and branched-chain amino acids during sustained exercise in man and their possible role in fatigue. Acta Physiol Scand. 1988 May;133(1):115-21.

Blomstrand E, Hassmen P, Ek S, Ekblom B, Newsholme EA. Influence of ingesting a solution of branched-chain amino acids on perceived exertion during exercise. Acta Physiol Scand. 1997 Jan;159(1):41-9.

Blomstrand E, Hassmen P, Ekblom B, Newsholme EA. Administration of branched-chain amino acids during sustained exercise—effects on performance and on plasma concentration of some amino acids. Eur J Appl Physiol Occup Physiol. 1991;63(2):83-8.

Castell LM, Yamamoto T, Phoenix J, Newsholme EA. The role of tryptophan in fatigue in different conditions of stress. Adv Exp Med Biol. 1999;467:697-704.

Davis JM. Carbohydrates, branched-chain amino acids, and endurance: The central fatigue hypothesis. Int J Sport Nutr. 1995 Jun;5 Suppl:S29-38.

Davis JM. Central and peripheral factors in fatigue. J Sports Sci. 1995 Summer;13 (Spec No):S49-53.

Davis JM, Alderson NL, Welsh RS. Serotonin and central nervous system fatigue: Nutritional considerations. Am J Clin Nutr. 2000 Aug;72(2 Suppl):573S-8S.

Davis JM, Bailey SP, Woods JA, Galiano FJ, Hamilton MT, Bartoli WP. Effects of carbohydrate feedings on plasma free tryptophan and branched-chain amino acids during prolonged cycling. Eur J Appl Physiol Occup Physiol. 1992;65(6):513-9.

Davis JM, Welsh RS, De Volve KL, Alderson NA. Effects of branched-chain amino acids and carbohydrate on fatigue during intermittent, high-intensity running. Int J Sports Med. 1999 Jul;20(5):309-14.

Gastmann UA, Lehmann MJ. Overtraining and the BCAA hypothesis. Med Sci Sports Exerc. 1998 Jul;30(7):1173-8.

Hassmen P, Blomstrand E, Ekblom B, Newsholme EA. Branched-chain amino acid supplementation during 30-km competitive run: Mood and cognitive performance. Nutrition. 1994 Sep-Oct;10(5):405-10.

Lehmann M, Huonker M, Dimeo F, Heinz N, Gastmann U, Treis N, Steinacker JM, Keul J, Kajewski R, Haussinger D. Serum amino acid concentrations in nine athletes before and after the 1993 Colmar ultra triathlon. Int J Sports Med. 1995 Apr;16(3):155-9.

Lehmann M, Mann H, Gastmann U, Keul J, Vetter D, Steinacker JM, Haussinger D. Unaccustomed high-mileage vs intensity training-related changes in performance and serum amino acid levels. Int J Sports Med. 1996 Apr;17(3):187-92.

Manner T, Wiese S, Katz DP, Skeie B, Askanazi J. Branched-chain amino acids and respiration. Nutrition. 1992 Sep-Oct;8(5):311-5.

Meeusen R, De Meirleir K. Exercise and brain neurotransmission. Sports Med. 1995 Sep;20(3):160-88.

Mittleman KD, Ricci MR, Bailey SP. Branched-chain amino acids prolong exercise during heat stress in men and women. Med Sci Sports Exerc. 1998 Jan;30(1):83-91.

Newsholme EA, Blomstrand E. Tryptophan, 5-hydroxytryptamine and a possible explanation for central fatigue. Adv Exp Med Biol. 1995;384:315-20.

Struder HK, Hollmann W, Platen P, Donike M, Gotzmann A, Weber K. Influence of paroxetine, branched-chain amino acids and tyrosine on neuroendocrine system responses and fatigue in humans. Horm Metab Res. 1998 Apr;30(4):188-94.

Tanaka H, West KA, Duncan GE, Bassett DR Jr. Changes in plasma tryptophan/branched chain amino acid ratio in responses to training volume variation. Int J Sports Med. 1997 May;18(4):270-5.

van Hall G, Raaymakers JS, Saris WH, Wagenmakers AJ. Ingestion of branched-chain amino acids and tryptophan during sustained exercise in man: Failure to affect performance. J Physiol. 1995 Aug 1;486(Pt 3):789-94.

Verger P, Aymard P, Cynobert L, Anton G, Luigi R. Effects of administration of branched-chain amino acids vs. glucose during acute exercise in the rat. Physiol Behav. 1994 Mar;55(3):523-6.

Wagenmakers AJ. Muscle amino acid metabolism at rest and during exercise: Role in human physiology and metabolism. Exerc Sport Sci Rev. 1998;26:287-314.

Williams C. Fatigue during prolonged exercise. Nutrition. 1996 Jul-Aug;12(7-8):553-4.

Williams MH. Facts and fallacies of purported ergogenic amino acid supplements. Clin Sports Med. 1999 Jul;18(3):633-49.

Yamamoto T, Castell LM, Botella J, Powell H, Hall GM, Young A, Newsholme EA. Changes in the albumin binding of tryptophan during postoperative recovery: A possible link with central fatigue? Brain Res Bull. 1997;43(1):43-6.

Yamamoto T, Newsholme EA. Diminished central fatigue by inhibition of the L-system transporter for the uptake of tryptophan. Brain Res Bull. 2000 May 1;52(1):35-8.

ANDROSTENEDIONE

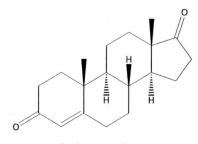

Androstenedione

What Is It?

Androstenedione is a prehormone, meaning that it is an inactive precursor of another hormone—in this case, a precursor of both female (estrogen) and male (testosterone) hormones.

Claims

- Increases testosterone levels
- Boosts libido (sex drive)
- Increases muscle mass and strength

Theory

In the body, androstenedione becomes active upon conversion to testosterone—the major male hormone responsible for muscle growth and other male characteristics such as growth of facial hair and development of a deep voice. Higher levels of testosterone are thought to help athletes exercise more intensely and recover faster. Use of androstenedione is banned in some sports, but not others. It is widely assumed that it may be consumed by some athletes to mask the fact that they are also taking anabolic steroids such as testosterone.

Scientific Support

Supplement makers claim that a 100 mg dose of androstenedione increases testosterone levels by 300 percent over a duration of two to four hours. Unfortunately, not much credible research supports this claim. In fact, the most recent studies suggest that androstenedione not only fails to increase testosterone levels in healthy young men, but appears to elevate estrogen levels—exactly the opposite effect that these weight lifters are looking for. In one study, an open-label randomized design was used to investigate the effect of androstenedione supplements in forty-two healthy men (twenty to forty years old). Subjects received either 100 mg per day (fifteen subjects) or 300 mg per day (fourteen subjects) of androstenedione, while thirteen subjects were used as controls (receiving no androstenedione) for seven days. Results showed that levels of testosterone in the blood were significantly higher (compared to the control group) in subjects consuming the 300 mg, but not the 100 mg dose of androstenedione. Interestingly, blood levels of estradiol (estrogen) were also significantly elevated in these young men by both the 100 mg and 300 mg doses of androstenedione.

In a similar study, twenty young men (ages nineteen to twenty-nine years) performed eight weeks of whole-body resistance training and consumed either 300 mg per day of androstenedione or a placebo. In another portion of the study, ten young men received a single 100 mg dose of androstenedione to determine the effects on serum testosterone and estrogen concentrations. Results showed that blood levels of testosterone were not affected by short- or long-term androstenedione consumption, but blood levels of estradiol were increased by more than 50 percent compared with presupplementation values. Following eight weeks of androstenedione consumption there were no differences between the placebo and androstenedione groups in terms of muscle strength, lean body mass, or fat mass. In the androstenedione group, however, blood levels of high-density lipoprotein (HDL) cholesterol (the "good" kind) was reduced after two weeks and remained low after five and eight weeks of training and supplementation. The overall conclusions of the study were that androstenedione supplementation does not increase serum testosterone concentrations or enhance muscle strength (in young men with normal testosterone levels)—but that it may result in adverse health consequences (increased estrogen levels and reduced HDL).

Safety

Although no long-term studies have been conducted on the safety of androstenedione as a dietary supplement, there is a fairly substantial body of literature concerning the adverse effects associated with other anabolic steroids such as testosterone. In particular, prolonged use of steroids can result in a number of dangerous side effects, such as blood lipid abnormalities (elevated LDL and reduced HDL cholesterol) that may increase the risk of heart disease, promotion of hormone-sensitive cancers such as breast and prostate cancer, and various liver abnormalities.

The psychological effects of anabolic steroid use are well known and include increased aggression ('roid rage), depression, and psychosis. From an appearance standpoint, steroid use will almost certainly result in increased muscle mass—provided that the right exercise program is being followed. On the down side, however are other cosmetic changes such as acne, premature hair loss (baldness) or excessive hair growth (in places that you don't want it), reduced testicle size, and breast growth in men. In teenagers, steroid use could fool the body into shutting off its normal hormone production and causing stunted growth.

Despite the clear evidence of the negative effects of anabolic steroid use in general, many androstenedione manufacturers claim that since no safety studies have been conducted specifically on it, we should not assume that it has the same adverse effects as excessive testosterone levels. The findings of adverse alterations in blood lipid profile, however, should be reason enough for intelligent consumers to avoid dietary supplements containing androstenedione unless specifically recommended by a nutritionally oriented physician.

Value

Due to the lack of positive research findings and the potential for serious health risks from anabolic steroids and altered hormone profiles, androstenedione supplements should be considered to be of low value for healthy individuals.

Dosage

Typical dosage recommendations are in the range of 50 to 200 mg. Competitive athletes should be aware of the potential for androstenedione supplementation to alter the testosterone-epitestosterone ratio so it exceeds the 6:1 limit set by both the International Olympic Committee and the NCAA in their screening for testosterone doping.

WORKS CONSULTED

King DS, Sharp RL, Vukovich MD, Brown GA, Reifenrath TA, Uhl NL, Parsons KA. Effect of oral androstenedione on serum testosterone and adaptations to resistance training in young men: A randomized controlled trial. JAMA. 1999 Jun 2;281(21):2020-8.

Leder BZ, Longcope C, Catlin DH, Ahrens B, Schoenfeld DA, Finkelstein JS. Oral androstenedione administration and serum testosterone concentrations in young men. JAMA. 2000 Feb 9;283(6):779-82.

DEHYDROEPIANDROSTERONE (DHEA)

What Is It?

DHEA is an androgenic hormone produced in the adrenal glands. In the body, DHEA is converted into other hormones such as testosterone, estrogen, progesterone, or cortisol. Some natural products include wild yams as a source of DHEA. A metabolic precursor to DHEA, DHEA-S (dehydroepiandrosterone-3-sulfate) can be converted to DHEA and vice versa. DHEA levels are known to decrease with age—particularly after the age of forty, but perhaps as early as ages twenty to thirty.

Claims

- Slows aging
- Improves memory
- Stimulates libido/increases sex drive
- Alleviates depression
- Boosts energy
- Promotes weight loss
- Builds muscle mass/increases strength

Theory

Because DHEA levels decline with age (up to 90 percent reduction) and function as a direct precursor to testosterone and estrogen, it is often promoted as a "fountain of youth" supplement. The theory is that by boosting blood DHEA levels, sex hormone levels can be elevated, and some of the conditions associated with aging can be alleviated. Such conditions as muscle wasting, bone loss, loss of strength and endurance, and reduced sex drive may be potential targets for DHEA supplementation.

Scientific Support

DHEA supplements, at 50 to 100 mg per day, have been shown to increase muscle mass and improve overall feelings of well-being among a group of forty- to seventy-year-old subjects who took the supplements for six months. Another small study (nine elderly men) showed a link between five months of DHEA supplementation (50 mg per day) and improvements in markers of immune system function (lymphocytes, natural killer cells, and immunoglobulins). Several studies have shown increased serum testosterone levels following regular DHEA supplementation (50 to 100 mg per day), and anorexic young women may be able to slow bone loss with DHEA supplements.

Safety

The FDA banned the sale of DHEA as a therapeutic drug in 1996 until its safety and value could be reviewed. DHEA products on the market as dietary supplements are regulated under DSHEA. Although it is difficult to show clear side effects from DHEA supplements, several publications have raised concerns regarding altered hormone profiles, liver abnormalities, increased cancer risk (prostate in men and breast in women), and other steroid-like effects (increased facial hair, acne, mood swings). Since DHEA is converted into testosterone, there have been concerns that chronic use in men might worsen prostate hyperplasia or even promote prostate cancer.

Of the potential adverse effects associated with high-dose DHEA supplements, virilization in women may result from increased testosterone levels, while gynecomastia may result in men from an elevation in estrogen levels. Because of these potential adverse effects, DHEA dosages should be limited to between 25 and 100 mg daily. If you take DHEA, you should inform your physician. It is important to note that although such concerns are certainly possible and logical, they are only suspected risks—which may not apply for all individuals who may derive benefits from DHEA supplements.

Value

DHEA supplements tend to be relatively inexpensive and widely available from a number of manufacturers. A recent publication, however, analyzed several DHEA products on the market and found a dramatic difference between the amount of DHEA stated on the supplement label and the amount actually present in the product. The range of actual DHEA present was zero to over 150 percent—and only seven of the sixteen products (44 percent) analyzed were found to have a DHEA content within 90 to 110 percent of the labeled claim. Of the remaining products, no DHEA was detected in one product, and trace amounts were detected in two other products. The latter two were labeled as containing naturally occurring DHEA, with no specific amount indicated on the label. This finding underscores the importance of choosing your supplements from a reputable manufacturer that you can trust to perform adequate quality control and ingredient analysis.

Dosage

Effective doses have ranged from 50 to 100 mg per day, depending on the condition under investigation. Based on the current positive findings with 50 mg dosages and the adverse effects that may be associated with excessive DHEA supplementation, a daily dose of 50 mg per day seems reasonable. Competitive athletes should be aware of the potential for DHEA supplementation to alter the testosterone-epitestosterone ratio to exceed the 6:1 limit set by both the International Olympic Committee and the NCAA in their screening for testosterone doping.

WORKS CONSULTED

Blue JG, Lombardo JA. Steroids and steroid-like compounds. Clin Sports Med. 1999 Jul;18(3):667-89.

Bosy TZ, Moore KA, Poklis A. The effect of oral dehydroepiandrosterone (DHEA) on the urine testosterone/epitestosterone (T/E) ratio in human male volunteers. J Anal Toxicol. 1998 Oct;22(6):455-9.

Brown GA, Vukovich MD, Sharp RL, Reifenrath TA, Parsons KA, King DS. Effect of oral DHEA on serum testosterone and adaptations to resistance training in young men. J Appl Physiol. 1999 Dec;87(6):2274-83.

Corrigan AB. Dehydroepiandrosterone and sport. Med J Aust. 1999 Aug 16; 171(4):206-8.

De Cree C. Androstenedione and dehydroepiandrosterone for athletes. Lancet. 1999 Aug 28;354(9180):779-80.

Dehennin L, Ferry M, Lafarge P, Peres G, Lafarge JP. Oral administration of dehydroepiandrosterone to healthy men: Alteration of the urinary androgen profile and consequences for the detection of abuse in sport by gas chromatography-mass spectrometry. Steroids. 1998 Feb;63(2):80-7.

Filaire E, Duche P, Lac G. Effects of amount of training on the saliva concentrations of cortisol, dehydroepiandrosterone and on the dehydroepiandrosterone: Cortisol concentration ratio in women over 16 weeks of training. Eur J Appl Physiol Occup Physiol. 1998 Oct;78(5):466-71.

Filaire E, Duche P, Lac G. Effects of training for two ball games on the saliva response of adrenocortical hormones to exercise in elite sportswomen. Eur J Appl Physiol Occup Physiol. 1998 Apr;77(5):452-6.

Filaire E, Lac G. Dehydroepiandrosterone (DHEA) rather than testosterone shows saliva androgen responses to exercise in elite female handball players. Int J Sports Med. 2000 Jan;21(1):17-20.

Filaire E, Le Scanff C, Duche P, Lac G. The relationship between salivary adrenocortical hormones changes and personality in elite female athletes during handball and volleyball competition. Res Q Exerc Sport. 1999 Sep;70(3):297-302.

Flynn MG, Pizza FX, Brolinson PG. Hormonal responses to excessive training: Influence of cross training. Int J Sports Med. 1997 Apr;18(3):191-6.

Hakkinen K, Pakarinen A, Kraemer WJ, Newton RU, Alen M. Basal concentrations and acute responses of serum hormones and strength development during heavy resistance training in middle-aged and elderly men and women. J Gerontol A Biol Sci Med Sci. 2000 Feb;55(2):B95-105.

Keizer H, Janssen GM, Menheere P, Kranenburg G. Changes in basal plasma testosterone, cortisol, and dehydroepiandrosterone sulfate in previously untrained males and females preparing for a marathon. Int J Sports Med. 1989 Oct;10 (Suppl 3):S139-45.

Kiraly CL. Androgenic-anabolic steroid effects on serum and skin surface lipids, on red cells, and on liver enzymes. Int J Sports Med. 1988 Aug;9(4):249-52.

Kreider RB. Dietary supplements and the promotion of muscle growth with resistance exercise. Sports Med. 1999 Feb;27(2):97-110.

Malarkey WB, Strauss RH, Leizman DJ, Liggett M, Demers LM. Endocrine effects in female weight lifters who self-administer testosterone and anabolic steroids. Am J Obstet Gynecol. 1991 Nov;165(5 Pt 1):1385-90.

Nair KS. Age-related changes in muscle. Mayo Clin Proc. 2000 Jan;75 Suppl:S14-8.

Ponjee GA, De Rooy HA, Vader HL. Androgen turnover during marathon running. Med Sci Sports Exerc. 1994 Oct;26(10):1274-7.

Ronkainen HR, Pakarinen AJ, Kauppila AJ. Adrenocortical function of female endurance runners and joggers. Med Sci Sports Exerc. 1986 Aug;18(4):385-9.

Ruokonen A, Alen M, Bolton N, Vihko R. Response of serum testosterone and its precursor steroids, SHBG and CBG to anabolic steroid and testosterone self-administration in man. J Steroid Biochem. 1985 Jul;23(1):33-8.

Shackleton CH, Roitman E, Phillips A, Chang T. Androstenediol and 5-androstenediol profiling for detecting exogenously administered dihydrotestosterone, epitestosterone, and dehydroepiandrosterone: Potential use in gas chromatography isotope ratio mass spectrometry. Steroids. 1997 Oct;62(10):665-73.

Sturmi JE, Diorio DJ. Anabolic agents. Clin Sports Med. 1998 Apr;17(2):261-82.

Tanaka H, Cleroux J, de Champlain J, Ducharme JR, Collu R. Persistent effects of a marathon run on the pituitary-testicular axis. J Endocrinol Invest. 1986 Apr;9(2):97-101.

Tegelman R, Aberg T, Pousette A, Carlstrom K. Effects of a diet regimen on pituitary and steroid hormones in male ice hockey players. Int J Sports Med. 1992 Jul;13(5):424-30.

Ueki M, Okano M. Analysis of exogenous dehydroepiandrosterone excretion in urine by gas chromatography/combustion/isotope ratio mass spectrometry. Rapid Commun Mass Spectrom. 1999;13(22):2237-43.

BETA-HYDROXY BETA-METHYLBUTYRATE (HMB)

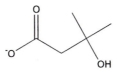

beta-hydroxy beta-methylbutyrate

What Is It?

HMB (beta-hydroxy beta-methylbutyrate) is a metabolite of the amino acid leucine. HMB is found in the diet in small amounts in some protein-rich foods such as fish and milk. Depending on total protein and leucine intake, HMB production in the body may average about .25 to 1 g per day.

Claims

- Increases protein synthesis/builds muscle
- Decreases muscle breakdown/prevents muscle catabolism
- Enhances fat burning

Theory

HMB is thought to be the active form of leucine—an amino acid that plays a role in regulating protein metabolism. In theory, if you supply HMB as a supplement, you may be able to reduce muscle breakdown during intense exercise.

Scientific Support

There is some evidence that HMB reduces muscle catabolism and may protect against muscle damage. For example, creatine kinase, an indicator of muscle damage, is reduced following exercise in subjects consuming HMB. This may indicate a reduced level of muscle damage and could lead to improved muscle function. Research in animals (cattle, pigs, and poultry) and humans suggests that HMB can increase muscle mass and strength. Leucine is also a common additive to chicken feed (which is normally low in this amino acid) for the purpose of improving the muscle tissue and providing bigger chicken breasts for dinner.

HMB has also been tested by NASA as a dietary approach to preventing the muscle wasting associated with prolonged spaceflight. Supplementation with 1.5 to 3.0 g of HMB daily during weight training for three weeks increased muscle mass and strength and decreased the rise in exercise-induced muscle damage. In one study, untrained subjects lifted weights for four weeks with or without 1.5 to 3 g of HMB per day. The HMB supplements resulted in significant improvements in muscle mass and strength as well as significant decreases in muscle breakdown compared with placebo subjects. Even in trained athletes, HMB supplements of about 3 g per day resulted in a significant increase in muscle mass and strength as well as a decrease in body fat.

One study looked at the effects of HMB supplements (as a calcium salt) on muscle breakdown (catabolism), muscle strength, and body composition during a resistance training program (seven hours per week for four weeks). Subjects were forty experienced weight lifters who received either 3 or 6 g per day of calcium HMB (or a placebo). Results showed that HMB supplementation resulted in a significant increase in blood levels of HMB, but no significant difference in muscle anabolic/catabolic status, lean body or fat mass, or overall muscle strength. Another study looked at HMB supplements (versus placebo) in thirty-nine men and thirty-six women (aged twenty to forty years). Subjects received 3 g of HMB per day while training three times per week for four weeks. In the HMB group, blood levels of creatine phosphokinase (an indicator of muscle damage) were reduced compared to the placebo group, and both upper body strength and fat-free mass were increased. Overall, the study showed that a short-term period of HMB supplementation can increase upper body strength and minimize muscle damage when combined with an exercise program in both men and women.

Safety

No side effects have been reported in animal studies (which have used large doses of HMB for several weeks) or in human studies of as much as 6 g per day.

Value

Athletes trying to minimize protein loss and muscle breakdown may want to consider HMB—particularly during very high intensity periods of training.

Dosage

Recommended dose depends on training intensity—from 1 g per day on rest days and easy days to about 3 g on heavy training days.

WORKS CONSULTED

Clark RH, Feleke G, Din M, Yasmin T, Singh G, Khan FA, Rathmacher JA. Nutritional treatment for acquired immunodeficiency virus-associated wasting using beta-hydroxy beta-methylbutyrate, glutamine, and arginine: A randomized, double-blind, placebo-controlled study. J Parenter Enteral Nutr. 2000 May-Jun; 24(3):133-9.

Clarkson PM, Rawson ES. Nutritional supplements to increase muscle mass. Crit Rev Food Sci Nutr. 1999 Jul;39(4):317-28.

Kreider RB. Dietary supplements and the promotion of muscle growth with resistance exercise. Sports Med. 1999 Feb;27(2):97-110.

Kreider RB, Ferreira M, Wilson M, Almada AL. Effects of calcium beta-hydroxy-beta-methylbutyrate (HMB) supplementation during resistance-training on markers of catabolism, body composition and strength. Int J Sports Med. 1999 Nov;20(8):503-9.

Mero A. Leucine supplementation and intensive training. Sports Med. 1999 Jun;27(6):347-58.

Nissen S, Sharp RL, Panton L, Vukovich M, Trappe S, Fuller JC Jr. Beta-hydroxy beta-methylbutyrate (HMB) supplementation in humans is safe and may decrease cardiovascular risk factors. J Nutr. 2000 Aug;130(8):1937-45.

Nissen S, Sharp R, Ray M, Rathmacher JA, Rice D, Fuller JC Jr, Connelly AS, Abumrad N. Effect of leucine metabolite beta-hydroxy-beta-methylbutyrate on muscle metabolism during resistance-exercise training. J Appl Physiol. 1996 Nov;81(5):2095-104.

Panton LB, Rathmacher JA, Baier S, Nissen S. Nutritional supplementation of the leucine metabolite beta-hydroxy-beta-methylbutyrate (hmb) during resistance training. Nutrition. 2000 Sep;16(9):734-9.

Papet I, Ostaszewski P, Glomot F, Obled C, Faure M, Bayle G, Nissen S, Arnal M, Grizard J. The effect of a high dose of beta-hydroxy beta-methylbutyrate on protein metabolism in growing lambs. Br J Nutr. 1997 Jun;77(6):885-96.

Slater GJ, Jenkins D. Beta-hydroxy-beta-methylbutyrate (HMB) supplementation and the promotion of muscle growth and strength. Sports Med. 2000 Aug;30(2):105-16.

TRIBULUS TERRESTRIS *(PUNCTURE VINE)*

What Is It?

Tribulus terrestris (puncture vine) is a vine that has been used as a general tonic (energy) and herbal treatment for impotence, but is found primarily in dietary supplements marketed for increasing testosterone levels in bodybuilders and power athletes.

Claims

- Increases testosterone production
- Increases muscle mass/strength

Theory

The idea behind tribulus is that it may increase testosterone levels indirectly by raising blood levels of another hormone, luteinizing hormone (LH). LH is a hormone produced by the pituitary gland that plays a role in regulating natural testosterone production and serum levels.

Scientific Support

The active ingredient in tribulus is unknown, but is thought to be a component known as furostanol saponins. Very little research has been conducted on the effectiveness of tribulus in elevating testosterone levels—the main claim made by bodybuilding products that contain the herb. In some cultures, the *Tribulus terrestris* plant has been used as a tonic to increase energy levels and treat sexual dysfunction (usually in males). In animals, tribulus may stimulate mounting behavior. Some European studies suggest that tribulus extract can increase testosterone levels 30 to 50 percent above baseline levels—which is still well within the normal range. Unfortunately, however, these same studies also suggest a similar increase in estradiol levels—not exactly what hard-core muscle builders should be interested in boosting.

If tribulus extract does indeed elevate testosterone levels somewhat, but keeps them within normal ranges, it may be an effective supplement for individuals with reduced testosterone levels, such as athletes at risk for overtraining syndrome, and individuals on a prolonged low-calorie diet. It will not, however, cause you to start sprouting muscles from all parts of your body, as many bodybuilding magazines would have you believe.

One of the few well-controlled studies to examine the effects of *Tribulus terrestris* on body composition and exercise performance looked at fifteen resistance-trained males. Subjects received either a placebo or a large dose of tribulus (1.5 mg per pound of body weight per day for two months). Results showed no changes in body weight, percentage of fat, total muscle mass, or muscle strength related to tribulus supplementation.

Safety

Although no significant side effects should be expected at doses of tribulus contained in commercial dietary supplements, animal studies have suggested the possibility of locomotor (muscle coordination) disturbances following ingestion of tribulus in large quantities. Sheep consuming tribulus for several months showed a neurological disease characterized by an irreversible, asymmetrical weakness of the hind limbs.

Value

Products containing tribulus are typically marketed to bodybuilders and athletes concerned with increasing muscle mass and strength. Although such products are typically combinations of ingredients that include tribulus, rather than tribulus alone, the scientific evidence for product effectiveness is typically lacking. At this time, tribulus extract (on its own) should not be viewed as a valuable dietary supplement for muscle building. As a support ingredient contained in a wider supplement blend, tribulus may provide some benefits to those individuals interested in maintaining testosterone levels in the normal range (overtrained athletes and dieters).

Dosage

A typical dosage of 250 to 1,500 mg of tribulus per day is fairly common, with extracts typically standardized for at least 30 to 45 percent steroidal saponins (furostanol).

WORKS CONSULTED

Antonio J, Uelmen J, Rodriguez R, Earnest C. The effects of Tribulus terrestris on body composition and exercise performance in resistance-trained males. Int J Sport Nutr Exerc Metab. 2000 Jun;10(2):208-15.

Arcasoy HB, Erenmemisoglu A, Tekol Y, Kurucu S, Kartal M. Effect of Tribulus terrestris L. saponin mixture on some smooth muscle preparations: A preliminary study. Boll Chim Farm. 1998 Dec;137(11):473-5.

Bourke CA. Hepatopathy in sheep associated with Tribulus terrestris. Aust Vet J. 1983 Jun;60(6):189.

Bourke CA. Staggers in sheep associated with the ingestion of Tribulus terrestris. Aust Vet J. 1984 Nov;61(11):360-3.

Duhan A, Chauhan BM, Punia D. Nutritional value of some non-conventional plant foods of India. Plant Foods Hum Nutr. 1992 Jul;42(3):193-200.

Wu G, Jiang S, Jiang F, Zhu D, Wu H, Jiang S. Steroidal glycosides from Tribulus terrestris. Phytochemistry. 1996 Aug;42(6):1677-81.

Xu YX, Chen HS, Liang HQ, Gu ZB, Liu WY, Leung WN, Li TJ. Three new saponins from Tribulus terrestris. Planta Med. 2000 Aug;66(6):545-50.

Yan W, Ohtani K, Kasai R, Yamasaki K. Steroidal saponins from fruits of Tribulus terrestris. Phytochemistry. 1996 Jul;42(5):1417-22.

CORDYCEPS SINENSIS

What Is It?

Cordyceps is a Chinese mushroom used in traditional Chinese medicine (TCM) for "lung protection" and "reproductive invigoration" as well as to balance the "Qi"—the "fundamental energy of life." Cordyceps is also known as the Chinese caterpillar fungus because it is a parasitic organism that grows on a rare Tibetan caterpillar until the caterpillar dies and the mushroom sprouts from the caterpillar's head (yuck!). Luckily, the source of cordyceps used in most modern supplements is not pulverized caterpillar heads, but a strain grown on soybeans or another less disgusting nutrient source.

Claims

- Relieves asthma
- Increases lung function
- Boosts libido and sexual function
- Improves athletic performance

Theory

Many of the claims for cordyceps parallel those of ginseng due to its reported effects on increasing energy levels, sex drive, and endurance performance. You may remember mention of cordyceps in the news a few years ago when several Chinese athletes came from out of nowhere to break world records in swimming and running. It turns out that the athletes were following a supplementation regimen that included cordyceps (along with turtle blood soup and anabolic steroids). Although the pharmacologically active components of cordyceps remain unknown, at least two chemical constituents, cordycepin (deoxyadenosine) and cordycepic acid (mannitol), have been identified and suggested as being the active compounds in improving lung function and increasing energy levels and sex drive.

Scientific Support

Although a number of studies have been conducted on cordyceps in China, relatively little information is available from U.S.-based scientists. A few animal studies have shown cordyceps feeding to increase the ratio of adenosine triphosphate (ATP) to inorganic phosphate (Pi) in the liver by about 50 percent—an effect that may be viewed as beneficial in terms of energy state and potential for enhancement of athletic performance. Furthermore, mice fed cordyceps and subjected to an extreme low-oxygen environment were able to utilize oxygen more efficiently (30 to 50 percent increase), better tolerate acidosis and hypoxia (lack of oxygen), and live two to three times longer than a control group.

In a number of Chinese clinical studies, primarily conducted in elderly patients with fatigue, cordyceps-treated patients reported significant improvements in their level of fatigue, ability to tolerate cold temperatures, memory and cognitive capacity, and sex drive. Patients with respiratory diseases also reported feeling physically stronger. Overall, the efficacy rate for cordyceps in alleviating fatigue in elderly subjects was 80 to 90 percent (possibly due to the adenosine content of cordyceps). At least one study in humans suggests that the increased libido reported in elderly subjects may be due to an increase in DHEA levels from low ranges back to normal (DHEA is a precursor to testosterone in both men and women).

Recently, a handful of small studies presented at sports medicine and nutrition meetings (1999-2001) showed that cordyceps-based supplements significantly increase maximal oxygen uptake and anaerobic threshold, which may lead to improved exercise capacity and resistance to fatigue.

Safety

Dietary supplements of *Cordyceps sinensis* are not associated with any significant side effects, although the possibility for a slight blood-thinning effect that could reduce blood clotting exists.

Value

At about $25 for a 120 capsule bottle, cordyceps will cost you around a dollar a day (usually two to six capsules)—not too bad for something that appears effective in alleviating fatigue and giving your libido a little nudge.

Dosage

Two to four grams per day of *Cordyceps sinensis* have been associated with increased energy levels, reduced fatigue, and an enhanced ability to use oxygen.

WORKS CONSULTED

Bao TT, Wang GF, Yang JL. Pharmacological actions of Cordyceps sinensis. Chung Hsi I Chieh Ho Tsa Chih. 1988 Jun;8(6):352-4, 325-6.

Bok JW, Lermer L, Chilton J, Klingeman HG, Towers GH. Antitumor sterols from the mycelia of Cordyceps sinensis. Phytochemistry. 1999 Aug;51(7):891-8.

Bucci LR. Selected herbals and human exercise performance. Am J Clin Nutr. 2000 Aug;72(2 Suppl):624S-36S.

Chiou WF, Chang PC, Chou CJ, Chen CF. Protein constituent contributes to the hypotensive and vasorelaxant activities of Cordyceps sinensis. Life Sci. 2000 Feb 25;66(14):1369-76.

Kaczka EA, Trenner NR, Arison B, Walker RW, Folkers K. Identification of cordycepin, a metabolite of Cordyceps militaris, as 3'-deoxyadenosine. Biochem Biophys Res Commun. 1964;14:456-7.

Kuo YC, Tsai WJ, Shiao MS, Chen CF, Lin CY. Cordyceps sinensis as an immunomodulatory agent. Am J Chin Med. 1996;24(2):111-25.

Manabe N, Azuma Y, Sugimoto M, Uchio K, Miyamoto M, Taketomo N, Tsuchita H, Miyamoto H. Effects of the mycelial extract of cultured Cordyceps sinensis on in vivo hepatic energy metabolism and blood flow in dietary hypoferric anaemic mice. Br J Nutr. 2000 Feb;83(2):197-204.

Manabe N, Sugimoto M, Azuma Y, Taketomo N, Yamashita A, Tsuboi H, Tsunoo A, Kinjo N, Nian-Lai H, Miyamoto H. Effects of the mycelial extract of cultured Cordyceps sinensis on in vivo hepatic energy metabolism in the mouse. Jpn J Pharmacol. 1996 Jan;70(1):85-8.

Wang SM, Lee LJ, Lin WW, Chang CM. Effects of a water-soluble extract of Cordyceps sinensis on steroidogenesis and capsular morphology of lipid droplets in cultured rat adrenocortical cells. J Cell Biochem. 1998 Jun 15;69(4):483-9.

Xu WH. Water-soluble constituents of Cordyceps sinenses (Berk.) Sacc.—the nucleosides. Chung Yao Tung Pao. 1988 Apr;13(4):34-6, 63.

Zhang SS, Zhang DS, Zhu TJ, Chen XY. A pharmacological analysis of the amino acid components of Cordyceps sinensis Sacc. Yao Hsueh Hsueh Pao. 1991;26(5):326-30.

Zhao-Long W, Xiao-Xia W, Wei-Ying C. Inhibitory effect of Cordyceps sinensis and Cordyceps militaris on human glomerular mesangial cell proliferation induced by native LDL. Cell Biochem Funct. 2000 Jun;18(2):93-7.

Zhu JS, Halpern GM, Jones K. The scientific rediscovery of an ancient Chinese herbal medicine: Cordyceps sinensis: Part I. J Altern Complement Med. 1998 Fall;4(3):289-303.

Zhu JS, Halpern GM, Jones K. The scientific rediscovery of a precious ancient Chinese herbal regimen: Cordyceps sinensis: Part II. J Altern Complement Med. 1998 Winter;4(4):429-57.

GLYCEROL

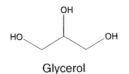

Glycerol

What Is It?

Glycerol, also known as glycerin, is an alcohol compound most commonly found in the diet as a component of fat or triglycerides. The glycerol serves as the backbone onto which fatty acid molecules are attached. Commercial preparation of glycerol can be obtained by hydrolysis (removal) of the fatty acids from the glycerol molecule.

Claims

- Increases blood volume
- Increases water-holding capacity of cells
- Enhances temperature regulation
- Improves exercise performance in the heat
- Reduces dehydration

Theory

Glycerol is proposed to help "hyperhydrate" the body by increasing blood volume levels and helping to delay dehydration.

Scientific Support

At least a few studies support the theory that glycerol added to fluids will increase tissue hydration compared to drinking fluid without glycerol added. Following glycerol consumption, heart rate and body core temperature are lower during exercise in the heat, suggesting an ergogenic (performance-enhancing) effect. In long-duration activities, a larger supply of stored water may lead to a delay in dehydration and exhaustion.

Safety

Straight (undiluted) glycerin is not recommended for internal consumption, but no significant adverse side effects are associated with glycerin diluted with fluids. In some subjects, glycerol consumption may lead to headaches or nausea. Individuals in whom increased blood volume may be undesirable, including conditions such as pregnancy, high blood pressure, diabetes, and kidney disease, should avoid glycerol supplementation.

Value

For endurance athletes engaged in strenuous training or competition in hot environments, consumption of glycerol-containing beverages may help hydrate tissues, increase blood volume, and delay fatigue and exhaustion associated with dehydration.

Dosage

Glycerol dosage relates to the amount of total body water—so bigger people have more body water and require more glycerol to obtain the desired effect. Approximately 1 g of glycerin per kilogram (2.2 lb) of body weight is diluted in 20 to 25 ml of liquid. A 70 kg man (154 lb), therefore, would need 70 g of glycerin diluted in 1,400 to 1,750 ml of fluid (about 1 to 2 liters of fluid). The mixture should be consumed slowly over the course of one to two hours prior to exercise in the heat.

WORKS CONSULTED

Arnall DA, Goforth HW Jr. Failure to reduce body water loss in cold-water immersion by glycerol ingestion. Undersea Hyperb Med. 1993 Dec;20(4):309-20.

Boulay MR, Song TM, Serresse O, Theriault G, Simoneau JA, Bouchard C. Changes in plasma electrolytes and muscle substrates during short-term maximal exercise in humans. Can J Appl Physiol. 1995 Mar;20(1):89-101.

Inder WJ, Swanney MP, Donald RA, Prickett TC, Hellemans J. The effect of glycerol and desmopressin on exercise performance and hydration in triathletes. Med Sci Sports Exerc. 1998 Aug;30(8):1263-9.

Jimenez C, Melin B, Koulmann N, Allevard AM, Launay JC, Savourey G. Plasma volume changes during and after acute variations of body hydration level in humans. Eur J Appl Physiol Occup Physiol. 1999 Jun;80(1):1-8.

Meyer LG, Horrigan DJ Jr, Lotz WG. Effects of three hydration beverages on exercise performance during 60 hours of heat exposure. Aviat Space Environ Med. 1995 Nov;66(11):1052-7.

Mitchell JB, Braun WA, Pizza FX, Forrest M. Pre-exercise carbohydrate and fluid ingestion: Influence of glycemic response on 10-km treadmill running performance in the heat. J Sports Med Phys Fitness. 2000 Mar;40(1):41-50.

Montner P, Stark DM, Riedesel ML, Murata G, Robergs R, Timms M, Chick TW. Pre-exercise glycerol hydration improves cycling endurance time. Int J Sports Med. 1996 Jan;17(1):27-33.

Wagner DR. Hyperhydrating with glycerol: Implications for athletic performance. J Am Diet Assoc. 1999 Feb;99(2):207-12.

ORNITHINE ALPHA-KETOGLUTARATE (OKG)
OR ALPHA-KETOGLUTARATE (AKG)

What Is It?

Ornithine alpha-ketoglutarate (OKG) is a salt formed by combining two molecules of the amino acid ornithine and one molecule of alpha-ketoglutarate (AKG). Because OKG seems to be involved in amino acid recycling/synthesis and protein availability, many athletes supplement with OKG as a way to increase muscle mass and strength—although the evidence for its effectiveness in this regard is quite limited.

Claims

- Increases muscle size and strength
- Reduces body fat
- Stimulates the immune system

Theory

OKG has been used to treat patients suffering from burns, surgery, malnutrition, and other trauma. Although the precise mechanism is unknown, OKG treatment decreases muscle protein catabolism (breakdown) and/or increases protein synthesis, in addition to promoting wound healing. OKG may promote the secretion of anabolic hormones such as insulin and growth hormone and increase amino acid metabolism (glutamine and arginine), which may help explain some of the clinical findings.

Scientific Support

Arginine and ornithine are precursors of nitric oxide and polyamines, respectively—metabolites that participate in a number of physiological functions. OKG supplements have been shown to promote growth hormone and insulin secretion with anabolic effects in postoperative patients. Their intermediary metabolites (glutamine and proline) may also have beneficial effects in promoting recovery from trauma. In animal studies, OKG supplementation has been shown to increase levels of arginine and glutamine in skeletal muscles and stimulate immune system function compared to animals not receiving OKG. The immunomodulatory properties found with OKG supplementation suggest that it may enhance host-defense mechanisms, particularly during injury and acute stress.

OKG supplements (15 g per day for five months) have been shown to improve growth rates in small children. The OKG supplements resulted in elevated concentrations of anabolic (growth) hormones and amino acid metabolites, including insulin-like growth factor 1 (IGF1), glutamine, and glutamate. In another study of healthy men, OKG given at 10 g per day resulted in a 20 to 30 percent elevation in insulin (another anabolic hormone), which was not observed with supplementation of either ornithine or alpha-ketoglutarate alone.

A test tube study found that OKG induces a significant increase in growth of human fibroblasts—cells with similarities to muscle fiber cells. This effect was dose dependent, meaning that a more pronounced growth effect was noted with increasing levels of OKG (but not with increasing levels of ornithine or alpha-ketoglutarate alone).

In one study, the anticatabolic effects of OKG were investigated in fourteen multiple trauma patients who were highly catabolic and hypermetabolic. One group of subjects received 20 g of OKG per day and showed a significant increase in protein turnover as well as an increase in blood levels of insulin, growth hormone, and free amino acids (glutamine, proline, and ornithine) compared to subjects not receiving OKG supplements.

Safety

No apparent side effects have been noted with OKG supplementation at the doses studied (10 to 20 g per day), although there have been anecdotal reports of increased appetite—perhaps owing to elevated insulin levels and fluctuations in blood sugar levels.

Value

OKG supplements, taken at a dose shown to produce effects (10 to 15 g per day), are a fairly expensive regimen. At $30 to $35 per 100 capsule bottle (1,250 mg capsules), a one-month supply will cost over $100. For stimulating increases in muscle mass, other dietary supplements, such as creatine, may be able to provide the same end benefit—at a much lower cost per day.

Dosage

OKG has been used at doses of 10 to 20 g per day in healthy men, short-stature children, and multiple trauma patients.

WORKS CONSULTED

Cochard A, Guilhermet R, Bonneau M. Plasma growth hormone (GH), insulin and amino acid responses to arginine with or without aspartic acid in pigs. Effect of the dose. Reprod Nutr Dev. 1998 May-Jun;38(3):331-43.

Jeevanandam M, Petersen SR. Substrate fuel kinetics in enterally fed trauma patients supplemented with ornithine alpha ketoglutarate. Clin Nutr. 1999 Aug; 18(4):209-17.

GAMMA-ORYZANOL/FERULIC ACID/RICE BRAN OIL

What Is It?

Gamma-oryzanol, also known as rice bran oil, is a compound made up of a plant sterol (a fatlike substance) and ferulic acid. Animal studies have shown that less than 10 percent of the gamma-oryzanol taken in via the diet is actually absorbed. The small amounts that are absorbed travel to the liver, where the compound is separated into the sterol and the ferulic acid. The sterol portion gets excreted while the ferulic acid circulates in the blood and can be taken up by tissues in the body where it has a minor effect on hormone release. Dietary sources of gamma-oryzanol include rice bran oil (used in India) and rice. One cup of white rice contains approximately 4 mg of gamma-oryzanol while a cup of brown rice contains about 18 mg because of the higher fat content.

Claims

- A "natural alternative" to anabolic steroids
- Increases muscle strength, size, and definition
- Reduces fatigue and sensations of pain
- Lowers cholesterol levels
- Protects against cancer

Theory

The theory behind gamma-oryzanol supplementation is the effect it has on the body's hormonal system—specifically the ability to increase testosterone levels. Gamma-oryzanol is also thought to stimulate the hypothalamus to secrete growth hormone releasing hormone (GHRH), which stimulates the release of growth hormone (GH). Both testosterone and growth hormone have muscle-building effects. Gamma-oryzanol may also have an effect on endorphins (the "feel good" chemicals), which are released during exercise and help reduce feelings of pain and fatigue.

Scientific Support

Two studies published in 1990 suggested that ferulic acid supplements may be beneficial for athletes. In the first study, six trained weight lifters received 30 mg per day of ferulic acid for eight weeks while four lifters received a placebo. Body weight and strength (measured by one maximum lift) increased in the group receiving the supplements. The authors concluded that some aspects of weight training might be helped by ferulic acid supplementation. The second study measured hormone levels in six trained male endurance runners who took 50 mg per day of ferulic acid for three days. Levels of endorphins were greater when the athletes were taking the supplements than when they took the placebo.

A more recent study (1997) tested the effect of gamma-oryzanol supplements during resistance (strength) training in twenty-two college-age males who had been weight training for more than one year. The subjects were divided into two groups. One group took a 500 mg gamma-oryzanol supplement daily for nine weeks. The second group took a placebo. Both groups completed the same weight-training program. The researchers measured body composition, muscle strength, power, heart rate, blood pressure, hormones such as testosterone, and blood lipids such as cholesterol. Measurements were taken after four and nine weeks. Both groups benefited from the weight-training program, but the group who received the gamma-oryzanol did not show any additional benefits. The researchers concluded that the gamma-oryzanol supplements did not help in any way.

The authors of the earlier studies (1990) thought the results were promising but in need of more research. The 1997 study measured more aspects in a larger number of people and is considered the strongest study. The results of that study would not support the use of gamma-oryzanol as a performance enhancer. It is interesting to note that in rat studies where gamma-oryzanol was injected, growth hormone manufacture and release was *decreased*—not increased as many supplements claim. The reason for the decrease is not known.

Safety

Gamma-oryzanol and ferulic acid appear to be nontoxic. Side effects have not been reported in animal studies using doses of up to 1,000 to 1,500 mg per day of gamma-oryzanol or ferulic acid. Poor absorption appears to be the reason for the lack of side effects associated with higher doses.

Value

Early studies would suggest that ferulic acid supplementation holds some promise, but the more recent studies would not support any of the claims made for gamma-oryzanol.

Dosage

Supplemental doses of gamma-oryzanol typically range from 100 to 500 mg per day. Absorption is poor (less than 10 percent) but can be improved if emulsified. The active ingredient, ferulic acid, may be sold separately—with absorption claimed to be approximately 90 percent. Ferulic acid supplements used in research studies ranged from 30 to 50 mg per day.

WORKS CONSULTED

Fry AC, Bonner E, Lewis DL, Johnson RL, Stone MH, Kraemer WJ. The effects of gamma-oryzanol supplementation during resistance exercise training. Int J Sport Nutr. 1997 Dec;7(4):318-29.

Grunewald KK, Bailey RS. Commercially marketed supplements for bodybuilding athletes. Sports Med. 1993 Feb;15(2):90-103.

Hiramatsu K, Tani T, Kimura Y, Izumi S, Nakane PK. Effect of gamma-oryzanol on atheroma formation in hypercholesterolemic rabbits. Tokai J Exp Clin Med. 1990 Jul;15(4):299-305.

Hirose M, Fukushima S, Imaida K, Ito N, Shirai T. Modifying effects of phytic acid and gamma-oryzanol on the promotion stage of rat carcinogenesis. Anticancer Res. 1999 Sep-Oct;19(5A):3665-70.

Ishihara M, Ito Y, Nakakita T, Maehama T, Hieda S, Yamamoto K, Ueno N. Clinical effect of gamma-oryzanol on climacteric disturbance on serum lipid peroxides. Nippon Sanka Fujinka Gakkai Zasshi. 1982 Feb;34(2):243-51.

Nakayama S, Manabe A, Suzuki J, Sakamoto K, Inagaki T. Comparative effects of two forms of gamma-oryzanol in different sterol compositions on hyperlipidemia induced by cholesterol diet in rats. Jpn J Pharmacol. 1987 Jun;44(2):135-43.

Rong N, Ausman LM, Nicolosi RJ. Oryzanol decreases cholesterol absorption and aortic fatty streaks in hamsters. Lipids. 1997 Mar;32(3):303-9.

Rosenbloom C, Millard-Stafford M, Lathrop J. Contemporary ergogenic aids used by strength/power athletes. J Am Diet Assoc. 1992 Oct;92(10):1264-6.

Rukmini C, Raghuram TC. Nutritional and biochemical aspects of the hypolipidemic action of rice bran oil: A review. J Am Coll Nutr. 1991 Dec;10(6):593-601.

Scavariello EM, Arellano DB. Gamma-oryzanol: An important component in rice brain oil. Arch Latinoam Nutr. 1998 Mar;48(1):7-12.

Seetharamaiah GS, Chandrasekhara N. Effect of oryzanol on fructose induced hypertriglyceridaemia in rats. Indian J Med Res. 1988 Sep;88:278-81.

Seetharamaiah GS, Chandrasekhara N. Studies on hypocholesterolemic activity of rice bran oil. Atherosclerosis. 1989 Aug;78(2-3):219-23.

Seetharamaiah GS, Krishnakantha TP, Chandrasekhara N. Influence of oryzanol on platelet aggregation in rats. J Nutr Sci Vitaminol (Tokyo). 1990 Jun;36(3):291-7.

Shimomura Y, Kobayashi I, Maruto S, Ohshima K, Mori M, Kamio N, Fukuda H. Effect of gamma-oryzanol on serum TSH concentrations in primary hypothyroidism. Endocrinol Jpn. 1980 Feb;27(1):83-6.

Sugano M, Koba K, Tsuji E. Health benefits of rice bran oil. Anticancer Res. 1999 Sep-Oct;19(5A):3651-7.

Sugano M, Tsuji E. Rice bran oil and cholesterol metabolism. J Nutr. 1997 Mar;127(3):521S-4S.

Tamagawa M, Otaki Y, Takahashi T, Otaka T, Kimura S, Miwa T. Carcinogenicity study of gamma-oryzanol in B6C3F1 mice. Food Chem Toxicol. 1992 Jan;30(1):49-56.

Tamagawa M, Shimizu Y, Takahashi T, Otaka T, Kimura S, Kadowaki H, Uda F, Miwa T. Carcinogenicity study of gamma-oryzanol in F344 rats. Food Chem Toxicol. 1992 Jan;30(1):41-8.

Tsushimoto G, Shibahara T, Awogi T, Kaneko E, Sutou S, Yamamoto K, Shirakawa H. DNA-damaging, mutagenic, clastogenic and cell-cell communication inhibitory properties of gamma-oryzanol. J Toxicol Sci. 1991 Nov;16(4):191-202.

Wheeler KB, Garleb KA. Gamma oryzanol-plant sterol supplementation: Metabolic, endocrine, and physiologic effects. Int J Sport Nutr. 1991 Jun;1(2):170-7.

Yamauchi J, Takahara J, Uneki T, Ofuki T. Inhibition of LH secretion by gamma-oryzanol in rat. Horm Metab Res. 1981 Mar;13(3):185.

Yasukawa K, Akihisa T, Kimura Y, Tamura T, Takido M. Inhibitory effect of cycloartenol ferulate, a component of rice bran, on tumor promotion in two-stage carcinogenesis in mouse skin. Biol Pharm Bull. 1998 Oct;21(10):1072-6.

MEDIUM-CHAIN TRIGLYCERIDES (MCTs)

What Is It?

Medium-chain triglycerides (MCTs) are fats that contain six, eight, ten, or twelve carbons. The number of carbons distinguishes them from long-chain (fourteen or more carbons) or short-chain (two or four carbons) fats. The length of the carbon chain affects function in the body. MCTs are absorbed rapidly and burned for immediate energy, whereas other fats are absorbed and metabolized slowly. Supplements are typically sold as MCT oil, either fruit-flavored or unflavored.

Claims

- Improves endurance performance
- Promotes fat burning
- Spares muscle glycogen
- Increases metabolic rate
- Maintains muscle mass

Theory

It is theorized that the ingestion of medium-chain triglycerides, because of their rapid absorption and metabolism, provides the athlete with a fuel source that helps to spare the use of muscle glycogen (stored carbohydrate). Because depletion of muscle glycogen is a factor in fatigue, ingestion of MCT oil could provide the body with an immediate source of fat that is rapidly broken down for energy—thus muscle glycogen stores are not used up as quickly and the onset of fatigue is delayed.

MCTs are also thought to increase metabolic rate. Assuming that diet (calorie intake) and exercise (calorie output) remains the same, any increase in metabolic rate could result in a small, slow loss of body fat. MCTs are thought to be burned immediately for energy rather than being stored as body fat and used for energy at a later time. In theory, MCTs help to maintain muscle mass because they produce ketone bodies, which are used for energy before the amino acids in muscle are used for energy.

Scientific Support

Because the length of the carbon chain affects absorption and medium-chain triglycerides are rapidly absorbed, they are transported directly to the liver and are quickly oxidized (broken down). Their rapid transport and oxidation is more similar to carbohydrate than to other fats, and MCTs have less of a tendency to be stored as body fat. In contrast, the long-chain fats, the most prevalent type of fat in the diet, are slowly absorbed and oxidized and often stored as body fat. Most MCTs are metabolized by the liver and provide energy, although some ketone bodies will also be produced by MCT metabolism. Ketone bodies may be eliminated in the urine or used as an alternative fuel source by the muscles and the brain when the body is in a starvation state.

The majority of MCT studies have looked at endurance cyclists to determine effectiveness in increasing endurance performance. Researchers have studied both the use of muscle glycogen when MCTs are consumed and the effect of MCTs on cycling times. In these studies, endurance cyclists engage in moderate to intense exercise while ingesting an MCT supplement, an MCT supplement plus a carbohydrate supplement, or a placebo. The results of these studies suggest that MCT oil does not reduce the use of muscle glycogen or improve endurance performance.

Despite the frequent claims for the benefits of MCTs in bodybuilding (increased metabolic rate, reduced body fat, and preservation of muscle mass), there are no published scientific studies that have examined MCT use by bodybuilders. The claims for MCTs are based on individual scientific studies that look at the use of MCTs in nonathletic populations. For example, a 1986 study found that the metabolic rate of seven healthy men increased by 12 percent with MCT ingestion versus only 4 percent with long-chain fats. The authors speculated that weight loss would occur if MCTs were substituted for long-chain fats and total calories remained the same.

There is clearly a need for more research regarding the role of MCTs in athletic performance. Some athletes have been experimenting with lower-carbohydrate, higher-fat "Zone"-type diets (40 percent carbohydrate, 30 percent protein, and 30 percent fat). It has been suggested that modifying a 40-30-30 diet by substituting MCTs for long-chain fatty acids may help further reduce body fat, but no scientific studies of athletes have been published to support this theory.

Safety

Consumption of MCT oil by humans is safe up to levels of 1 g per kilogram of body weight (e.g., 50 g in a 110 lb person). A by-product of MCT metabolism is ketone bodies, and the use of MCT oil by diabetics is not recommended unless it is part of medically supervised treatment. People with liver disease should not use MCT oil because MCTs are delivered rapidly to the liver, and their presence would put additional stress on the liver. Medium-chain triglycerides supplements do not contain any essential fatty acids, but this would not present a problem unless MCTs were the only source of fat in the diet. In one study, the use of 85 g of MCT oil (a large dose) was associated with intestinal cramping, whereas smaller quantities of MCT oil did not affect gastrointestinal function.

Value

The results of recent (1998-2000) well-controlled studies in endurance athletes do not support the use of MCT oil to spare muscle glycogen or enhance performance. Although a 1996 study seemed promising, the results of that study have not been replicated. At present, MCT supplements do not appear to be an effective way to increase endurance cycling performance. In the absence of any scientific study of MCT use and bodybuilders, MCT oil cannot be recommended as an effective supplement for reducing body fat and maintaining muscle mass.

General claims that MCTs act more like carbohydrates than short- or long-chain fats in the body, are a concentrated energy source, and do not contribute to heart disease are true. Any athlete who is having trouble consuming enough calories will find that 1 tablespoon of MCT oil provides approximately 110 calories. This concentrated energy source may be valuable for the athlete who chronically has trouble ingesting sufficient calories.

Dosage

The usual recommended dose is 1 to 2 tablespoons per day. Initial doses should be small (e.g., ½ tablespoon per day) to make sure there are no gastrointestinal side effects. One tablespoon of MCT oil contains 14 g of fat. MCT oil is often used as a substitute for salad dressing but should not be used for frying, as the high temperature negatively affects the taste.

WORKS CONSULTED

Angus DJ, Hargreaves M, Dancey J, Febbraio MA. Effect of carbohydrate or carbohydrate plus medium-chain triglyceride ingestion on cycling time trial performance. J Appl Physiol. 2000;88:113-9.

Bach AC, Ingenbleek Y, Frey A. The usefulness of dietary medium-chain triglycerides in body weight control: Fact or fancy? J Lipid Res. 1996;37:708-26.

Bell SJ, Bradley D, Forse RA, Bistrian BR. The new dietary fats in health and disease. J Am Dietetic Assoc. 1997;97:280-6.

Goedecke JH, Christie C, Wilson G, Dennis SC, Noakes TD, Hopkins WG, Lambert EV. Metabolic adaptations to a high-fat diet in endurance cyclists. Metabolism. 1999;48:1509-17.

Goedecke JH, Elmer-English R, Dennis SC, Schloss I, Noakes TD, Lambert EV. Effects of medium-chain triaclyglycerol ingested with carbohydrate on metabolism and exercise performance. Int J Sport Nutr. 1999;9:35-47.

Hawley JA, Brouns F, Jeukendrup A. Strategies to enhance fat utilisation during exercise. Sports Med. 1998;25:241-57.

Horowitz JF, Mora-Rodriguez R, Byerley LO, Coyle EF. Preexercise medium-chain triglyceride ingestion does not alter muscle glycogen use during exercise. J Appl Physiol. 2000;88:219-25.

Jeukendrup AE. Dietary fat and physical performance. Curr Opin Clin Nutri Metab Care. 1999;2:521-26.

Jeukendrup AE, Saris WH, Schrauwen P, Brouns F, Wagenmakers AJ. Metabolic availability of medium-chain triglycerides coingested with carbohydrates during prolonged exercise. J Appl Physiol. 1995;79:756-62.

Jeukendrup AE, Saris WH, Wagenmakers AJ. Fat metabolism during exercise: A review—Part III: Effects of nutritional interventions. Int J Sports Med. 1998; 19:371-79.

Jeukendrup AE, Thielen JJ, Wagenmakers AJ, Brouns F, Saris WH. Effect of medium-chain triacylglycerol and carbohydrate ingestion during exercise on substrate utilization and subsequent cycling performance. Am J Clin Nutr. 1998; 67:397-404.

Lambert EV, Hawley JA, Goedecke J, Noakes TD, Dennis SC. Nutritional strategies for promoting fat utilization and delaying the onset of fatigue during prolonged exercise. J Sports Sci. 1997;15:315-24.

Seaton TB, Welle SL, Warenko MK, Campbell RG. Thermic effect of medium-chain and long-chain triglycerides in man. Am J Clin Nutr. 1986;44:630-34.

Traul KA, Driedger A, Ingle DL, Nakhasi D. Review of the toxicologic properties of medium-chain triglycerides. Food Chem Toxicol. 2000;38:79-98.

Van Zyl CG, Lambert EV, Hawley JA, Noakes TD, Dennis SC. Effects of medium-chain triglyceride ingestion on fuel metabolism and cycling performance. J Appl Physiol. 1996;80:2217-25.

SODIUM BICARBONATE

What Is It?

Sodium bicarbonate is referred to as an "alkaline" salt—meaning that it has the ability to neutralize or counteract acids. Many people understand alkaline solutions as a remedy for combating the acidic stomach associated with heartburn. As an ergogenic aid, sodium bicarbonate has been used by athletes in sports such as sprinting to combat the fatiguing effects of another acid—lactic acid.

Claims

- Reduces lactic acid accumulation
- Improves endurance and sprint performance
- Increases power output

Theory

During very intense exercise, lactic acid accumulation in the muscle cell can lead to premature fatigue and compromised athletic performance. Within the muscle cell, the accumulation of lactate and hydrogen ions is thought to inhibit the activity of several enzymes involved with energy generation. A higher concentration of alkali—such as sodium bicarbonate—might promote the removal of lactate and hydrogen ions from the muscle cells into the bloodstream. In theory, this would reduce the lactate concentration within the muscle cell and prevent the premature fatigue associated with lactic acid accumulation.

Scientific Support

A number of studies have tested and confirmed the benefits of sodium bicarbonate loading as an effective ergogenic aid for athletes competing in high-intensity activities. In general, events in which lactic acid accumulation is typically a limiting factor seem to respond well to bicarbonate loading. Athletes competing in running events from 400 to 1,500 meters, swimming events of 100 to 200 meters, track cycling (1 to 5 kilometers), and rowing (2,000 meters) have all shown significant improvements in performance following pre-event loading with sodium bicarbonate.

Safety

At recommended doses, sodium bicarbonate is safe. Some individuals, however, may experience mild to moderate side effects such as gastrointestinal upset, nausea, bloating, and diarrhea.

Value

Basic sodium bicarbonate solutions are inexpensive and can be made at home (see Dosage). It is highly advisable to perform a practice run of bicarbonate loading prior to using it in actual competition, just to see how your body will tolerate the high alkali load. Several alkalizing dietary supplements are marketed to athletes as performance aids.

Dosage

About 300 mg of sodium bicarbonate per kilogram of body weight *or* 4 to 6 rounded teaspoons of baking soda mixed into approximately 1 liter of sports drink. Consume one to two hours prior to competition.

WORKS CONSULTED

Coppoolse R, Barstow TJ, Stringer WW, Carithers E, Casaburi R. Effect of acute bicarbonate administration on exercise responses of COPD patients. Med Sci Sports Exerc. 1997 Jun;29(6):725-32.

Ferrante PL, Kronfeld DS, Taylor LE, Meacham TN. Plasma [H+] responses to exercise in horses fed a high-fat diet and given sodium bicarbonate. J Nutr. 1994 Dec;124(12 Suppl):2736S-7S.

Ferrante PL, Menninger JH, Spencer PA, Kronfeld DS. Metabolic response of horses to a high soluble carbohydrate diet: Effects of low-intensity submaximal exercise and sodium bicarbonate supplementation. Am J Vet Res. 1992 Mar;53(3):321-5.

Ferrante PL, Taylor LE, Kronfeld DS, Meacham TN. Blood lactate concentration during exercise in horses fed a high-fat diet and administered sodium bicarbonate. J Nutr. 1994 Dec;124(12 Suppl):2738S-9S.

Gaitanos GC, Nevill ME, Brooks S, Williams C. Repeated bouts of sprint running after induced alkalosis. J Sports Sci. 1991 Winter;9(4):355-70.

Granier PL, Dubouchaud H, Mercier BM, Mercier JG, Ahmaidi S, Prefaut CG. Effect of NaHCO3 on lactate kinetics in forearm muscles during leg exercise in man. Med Sci Sports Exerc. 1996 Jun;28(6):692-7.

Greenhaff PL, Harris RC, Snow DH, Sewell DA, Dunnett M. The influence of metabolic alkalosis upon exercise metabolism in the thoroughbred horse. Eur J Appl Physiol Occup Physiol. 1991;63(2):129-34.

Heck KL, Potteiger JA, Nau KL, Schroeder JM. Sodium bicarbonate ingestion does not attenuate the VO2 slow component during constant-load exercise. Int J Sport Nutr. 1998 Mar;8(1):60-9.

Hirakoba K, Maruyama A, Misaka K. Effect of acute sodium bicarbonate ingestion on excess CO2 output during incremental exercise. Eur J Appl Physiol Occup Physiol. 1993;66(6):536-41.

Hollidge-Horvat MG, Parolin ML, Wong D, Jones NL, Heigenhauser GJ. Effect of induced metabolic alkalosis on human skeletal muscle metabolism during exercise. Am J Physiol Endocrinol Metab. 2000 Feb;278(2):E316-29.

Holloway SA, Sundstrom D, Senior DF. Effect of acute induced metabolic alkalosis on the acid/base responses to sprint exercise of six racing greyhounds. Res Vet Sci. 1996 Nov;61(3):245-51.

Hyyppa S, Poso AR. Fluid, electrolyte, and acid-base responses to exercise in racehorses. Vet Clin North Am Equine Pract. 1998 Apr;14(1):121-36.

Kayser B, Ferretti G, Grassi B, Binzoni T, Cerretelli P. Maximal lactic capacity at altitude: Effect of bicarbonate loading. J Appl Physiol. 1993 Sep;75(3):1070-4.

Kozak-Collins K, Burke ER, Schoene RB. Sodium bicarbonate ingestion does not improve performance in women cyclists. Med Sci Sports Exerc. 1994 Dec;26(12):1510-5.

Lambert CP, Greenhaff PL, Ball D, Maughan RJ. Influence of sodium bicarbonate ingestion on plasma ammonia accumulation during incremental exercise in man. Eur J Appl Physiol Occup Physiol. 1993;66(1):49-54.

Light RW, Peng MJ, Stansbury DW, Sassoon CS, Despars JA, Mahutte CK. Effects of sodium bicarbonate administration on the exercise tolerance of normal subjects breathing through dead space. Chest. 1999 Jan;115(1):102-8.

Linderman J, Fahey TD. Sodium bicarbonate ingestion and exercise performance. An update. Sports Med. 1991 Feb;11(2):71-7.

Linderman J, Kirk L, Musselman J, Dolinar B, Fahey TD. The effects of sodium bicarbonate and pyridoxine-alpha-ketoglutarate on short-term maximal exercise capacity. J Sports Sci. 1992 Jun;10(3):243-53.

Linderman JK, Gosselink KL. The effects of sodium bicarbonate ingestion on exercise performance. Sports Med. 1994 Aug;18(2):75-80.

Lloyd DR, Evans DL, Hodgson DR, Suann CJ, Rose RJ. Effects of sodium bicarbonate on cardiorespiratory measurements and exercise capacity in thoroughbred horses. Equine Vet J. 1993 Mar;25(2):125-9.

Matson LG, Tran ZV. Effects of sodium bicarbonate ingestion on anaerobic performance: A meta-analytic review. Int J Sport Nutr. 1993 Mar;3(1):2-28.

McNaughton L, Backx K, Palmer G, Strange N. Effects of chronic bicarbonate ingestion on the performance of high-intensity work. Eur J Appl Physiol Occup Physiol. 1999 Sep;80(4):333-6.

McNaughton L, Dalton B, Palmer G. Sodium bicarbonate can be used as an ergogenic aid in high-intensity, competitive cycle ergometry of 1 h duration. Eur J Appl Physiol Occup Physiol. 1999 Jun;80(1):64-9.

McNaughton LR. Bicarbonate ingestion: Effects of dosage on 60 s cycle ergometry. J Sports Sci. 1992 Oct;10(5):415-23.

McNaughton LR. Sodium bicarbonate ingestion and its effects on anaerobic exercise of various durations. J Sports Sci. 1992 Oct;10(5):425-35.

Pierce EF, Eastman NW, Hammer WH, Lynn TD. Effect of induced alkalosis on swimming time trials. J Sports Sci. 1992 Jun;10(3):255-9.

Portington KJ, Pascoe DD, Webster MJ, Anderson LH, Rutland RR, Gladden LB. Effect of induced alkalosis on exhaustive leg press performance. Med Sci Sports Exerc. 1998 Apr;30(4):523-8.

Potteiger JA, Webster MJ, Nickel GL, Haub MD, Palmer RJ. The effects of buffer ingestion on metabolic factors related to distance running performance. Eur J Appl Physiol Occup Physiol. 1996;72(4):365-71.

Tiryaki GR, Atterbom HA. The effects of sodium bicarbonate and sodium citrate on 600 m running time of trained females. J Sports Med Phys Fitness. 1995 Sep;35(3):194-8.

Verbitsky O, Mizrahi J, Levin M, Isakov E. Effect of ingested sodium bicarbonate on muscle force, fatigue, and recovery. J Appl Physiol. 1997 Aug;83(2):333-7.

Webster MJ, Webster MN, Crawford RE, Gladden LB. Effect of sodium bicarbonate ingestion on exhaustive resistance exercise performance. Med Sci Sports Exerc. 1993 Aug;25(8):960-5.

Williams MH. Ergogenic and ergolytic substances. Med Sci Sports Exerc. 1992 Sep;24(9 Suppl):S344-8.

Zoladz JA, Duda K, Majerczak J, Domanski J, Emmerich J. Metabolic alkalosis induced by pre-exercise ingestion of NaHCO3 does not modulate the slow component of VO2 kinetics in humans. J Physiol Pharmacol. 1997 Jun;48(2):211-23.

PROTEIN SUPPLEMENTS

What Is It?

There is no denying that protein is a vital nutrient for general health and hundreds of specific functions in the body. There's an old saying in nutrition research that the body contains no extra protein—which means that every single protein in the body was assembled to carry out a specific function. There is no storage form of protein in the body. The recommended dietary allowance (RDA) for protein is 0.8 g per kilogram of body weight for adults (0.36 g per pound)—with growing kids, adolescents, and both power and endurance athletes needing slightly more (see Dosage). By RDA standards, a 70 kg adult (154 lb) would need about 56 g per day (about the amount provided in 8 oz of lean meat).

Claims

- Builds muscle/increases strength
- Controls appetite/aids weight loss
- Improves endurance
- Boosts energy levels
- Promotes immune function

Theory

Protein is one of the primary nutrients involved in growth, development, and repair of virtually all tissues in the body. Through protein-based molecules called enzymes, protein plays a vital role in regulating many of the metabolic processes in the body. In some cases, such as extreme endurance exercise, protein can also serve as an important source of energy, particularly when energy stores of carbohydrates in muscle and liver become exhausted. Following strenuous exercise, protein supplements are theorized to help speed repair and regeneration of damaged tissues by providing an additional source of amino acids needed to synthesize tissue structures. As a weight loss aid, elevated protein intakes have been associated with a more gradual rise in blood sugar and a heightened sense of satiety compared to meals higher in carbohydrates.

Scientific Support

There is very good evidence that protein needs are elevated by exercise training, infection, and other periods of acute and chronic stress. Some of the best evidence comes from studies of competitive athletes, in whom protein needs are nearly doubled during periods of intense training and competition. Athletes competing in power or strength sports probably require about 1.6 g of protein per kilogram of body weight, while endurance-trained athletes may need about 1.3 g per kilogram. For athletes, who also need to replenish bodily stores of carbohydrates and fluids in addition to protein, a postexercise recovery drink is often the most convenient and effective form of supplement.

Safety

Although protein is a major dietary component, excess intake could lead to imbalances in other aspects of the diet. Protein intake should probably be kept below 2.0 g per kilogram of body weight because no scientific evidence supports beneficial effects above this level. Concerns have been raised for several years regarding a possible strain put on the liver and kidneys by excessive protein intake. Although this may be a very real concern for individuals at risk for liver or kidney disease (where high-protein diets may accelerate tissue damage), there is no strong evidence indicating a safety concern for healthy individuals.

Value

A wide variety of protein supplements exist—complete with their own set of claims of superiority versus the competition (see whey protein summary in this chapter and soy protein summary in Chapter 10). Various mixtures from protein sources such as milk, eggs, and soy are among the most popular—but the cost varies considerably across the wide range of choices. In terms of convenience, isolated and/or concentrated protein mixtures make a lot of sense for many individuals.

Dosage

- For sedentary individuals the protein RDA is 0.8 g per kilogram of body weight.
- For strength athletes, protein intake should approximate 1.6 g per kilogram of body weight.
- For endurance athletes, protein intake of 1.3 g per kilogram of body weight is recommended.

WORKS CONSULTED

Applegate EA. Nutritional considerations for ultraendurance performance. Int J Sport Nutr. 1991 Jun;1(2):118-26.

Beltz SD, Doering PL. Efficacy of nutritional supplements used by athletes. Clin Pharm. 1993 Dec;12(12):900-8.

Economos CD, Bortz SS, Nelson ME. Nutritional practices of elite athletes. Practical recommendations. Sports Med. 1993 Dec;16(6):381-99.

Evans WJ. Muscle damage: Nutritional considerations. Int J Sport Nutr. 1991 Sep; 1(3):214-24.

Holt WS Jr. Nutrition and athletes. Am Fam Physician. 1993 Jun;47(8):1757-64.

Lemon PW. Effect of exercise on protein requirements. J Sports Sci. 1991 Summer;9 (Spec No):53-70.

Lemon PW. Is increased dietary protein necessary or beneficial for individuals with a physically active lifestyle? Nutr Rev. 1996 Apr;54(4 Pt 2):S169-75.

Lemon PW. Protein and amino acid needs of the strength athlete. Int J Sport Nutr. 1991 Jun;1(2):127-45.

Lemon PW, Proctor DN. Protein intake and athletic performance. Sports Med. 1991 Nov;12(5):313-25.

Maffucci DM, McMurray RG. Towards optimizing the timing of the pre-exercise meal. Int J Sport Nutr Exerc Metab. 2000 Jun;10(2):103-13.

Millward DJ. Optimal intakes of protein in the human diet. Proc Nutr Soc. 1999 May;58(2):403-13.

Nieman DC. Physical fitness and vegetarian diets: Is there a relation? Am J Clin Nutr. 1999 Sep;70(3 Suppl):570S-5S.

Nuviala Mateo RJ, Lapieza Lainez MG. The intake of proteins and essential amino acids in top-competing women athletes. Nutr Hosp. 1997 Mar-Apr;12(2):85-91.

Phillips SM, Atkinson SA, Tarnopolsky MA, MacDougall JD. Gender differences in leucine kinetics and nitrogen balance in endurance athletes. J Appl Physiol. 1993 Nov;75(5):2134-41.

Poortmans JR, Dellalieux O. Do regular high protein diets have potential health risks on kidney function in athletes? Int J Sport Nutr Exerc Metab. 2000 Mar;10(1):28-38.

Probart CK, Bird PJ, Parker KA. Diet and athletic performance. Med Clin North Am. 1993 Jul;77(4):757-72.

Shephard RJ, Shek PN. Immunological hazards from nutritional imbalance in athletes. Exerc Immunol Rev. 1998;4:22-48.

Tarnopolsky MA, Atkinson SA, MacDougall JD, Chesley A, Phillips S, Schwarcz HP. Evaluation of protein requirements for trained strength athletes. J Appl Physiol. 1992 Nov;73(5):1986-95.

Tarnopolsky MA, Bosman M, Macdonald JR, Vandeputte D, Martin J, Roy BD. Postexercise protein-carbohydrate and carbohydrate supplements increase muscle glycogen in men and women. J Appl Physiol. 1997 Dec;83(6):1877-83.

Williams C. Macronutrients and performance. J Sports Sci. 1995 Summer;13 (Spec No):S1-10.

WHEY PROTEIN

What Is It?

Whey is one of the proteins found in milk (the other is casein). Whey protein accounts for only about 20 percent of the total protein found in milk, while casein makes up about 80 percent. Long considered a useless by-product of dairy (cheese) manufacturing, whey protein is enjoying increased interest as a protein supplement. Whey has a long history of use as a cheap protein source for low-cost protein powders. Recent claims of the high biological activity of whey protein, and the profits to be made by selling something that used to be thrown away, have encouraged dairy processing plants to begin processing and spray-drying whey in various ways to enhance its benefits in commercial protein powders.

Claims

- Enhances immune function
- Increases protein synthesis
- More biologically active than other proteins
- Associated with greater nitrogen retention

Theory

Whey protein is rich in certain amino acids and low in fat. The key amino acids, the branched-chain amino acids (BCAAs, leucine, valine, and isoleucine), may help delay fatigue during endurance exercise. Another amino acid, cysteine, can be found in relatively high amounts in whey protein—compared to other protein sources such as soy or gelatin in which cysteine is lacking. Various protein groups (immunoglobulins) found in whey protein have been cited as immune stimulators.

Scientific Support

Whey proteins can differ dramatically from one another depending on the processing method and the total protein content. For example, whey protein can exist as simple whey powder (30 percent or less total protein content), whey protein concentrate (30 to 85 percent protein) or whey protein isolate (90 percent or higher protein content). In the case of whey protein isolates (the most expensive type), two key processing methods, ion exchange filtration and cross-flow microfiltration, can remove different components of the total whey protein, resulting in end products with different taste, texture, and functional properties. Whey proteins processed using the ion exchange methodology appear to retain the majority of the functional benefits associated with immune system maintenance. Enhanced resistance to infection and elevated glutathione levels (an antioxidant enzyme containing cysteine) have been noted in subjects consuming concentrated whey protein. Whey protein also contains lactoferrin, a protein that has been shown to possess bacteriostatic and bactericidal activity against microorganisms that can cause gastroenteric infections and food poisoning.

Whey protein has been used in a number of animal and human feeding studies, where it has shown benefits in promoting weight gain, elevating glutathione levels (an antioxidant), and preventing metabolic acidosis (although the same can be claimed for virtually any high-quality protein source). Whether the minor content differences between various whey proteins actually result in any appreciable differences in muscle gain in humans (their primary claim) has never been demonstrated.

Safety

No adverse side effects are associated with whey protein aside from the obvious potential for allergic and digestive reactions in individuals sensitive to dairy products.

Value

Whey protein can be used as a general source of high-quality, low-fat protein in any diet. Individuals who also want the supposed immune system benefits of whey protein may want to consider the more expensive whey isolates produced by ion exchange filtration—be aware, however, that these claims are largely speculative and have not yet been adequately proven in human subjects. Individuals in this category may include athletes at risk for infection (during intense training or recovery) or anybody recovering from injury or illness. Those individuals simply looking for a high-quality protein source to supplement their diet may want to consider one of the less expensive protein concentrates currently available, such as casein, egg, or soy.

Dosage

Intake levels should be based on total caloric requirements, body weight, and period of training. During intense training or recovery, you may want as much as 50 percent of your protein requirements to come from whey protein or another source of concentrated low-fat protein (approximately 40 g per day for a 160 lb man). As a general daily supplement, however, lower doses of whey, perhaps 10 to 20 g per day, as part of an adequate intake combined with other protein sources, may be sufficient to deliver the biological benefits of whey. A useful combination strategy is to split protein intake evenly between high-quality sources such as whey, egg, casein, and soy proteins.

WORKS CONSULTED

Alexander JW, Gottschlich MM. Nutritional immunomodulation in burn patients. Crit Care Med. 1990 Feb;18(2 Suppl):S149-53.

Barth CA, Behnke U. Nutritional physiology of whey and whey components. Nahrung. 1997 Feb;41(1):2-12.

Bernbaum JC, Sasanow SR, Churella HR, Daft A. Growth and metabolic response of premature infants fed whey- or casein-dominant formulas after hospital discharge. J Pediatr. 1989 Oct;115(4):652-6.

Bounous G, Batist G, Gold P. Immunoenhancing property of dietary whey protein in mice: Role of glutathione. Clin Invest Med. 1989 Jun;12(3):154-61.

Graham GG, MacLean WC Jr, Brown KH, Morales E, Lembcke J, Gastanaduy A. Protein requirements of infants and children: Growth during recovery from malnutrition. Pediatrics. 1996 Apr;97(4):499-505.

Hanning RM, Paes B, Atkinson SA. Protein metabolism and growth of term infants in response to a reduced-protein, 40:60 whey:casein formula with added tryptophan. Am J Clin Nutr. 1992 Dec;56(6):1004-11.

Kawase M, Hashimoto H, Hosoda M, Morita H, Hosono A. Effect of administration of fermented milk containing whey protein concentrate to rats and healthy men on serum lipids and blood pressure. J Dairy Sci. 2000 Feb;83(2):255-63.

Lonnerdal B. Effects of milk and milk components on calcium, magnesium, and trace element absorption during infancy. Physiol Rev. 1997 Jul;77(3):643-69.

Markus CR, Olivier B, Panhuysen GE, Van Der Gugten J, Alles MS, Tuiten A, Westenberg HG, Fekkes D, Koppeschaar HF, de Haan EE. The bovine protein alpha-lactalbumin increases the plasma ratio of tryptophan to the other large neutral amino acids, and in vulnerable subjects raises brain serotonin activity, reduces cortisol concentration, and improves mood under stress. Am J Clin Nutr. 2000 Jun;71(6):1536-44.

Nessmith WB Jr, Nelssen JL, Tokach MD, Goodband RD, Bergstrom JR. Effects of substituting deproteinized whey and(or) crystalline lactose for dried whey on weanling pig performance. J Anim Sci. 1997 Dec;75(12):3222-8.

Poullain MG, Cezard JP, Roger L, Mendy F. Effect of whey proteins, their oligopeptide hydrolysates and free amino acid mixtures on growth and nitrogen retention in fed and starved rats. J Parenter Enteral Nutr. 1989 Jul-Aug;13(4): 382-6.

Takada Y, Kobayashi N, Kato K, Matsuyama H, Yahiro M, Aoe S. Effects of whey protein on calcium and bone metabolism in ovariectomized rats. J Nutr Sci Vitaminol (Tokyo). 1997 Apr;43(2):199-210.

Terosky TL, Heinrichs AJ, Wilson LL. A comparison of milk protein sources in diets of calves up to eight weeks of age. J Dairy Sci. 1997 Nov;80(11):2977-83.

Tsuda H, Sekine K, Ushida Y, Kuhara T, Takasuka N, Iigo M, Han BS, Moore MA. Milk and dairy products in cancer prevention: Focus on bovine lactoferrin. Mutat Res. 2000 Apr;462(2-3):227-33.

Wong CW, Watson DL. Immunomodulatory effects of dietary whey proteins in mice. J Dairy Res. 1995 May;62(2):359-68.

CARNOSINE

What Is It?

Carnosine is a dipeptide—meaning that it is a compound comprising two amino acids linked together (alanine and histidine). Carnosine is found in high concentrations in skeletal muscles.

Claims

- Antioxidant
- Enhances wound healing
- Reduces lactic acid accumulation
- Promotes muscle recovery
- Enhances muscle contraction

Theory

Although no definite metabolic role has been ascribed to carnosine, it has been implicated in a variety of physiological processes. Perhaps the best-described function of carnosine is as a broad-spectrum antioxidant, where it has been shown to interact with several free radical species including singlet oxygen, hydrogen peroxide, and both peroxyl and hydroxyl radicals. In addition, carnosine is able to inhibit cellular damage induced by iron, copper, and zinc radicals. Carnosine also appears to play a role in activating the enzymes responsible for generating muscle contractions (myofibrillar-ATPase) as well as serving as an intramuscular buffering agent to retard accumulation of lactic acid. Among athletes, muscle carnosine levels are known to be highest in those with high anaerobic demands (rowers and track sprinters), but levels are also elevated in endurance athletes (marathon runners) when compared to untrained subjects. For the *potential* therapeutic actions of carnosine, including antihypertensive effects, immunomodulation, wound healing, and antitumor/chemopreventive effects, there is some laboratory and preclinical evidence to suggest benefits, but most of these claims have not been convincingly documented nor subjected to rigorous clinical evaluation.

Scientific Support

Carnosine is absorbed intact in the small intestine (jejunum) by a specific active transport mechanism. It circulates in the blood for transport to the kidney, liver, and muscle (where the highest concentrations are found).

Carnosine is either used by these tissues or is hydrolyzed (broken down) into alanine and histidine by the enzyme carnosinase (which is found in blood, liver, and kidney).

As a water-soluble antioxidant, carnosine is capable of decreasing cell membrane oxidation caused by iron, zinc, copper, hydrogen peroxide, singlet oxygen, and both peroxyl and hydroxyl free radicals. The antioxidant effect of carnosine appears to be far greater than the individual or combined activity of its constituent amino acids—indicating that the peptide linkage between alanine and histidine is involved in some unique way in the overall antioxidant activity of carnosine. In animal and test-tube experiments, carnosine has been shown to inhibit oxidation of LDL cholesterol (a possible benefit in preventing heart disease) and reduce development of breast cancer (in rats). High doses of carnosine may also possess some immune-stimulating activity, as shown by animal experiments in which survival time in X-ray irradiated mice was increased by about 50 percent following carnosine intake (50 to 200 mg/kg per day—a very large dose). Carnosine appears to promote wound healing, as shown by animal experiments in which 6 to 20 mg/kg per day for two weeks reduced the size and depth of gastric ulcers and accelerated regeneration of the damaged tissue.

It has been calculated that the pool of muscle dipeptides (mainly carnosine) can account for about 10 to 40 percent of the pH-buffering capacity of muscle tissue. During intense exercise, carnosine may play an important role in preventing the reduction in pH caused by lactic acid accumulation—thereby improving exercise performance. Although this theory has not been evaluated in clinical studies, studies in racehorses have shown that carnosine concentrations are higher in muscles with a high percentage of fast-twitch glycolytic fibers and lower in muscles with predominantly slower-twitch oxidative fiber types. In addition to its potential effects on anaerobic metabolism (lactic acid), carnosine may enhance oxidative (aerobic) metabolism by increasing the efficiency of mitochondria in producing cellular energy.

Safety

Although no long-term safety studies have been conducted in humans, carnosine is not expected to result in any significant side effects when consumed at levels found in most commercial dietary supplements. Rodent experiments have suggested that carnosine is extremely safe—no adverse toxic effects are noted even at doses up to 500 mg per kilogram of body weight (about 35 g for an average-sized man).

Value

Given the potential physiological benefits of carnosine, its use as a dietary supplement is generally slanted toward sports nutrition. Its possible roles in delaying fatigue, reducing stress, buffering acid buildup, healing wounds, improving muscle contraction, and protecting cells from oxidative damage position carnosine as both an ergogenic aid and a general tonic.

Dosage

The average daily intake of carnosine from foods is probably in the range of 50 to 250 mg (based on a diet containing at least one serving, 3 to 4 oz, of beef, pork, or chicken). Given that carnosine is fairly well absorbed (up to 15 percent of ingested dose), circulates in the blood and is quickly used by peripheral tissues, metabolized to its constituent amino acids (alanine and histidine), or filtered to the urine by the kidneys, supplements should be consumed in several divided doses throughout the day. Oral doses of 1 to 3 g per day have been used with success in managing immune system function in cancer patients.

WORKS CONSULTED

Alabovskii VV, Boldyrev AA, Vinokurov AA, Gallant S, Chesnokov DN. Comparison of protective effects of carnosine and acetylcarnosine during cardioplegia. Biull Eksp Biol Med. 1999 Mar;127(3):290-4.

Bakardjiev A, Bauer K. Biosynthesis, release, and uptake of carnosine in primary cultures. Biochemistry (Mosc). 2000 Jul;65(7):779-82.

Dadmarz M, van der Burg C, Milakofsky L, Hofford JM, Vogel WH. Effects of stress on amino acids and related compounds in various tissues of fasted rats. Life Sci. 1998;63(16):1485-91.

Decker EA, Livisay SA, Zhou S. A re-evaluation of the antioxidant activity of purified carnosine. Biochemistry (Mosc). 2000 Jul;65(7):766-70.

Deev LI, Goncharenko EN, Baizhumanov AA, Akhalaia MIA, Antonova SV, Shestakova SV. Protective effect of carnosine in hyperthermia. Biull Eksp Biol Med. 1997 Jul;124(7):50-2.

Gutierrez A, Anderstam B, Alvestrand A. Amino acid concentration in the interstitium of human skeletal muscle: A microdialysis study. Eur J Clin Invest. 1999 Nov;29(11):947-52.

Lee JW, Miyawaki H, Bobst EV, Hester JD, Ashraf M, Bobst AM. Improved functional recovery of ischemic rat hearts due to singlet oxygen scavengers histidine and carnosine. J Mol Cell Cardiol. 1999 Jan;31(1):113-21.

Mzhel'skaia TI, Boldyrev AA. The biological role of carnosine in excitable tissues. Zh Obshch Biol. 1998 May-Jun;59(3):263-78.

Preedy VR, Patel VB, Reilly ME, Richardson PJ, Falkous G, Mantle D. Oxidants, antioxidants and alcohol: Implications for skeletal and cardiac muscle. Front Biosci. 1999 Aug 1;4:e58-66.

Quinn PJ, Boldyrev AA, Formazuyk VE. Carnosine: Its properties, functions and potential therapeutic applications. Mol Aspects Med. 1992;13(5):379-444.

Roberts PR, Zaloga GP. Cardiovascular effects of carnosine. Biochemistry (Mosc). 2000 Jul;65(7):856-61.

Stuerenburg HJ. The roles of carnosine in aging of skeletal muscle and in neuro-muscular diseases. Biochemistry (Mosc). 2000 Jul;65(7):862-5.

Swearengin TA, Fitzgerald C, Seidler NW. Carnosine prevents glyceraldehyde 3-phosphate-mediated inhibition of aspartate aminotransferase. Arch Toxicol. 1999 Aug;73(6):307-9.

Zaloga GP, Roberts PR, Black KW, Lin M, Zapata-Sudo G, Sudo RT, Nelson TE. Carnosine is a novel peptide modulator of intracellular calcium and contractility in cardiac cells. Am J Physiol. 1997 Jan;272(1 Pt 2):H462-8.

PROTEOLYTIC ENZYMES

What Is It?

"Proteolytic" is a catchall term referring to enzymes that digest protein. Supplemental forms can incorporate any of a wide variety of enzymes including trypsin, chymotrypsin, pancreatin, bromelain, papain, and a range of fungal proteases. In the body, proteolytic digestive enzymes are produced in the pancreas, but supplemental forms of enzymes may come from fungal or bacterial sources, extracted from the pancreas of livestock animals (trypsin/chymotrypsin) or from plants (such as papain from papayas and bromelain from pineapples). The primary uses of proteolytic enzymes in dietary supplements are as digestive enzymes, anti-inflammatory agents, and pain relievers.

Claims

- Speeds recovery after exercise and accelerates healing of wounds and other minor injuries
- Aids digestion and reduces flatulence
- Anti-inflammatory
- Reduces pain and stiffness of arthritis
- Reduces symptoms of allergies and hay fever

Theory

It is quite logical that proteolytic enzymes would help alleviate a suboptimal production of the body's own digestive enzymes (which can occur in various pancreatic conditions). As such, supplemental enzymes can help alleviate gastrointestinal complaints such as gas and bloating, diarrhea, and cramps associated with inefficient or incomplete digestion. There is also some evidence that a small percentage of supplemental enzymes may be absorbed intact (and active) into the systemic circulation, where they appear to have anti-inflammatory and pain-relieving actions that can benefit athletes recovering from exercise or injury and patients recovering from surgery.

Scientific Support

A number of clinical trials have shown the benefit of using oral proteolytic enzymes as a digestive aid. Proteolytic enzymes are also theorized to help reduce symptoms of food allergies and to treat rheumatoid arthritis and other autoimmune diseases (which are thought by some alternative medicine practitioners to be caused by whole proteins from foods leaking into the blood and causing an immune reaction—sometimes called "leaky gut"). Unfortunately, not a great deal of scientific evidence, either from laboratory or clinical studies, supports the use of enzymes for treating allergies or autoimmune conditions.

Perhaps the strongest evidence for benefits of proteolytic enzyme supplements comes from the numerous European studies showing various enzyme blends to be effective in accelerating recovery from exercise and injury in athletes as well as promoting tissue repair in patients following surgery. In one study of football players suffering from ankle injuries, proteolytic enzyme supplements accelerated healing and got players back on the field about 50 percent faster than athletes assigned to receive a placebo tablet. A handful of other small trials in athletes have shown enzymes can help reduce inflammation, speed healing of bruises and other tissue injuries (including fractures), and reduce overall recovery time compared to a placebo. In patients recovering from facial and various reconstructive surgery, treatment with proteolytic enzymes significantly reduced swelling, bruising, and stiffness compared to placebo groups.

In one double-blind study, the pain-relieving effects of an enzyme blend (Wobenzym) were compared to those of a common analgesic drug (diclofenac) in eighty patients suffering from osteoarthritis of the knee. The study lasted two months, with a twenty-eight-day treatment period followed by a treatment-free period of another twenty-eight days. Pain measurements (at rest, on motion, on walking, and at night) showed a significant improvement after treatment in both groups, with a tendency to relapse in the treatment-free period. Of particular interest was the finding of no significant difference between the treatment groups—meaning that the enzyme blend was just as effective as the drug in relieving the pain and stiffness of arthritis. Similar findings have been reported for other painful or inflammatory conditions including carpal tunnel syndrome, fibromyalgia, facial bruising, ankle sprains, muscle soreness, and others.

Safety

Proteolytic enzymes are generally considered quite safe, although mild gastrointestinal side effects (heartburn) may result in some individuals. Individuals at risk for gastric or duodenal ulcers may want to avoid enzyme supplements, which may aggravate ulcerated tissues. In addition, because proteolytic enzyme supplements also tend to produce a modest anticoagulant (blood-thinning) effect, they should probably not be used in conjunction with warfarin or other blood-thinning agents.

Value

The scientific evidence supports the use of proteolytic enzyme supplements for enhancing digestive function and for speeding recovery from injury or surgery and reducing swelling and bruising. The benefits in autoimmune diseases and food allergies are less substantial and await further study. Thus, the moderate price of most proteolytic enzyme supplements ($10 to $30 per month) would appear to represent a good value for athletes wishing to enhance recovery from exercise or injury and for patients recovering from surgery.

Dosage

The dosage or strength of an enzyme supplement is typically expressed in "activity units" that refer to the enzyme's ability to digest a certain amount of protein. Because the same milligram amount of a particular enzyme may have different activity units based on its processing and blending, it may be advisable to select an enzyme supplement that employs a combination of enzymes with activity at different pH levels. Also, look for a brand that is "enteric coated"—meaning that the formulation is protected from digestion in the stomach for optimal delivery of the enzymes to the intestines where they can perform their actions.

WORKS CONSULTED

Adamek J, Prausova J, Wald M. Enzyme therapy in the treatment of lymphedema in the arm after breast carcinoma surgery. Rozhl Chir. 1997 Apr;76(4):203-4.

Buck JE, Phillips N. Trial of Chymoral in professional footballers. Br J Clin Pract. 1970 Sep;24(9):375-7.

Craig RP. The quantitative evaluation of the use of oral proteolytic enzymes in the treatment of sprained ankles. Injury. 1975 May;6(4):313-6.

Desser L, Rehberger A, Kokron E, Paukovits W. Cytokine synthesis in human peripheral blood mononuclear cells after oral administration of polyenzyme preparations. Oncology. 1993 Nov-Dec;50(6):403-7.

Duskova M, Wald M. Orally administered proteases in aesthetic surgery. Aesthetic Plast Surg. 1999 Jan-Feb;23(1):41-4.

Fisher JD, Weeks RL, Curry WM, Hrinda ME, Rosen LL. Effects of an oral enzyme preparation, Chymoral, upon serum proteins associated with injury (acute phase reactants) in man. J Med. 1974;5(5):258-73.

France LH. Treatment of injuries with orally administered Varidase as compared to Chymoral and Tanderil. Praxis. 1968 May 14;57(19):683-5.

Gal P, Tecl F, Skotakova J, Mach V. Systemic enzyme therapy in the treatment of supracondylar fractures of the humerus in children. Rozhl Chir. 1998 Dec;77(12):574-6.

Gubareva AA. The use of enzymes in treating patients with malignant lymphoma with a large tumor mass. Lik Sprava. 1998 Aug;(6):141-3.

Hingorani K. Oral enzyme therapy in severe back pain. Br J Clin Pract. 1968 May 5;22(5):209-10.

Hoernecke R, Doenicke A. Perioperative enzyme therapy. A significant supplement to postoperative pain therapy? Anaesthesist. 1993 Dec;42(12):856-61.

Kolomoiets MI, Shorikov II. The effect of the preparation Wobenzym on the antioxidant protection indices and on the functional-morphological properties of the erythrocytes in a toxic lesion of the liver. Lik Sprava. 1999 Jul;(5):124-8.

Korpan MI, Korpan NN, Chekman IS, Fialka V. The pharmacological action of wobenzym on blood coagulability. Lik Sprava. 1997 Jul-Aug;(4):70-2.

Kullich W, Schwann H. Circulating immune complexes and complement fragment iC3b in chronic polyarthritis during 12 months therapy with oral enzymes in comparison with oral gold. Wien Med Wochenschr. 1992;142(22):493-7.

Lie KK, Larsen RD, Posch JL. Therapeutic value of oral proteolytic enzymes following hand surgery. Arch Surg. 1969 Jan;98(1):103-4.

Love JW. The effect of orally administered proteolytic enzymes on the postoperative course of periodontal surgery. J Periodontol. 1968 Nov;39(6):337-40.

Martynenko AV. Wobenzym in the combined pathogenetic therapy of chronic urethrogenic prostatitis. Lik Sprava. 1998 Aug;(6):118-20.

McCue FC 3d, Webster TM, Gieck J. Clinical effects of proteolytic enzymes after reconstructive hand surgery. A double-blind evaluation of oral trypsin-chymotrypsin. Int Surg. 1972 Jun;57(6):479-82.

Neverov VA, Klimov AV. The pathogenetic basis for and clinical use of systemic enzyme therapy in traumatology and orthopedics. Vestn Khir Im I I Grek. 1999;158(1):41-4.

Rammer E, Friedrich F. Enzyme therapy in treatment of mastopathy. A randomized double-blind clinical study. Wien Klin Wochenschr. 1996;108(6):180-3.

Rathgeber WF. The use of proteolytic enzymes (chymoral) in sporting injuries. S Afr Med J. 1971 Feb 13;45(7):181-3.

Sakalova A, Kunze R, Holomanova D, Hapalova J, Chorvath B, Mistrik M, Sedlak J. Density of adhesive proteins after oral administration of proteolytic enzymes in multiple myeloma. Vnitr Lek. 1995 Dec;41(12):822-6.

Salisbury RE, Hunter JM. Evaluation of oral trypsin-chymotrypsin for prevention of swelling after hand surgery. Plast Reconstr Surg. 1972 Feb;49(2):171-5.

Sarkisov KR, Protasevich AI. On the use of proteolytic enzymes in the treatment of fractures of the mandible by extraoral supporting ligaments. Vestn Khir Im I I Grek. 1966 Apr;96(4):91-3.

Schwinger O. Results of oral enzyme therapy in wounds of muscles, tendons and bones after accidents. Wien Med Wochenschr. 1970 Sep 5;120(36):603-5.

Shaw PC. The use of a trypsin-chymotrypsin formulation in fractures of the hand. Br J Clin Pract. 1969 Jan 1;23(1):25-6.

Singer F, Oberleitner H. Drug therapy of activated arthrosis. On the effectiveness of an enzyme mixture versus diclofenac. Wien Med Wochenschr. 1996;146(3):55-8.

Steffen C, Menzel J. Basic studies on enzyme therapy of immune complex diseases. Wien Klin Wochenschr. 1985 Apr 12;97(8):376-85.

Steffen C, Menzel J, Smolen J. Intestinal resorption with 3H labeled enzyme mixture. Acta Med Austriaca. 1979;6(1):13-8.

Steffen C, Smolen J, Miehlke K, Horger I, Menzel J. Enzyme therapy in comparison with immune complex determinations in chronic polyarthritis. Z Rheumatol. 1985 Mar-Apr;44(2):51-6.

Strafun SS, Tovmasian VV. The use of vobenzym in the comprehensive treatment of patients with digital flexor tendon injury. Klin Khir. 2000;(4):39-40.

Suzdal'nitskii RS, Levando VA, Emel'ianov BA, Sokolov IA. The adaptational properties and immunoregulatory action of a preparation of proteolytic enzymes in experimental stress. Zh Mikrobiol Epidemiol Immunobiol. 1999 Sep-Oct;(5):103-6.

Tilscher H, Keusch R, Neumann K. Results of a double-blind, randomized comparative study of Wobenzym-placebo in patients with cervical syndrome. Wien Med Wochenschr. 1996;146(5):91-5.

Chapter 6

Supplements for Boosting Energy Levels

INTRODUCTION

The number one reason that most people report for a doctor visit is lack of energy. Relief from fatigue is also the top reason that most people turn to dietary supplements. There is certainly no shortage of products on the market—and with good reason. The lifestyles many of us lead these days are perfectly suited to draining our bodies of every last drop of energy. Many of us are up early to get the kids ready for school and maybe squeeze in a quick workout, or we're up late to finish a last-minute project. Never mind the sleep deprivation, because the major part of the day is full of meetings, errands, and soccer practices—leaving virtually no time for adequate nutrition. Skipped breakfasts, fast-food lunches, and take-out dinners are becoming the rule rather than the exception for many a harried family. It's no wonder that come Friday night, we can barely drag ourselves into bed.

It's often helpful for busy people to look at their hectic lifestyles from the viewpoint of an elite athlete. Olympic and professional athletes are up early every morning. Their day is typically chock-full of travel, practice sessions, meetings, drills, and interviews. Throughout the day, they need to concentrate on building and maintaining their strength and stamina, not to mention dealing with the stress that comes from knowing that their competition is doing exactly the same thing—and maybe a little bit better. A major difference between the hectic schedules of the elite athlete and Joe the Accountant is that Joe thinks he can work harder and longer to get more done by skipping breakfast, eating fast food for lunch, and losing sleep to work on more projects. Elite athletes, on the other hand, understand that they would only be spinning their wheels and setting themselves up for injury or illness if they didn't balance work with rest and proper nutrition.

Both athletes and regular Joes (and Janes) can see remarkable benefits from the simplest dietary strategy—power eating. For example, studies have conclusively shown that kids who eat breakfast before racing out the door to school do significantly better on a wide range of mental exercises—they are able to concentrate better and they get higher grades. Why shouldn't the same scenario hold true for adults and their physical and mental performance throughout the day and at work?

Before trying any of the energy supplements outlined in this chapter, take a couple of weeks to follow the tips in the next section to help get the rest of your diet in order. These eating strategies should do two things: (1) they'll make you feel better and more energetic because of the modest increase in metabolic rate that will occur, and (2) they'll put your body in the proper metabolic state to make the best use of any energy supplements that you choose to use in the future. Here goes.

DAILY EATING STRATEGIES

Breakfast

Let's start at the beginning—your first meal of the day. The most important rule to remember when it comes to breakfast is simple—*Eat It!* I know, it sounded corny when your mom told you, and it still sounds corny now, but breakfast *is* the most important meal of the day. If you don't eat breakfast, your metabolic rate drops slowly throughout the day, so you burn fewer and fewer fat calories while you're sitting at your desk listening to your stomach growl. Your blood sugar is also now at its lowest point, so your brain is being deprived of its primary fuel. Finally, by the time lunch rolls around, you'll be so famished that that triple cheeseburger with bacon (super-size it!) is going to look too good to pass up.

Do your body (and brain) a major favor by taking a measly ten minutes to have breakfast. Stay away from highly refined carbohydrates like those silly no-fat cereal bars—unless you want to be starving again by 10 a.m. Instead, grab something just as fast such as whole-grain oatmeal with a hard-boiled egg and a piece of fruit (300 calories). The trick here is to get a balanced intake of complex carbohydrates and protein—which will provide a continuous release of energy throughout the morning until your next pit stop at lunch.

Lunch

For your midday meal, we have another simple rule of thumb—don't be a pig! Nothing will put you to sleep faster than a big lunch. If at all possible, go for the salad. In most cases, you can practically eat your body weight in green salad without becoming drowsy. As always, watch the salad dressing, but don't avoid it completely because you can use a bit of fat to help slow the absorption of the carbs in your salad. As with breakfast, include a bit of protein with your salad—a few slices of turkey breast or some grilled fish would be perfect. The protein will do two things for you as the afternoon progresses: (1) it will maintain your level of alertness for the rest of the day by increasing the levels of neurotransmitters in the brain, and (2) it will help you avoid that mid-afternoon slump in energy levels that typically follows a carbohydrate-only lunch.

Dinner

Instead of thinking of dinner as some kind of gorge-fest, try to think of it simply as a somewhat larger lunch. The same rules apply—balance your carbs with lean protein, add some fat in the form of a yummy sauce or a buttered roll, and maybe treat yourself to a bit of dessert if you've had a good workout that day.

Snacks

Despite what your mother said about snacks before dinner ruining your appetite, don't be afraid to grab a piece of fruit for the commute home. There's little doubt that you can use the fiber, but it can also help curb hunger just enough so that you're not ravenous when you walk through the front door. Many people respond very nicely to six snacks or meals per day as opposed to the standard three-meal regimen. In that case, breakfast, lunch, and dinner follow the carbohydrate/protein balance described above but are reduced in size to allow two to three small (100 to 200 calories) snacks in between breakfast, lunch, dinner, and bedtime. Whatever works for you.

Beverages

Again, nutrition is simple when it comes to choosing what to drink throughout the day—drink more *water.* You've probably heard the old "eight cups a day" recommendation, to which I say, "Whatever." Just try to have a glass of water with each meal and snack followed by an extra one after your workout and another before bed. You may find yourself making a few more trips to the bathroom, but your body should get accustomed to your new hydration level in a week or so.

What about caffeine? A cup or two of coffee or tea in the morning isn't going to hurt you, but you may want to avoid it in the afternoon because it could interfere with a restful night of sleep and leave you feeling sleepy the next morning (a decidedly antienergy effect). Pregnant women may choose to completely eliminate caffeine from their diets due to concerns about an increased risk of miscarriage.

REST

One last thing before I discuss the actual herbs and supplements that can be effective in boosting energy levels. It never fails to amaze me how many people want to turn immediately to supplements as a quick fix for boosting their energy levels. The questions usually start off something like this: "Hi, I'm a lawyer who really needs more energy at work. I only get about four hours of sleep at night and I find myself losing steam by afternoon." A similar theme repeats itself from errand-running soccer moms to construction workers putting in eighteen-hour days. The only simple answer here is— *get more sleep!* You simply cannot make up for inadequate sleep with dietary supplements.

It's obvious that some people don't need as much sleep as others—so it is important to find out just how much sleep *you* need to function at 100 percent. For example, Bill Clinton only sleeps four hours each night, while both Jeff Bezos (the head of Amazon.com) and Bill Gates say that they need their full eight-hour allotment to be at top form. Top athletes such as Michael Johnson (200 meter world record holder) and Lance Armstrong (1999, 2000, 2001, and 2002 Tour de France cycling champion) report that they need as much as ten hours per night to fully recover during periods of intense training and competition.

Take this information for what it's worth—and do not expect any of the supplements outlined in this chapter to deliver significant benefits in energy levels or ability to concentrate until you have taken steps to consume a proper diet and get enough sleep.

SUPPLEMENTS

Among the many herbs promoted as energy boosters, ginseng is by far the most popular. Although the term "ginseng" actually encompasses a family of roots, *Panax ginseng,* the type grown in China, Korea, and Japan, is the type generally known for its energetic and antistress properties. In traditional Chinese medicine, *Panax ginseng* is used as a tonic herb with adaptogenic properties. In general terms, an adaptogen is a substance that boosts energy when you're fatigued and helps you combat stress and remain calm. The research on ginseng's benefits as a tonic and energy booster is equivocal. Some studies have shown increased energy levels in fatigued subjects, while the majority of studies on ginseng as an athletic performance aid have shown no effect. The differences between study results may have been due, in part, to the fact that many commercially available ginseng supplements actually contain little or no ginseng at all. The clearest indication that a supplement contains something other than real ginseng is the price—ginseng root is a very expensive ingredient, and "bargain" ginseng products are not what they're cracked up to be. Choose your ginseng supplements from a reputable manufacturer and insist that they guarantee the potency levels by using a standardized extract (this will be indicated on the label).

Siberian ginseng (eleuthero) is not truly ginseng but is a close enough cousin to deliver some of the same energetic benefits. Eleuthero is also known as ciwuja in popular sports products. The Siberian form of ginseng is generally a less expensive alternative to Asian or *Panax ginseng,* although it may have more of a stimulatory effect than an adaptogenic effect (not necessarily a bad thing if you just need a boost). Often promoted as an athletic performance enhancer, eleuthero may also possess mild to moderate benefits in promoting recovery following intense exercise—perhaps due in part to an enhanced delivery of oxygen to recovering muscles.

Ashwagandha, an herb from India, is sometimes called "Indian ginseng"—not because it is part of the ginseng family, but to suggest energy-promoting benefits similar to those attributed to the more well-known Asian and Siberian ginsengs. Although very little research has been done on ashwagandha, herbalists and natural medicine practitioners often recommend it to combat stress and fatigue.

Astragalus is an herb recommended as much for stimulation of the immune system as for its energy-promoting properties. Perhaps because chronic stress can both deplete energy levels and increase the risk of illness and infection, astragalus may be particularly beneficial in individuals who feel fatigued due to high levels of emotional and physical stress. Athletes in particular may benefit from astragalus supplementation because intense training and competition are often associated with an increased incidence of colds and other upper respiratory tract infections—conditions in which astragalus is thought to be most effective.

Cordyceps is a Chinese mushroom that has been used for centuries to reduce fatigue, increase stamina, and improve lung function. A few small-scale studies in the United States have confirmed the improvements in lung function and suggested that athletes may benefit from an increased ability to take up and use oxygen. At least one small study has suggested increased libido (sex drive), possibly due to elevated sex hormone levels, following cordyceps supplementation.

St. John's wort is not typically recommended specifically as an energy supplement, but rather as an herbal alternative to antidepressant medications. St. John's wort is effective in balancing mood and lifting spirits, and in many people it is also quite beneficial in relieving the fatigue that is often associated with mild to moderate depression. People who are depressed often lack the energy even to get themselves out of bed in the morning, and their day is a never-ending battle against fatigue. By correcting the neurotransmitter imbalance in the brain, St. John's wort can bring energy levels back to normal.

Finally, a general multivitamin/mineral supplement is always a good idea for anybody who needs more energy. Every energy-related reaction in your body relies in one way or another on vitamins and minerals as cofactors to make the reactions go. For example, B-complex vitamins are needed in protein/carbohydrate metabolism; chromium is involved in carbohydrate handling; magnesium and calcium are needed for proper muscle contraction; zinc and copper are required as enzyme cofactors in nearly 300 separate reactions; iron is needed to help shuttle oxygen in the blood—the list goes on and on. The supplements discussed in this chapter are listed in Table 6.1.

TABLE 6.1. Dietary Supplements for Boosting Energy Levels

Ingredient	Dose (per day)	Primary claim
B-complex vitamins	RDA levels and higher	Macronutrient metabolism
Bee pollen	1-3 g	Various energy claims
Brewer's yeast	1-3 tbsp	Various energy claims
Ginseng	100-300 mg	Adaptogen
Inosine	5-6 g	Enhances ATP production
NADH	2.5-15 mg	Reduces fatigue
Rhodiola	100-300 mg	Adaptogen
Royal jelly	50-100 mg	Various energy claims
Sea buckthorn	250-500 mg	Various energy claims
Vitamin B_1 (Thiamine)	1.5-15 mg	Carbohydrate metabolism
Vitamin B_2 (Riboflavin)	1.7-17 mg	Energy metabolism
Vitamin B_6 (Pyridoxine)	2-20 mg	Protein metabolism

GINSENG

What Is It?

Ginseng is a group of adaptogenic herbs from the plant family Araliaceae. Commonly, ginseng refers to "true" ginseng (*Panax ginseng* C. A. Meyer), as well as to a related plant called Siberian ginseng *(Eleutherococcus senticosus)* or eleuthero for short. Medicinal preparations are made from the roots of the plants. *Panax ginseng* has been used in traditional Chinese medicine for thousands of years for its beneficial effects on the central nervous system, protection from stress, antifatigue action, enhancement of sexual function, and acceleration of metabolism. Siberian ginseng did not really come into the picture as a botanical remedy until the twentieth century. Found in the northern regions of Russia, the roots of *Eleutherococcus senticosus* were sought out as a cheaper substitute for the expensive Oriental ginsengs. Soviet researchers found Siberian ginseng to be an excellent tonic to enhance athletic performance as well as to strengthen the body during times of stress. Several other "ginsengs" are used as adaptogenic tonics throughout the world; among them are *Panax quinquefolium* (also known as American ginseng) and ashwagandha, sometimes called Indian ginseng (although not a true ginseng). American ginseng is the most similar to "true" ginseng and is highly prized in the Orient, where it is thought to provide a "cooler" invigoration than the native ginseng.

Claims

- Increases energy levels
- Relieves stress
- Enhances athletic performance
- Tonic for well-being
- Immune enhancer
- Hypoglycemic (reduces blood sugar)
- Improves cognitive function

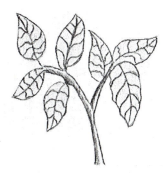

Theory

Ginseng, whether Siberian, *Panax,* or one of the other varieties, is termed an adaptogen. An adaptogen is defined as a therapeutic and restorative tonic generally considered to produce a "balancing" effect on the body. The properties generally attributed to adaptogens are a nonspecific increase in resistance to a wide range of stressors (including physical, chemical, and biological factors) as well as a "normalizing" action irrespective of the direction of the pathological changes. In general, an adaptogen can be thought of as a substance that helps the body to deal with stress.

The active components in Oriental and American ginseng are thought to be a family of triterpenoid saponins that are collectively referred to as ginsenosides. In general, most of the top-quality ginseng products, whether whole root or extract, are standardized for ginsenoside content. The active components in Siberian ginseng are considered to be a group of related compounds called eleutherosides. It has been theorized that ginseng's action in the body is due to its interaction within the hypothalamic-pituitary axis to balance secretion of adrenal corticotropic hormone (ACTH). ACTH has the ability to bind directly to brain cells and can affect a variety of stress-related processes in the body. These behaviors might include motivation, vitality, performance, and arousal.

Scientific Support

In a widely cited, although poorly conducted, study of student nurses on night duty, 1,200 mg of *Panax ginseng* appeared to improve general indices of stress and mood disturbances. Levels of free fatty acids, testosterone, and blood sugar, which were all elevated by night work, were significantly reduced to levels observed under day work. In another study, 2,700 mg per day of *Panax ginseng* was able to reduce blood sugar levels and insulin requirements in a group of diabetic subjects following three months of supplementation. One study of the effects of 200 mg per day of *Panax ginseng* extract for twelve weeks showed improvements over baseline values of mental performance (attention, mental processing, logical deduction, and both motor function and reaction time).

Over a period of several decades, German and Soviet researchers have studied the effects of *Panax ginseng* extract, typically standardized to 4 percent ginsenosides, on the performance of athletes. One study compared 200 mg per day of *Panax ginseng* extract in fourteen highly trained male athletes versus a placebo. The ginseng group showed an increase in their maximum oxygen uptake when compared to the placebo group as well as a statistically significant improvement in recovery time and lower serum lactate values. Other studies in various groups of young athletes have shown *Panax ginseng* extract to provide statistically significant improvements in performance measures such as forced vital capacity and maximum breathing capacity as compared to the placebo groups.

Unfortunately, the scientific evidence for ginseng is far from proven. For every study showing a positive benefit in terms of energy levels and/or physical or mental performance, there is at least one other study showing no benefits. Part of the discrepancy in results from well-controlled studies may have to do with differences between the ginseng extracts used in various studies (nonstandardized extracts with unknown quantities of active components).

Safety

For the most part, plants in the ginseng family are generally considered to be quite safe. There are no known drug interactions, contraindications, common allergic reactions, or toxicity to Siberian ginseng, *Panax ginseng,* or American ginseng, although it is recommended that a course of treatment with ginseng not exceed three months. A word of caution is recommended, however, for individuals with hypertension, as the stimulatory nature of some ginseng preparations has been reported to increase blood pressure. Additionally, individuals prone to hypoglycemia (low blood sugar) should use ginseng with caution due to the reported effects of ginseng to reduce blood sugar levels.

Value

Although the scientific evidence for the benefits of ginseng and its mechanisms of action can be considered inconclusive, the adaptogenic role of the various ginseng strains has proven beneficial for many thousands of years, and ginseng may, therefore, prove valuable as a "normalizing" substance during stressful conditions.

Dosage

Ginseng is one of the many herbal supplements that can be purchased readily as a whole root, a dried powder, or a standardized extract. The most precise approach would be to use a standardized extract to ensure that you are getting an effective product. Products should be standardized to contain 4 to 5 percent ginsenosides (for *Panax ginseng*) and 0.5 to 1.0 percent eleutherosides (for Siberian ginseng). Daily intake of 100 to 300 mg for three to six weeks is recommended to produce adaptogenic and energetic benefits. As a dried root, 1 to 2 g per day should be used in the case of American or Oriental ginseng or 2 to 3 g per day of Siberian ginseng.

WORKS CONSULTED

Avakian EV, Sugimoto RB, Taguchi S, Horvath SM. Effect of Panax ginseng extract on energy metabolism during exercise in rats. Planta Med. 1984 Apr;50(2):151-4.

Bruce A, Ekblom B, Nilsson I. The effect of vitamin and mineral supplements and health foods on physical endurance and performance. Proc Nutr Soc. 1985 Jul;44(2):283-95.

Dowling EA, Redondo DR, Branch JD, Jones S, McNabb G, Williams MH. Effect of Eleutherococcus senticosus on submaximal and maximal exercise performance. Med Sci Sports Exerc. 1996 Apr;28(4):482-9.

Grandhi A, Mujumdar AM, Patwardhan B. A comparative pharmacological investigation of Ashwagandha and Ginseng. J Ethnopharmacol. 1994 Dec;44(3):131-5.

Lewis WH, Zenger VE, Lynch RG. No adaptogen response of mice to ginseng and Eleutherococcus infusions. J Ethnopharmacol. 1983 Aug;8(2):209-14.

Martinez B, Staba EJ. The physiological effects of Aralia, Panax and Eleutherococcus on exercised rats. Jpn J Pharmacol. 1984 Jun;35(2):79-85.

Pieralisi G, Ripari P, Vecchiet L. Effects of a standardized ginseng extract combined with dimethylaminoethanol bitartrate, vitamins, minerals, and trace elements on physical performance during exercise. Clin Ther. 1991 May-Jun;13(3):373-82.

Ramachandran U, Divekar HM, Grover SK, Srivastava KK. New experimental model for the evaluation of adaptogenic products. J Ethnopharmacol. 1990 Jul;29(3):275-81.

Tadano T, Nakagawasai O, Niijima F, Tan-No K, Kisara K. The effects of traditional tonics on fatigue in mice differ from those of the antidepressant imipramine: A pharmacological and behavioral study. Am J Chin Med. 2000;28(1):97-104.

Wang BX, Cui JC, Liu AJ, Wu SK. Studies on the anti-fatigue effect of the saponins of stems and leaves of panax ginseng (SSLG). J Tradit Chin Med. 1983 Jun;3(2):89-94.

Wang LC, Lee TF. Effect of ginseng saponins on exercise performance in non-trained rats. Planta Med. 1998 Mar;64(2):130-3.

Yokozawa T, Oura H. Increased hepatic adenine nucleotide content by ginseng. J Ethnopharmacol. 1991 Aug;34(1):79-82.

Ziemba AW, Chmura J, Kaciuba-Uscilko H, Nazar K, Wisnik P, Gawronski W. Ginseng treatment improves psychomotor performance at rest and during graded exercise in young athletes. Int J Sport Nutr. 1999 Dec;9(4):371-7.

ROYAL JELLY

What Is It?

Royal jelly, unlike many supplements, is not the product of a plant. Instead, it is literally the food that creates queens—bees, that is. Worker bees secrete this milky white substance from glands on their heads. Royal jelly is a combination of flower nectar, sugars, proteins, and bee glandular secretions. For the first three days of a larval bee's life, it is fed royal jelly. After three days, however, royal jelly is fed only to the larva that is destined to be the queen. As a result of this royal diet, the queen bee is nearly 50 percent larger than her dutiful servants, and she lives an average of six years, compared to the six-week lifespan of those in her kingdom. Although laboratory studies have found that this mysterious food is a combination of well-known vitamins and nutrients, because of its effect on bee longevity it has traditionally been used as a health food in many cultures for everything from weight loss to liver disease to a fountain of eternal youth.

Claims

- Combats fatigue and insomnia
- Reduces atherosclerosis and high cholesterol
- Slows aging
- Treats failure to thrive in newborns
- Boosts immune system and prevents rheumatoid arthritis and multiple sclerosis

Theory

Because royal jelly is the food that sets worker bees and drones apart from the large and long-living queen bee, it is claimed that royal jelly could promote longevity in humans as well. Despite all of the grandiose claims, however, very little scientific support exists to substantiate the abundance of anecdotal evidence promoting its use.

Scientific Support

Royal jelly's mysterious composition is actually not so mysterious after scientific analysis. It is a concoction of water, amino acids and protein, sugars, fatty acids, some of the B vitamins, potassium, zinc, iron, copper, and manganese.

Despite the various claims, only one scientific study is available on anything other than the safety risks associated with royal jelly supplementation in humans. One review paper found that royal jelly significantly decreased total lipids and cholesterol in the blood and liver of rats and rabbits (rabbits being the standard animal model of atherosclerosis). Additionally, royal jelly slowed the formation of aortic plaques in rabbits fed a diet high in fats and cholesterol. Analysis of human trials revealed that in those with hyperlipidemia (too much fat in their blood), treatment with 50 to 100 mg per day of royal jelly was associated with a significant reduction in total serum lipids (10 percent) and cholesterol (14 percent). Furthermore, HDL (bad cholesterol) and LDL (good cholesterol) levels were normalized after treatment with royal jelly. It is not clear whether any of these unpublished reports were controlled for diet, exercise, or any other factors that could have also explained these favorable results.

More recent findings have shown that in rats and mice, royal jelly supplementation increased proliferation of immune cells, although without any human studies to bolster this finding, the results are of little value. Whether royal jelly would aid those with autoimmune diseases such as rheumatoid arthritis or multiple sclerosis needs to be explored, as the results of one animal study are only a basis for an initial hypothesis and not a substantiated claim.

Regarding speculation that taking royal jelly could combat fatigue and insomnia as well as reverse failure to thrive in newborns who do not grow sufficiently, a balanced diet with a high concentration of vital nutrients (whether from royal jelly or other supplements) could also help these conditions. It is well established that a lack of several nutrients in the diet can result in fatigue. For example, one popular claim is that women who take royal jelly note an energy boost more than men do. Because royal jelly contains iron, a mineral in which many women are deficient, and because a major symptom of iron deficiency is fatigue, the benefit of royal jelly in this case may be simply as a source of dietary iron. Conceivably, a study comparing the supplementation of iron-deficient women either with iron or with royal jelly while both groups are on a controlled diet may address the usefulness of taking royal jelly.

Safety

The safety profile for royal jelly is quite discouraging for certain populations. For those with a history of allergies or asthma, taking royal jelly has caused bronchial spasms, acute asthma, anaphylactic shock, and, in rare cases, death. It is therefore imperative that anyone who is considering supplementing with royal jelly consult with his or her physician, especially those who are allergic to bee stings or honey, or who have asthma. A special caution should be noted for pregnant and/or lactating women as well as for small children.

Value

Royal jelly is sold in tablet, capsule, and liquid form, and because it has a slightly bitter taste, it is also sold as a mixture with honey. Royal jelly formulations are generally sold in concentrations of 300 to 2,000 mg—with a one-month supply selling for about $11. Considering the lack of solid scientific evidence along with the fact that royal jelly may induce severe allergic reactions, the value of taking royal jelly appears to be quite limited. Those with high cholesterol or hyperlipidemia would probably benefit more from an increase in dietary fiber and exercise, and those with a diet poor in nutrients should spend their money on more varied foods or, if necessary, multivitamins.

Dosage

Studies showing any efficacy for royal jelly used doses of 50 to 100 mg per day. Although many formulations of royal jelly contain up to forty times the suggested dose, more has not been shown to be better. Thus, spreading a small amount of a honey-based royal jelly formulation onto some whole-grain bread may be the smartest, safest, and most cost-effective option.

WORKS CONSULTED

Albert S, Bhattacharya D, Klaudiny J, Schmitzova J, Simuth J. The family of major royal jelly proteins and its evolution. J Mol Evol. 1999 Aug;49(2):290-7.

Bullock RJ, Rohan A, Straatmans JA. Fatal royal jelly-induced asthma. Med J Aust. 1994 Jan 3;160(1):44.

Fleche C, Clement MC, Zeggane S, Faucon JP. Contamination of bee products and risk for human health: Situation in France. Rev Sci Tech. 1997 Aug;16(2):609-19.

Fujii A, Kobayashi S, Kuboyama N, Furukawa Y, Kaneko Y, Ishihama S, Yamamoto H, Tamura T. Augmentation of wound healing by royal jelly (RJ) in streptozotocin-diabetic rats. Jpn J Pharmacol. 1990 Jul;53(3):331-7.

Hamerlinck FF. Neopterin: A review. Exp Dermatol. 1999 Jun;8(3):167-76.

Harwood M, Harding S, Beasley R, Frankish PD. Asthma following royal jelly. N Z Med J. 1996 Aug 23;109(1028):325.

Laporte JR, Ibaanez L, Vendrell L, Ballarin E. Bronchospasm induced by royal jelly. Allergy. 1996 Jun;51(6):440.

Leung R, Ho A, Chan J, Choy D, Lai CK. Royal jelly consumption and hypersensitivity in the community. Clin Exp Allergy. 1997 Mar;27(3):333-6.

Lombardi C, Senna GE, Gatti B, Feligioni M, Riva G, Bonadonna P, Dama AR, Canonica GW, Passalacqua G. Allergic reactions to honey and royal jelly and their relationship with sensitization to compositae. Allergol Immunopathol (Madr). 1998 Nov-Dec;26(6):288-90.

Morris DH, Stare FJ. Unproven diet therapies in the treatment of the chronic fatigue syndrome. Arch Fam Med. 1993 Feb;2(2):181-6.

Peacock S, Murray V, Turton C. Respiratory distress and royal jelly. Br Med J. 1995 Dec 2;311(7018):1472.

Shaw D, Leon C, Kolev S, Murray V. Traditional remedies and food supplements. A 5-year toxicological study (1991-1995). Drug Saf. 1997 Nov;17(5):342-56.

Sver L, Orsolic N, Tadic Z, Njari B, Valpotic I, Basic I. A royal jelly as a new potential immunomodulator in rats and mice. Comp Immunol Microbiol Infect Dis. 1996 Jan;19(1):31-8.

Thien FC, Leung R, Baldo BA, Weiner JA, Plomley R, Czarny D. Asthma and anaphylaxis induced by royal jelly. Clin Exp Allergy. 1996 Feb;26(2):216-22.

Thien FC, Leung R, Plomley R, Weiner J, Czarny D. Royal jelly-induced asthma. Med J Aust. 1993 Nov 1;159(9):639.

Vittek J. Effect of royal jelly on serum lipids in experimental animals and humans with atherosclerosis. Experientia. 1995 Sep 29;51(9-10):927-35.

BEE POLLEN

What Is It?

The precise chemical analysis and composition of items sold as bee pollen is unclear. Bee pollen is harvested from beehives and may contain a widely variable mixture of vitamins, minerals, amino acids, carbohydrates, and several trace minerals.

Claims

- Increases energy
- Prolongs endurance
- Promotes weight loss
- Immune system stimulation

Theory

Anecdotal reports abound for the use of bee pollen as a natural "energy food"—probably due to its combination of small amounts of various vitamins and minerals involved in energy metabolism.

Scientific Support

No credible studies support the claimed effects of bee pollen as an energy food. Studies that have examined the effects of bee pollen on exercise performance have failed to show any beneficial effects of the supplement on parameters such as endurance capacity and maximal oxygen uptake.

Safety

Bee pollen tends to be a fairly innocuous mixture of small amounts of several nutrients, so there is little or no risk of consuming toxic levels of any specific nutrient. Because of the widely variable composition, however, consumers should purchase from a reliable manufacturer. Individuals with allergic reactions to bee stings should proceed with caution when consuming bee pollen, as several reports of adverse allergic reactions have been documented among susceptible individuals.

Value

Little to no scientific data supports the claimed benefits of dietary supplementation with bee pollen. Bee pollen is not recommended as a dietary supplement.

Dosage

Bee pollen is available in a number of commercial capsule products with recommended doses of 1 to 3 g daily. Dosage is variable based on product composition and manufacturer recommendations.

WORKS CONSULTED

Dudov IA, Morenets AA, Artiukh VP, Starodub NF. Immunomodulatory effect of honeybee flower pollen load. WMJ. 1994 Nov-Dec;66(6):91-3.

Dudov IA, Starodub NF. Antioxidant system of rat erythrocytes under conditions of prolonged intake of honeybee flower pollen load. WMJ. 1994 Nov-Dec;66(6):94-6.

Mahan LK. Nutrition and the allergic athlete. J Allergy Clin Immunol. 1984 May;73(5 Pt 2):728-34.

Qian B, Zang X, Liu X. Effects of bee pollen on lipid peroxides and immune response in aging and malnourished mice. Chung Kuo Chung Yao Tsa Chih. 1990 May;15(5):301-3, 319.

Xie Y, Wan B, Li W. Effect of bee pollen on maternal nutrition and fetal growth. Hua Hsi I Ko Ta Hsueh Hsueh Pao. 1994 Dec;25(4):434-7.

B-COMPLEX VITAMINS

The term "B complex" simply refers to a mixture or combination of the eight essential B vitamins (thiamine/B_1, riboflavin/B_2, niacin/B_3, pyridoxine/B_6, pantothenic acid, folic acid, cyanocobalamin/B_{12}, biotin). Most of the B vitamins play a critical role as cofactors in cellular energy metabolism. Cofactors can be thought of as "helper nutrients" that assist chemical reactions. For example, the process of glycolysis, which converts energy stored as glycogen into glucose molecules, requires vitamin B_6 and biotin. The conversion of pyruvate (a metabolite of glucose) to acetyl coenzyme A (the first step in the Krebs cycle in energy metabolism) requires pantothenic acid, and further metabolism requires biotin, riboflavin, and niacin. Lack of any of the B vitamins can cause fatigue and lethargy—which is why B-complex supplements are often promoted as energy boosters and stress formulas.

Virtually every multivitamin/mineral supplement available contains the full complement of B-complex vitamins at RDA or higher levels. It is often a better value to get your B vitamins as part of your daily multivitamin than as a separate B-complex supplement. This chapter on energy supplements contains information on Vitamins B_1 and B_2, while other B vitamins such as niacin, folic acid, B_6 and B_{12} are covered in Chapter 10 (Heart Health).

WORKS CONSULTED

Dreon DM, Butterfield GE. Vitamin B6 utilization in active and inactive young men. Am J Clin Nutr. 1986 May;43(5):816-24.

Eisinger J, Clairet D, Brue F, Ayavou T. Absence of correlation between magnesium and riboflavin status. Magnes Res. 1993 Jun;6(2):165-6.

Fogelholm M, Rehunen S, Gref CG, Laakso JT, Lehto J, Ruokonen I, Himberg JJ. Dietary intake and thiamin, iron, and zinc status in elite Nordic skiers during different training periods. Int J Sport Nutr. 1992 Dec;2(4):351-65.

Gray ME, Titlow LW. The effect of pangamic acid on maximal treadmill performance. Med Sci Sports Exerc. 1982;14(6):424-7.

Kopp-Woodroffe SA, Manore MM, Dueck CA, Skinner JS, Matt KS. Energy and nutrient status of amenorrheic athletes participating in a diet and exercise training intervention program. Int J Sport Nutr. 1999 Mar;9(1):70-88.

Leklem JE, Shultz TD. Increased plasma pyridoxal 5'-phosphate and vitamin B6 in male adolescents after 4500-meter run. Am J Clin Nutr. 1983 Oct;38(4):541-8.

Manore MM. Effect of physical activity on thiamine, riboflavin, and vitamin B-6 requirements. Am J Clin Nutr. 2000 Aug;72(2 Suppl):598S-606S.

Manore MM. Vitamin B6 and exercise. Int J Sport Nutr. 1994 Jun;4(2):89-103.

Rokitzki L, Sagredos A, Keck E, Sauer B, Keul J. Assessment of vitamin B2 status in performance athletes of various types of sports. J Nutr Sci Vitaminol (Tokyo). 1994 Feb;40(1):11-22.

Rokitzki L, Sagredos A, Reuss F, Petersen G, Keul J. Pantothenic acid levels in blood of athletes at rest and after aerobic exercise. Z Ernahrungswiss. 1993 Dec;32(4):282-8.

Rokitzki L, Sagredos AN, Reuss F, Buchner M, Keul J. Acute changes in vitamin B6 status in endurance athletes before and after a marathon. Int J Sport Nutr. 1994 Jun;4(2):154-65.

Rokitzki L, Sagredos AN, Reuss F, Cufi D, Keul J. Assessment of vitamin B6 status of strength and speedpower athletes. J Am Coll Nutr. 1994 Feb;13(1):87-94.

Suzuki M, Itokawa Y. Effects of thiamine supplementation on exercise-induced fatigue. Metab Brain Dis. 1996 Mar;11(1):95-106.

Tonda ME, Hart LL. N,N dimethylglycine and L-carnitine as performance enhancers in athletes. Ann Pharmacother. 1992 Jul-Aug;26(7-8):935-7.

VITAMIN B₁ (THIAMINE)

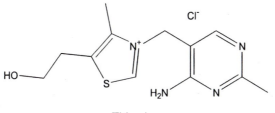

Thiamine

What Is It?

Thiamine is a water-soluble vitamin. The active form is a phosphorylated form of thiamine called thiamine pyrophosphate (TPP), which functions in carbohydrate metabolism to help convert pyruvate to acetyl CoA for entry to the Krebs cycle and subsequent steps to generate ATP. Thiamine also functions in maintaining nervous system and heart muscle health. Food sources include nuts, liver, brewer's yeast, and pork.

Claims

- Increases energy production
- Maintains memory
- Improves carbohydrate tolerance

Theory

Because of thiamine's role in carbohydrate metabolism and nerve function, supplements have been promoted for increasing energy and maintaining memory. Thiamine does seem to be involved in the release of acetylcholine, a neurotransmitter, from nerve cells, and thiamine deficiency is associated with generalized muscle weakness and mental confusion.

Scientific Support

Because dietary thiamine requirements are based on caloric intake, individuals who consume more calories, such as athletes, are likely to require a higher than average intake of thiamine to help process the extra carbohydrates into energy. During acute periods of stress, thiamine needs may be temporarily elevated, but outright thiamine deficiencies are rare except in individuals consuming a severely restricted diet.

Safety

No adverse side effects are known with thiamine intakes at RDA levels or even at levels several times the RDA.

Value

Virtually every multivitamin contains thiamine at 100 percent daily value (DV) levels (1.5 mg) or higher. Isolated supplements of thiamine are not necessary.

Dosage

The DV for thiamine is 1.5 mg.

WORKS CONSULTED

Fogelholm M, Rehunen S, Gref CG, Laakso JT, Lehto J, Ruokonen I, Himberg JJ. Dietary intake and thiamin, iron, and zinc status in elite Nordic skiers during different training periods. Int J Sport Nutr. 1992 Dec;2(4):351-65.

Kopp-Woodroffe SA, Manore MM, Dueck CA, Skinner JS, Matt KS. Energy and nutrient status of amenorrheic athletes participating in a diet and exercise training intervention program. Int J Sport Nutr. 1999 Mar;9(1):70-88.

Manore MM. Effect of physical activity on thiamine, riboflavin, and vitamin B-6 requirements. Am J Clin Nutr. 2000 Aug;72(2 Suppl):598S-606S.

Suzuki M, Itokawa Y. Effects of thiamine supplementation on exercise-induced fatigue. Metab Brain Dis. 1996 Mar;11(1):95-106.

VITAMIN B₂ (RIBOFLAVIN)

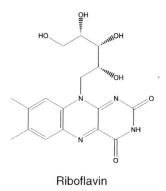

Riboflavin

What Is It?

Vitamin B$_2$, or riboflavin, is a water-soluble vitamin. It functions primarily as a coenzyme for many metabolic processes in the body such as red blood cell formation and nervous system function. Riboflavin is involved in energy production as part of the electron transport chain that produces cellular energy. As a building block for FAD (flavin adenine dinucleotide), riboflavin is a crucial component in converting food into energy. FAD is required for electron transport and ATP production in the Krebs cycle. Liver, dairy products, dark green vegetables, and many seafoods are good sources of riboflavin.

Claims

- Increases energy levels
- Reduces chronic fatigue
- Improves concentration and mood

Theory

Requirements for riboflavin, like most B vitamins, are related to calorie intake—so the more food you eat, the more riboflavin you need to support the metabolic processes which will convert that food into usable energy. Women should be aware that riboflavin needs are elevated during pregnancy and lactation as well as by the use of oral contraceptives (birth control pills). Athletes may require more riboflavin due both to increased caloric intake and increased needs of exercise.

Scientific Support

There is no strong support for the efficacy of isolated riboflavin supplements in promoting health outside of correcting a nutrient deficiency. Despite the role of riboflavin in a variety of energy-generating processes, a supplement is unlikely to improve energy levels in a well-nourished person.

Safety

No serious side effects have been reported for supplementation with riboflavin at levels several times above the DV of 1.7 mg. Because the body excretes excess riboflavin in the urine, high supplemental levels are likely to result in brightly colored urine (fluorescent yellow).

Value

Isolated riboflavin supplements are not necessary. Virtually all multivitamins and B-complex formulas contain riboflavin at RDA or higher levels.

Dosage

The DV for riboflavin is 1.7 mg.

WORKS CONSULTED

Eisinger J, Clairet D, Brue F, Ayavou T. Absence of correlation between magnesium and riboflavin status. Magnes Res. 1993 Jun;6(2):165-6.

Kopp-Woodroffe SA, Manore MM, Dueck CA, Skinner JS, Matt KS. Energy and nutrient status of amenorrheic athletes participating in a diet and exercise training intervention program. Int J Sport Nutr. 1999 Mar;9(1):70-88.

Manore MM. Effect of physical activity on thiamine, riboflavin, and vitamin B-6 requirements. Am J Clin Nutr. 2000 Aug;72(2 Suppl):598S-606S.

Rokitzki L, Sagredos A, Keck E, Sauer B, Keul J. Assessment of vitamin B2 status in performance athletes of various types of sports. J Nutr Sci Vitaminol (Tokyo). 1994 Feb;40(1):11-22.

RHODIOLA

What Is It?

Rhodiola *(Rhodiola rosea/Rhodiola crenulata)* comprises several species of plants in the Crassulaceae family and is generally found in the arctic mountain regions of Siberia. The root of the plant is used medicinally and is also known as Arctic root or golden root and more recently as crenulin. Rhodiola has been used for centuries to treat cold and flulike symptoms, promote longevity, and increase the body's resistance to physical and mental stresses.

Claims

- Promotes weight loss
- Aphrodisiac
- Relieves stress and depression
- Enhances athletic performance
- Immune enhancer
- Improves cognitive function

Theory

Rhodiola is typically considered to be an adaptogen (like ginseng) and is believed to invigorate the body and mind to increase resistance to a multitude of stresses. The key active constituents in rhodiola are believed to be rosavin, rosarin, rosin, and salidroside.

Scientific Support

In a placebo-controlled study of *Rhodiola rosea's* ability to mobilize fatty acids from adipose tissue, 121 subjects were given either *Rhodiola rosea* extract or a placebo, and their serum lipid levels were tested at rest and after one hour of exercise. The rhodiola group had 6 percent greater serum fatty acid levels than the placebo group at rest and 44 percent greater levels after one hour of exercise. This difference is presumably due to *Rhodiola rosea's* ability to activate adipose lipase, a key enzyme required to break down the body's fat stores.

In an open clinical trial of *Rhodiola rosea's* ability to alleviate symptoms of depression, 128 patients were given extract of *Rhodiola rosea.* The *Rhodiola rosea* extract was effective in reducing or removing symptoms of depression in 65 percent of the patients. In another open-label study, twenty-six out of thirty-five men suffering from weak erections or premature ejaculation reported improvements in sexual function following treatment with 100 to 150 mg of *Rhodiola rosea* extract for three months.

A placebo-controlled study of *Rhodiola rosea* extract's effects on intellectual performance showed a significant improvement in reading scores between rhodiola or placebo groups.

Safety

Rhodiola rosea extract is thought to be quite safe. There are no known contraindications or interactions with other drugs or herbs, but there is some potential for mild allergic reactions (rashes) in some individuals.

Value

Rhodiola rosea extract appears to be valuable as an adaptogen, to increase the body's ability to deal with a number of psychological and physiological stresses. Of particular value is the theoretical role for rhodiola in increasing the body's ability to take up and utilize oxygen—an effect similar to that of cordyceps, which may explain some of the nonstimulant energizing effects attributed to the plant. Rhodiola is often called the "poor man's cordyceps" because of ancient stories in which "commoners" used rhodiola for energy because the plants grew wild throughout the countryside, while only the emperor and his immediate family (and concubines) were allowed access to the rare cordyceps mushroom (which was harvested in the spring at elevations above 14,000 feet).

Dosage

General dosage recommendations for *Rhodiola rosea* extract are typically in the range of 100 to 300 mg per day.

WORKS CONSULTED

Linh PT, Kim YH, Hong SP, Jian JJ, Kang JS. Quantitative determination of salidroside and tyrosol from the underground part of Rhodiola rosea by high performance liquid chromatography. Arch Pharm Res. 2000 Aug;23(4):349-52.

Lishmanov IB, Naumova AV, Afanas'ev SA, Maslov LN. Contribution of the opioid system to realization of inotropic effects of Rhodiola rosea extracts in ischemic and reperfusion heart damage in vitro. Eksp Klin Farmakol. 1997 May-Jun;60(3):34-6.

Maslova LV, Kondrat'ev BI, Maslov LN, Lishmanov IB. The cardioprotective and antiadrenergic activity of an extract of Rhodiola rosea in stress. Eksp Klin Farmakol. 1994 Nov-Dec;57(6):61-3.

Rege NN, Thatte UM, Dahanukar SA. Adaptogenic properties of six rasayana herbs used in Ayurvedic medicine. Phytother Res. 1999 Jun;13(4):275-91.

Spasov AA, Wikman GK, Mandrikov VB, Mironova IA, Neumoin VV. A double-blind, placebo-controlled pilot study of the stimulating and adaptogenic effect of Rhodiola rosea SHR-5 extract on the fatigue of students caused by stress during an examination period with a repeated low-dose regimen. Phytomedicine. 2000 Apr;7(2):85-9.

Wang S, Wang FP. Studies on the chemical components of Rhodiola crenulata. Yao Hsueh Hsueh Pao. 1992;27(2):117-20.

Wang S, You XT, Wang FP. HPLC determination of salidroside in the roots of Rhodiola genus plants. Yao Hsueh Hsueh Pao. 1992;27(11):849-52.

Xu J, Xie J, Feng P, Su Z. Oxygen transfer characteristics in the compact callus aggregates of Rhodiola sachalinensis. Chin J Biotechnol. 1998;14(2):99-107.

Yoshikawa M, Shimada H, Horikawa S, Murakami T, Shimoda H, Yamahara J, Matsuda H. Bioactive constituents of Chinese natural medicines. IV. Rhodiolae radix. Chem Pharm Bull (Tokyo). 1997 Sep;45(9):1498-503.

Zhang S, Wang J, Zhang H. Chemical constituents of Tibetan medicinal herb Rhodiola kirilowii. Chung Kuo Chung Yao Tsa Chih. 1991 Aug;16(8):483, 512.

Zong Y, Lowell K, Ping JA, Che CT, Pezzuto JM, Fong HH. Phenolic constituents of Rhodiola coccinea, a Tibetan folk medicine. Planta Med. 1991 Dec;57(6):589.

NICOTINAMIDE ADENINE DINUCLEOTIDE (NADH)

What Is It?

NADH is the abbreviation for a molecule with the tongue-twisting name nicotinamide adenine dinucleotide (NAD), with the "H" indicating the reduced form (with an extra hydrogen atom). NADH functions as a coenzyme, meaning that it is a required cofactor for a metabolic process. Without the coenzyme, the reaction will not happen (or it may happen very slowly). In the case of NADH, coenzyme functions include roles in energy generation and production of neurotransmitters such as dopamine and norepinephrine.

Claims

- Increases energy levels
- Reduces chronic fatigue
- Stimulates cognitive function
- Enhances memory and reaction time
- Improves mood and emotional balance

Theory

The precise cause of chronic fatigue syndrome (CFS) is unknown. Symptoms include prolonged, debilitating fatigue, inability to concentrate, flu-like symptoms, muscle weakness, joint pain, headaches, and sleep disturbances. CFS affects about 500,000 Americans—but no effective treatment is known. Researchers theorize that CFS stems from a lack of the chemical responsible for cellular energy, adenosine triphosphate (ATP). One theory posits that both infections and stress may deplete cellular ATP levels and lead to chronic fatigue, but that supplemental levels of NADH can stimulate ATP production and provide benefits to people suffering from fatigue and cognitive dysfunction. Further benefits from NADH may stem from its role in stimulating the production of the neurotransmitters dopamine and norepinephrine (involved in brain function and memory) as well as from the stimulation of tyrosine hydroxylase (an enzyme involved in synthesizing neurotransmitters).

Scientific Support

Because NADH is thought to stimulate ATP generation, it may also increase energy levels and reduce fatigue. In a handful of small studies, 30 to

50 percent of patients receiving 10 mg per day of NADH for four weeks responded favorably by reporting a significant lessening of their chronic fatigue symptoms. More recent studies of NADH supplementation have shown a modest benefit in combating the deficits in energy and concentration associated with disrupted sleep and jet lag.

Safety

Some individuals report mild side effects such as nervousness and loss of appetite in the first few days of taking NADH. No serious side effects are documented.

Value

NADH supplements typically cost approximately $1 per 5 mg dose—meaning that an effective dose of the supplement may cost between $1 and $3 per day. Based on the lack of a reliable treatment for chronic fatigue syndrome and the preliminary positive results from pilot studies, individuals affected with this debilitating condition may want to consider investing $30 to $90 for a monthly supply.

Dosage

NADH is found in small amounts in most foods, with meat and poultry providing the highest levels at about 4 to 5 mg per 4 oz serving (but cooking may destroy NADH). The leading brand of NADH supplement, Enada, is available in 2.5 mg and 5 mg tablets. Suggested dosage ranges from 2.5 to 15 mg per day, depending on individual requirements (e.g., therapy or maintenance).

WORKS CONSULTED

Birkmayer JG. Coenzyme nicotinamide adenine dinucleotide: New therapeutic approach for improving dementia of the Alzheimer type. Ann Clin Lab Sci. 1996 Jan-Feb;26(1):1-9.

Calabrese L, Danao T, Camara E, Wilke W. Chronic fatigue syndrome. Am Fam Physician. 1992 Mar;45(3):1205-13.

Chester AC. Chronic fatigue syndrome criteria in patients with other forms of unexplained chronic fatigue. J Psychiatr Res. 1997 Jan-Feb;31(1):45-50.

Clark JB, Hayes DJ, Morgan-Hughes JA, Byrne E. Mitochondrial myopathies: Disorders of the respiratory chain and oxidative phosphorylation. J Inherit Metab Dis. 1984;7(Suppl 1):62-8.

Colquhoun D, Senn S. Is NADH effective in the treatment of chronic fatigue syndrome? Ann Allergy Asthma Immunol. 2000 Jun;84(6):639-40.

Forsyth LM, Preuss HG, MacDowell AL, Chiazze L Jr, Birkmayer GD, Bellanti JA. Therapeutic effects of oral NADH on the symptoms of patients with chronic fatigue syndrome. Ann Allergy Asthma Immunol. 1999 Feb;82(2):185-91.

Gantz NM, Holmes GP. Treatment of patients with chronic fatigue syndrome. Drugs. 1989 Dec;38(6):855-62.

Houde SC, Kampfe-Leacher R. Chronic fatigue syndrome: An update for clinicians in primary care. Nurse Pract. 1997 Jul;22(7):30, 35-6, 39-40 passim.

Klonoff DC. Chronic fatigue syndrome. Clin Infect Dis. 1992 Nov;15(5):812-23.

Komaroff AL, Buchwald D. Symptoms and signs of chronic fatigue syndrome. Rev Infect Dis. 1991 Jan-Feb;13(Suppl 1):S8-11.

Lewis SF, Haller RG. The pathophysiology of McArdle's disease: Clues to regulation in exercise and fatigue. J Appl Physiol. 1986 Aug;61(2):391-401. Review.

Lieb K, Dammann G, Berger M, Bauer J. Chronic fatigue syndrome. Definition, diagnostic measures and therapeutic possibilities. Nervenarzt. 1996 Sep;67(9): 711-20.

Sussman KE, Alfrey A, Kirsch WM, Zweig P, Felig P, Messner F. Chronic lactic acidosis in an adult. A new syndrome associated with an altered redox state of certain NAD-NADH coupled reactions. Am J Med. 1970 Jan;48(1):104-12.

Wearden AJ, Morriss RK, Mullis R, Strickland PL, Pearson DJ, Appleby L, Campbell IT, Morris JA. Randomised, double-blind, placebo-controlled treatment trial of fluoxetine and graded exercise for chronic fatigue syndrome. Br J Psychiatry. 1998 Jun;172:485-90.

SEA BUCKTHORN

What Is It?

Sea buckthorn *(Hippophae rhamnoides)*, also known as Siberian pine-apple, is a small shrub native to Europe and Asia. The berries have been used since the days of ancient Greece as a remedy for promoting weight gain and a shiny coat in horses. In traditional Chinese medicine, sea buckthorn is used for "invigoration" and increasing energy levels. In Russia, sea buckthorn has been used in creams to help protect cosmonauts from radiation damage. A number of cosmetics companies in the United States add sea buckthorn to their skin creams as a wound healer and skin protectant. In China, a number of sea buckthorn–based sports drinks have been used by athletes as a training and performance aid.

Claims

- Increases energy levels
- Promotes wound healing
- Protects skin from UV damage

Theory

Biochemical analysis of sea buckthorn berries reveal them as a rich source of vitamins C and E, carotenoids, and flavonoids as well as glucose, fructose, and several amino acids and fatty acids (like all other berries).

Scientific Support

There are a handful of preliminary studies on the wound-healing and tissue-protecting ability of sea buckthorn extracts, but no published reports support its use to improve energy levels. In animal studies, sea buckthorn has been shown to strengthen cardiac pump function and myocardial contractility in dogs with heart failure. It also appears to improve the heart's ability to use oxygen (in dogs and in test-tube cultures of heart cells from rats and guinea pigs).

Safety

No known side effects are associated with topical or internal use of sea buckthorn, but there are also no studies showing long-term safety.

Value

Preparations of sea buckthorn oils are generally recommended for external use in the case of burns and other skin damage as well as internally for the treatment of stomach and duodenal ulcers. There have also been anecdotal reports of using sea buckthorn extracts to reduce tumor growth and treat high cholesterol and high blood pressure. Sea buckthorn oils contain high concentrations of palmitoleic acid. This relatively rare fatty acid is a component of skin fat and can support cell tissue and wound healing. It is generally accepted in the cosmetic industry that sea buckthorn oils have unique antiaging properties. As a result, they are becoming an important component of many facial creams.

Dosage

Due to the lack of solid scientific evidence for the proposed benefits of sea buckthorn, it is difficult to make a definitive dosage recommendation. In general, typical usage of sea buckthorn may range from 250 to 500 mg orally as an energy promoter to gram quantities as a topical skin protectant and healer.

WORKS CONSULTED

Cheng TJ. Protective action of seed oil of Hippophae rhamnoides L. (HR) against experimental liver injury in mice. Chung Hua Yu Fang I Hsueh Tsa Chih. 1992 Jul;26(4):227-9.

Cheng TJ, Pu JK, Wu LW, Ma ZR, Cao Z, Li TJ. An preliminary study on hepatoprotective action of seed oil of Hippophae rhamnoides L. (HR) and mechanism of the action. Chung Kuo Chung Yao Tsa Chih. 1994 Jun;19(6):367-70, 384.

Fu G, Zhao S, Feng R, Xiao P. Determination of flavonoids in the leaves of Hippophae L. by HPLC. Chung Kuo Chung Yao Tsa Chih. 1997 May;22(5):299-300, 320.

Ianev E, Radev S, Balutsov M, Klouchek E, Popov A. The effect of an extract of sea buckthorn (Hippophae rhamnoides L.) on the healing of experimental skin wounds in rats. Khirurgiia (Sofiia). 1995;48(3):30-3.

Khizhazi AA. The therapeutic and prophylactic anti-ulcerogenic action of marigold (Tagetes patula L.) and sea buckthorn (Hippophae) oils in neurogenic ulcerative lesions caused by immobilization, noise and vibration. Lik Sprava. 1998 Jan-Feb;(1):172-6.

Liu FM, Li ZX, Shi S. Effects of total flavones of Hippophae rhamnoides L on cultured rat heart cells and on cAMP level and adenylate cyclase in myocardium. Chung Kuo Yao Li Hsueh Pao. 1988 Nov;9(6):539-42.

Nikulin AA, Iakusheva EN, Zakharova NM. A comparative pharmacological evaluation of sea buckthorn, rose and plantain oils in experimental eye burns. Eksp Klin Farmakol. 1992 Jul-Aug;55(4):64-6.

Wu J, Yu XJ, Ma X, Li XG, Liu D. Electrophysiologic effects of total flavones of Hippophae rhamnoides L on guinea pig papillary muscles and cultured rat myocardial cells. Chung Kuo Yao Li Hsueh Pao. 1994 Jul;15(4):341-3.

Wu Y, Wang Y, Wang B, Lei H, Yang Y. Effects of total flavones of fructus Hippophae (TFH) on cardiac function and hemodynamics of anesthetized open-chest dogs with acute heart failure. Chung Kuo Chung Yao Tsa Chih. 1997 Jul;22(7):429-31, 448.

Zhang MS. A control trial of flavonoids of Hippophae rhamnoides L. in treating ischemic heart disease. Chung Hua Hsin Hsueh Kuan Ping Tsa Chih. 1987 Apr;15(2):97-9.

BREWER'S YEAST

What Is It?

Brewer's yeast *(Saccharomyces cerevisiae)* is just what it sounds like—the yeast that brewers use to make beer. Brewer's yeast is different from *baker's* yeast (which causes bread to rise) and is not related to the species that causes yeast infections, *Candida albicans*. Most of the supplemental forms of brewer's yeast on the market are a by-product of beer making—so many of the raw forms may have quite a bitter taste.

Claims

- Lowers cholesterol
- Increases energy levels
- Boosts exercise performance
- Reduces blood sugar

Theory

Brewer's yeast tends to be a fairly good source of many vitamins and minerals, including thiamine (B_1), riboflavin (B_2), niacin (B_3), folic acid, pyridoxine (B_6), B_{12}, chromium, copper, iron, and zinc—all of which have widespread functions in many areas of metabolism and health.

Scientific Support

There really aren't any credible scientific reports showing the efficacy of brewer's yeast on any of the health claims made by manufacturers. Aside from using it as a source of B vitamins, the evidence for brewer's yeast as an effective dietary supplement is weak.

Safety

Only mild gastrointestinal side effects are noted—usually occurring in the first few days as your body gets used to the yeast intake.

Value

Because the exact nutrient content of brewer's yeast will vary depending on how it is grown and processed, make sure you check the label for precise nutrient levels. Brewer's yeast products, depending on the other nutrients that it may be mixed with, tend to cost in the range of $20 to $30 per month. There are certainly less expensive and more pure sources of vitamins and minerals to choose from.

Dosage

If you decide to give brewer's yeast a try, it is suggested to start with about ¼ teaspoon per day, slowly increasing your intake to 1 to 3 tablespoons per day (check the supplement facts panel for recommended serving sizes of specific products).

WORKS CONSULTED

Alic M. Baker's yeast in Crohn's disease—can it kill you? Am J Gastroenterol. 1999 Jun;94(6):1711.

Dorant E, van den Brandt PA, Hamstra AM, Feenstra MH, Goldbohm RA, Hermus RJ, Sturmans F. The use of vitamins, minerals and other dietary supplements in The Netherlands. Int J Vitam Nutr Res. 1993;63(1):4-10.

McKenzie H, Main J, Pennington CR, Parratt D. Antibody to selected strains of Saccharomyces cerevisiae (baker's and brewer's yeast) and Candida albicans in Crohn's disease. Gut. 1990 May;31(5):536-8.

Warin RP. Food factors in urticaria. J Hum Nutr. 1976 Jun;30(3):179-86.

INOSINE

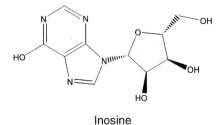

Inosine

What Is It?

Inosine is a nucleoside involved in the formation of purines and has possible roles in energy metabolism.

Claims

- Increases energy levels and endurance performance
- Enhances ATP production
- Reduces lactic acid accumulation

Theory

Many of the effects attributed to inosine stem from its potential role in increasing levels of a compound known as 2,3 DPG in red blood cells. An enhanced 2,3 DPG level would allow an easier release of oxygen from the blood cells to the tissues and, in theory, an enhancement of energy generation, ability to remove lactic acid, and an overall improvement in exercise performance.

Scientific Support

Several studies have investigated the effects of inosine supplementation on aerobic performance in athletes, yet none have shown convincing benefits associated with the supplement. In at least two studies, a potential for inosine to *interfere* with energy metabolism was suggested, particularly in high-intensity events such as sprinting.

Safety

In general, supplemental inosine appears to be safe at doses of as much as 5 to 6 g for several weeks. In susceptible individuals, however, inosine supplementation may lead to buildup of uric acid levels. Uric acid is a by-product of inosine metabolism and may lead to painful symptoms of gout such as arthritic joints and toes due to deposits of uric acid crystals.

Value

Because no convincing studies demonstrate the beneficial effects of inosine as a dietary supplement, it is not recommended as a stand-alone dietary aid. Inosine is commonly part of a mixture of ingredients in dietary supplements that may contribute to energy metabolism.

Dosage

Doses of 5 to 6 g over approximately one week have failed to show consistent beneficial effects. Using inosine as part of a more diverse mixture of energy-promoting supplements may be a more logical approach.

WORKS CONSULTED

Bianchi GP, Grossi G, Bargossi AM, Fiorella PL, Marchesini G. Can oxypurines plasma levels classify the type of physical exercise? J Sports Med Phys Fitness. 1999 Jun;39(2):123-7.

Febbraio MA, Dancey J. Skeletal muscle energy metabolism during prolonged, fatiguing exercise. J Appl Physiol. 1999 Dec;87(6):2341-7.

Febbraio MA, Flanagan TR, Snow RJ, Zhao S, Carey MF. Effect of creatine supplementation on intramuscular TCr, metabolism and performance during intermittent, supramaximal exercise in humans. Acta Physiol Scand. 1995 Dec; 155(4):387-95.

Green H, Roy B, Grant S, Otto C, Pipe A, McKenzie D, Johnson M. Human skeletal muscle exercise metabolism following an expedition to Mount Denali. Am J Physiol Regul Integr Comp Physiol. 2000 Nov;279(5):R1872-9.

Iwasa Y, Iwasa M, Omori Y, Toki T, Yamamoto A, Maeda H, Kume M, Ogoshi S. The well-balanced nucleoside-nucleotide mixture "OG-VI" for special medical purposes. Nutrition. 1997 Apr;13(4):361-4.

Jabs CM, Sigurdsson GH, Neglen P. Plasma levels of high-energy compounds compared with severity of illness in critically ill patients in the intensive care unit. Surgery. 1998 Jul;124(1):65-72.

Norman B. Inosine monophosphate accumulation in energy-deficient human skeletal muscle with reference to substrate availability, fibre types and AMP deaminase activity. Scand J Clin Lab Invest. 1995 Dec;55(8):733-41.

Norman B, Heden P, Jansson E. Small accumulation of inosine monophosphate (IMP) despite high lactate levels in latissimus dorsi during transplantation. Clin Physiol. 1991 Jul;11(4):375-84.

Norman B, Sollevi A, Kaijser L, Jansson E. ATP breakdown products in human skeletal muscle during prolonged exercise to exhaustion. Clin Physiol. 1987 Dec;7(6):503-10.

Pouw EM, Schols AM, van der Vusse GJ, Wouters EF. Elevated inosine monophosphate levels in resting muscle of patients with stable chronic obstructive pulmonary disease. Am J Respir Crit Care Med. 1998 Feb;157(2):453-7.

Sahlin K. Metabolic factors in fatigue. Sports Med. 1992 Feb;13(2):99-107.

Sahlin K, Broberg S. Adenine nucleotide depletion in human muscle during exercise: Causality and significance of AMP deamination. Int J Sports Med. 1990 May;11(Suppl 2):S62-7.

Smolenski RT, Lachno DR, Yacoub MH. Adenine nucleotide catabolism in human myocardium during heart and heart-lung transplantation. Eur J Cardiothorac Surg. 1992;6(1):25-30.

Tavazzi B, Di Pierro D, Amorini AM, Fazzina G, Tuttobene M, Giardina B, Lazzarino G. Energy metabolism and lipid peroxidation of human erythrocytes as a function of increased oxidative stress. Eur J Biochem. 2000 Feb;267(3):684-9.

Wagner DR, Gresser U, Zollner N. Effects of oral ribose on muscle metabolism during bicycle ergometer in AMPD-deficient patients. Ann Nutr Metab. 1991; 35(5):297-302.

Chapter 7

Supplements for Bone Health

INTRODUCTION

If you don't think that osteoporosis is a disease that you should be concerned about, think again. While most women are concerned about their risk for breast cancer and many men are concerned about prostate cancer, they really should be concerned about their risk for developing osteoporosis later in life. Why? Because the lifetime risk of hip fracture in white women is 15 percent—as great as that of breast, endometrial, and ovarian cancer *combined*. For men, the lifetime risk of hip fracture (5 percent) is as great as the risk of developing prostate cancer. For men and women alike, promoting and maintaining optimal bone health is an important consideration at any age.

Osteoporosis, which literally means "porous bones," occurs when the amount of mineral in the bones drops to a level low enough to permit fractures to occur after minimal trauma. The mineral content of the bones (called bone mineral density or BMD) drops gradually throughout life as a normal process of aging. In women, who are at a higher risk for osteoporosis, BMD begins to decline slowly around age thirty-five. For three to five years before and three to five years after menopause (which occurs, on average, around age fifty) bone loss speeds up dramatically due to the loss of estrogen production by the ovaries. Bone continues to be lost at a slower rate after this rapid phase and continues to be lost slowly as we age. If the BMD drops too fast or gets too low, however, the risk for fractures is increased.

Although more than 25 million Americans suffer from osteoporosis, the stereotypical osteoporotic patient is a postmenopausal white female, often with a history of low body weight, low calcium intake, and a sedentary lifestyle. Each of these factors (gender, age, hormonal status, nutritional intake, and physical activity) can influence the risk for developing osteoporosis. As such, osteoporosis is considered a multifactorial disease—meaning that it is caused by a number of factors and cannot be "cured" by changing any single factor.

FACTORS ASSOCIATED WITH SKELETAL HEALTH

Nutrition

The primary role of adequate nutrition for skeletal health is that it allows development of the largest possible skeleton during growth, thus protecting against calcium loss in old age. Large population studies have shown that if we could ensure a fully adequate intake of calcium and vitamin D for every member of the North American and European populations, we could eradicate as much as 50 percent of the worldwide osteoporosis burden.

When calcium intake is restricted during growth, the body tries to spread the inadequate amount of calcium over as much of the skeleton as possible. The result is not stunted growth, but normal growth accompanied by a reduced amount of bone tissue overall. The bone is normal in every way, but it tends to be flimsy, thin, and weak. Such bone will not only not serve the structural needs under conditions of high mechanical stress, but will also not serve as much of a calcium reservoir in later years, when calcium stores are drawn upon with greater frequency.

Chronically low calcium intake results in a chronic drain on the body's calcium reserve. There is an old analogy about your skeleton being a bank vault for calcium storage. When you are getting enough calcium in your diet, you are able to store some of it—to make "deposits" in the vault. During times of low calcium intake, you can draw on these savings to pay your "bills"—which in this case are the other functions for which the body uses calcium (electrolyte balance, nerve conduction, muscle contraction).

Hormonal Status

Whenever women lose ovarian hormones (menopause), or men lose testosterone (andropause), the skeleton seems to sense that it has more bone than it needs. The result is an increase in bone resorption (breakdown) to get rid of what the body thinks it doesn't need. A woman can expect to lose approximately 15 percent of her peak bone mass during menopause. No amount of increased calcium intake or increased exercise will substantially influence this change due to hormones.

Exercise

Bones have the unique ability to adjust their mass in response to stress. Normal deformation of living bones is in the range of 0.1 percent to 0.15 percent. This means that when a force is applied to a bone—say, by exercise—the bone will bend slightly. When a bone encounters a force that causes a deformation greater than this range (more bending than it wants to do), the skeleton responds by depositing more bone to the area. When less deformation is "sensed" by the skeleton, bone is removed from the area. Thus, the more stress is delivered to the skeleton, the more bone is deposited to maintain a set level of deformation. The less exercise, the less strain, and the less bone that is needed, so the body gets rid of the excess bone by increasing the rate of bone resorption.

Body Weight

Body weight is a strong predictor of bone mass and density. Overweight women are known to have more bone and less bone loss at menopause and have been shown to absorb calcium with greater efficiency. Each of these factors may be due to somewhat higher estrogen levels in heavier women. Thin women tend to have a greater risk of osteoporotic fractures. This increased fracture risk in thin women is partly due to lower bone mass and also partly due to having less soft tissue around their bones to absorb the shock of a fall.

Two factors that interact to help determine body weight—dietary intake and physical activity—also have a strong influence on overall bone mass. For example, a thin woman may be at a higher risk for osteoporosis because of low body weight, but if her low weight was achieved through a program of rigorous exercise, then perhaps her risk is not as high as we would expect based on body weight alone. On the other hand, suppose another woman achieves her low body weight through chronic dietary restriction. Chances are that her diet is also lacking in important nutrients such as calcium, phosphorous, magnesium, vitamin K, boron, and zinc, which are needed to support proper bone health.

Other Factors

When most people think of bone health and nutrition, they immediately think of calcium. Although calcium intake is certainly a critical component of achieving and maintaining healthy bones, there is much more to the optimal nutrition of bones than just calcium. Many nutritional factors can interact to influence calcium absorption, bone breakdown, and bone formation. For example, high levels of both sodium and protein in the diet can increase the amount of calcium lost each day in the urine, while both fiber and caffeine slightly reduce the absorption of calcium from the diet. For example, because of dietary fiber content, the calcium in beans is only about half as available as the calcium found in milk, while calcium from spinach is almost totally unavailable to the body.

Major Risk Factors for Osteoporosis

- White or Asian ethnicity
- Family history (genetic causes)
- Small body frame/low body weight (less than 130 lb)
- Low dietary calcium intake
- Amenorrhea, irregular menstrual cycles, or early natural menopause
- Sedentary lifestyle
- Cigarette smoking
- Medications that increase bone loss (corticosteroids)

DIETARY SUPPLEMENTS FOR HEALTHY BONES

Calcium supplements are the king (queen) of the hill when it comes to bone health—but it's important to remember that bones are a lot more than just sticks of calcium (that's what chalk is). Although calcium supplements have been clearly shown to help reduce bone loss and increase bone density at doses of 500 to 1,500 mg per day, a number of additional nutrients are crucial for the optimal utilization of calcium. For example, vitamin D is needed for optimal absorption of calcium from the intestines as well as for proper maintenance of calcium levels within the blood and bone tissue. Elderly people are most at risk for vitamin D deficiency because production is reduced as we age. Vitamin D supplements of 200 to 400 IU can help maintain calcium absorption. Vitamin K status has been linked to overall bone health in elderly subjects, with those having low vitamin K levels also showing reduced bone density. Because vitamin K functions in coordinating the proper deposition of calcium crystals in bone tissue, it works in conjunction with vitamin D to get calcium from the gastrointestinal tract into the blood and then into the bones in a coordinated fashion. Likewise, the absorption of calcium is also tied to adequate levels of magnesium and zinc in the diet. As with calcium, both minerals are found at high concentrations in bones and are thought to help maintain optimal bone metabolism. Supplemental intakes of 15 to 30 mg of zinc and 200 to 400 mg of magnesium are often combined with calcium preparations.

Occasionally, bone supplements also contain varying levels of trace minerals involved in bone metabolism. For example, copper is involved in the synthesis of a protein called collagen, which forms the major nonmineral structural portion of bones. Levels of copper up to 1 to 3 mg per day seem to be well tolerated and may help maintain bone health by supporting collagen production. Other minerals such as boron, silicon, and manganese may play a supporting role in bone metabolism, but isolated supplements are generally not needed as most are available in multivitamin/mineral supplements.

Last, but certainly not least, are dietary supplements containing isoflavones—usually from soybeans, red clover, or another plant source (also called "phytoestrogens"). The chemical structure of isoflavone compounds is similar enough to estrogen to permit some of the good effects of estrogen (such as bone building) without many of the bad side effects (such as increased breast cancer risk). Most of the time, the isoflavones in dietary supplements are a mixture of the primary soy extracts genistein and daidzein, but synthetic isoflavones, such as ipriflavone, are also available in many dietary supplements. The isoflavones appear to be safe and effective in reducing bone loss during menopause, so much so that they are frequently included in mainstream calcium supplements. A summary of supplements for bone health appears in Table 7.1.

TABLE 7.1. Dietary Supplements for Bone Health

Ingredient	Dose (per day)	Primary claims
Boron	1-2 mg	Builds bone
Calcium	500-1,500 mg	Slows bone loss and builds bone
Isoflavones	25-50 mg	Slows bone loss
Magnesium	250-750 mg	Promotes calcium absorption
Vitamin D	200-500 IU	Increases calcium absorption
Vitamin K	10-120 mcg	Promotes bone formation

CALCIUM

What Is It?

Calcium is the most abundant mineral in the human body. The average adult has about 2 to 3 lb of calcium, with about 99 percent in the bones and teeth. The remaining 1 percent of body calcium is found in the blood and within cells, where calcium helps with dozens of metabolic processes. This 1 percent of blood and cellular calcium is so tightly maintained within normal ranges that the body will draw on calcium stores in the bones to get it—even at the expense of causing osteoporosis. Good dietary sources of calcium include all dairy products and several vegetables such as broccoli, bok choy, and kale. A cup of milk contains about 300 mg of calcium.

Claims

- Promotes strong bones
- Lowers blood pressure
- Reduces risk of colon cancer
- Reduces symptoms of premenstrual syndrome (PMS)

Theory

More than 99 percent of the body's calcium is stored in bones, where it serves both a structural and physiological role. The most obvious need for calcium is to help build and maintain strong bones, but calcium is also important for blood clotting, muscle contraction, nerve transmission, and maintenance of normal blood pressure. There is also some evidence that calcium supplements may be helpful in reducing the risk of colon cancer, regulating heart rhythms, and treating PMS.

Scientific Support

For decades, we have known about the important role that calcium plays in achieving and maintaining strong bones—and helping to prevent osteoporosis. More recent research, much of it conducted over the past five years, has suggested a number of other beneficial health effects of getting adequate calcium in the diet. Among the more exciting research, scientists have recently shown that eating more calcium-rich foods reduces the risk of colon cancer in men and that women who take daily calcium supplements can cut premenstrual symptoms in half (pain, bloating, mood swings, and food cravings). In other studies, researchers found that adequate calcium intake (along with vitamin D) can reduce blood pressure in women with mild hypertension and in black teenagers (two groups who rarely consume enough calcium). The hypertensive effects of a high-salt diet tend to be most pronounced among people whose diets are low in calcium. In addition, women who take calcium supplements during pregnancy tend to give birth to children with healthier blood pressure levels (lower than average for the first seven years of life)—which may reduce the child's risk of developing high blood pressure later in life.

If that weren't enough evidence that calcium supplements might be a good idea, there is also some evidence that calcium can even influence mood and behavior. The suggestion comes from a space shuttle study in which hypertensive rats became agitated when consuming a low-calcium diet, but were more calm and relaxed when their diets contained adequate calcium levels.

Additional functions in which calcium plays a role:

- Transmission of nerve impulses and control of muscle contractions
- Release of chemical messengers for communication between nerves
- Chemical signaling between cells
- Regulation of hormone and enzyme production and activity (regulation of digestion, fat metabolism, energy production)
- Hormone secretion
- Blood clotting
- Wound healing

Safety

Side effects from calcium supplements are rare, but may be possible at extremely high intakes. The upper intake level (UL) for calcium is 2,500 mg per day. Intakes above 1,500 mg per day have not been associated with any greater benefits than more moderate intakes in the 1,200 to 1,500 mg per day range.

Value

Calcium—it's not just for bones anymore. The body's calcium stores are much more than idle calcium warehouses—they are actually a very active site of continuous mineral exchange between the bones and the blood. The bones continuously release calcium and other minerals into the circulation, where calcium plays a role in controlling blood pressure, easing PMS, and fighting colon cancer. Calcium is cheap, easily available, and well tolerated as a supplement. Practically nobody consumes enough calcium in their daily diet, so calcium is one of the nutrients for which supplementation is highly recommended.

Dosage

The daily reference intakes (DRIs) are reference values for nutrients that are intended to replace the older recommended dietary allowances (RDAs) for use in diet planning and assessment. The DRIs reflect a shift in emphasis from preventing deficiency to decreasing the risk of chronic disease through nutrition. The RDAs focused on the amount of a specific nutrient needed to prevent certain deficiency diseases, while the DRIs will identify nutrient levels that can help prevent diet-related chronic diseases.

The daily reference intakes (DRI) recommend the following daily intakes for calcium:

- 1,300 mg for ages nine to eighteen
- 1,000 mg for adults ages nineteen to fifty
- 1,200 mg for older adults
- 1,500 mg for postmenopausal women not taking hormone replacement therapy

WORKS CONSULTED

Abrams SA. Bone turnover during lactation—can calcium supplementation make a difference? J Clin Endocrinol Metab. 1998 Apr;83(4):1056-8.

Bonjour JP, Rizzoli R. The property of calcium in the child and the adolescent: Importance in the acquisition of bone mineral density. Arch Pediatr. 1999;6 (Suppl 2):155s-7s.

Brooks ER, Howat PM, Cavalier DS. Calcium supplementation and exercise increase appendicular bone density in anorexia: A case study. J Am Diet Assoc. 1999 May;99(5):591-3.

Celotti F, Bignamini A. Dietary calcium and mineral/vitamin supplementation: A controversial problem. J Int Med Res. 1999 Jan-Feb;27(1):1-14.

Dawson-Hughes B. Vitamin D and calcium: Recommended intake for bone health. Osteoporos Int. 1998;8(Suppl 2):S30-4.

de Jong N, Paw MJ, de Groot LC, Hiddink GJ, van Staveren WA. Dietary supplements and physical exercise affecting bone and body composition in frail elderly persons. Am J Public Health. 2000 Jun;90(6):947-54.

Dibba B, Prentice A, Ceesay M, Stirling DM, Cole TJ, Poskitt EM. Effect of calcium supplementation on bone mineral accretion in Gambian children accustomed to a low-calcium diet. Am J Clin Nutr. 2000 Feb;71(2):544-9.

Fardellone P, Brazier M, Kamel S, Gueris J, Graulet AM, Lienard J, Sebert JL. Biochemical effects of calcium supplementation in postmenopausal women: Influence of dietary calcium intake. Am J Clin Nutr. 1998 Jun;67(6):1273-8.

Feit JM. Calcium and vitamin D supplements for elderly patients. J Fam Pract. 1997 Dec;45(6):471-2.

Ferrari SL, Rizzoli R, Slosman DO, Bonjour JP. Do dietary calcium and age explain the controversy surrounding the relationship between bone mineral density and vitamin D receptor gene polymorphisms? J Bone Miner Res. 1998 Mar;13(3):363-70.

Heaney RP. Calcium, dairy products and osteoporosis. J Am Coll Nutr. 2000 Apr;19(2 Suppl):83S-99S.

Ilich-Ernst JZ, McKenna AA, Badenhop NE, Clairmont AC, Andon MB, Nahhas RW, Goel P, Matkovic V. Iron status, menarche, and calcium supplementation in adolescent girls. Am J Clin Nutr. 1998 Oct;68(4):880-7.

Juby A. Managing elderly people's osteoporosis. Why? Who? How? Can Fam Physician. 1999 Jun;45:1526-36.

Kalkwarf HJ, Specker BL, Ho M. Effects of calcium supplementation on calcium homeostasis and bone turnover in lactating women. J Clin Endocrinol Metab. 1999 Feb;84(2):464-70.

Kleerekoper M. Osteoporosis: Protecting bone mass with fundamentals and drug therapy. Geriatrics. 1999 Jul;54(7):38-43.

Koo WW, Walters JC, Esterlitz J, Levine RJ, Bush AJ, Sibai B. Maternal calcium supplementation and fetal bone mineralization. Obstet Gynecol. 1999 Oct;94(4):577-82.

Lamke B, Engfeldt B, Sjoberg HE. Bone mineral content in women with vertebral fractures. Acta Med Scand. 1980;207(1-2):71-2.

Lesser GT. Long-term prevention of bone loss. Ann Intern Med. 2000 Jul 4;133(1):72-3.

Meunier PJ. Calcium, vitamin D and vitamin K in the prevention of fractures due to osteoporosis. Osteoporos Int. 1999;9(Suppl 2):S48-52.

Pfeifer M, Begerow B, Minne HW, Abrams C, Nachtigall D, Hansen C. Effects of a short-term vitamin D and calcium supplementation on body sway and secondary hyperparathyroidism in elderly women. J Bone Miner Res. 2000 Jun;15(6):1113-8.

Pines A, Katchman H, Villa Y, Mijatovic V, Dotan I, Levo Y, Ayalon D. The effect of various hormonal preparations and calcium supplementation on bone mass in early menopause. Is there a predictive value for the initial bone density and body weight? J Intern Med. 1999 Oct;246(4):357-61.

Prentice A. Maternal calcium metabolism and bone mineral status. Am J Clin Nutr. 2000 May;71(5 Suppl):1312S-6S.

Prentice A, Jarjou LM, Stirling DM, Buffenstein R, Fairweather-Tait S. Biochemical markers of calcium and bone metabolism during 18 months of lactation in Gambian women accustomed to a low calcium intake and in those consuming a calcium supplement. J Clin Endocrinol Metab. 1998 Apr;83(4):1059-66.

Recker RR, Davies KM, Dowd RM, Heaney RP. The effect of low-dose continuous estrogen and progesterone therapy with calcium and vitamin D on bone in elderly women. A randomized, controlled trial. Ann Intern Med. 1999 Jun 1;130(11):897-904.

Ricci TA, Chowdhury HA, Heymsfield SB, Stahl T, Pierson RN Jr, Shapses SA. Calcium supplementation suppresses bone turnover during weight reduction in postmenopausal women. J Bone Miner Res. 1998 Jun;13(6):1045-50.

Riggs BL, O'Fallon WM, Muhs J, O'Connor MK, Kumar R, Melton LJ 3rd. Long-term effects of calcium supplementation on serum parathyroid hormone level, bone turnover, and bone loss in elderly women. J Bone Miner Res. 1998 Feb;13(2):168-74.

Rodriguez JA, Novik V. Calcium intake and bone density in menopause. Data of a sample of Chilean women followed-up for 5 years with calcium supplementation. Rev Med Chil. 1998 Feb;126(2):145-50.

Schaafsma A, Pakan I. Short-term effects of a chicken egg shell powder enriched dairy-based products on bone mineral density in persons with osteoporosis or osteopenia. Bratisl Lek Listy. 1999 Dec;100(12):651-6.

Scopacasa F, Horowitz M, Wishart JM, Need AG, Morris HA, Wittert G, Nordin BE. Calcium supplementation suppresses bone resorption in early postmenopausal women. Calcif Tissue Int. 1998 Jan;62(1):8-12.

Setnikar I, Rovati LC, Schmid K, Vens-Cappell B, Barkworth MF. Bioavailability and pharmacokinetic characteristics of two monofluorophosphate preparations with calcium supplement. Arzneimittelforschung. 1998 Dec;48(12):1172-8.

Singh MA. Combined exercise and dietary intervention to optimize body composition in aging. Ann N Y Acad Sci. 1998 Nov 20;854:378-93.

Stallings VA. Calcium and bone health in children: A review. Am J Ther. 1997 Jul-Aug;4(7-8):259-73.

Storm D, Eslin R, Porter ES, Musgrave K, Vereault D, Patton C, Kessenich C, Mohan S, Chen T, Holick MF, Rosen CJ. Calcium supplementation prevents seasonal bone loss and changes in biochemical markers of bone turnover in elderly New England women: A randomized placebo-controlled trial. J Clin Endocrinol Metab. 1998 Nov;83(11):3817-25.

Swaminathan R. Nutritional factors in osteoporosis. Int J Clin Pract. 1999 Oct-Nov;53(7):540-8.

Zerwekh JE, Pak CY. Lack of skeletal lead accumulation during calcium citrate supplementation. Clin Chem. 1998 Feb;44(2):353-4.

MAGNESIUM

What Is It?

Magnesium is a mineral that functions as a coenzyme (part of about 100 enzymes) for nerve and muscle function, regulation of body temperature, energy metabolism, DNA/RNA synthesis, and the formation of bones. The majority of the body's magnesium (60 percent) is found in the bones. Food sources include artichokes, nuts, beans, whole grains, and shellfish. Too much can cause nausea, vomiting, and diarrhea.

Claims

- Builds bone
- Increases energy levels
- Promotes heart health
- Enhances protein synthesis (muscle building)

Theory

Because magnesium is needed as a cofactor for several enzymes to help convert carbohydrates, protein, and fat into energy, magnesium supplements may play a role in energy metabolism. Due to the role of magnesium in conducting nerve impulses, numerous magnesium-based supplements have been promoted for support of heart function. Magnesium's role in bone health stems from its primary location in bone tissue and its ability to help increase calcium absorption.

Scientific Support

The scientific support for magnesium as an adjunct to calcium supplements is fairly well founded. Magnesium can help improve calcium absorption and may help maintain bone density in individuals at risk for excessive bone loss. A few studies have suggested a potential role for magnesium supplements in energy metabolism by showing increased exercise efficiency in endurance athletes. In general, however, no overwhelming evidence suggests any increases in muscular strength or elevated energy levels following magnesium supplementation.

Safety

Excessive magnesium intake can cause diarrhea and general gastrointestinal distress as well as interfere with calcium absorption and bone metabolism. Since there are no known benefits associated with consuming more than 600 mg per day of magnesium, higher intakes should be avoided.

Value

Since nearly three-quarters of the American population fails to consume enough magnesium from the diet, supplements may be warranted in some cases, particularly those in which bone metabolism are concerned.

Dosage

The daily value for magnesium is 400 mg per day, but requirements may be elevated somewhat by stressors such as exercise and when taking calcium supplements for bone building or prevention of bone loss.

WORKS CONSULTED

Altura BM, Altura BT. New perspectives on the role of magnesium in the pathophysiology of the cardiovascular system. Clinical aspects. Magnesium. 1985;4(5-6):226-44.

Altura BM, Gebrewold A, Altura BT, Brautbar N. Magnesium depletion impairs myocardial carbohydrate and lipid metabolism and cardiac bioenergetics and raises myocardial calcium content in-vivo: Relationship to etiology of cardiac diseases. Biochem Mol Biol Int. 1996 Dec;40(6):1183-90.

Chang C, Varghese PJ, Downey J, Bloom S. Magnesium deficiency and myocardial infarct size in the dog. J Am Coll Cardiol. 1985 Feb;5(2 Pt 1):280-9.

Clandinin MT, Yamashiro S. Dietary factors affecting the incidence of dietary fat-induced myocardial lesions. J Nutr. 1982 Apr;112(4):825-8.

Ericsson Y, Luoma H, Ekberg O. Effects of calcium, fluoride and magnesium supplementations on tissue mineralization in calcium- and magnesium-deficient rats. J Nutr. 1986 Jun;116(6):1018-27.

Freedman AM, Atrakchi AH, Cassidy MM, Weglicki WB. Magnesium deficiency-induced cardiomyopathy: Protection by vitamin E. Biochem Biophys Res Commun. 1990 Aug 16;170(3):1102-6.

Freedman AM, Cassidy MM, Weglicki WB. Magnesium-deficient myocardium demonstrates an increased susceptibility to an in vivo oxidative stress. Magnes Res. 1991 Sep-Dec;4(3-4):185-9.

Hustler BI, Singh J, Waring JJ, Howarth FC. Dietary and physiological studies involving magnesium homeostasis in the heart. Ann N Y Acad Sci. 1996 Sep 30;793:473-8.

Kurantsin-Mills J, Cassidy MM, Stafford RE, Weglicki WB. Marked alterations in circulating inflammatory cells during cardiomyopathy development in a magnesium-deficient rat model. Br J Nutr. 1997 Nov;78(5):845-55.

Paddle BM, Haugaard N. Role of magnesium in effects of epinephrine on heart contraction and metabolism. Am J Physiol. 1971 Oct;221(4):1178-84.

Rayssiguier Y, Gueux E, Bussiere L, Durlach J, Mazur A. Dietary magnesium affects susceptibility of lipoproteins and tissues to peroxidation in rats. J Am Coll Nutr. 1993 Apr;12(2):133-7.

Savabi F, Gura V, Bessman S, Brautbar N. Effects of magnesium depletion on myocardial high-energy phosphates and contractility. Biochem Med Metab Biol. 1988 Apr;39(2):131-9.

Singh J, Hustler BI, Waring JJ, Howarth FC. Dietary and physiological studies to investigate the relationship between calcium and magnesium signalling in the mammalian myocardium. Mol Cell Biochem. 1997 Nov;176(1-2):127-34.

Truswell AS. ABC of nutrition. Reducing the risk of coronary heart disease. Br Med J (Clin Res Ed). 1985 Jul 6;291(6487):34-7.

van den Broek FA, Beynen AC. The influence of dietary phosphorus and magnesium concentrations on the calcium content of heart and kidneys of DBA/2 and NMRI mice. Lab Anim. 1998 Oct;32(4):483-91.

Wutzen J. Effect of low-magnesium diet on the histology and the activity of certain enzymes of rat myocardium. Pol Med Sci Hist Bull. 1975 Sep-Dec;15(5-6):531-8.

Zimmermann P, Weiss U, Classen HG, Wendt B, Epple A, Zollner H, Temmel W, Weger M, Porta S. The impact of diets with different magnesium contents on magnesium and calcium in serum and tissues of the rat. Life Sci. 2000 Jul 14;67(8):949-58.

BORON

What Is It?

Boron is a trace element that influences calcium and magnesium metabolism. Although no recommended dietary allowance (RDA) has been established for boron, the average daily intake is highly variable, having been estimated at between 0.5 and 7 mg per day. Boron is found in most tissues, but is concentrated in the bone, spleen, and thyroid—indicating boron's functions in bone metabolism and suggesting a potential role for boron in hormone metabolism. Boron is found in relatively high levels in foods of plant origin, such as dried fruits, nuts, dark green leafy vegetables, applesauce, grape juice, and cooked dried beans and peas. Meat and fish are poor dietary sources of boron.

Claims

- Increases muscle mass/strength
- Maintains bone density/improves calcium absorption

Theory

Low-boron diets have been associated with reduced testosterone levels, and boron supplements have been shown to increase serum levels of testosterone in postmenopausal women. This finding has spawned a number of boron supplements targeting athletes and bodybuilders and touting the benefits of boron for boosting testosterone levels, strength, and muscle mass.

Scientific Support

The claims that boron boosts testosterone were based on a USDA study of boron-deprived postmenopausal women—in whom boron supplements increased testosterone levels. Serum testosterone levels in postmenopausal women, however, are more than ten times lower than those found in normal men and in strength athletes. No studies suggest that boron supplementation alone will augment testosterone production or promote muscle growth in healthy men. In fact, a number of studies have shown no effect of boron supplements on serum testosterone in either men or women consuming a typical diet. Studies among bodybuilders have yielded similar "noneffects" of boron supplements on measures of lean body mass, body fat, and strength.

In one study of boron supplementation in nineteen male bodybuilders (ages twenty to twenty-seven years), ten subjects received 2.5 mg of boron per day for seven weeks (nine received a placebo). Although blood levels of boron were significantly elevated in the supplement group, boron supplementation had no significant effects on testosterone levels, lean body mass, or muscle strength.

In another study of boron supplementation in twelve postmenopausal women (ages forty-eight to eighty-two years) consuming a low-boron diet (0.25 mg per day), the addition of a 3 mg per day boron supplement was shown to reduce the urinary excretion of calcium and magnesium (a possible bone-health benefit) and to increase blood levels of estrogen (17 beta-estradiol) and testosterone. Another study also looked at the benefits of boron supplements (3 mg per day for three weeks) on bone health—finding no effect on urinary markers of bone breakdown (pyridinium cross-links), but an increase in calcium absorption.

Safety

Boron consumption of 1 to 10 mg per day is considered safe, but caution is warranted at higher intake levels, as consumption of 50 mg or more has been linked to toxicity, loss of appetite, nausea, vomiting, skin rashes, lethargy, and diarrhea.

Value

As part of a balanced multivitamin/mineral supplement, boron may have beneficial effects on maintaining adequate calcium and magnesium metabolism for optimal bone health. Athletes looking to boron supplements to increase serum testosterone levels and improve muscle mass and strength should look elsewhere.

Dosage

Daily needs for boron probably fall somewhere around 1 mg—which is about the amount found in the following foods:

- 1.5 oz of raisins or prunes
- 2 oz of almonds or peanuts
- 4 oz of red wine

WORKS CONSULTED

Beattie JH, Peace HS. The influence of a low-boron diet and boron supplementation on bone, major mineral and sex steroid metabolism in postmenopausal women. Br J Nutr. 1993 May;69(3):871-84.

Benderdour M, Bui-Van T, Dicko A, Belleville F. In vivo and in vitro effects of boron and boronated compounds. J Trace Elem Med Biol. 1998 Mar;12(1):2-7.

Clarkson PM, Rawson ES. Nutritional supplements to increase muscle mass. Crit Rev Food Sci Nutr. 1999 Jul;39(4):317-28.

Ferrando AA, Green NR. The effect of boron supplementation on lean body mass, plasma testosterone levels, and strength in male bodybuilders. Int J Sport Nutr. 1993 Jun;3(2):140-9.

Green NR, Ferrando AA. Plasma boron and the effects of boron supplementation in males. Environ Health Perspect. 1994 Nov;102(Suppl 7):73-7.

Hunt CD. Regulation of enzymatic activity: one possible role of dietary boron in higher animals and humans. Biol Trace Elem Res. 1998 Winter;66(1-3):205-25.

Hunt CD, Herbel JL, Nielsen FH. Metabolic responses of postmenopausal women to supplemental dietary boron and aluminum during usual and low magnesium intake: boron, calcium, and magnesium absorption and retention and blood mineral concentrations. Am J Clin Nutr. 1997 Mar;65(3):803-13.

Kreider RB. Dietary supplements and the promotion of muscle growth with resistance exercise. Sports Med. 1999 Feb;27(2):97-110.

Meacham SL, Hunt CD. Dietary boron intakes of selected populations in the United States. Biol Trace Elem Res. 1998 Winter;66(1-3):65-78.

Naghii MR. The significance of dietary boron, with particular reference to athletes. Nutr Health. 1999;13(1):31-7.

Naghii MR, Samman S. The effect of boron supplementation on its urinary excretion and selected cardiovascular risk factors in healthy male subjects. Biol Trace Elem Res. 1997 Mar;56(3):273-86.

Naghii MR, Samman S. The role of boron in nutrition and metabolism. Prog Food Nutr Sci. 1993 Oct-Dec;17(4):331-49.

Naghii MR, Wall PM, Samman S. The boron content of selected foods and the estimation of its daily intake among free-living subjects. J Am Coll Nutr. 1996 Dec;15(6):614-9.

Nielsen FH. Biochemical and physiologic consequences of boron deprivation in humans. Environ Health Perspect. 1994 Nov;102(Suppl 7):59-63.

Nielsen FH. The justification for providing dietary guidance for the nutritional intake of boron. Biol Trace Elem Res. 1998 Winter;66(1-3):319-30.

Nielsen FH, Hunt CD, Mullen LM, Hunt JR. Effect of dietary boron on mineral, estrogen, and testosterone metabolism in postmenopausal women. FASEB J. 1987 Nov;1(5):394-7.

Rainey C, Nyquist L. Multicountry estimation of dietary boron intake. Biol Trace Elem Res. 1998 Winter;66(1-3):79-86.

Rainey CJ, Nyquist LA, Christensen RE, Strong PL, Culver BD, Coughlin JR. Daily boron intake from the American diet. J Am Diet Assoc. 1999 Mar;99(3):335-40.

Samman S, Naghii MR, Lyons Wall PM, Verus AP. The nutritional and metabolic effects of boron in humans and animals. Biol Trace Elem Res. 1998 Winter;66(1-3):227-35.

Sutherland B, Strong P, King JC. Determining human dietary requirements for boron. Biol Trace Elem Res. 1998 Winter;66(1-3):193-204.

VITAMIN D

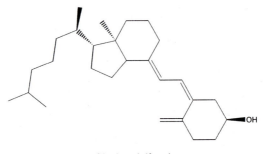

Cholecalciferol

What Is It?

Although vitamin D (calciferol/cholecalciferol) is typically classified as a fat-soluble vitamin, it actually functions as a hormone in the body. Because it can be manufactured by the body (formed in the skin following exposure to the ultraviolet rays of the sun), vitamin D is not technically classified as an essential nutrient at all. In the skin, exposure to ultraviolet rays converts vitamin D precursors (compounds with structures similar to cholesterol) into an inactive form of vitamin D. This inactive form is then converted to the active form by enzymes located in the liver and kidneys. Regular sunlight exposure is the primary way that most of us get our vitamin D. Food sources of vitamin D include only a few, such as vitamin D-fortified milk (100 IU per cup), cod liver oil, and fatty fish such as salmon. Small amounts of vitamin D are also found in egg yolks and liver.

Claims

- Prevents osteoporosis
- Increases bone strength
- Increases calcium absorption
- Treats psoriasis

Theory

The primary effect of vitamin D is to maintain calcium levels in the blood. To do this, vitamin D promotes both the absorption of calcium from the intestines into the blood and the removal of calcium from the bones into the blood. Vitamin D also reduces calcium loss in the urine. In most cases, the increased calcium absorption results in an increase in bone density and bone strength, which can help reduce the risk of osteoporosis.

Scientific Support

It is well accepted that adequate vitamin D levels are crucial for healthy bone development, maintenance of bone density and bone strength, and the prevention of osteoporosis. Vitamin D deficiency results in rickets (in children) and osteomalacia (in adults), both of which are characterized by a reduced level of calcium being deposited in bones and a weakening of bone strength.

A number of studies have clearly demonstrated that supplemental vitamin D intake (200 to 1,000 IU per day), usually combined with calcium, increases bone density and helps prevent osteoporosis. In one study, 240 healthy postmenopausal women consumed calcium (900 mg per day) and vitamin D (200 IU per day) for two years. Results showed a reduced loss of calcium in the urine and an increase of almost 2 percent in lumbar spine bone mineral density (a highly significant increase). Another study, also in postmenopausal women, included supplements containing 1,000 mg of calcium (as calcium carbonate) and 500 IU of vitamin D and showed a positive effect on bone density—even though initial calcium and vitamin D status was adequate.

Safety

Because vitamin D is fat-soluble, it is stored in the body and has the potential to reach toxic levels if taken in high doses for prolonged periods of time. Intakes over 1,000 IU (nearly three times the daily value) can cause nausea, diarrhea, skin rash, headaches, muscle weakness, calcium deposits, and kidney stones. Prolonged sunlight exposure does not cause buildup of vitamin D, as the body reduces its production when levels are adequate.

Value

For most people, there is no reason to take more than the recommended daily value (400 IU) of vitamin D. During the winter months, synthesis of vitamin D in the skin is severely reduced due to reduced exposure to sunlight. In some parts of the country (northern latitudes such as Boston or Seattle), virtually no vitamin synthesis occurs in skin during the winter months. Thus, vitamin D supplementation should be considered for people living in northern cities as well as by those who are not exposed to sunlight on a regular basis. In addition, elderly individuals should consider vitamin D supplements, as the skin loses its ability to adequately synthesize vitamin D as we age. Frequent sunblock users may also consider a vitamin D supplement, as sunblocks can reduce the skin's ability to produce vitamin D.

Dosage

The daily value for vitamin D is 400 IU, and supplements at this level have been shown to be safe and effective in reducing calcium loss and maintaining bone density in postmenopausal women. Dietary supplements are not necessary in healthy, young individuals who are frequently exposed to moderate amounts of sunlight (15 minutes or so per day). In dietary supplements, vitamin D and calcium do not have to be taken together to be effective, but many calcium/vitamin D combinations are available and may be more convenient than taking separate tablets.

WORKS CONSULTED

Backstrom MC, Maki R, Kuusela AL, Sievanen H, Koivisto AM, Ikonen RS, Kouri T, Maki M. Randomised controlled trial of vitamin D supplementation on bone density and biochemical indices in preterm infants. Arch Dis Child Fetal Neonatal Ed. 1999 May;80(3):F161-6.

Backstrom MC, Maki R, Kuusela AL, Sievanen H, Koivisto AM, Koskinen M, Ikonen RS, Maki M. The long-term effect of early mineral, vitamin D, and breast milk intake on bone mineral status in 9- to 11-year-old children born prematurely. J Pediatr Gastroenterol Nutr. 1999 Nov;29(5):575-82.

Celotti F, Bignamini A. Dietary calcium and mineral/vitamin supplementation: A controversial problem. J Int Med Res. 1999 Jan-Feb;27(1):1-14.

Davies PS, Bates CJ, Cole TJ, Prentice A, Clarke PC. Vitamin D: Seasonal and regional differences in preschool children in Great Britain. Eur J Clin Nutr. 1999 Mar;53(3):195-8.

Dawson-Hughes B. Vitamin D and calcium: Recommended intake for bone health. Osteoporos Int. 1998;8(Suppl 2):S30-4.

Feit JM. Calcium and vitamin D supplements for elderly patients. J Fam Pract. 1997 Dec;45(6):471-2.

Ferrari SL, Rizzoli R, Slosman DO, Bonjour JP. Do dietary calcium and age explain the controversy surrounding the relationship between bone mineral density and vitamin D receptor gene polymorphisms? J Bone Miner Res. 1998 Mar;13(3):363-70.

Gillespie WJ, Henry DA, O'Connell DL, Robertson J. Vitamin D and vitamin D analogues for preventing fractures associated with involutional and post-menopausal osteoporosis. Cochrane Database Syst Rev. 2000;(2):CD000227.

Juby A. Managing elderly people's osteoporosis. Why? Who? How? Can Fam Physician. 1999 Jun;45:1526-36.

Kleerekoper M. Osteoporosis: Protecting bone mass with fundamentals and drug therapy. Geriatrics. 1999 Jul;54(7):38-43.

Kobayashi T. Nutritional and biochemical studies on vitamin D and its active derivatives. Yakugaku Zasshi. 1996 Jun;116(6):457-72.

Kyriakidou-Himonas M, Aloia JF, Yeh JK. Vitamin D supplementation in postmenopausal black women. J Clin Endocrinol Metab. 1999 Nov;84(11):3988-90.

Lamke B, Engfeldt B, Sjoberg HE. Bone mineral content in women with vertebral fractures. Acta Med Scand. 1980;207(1-2):71-2.

Lesser GT. Long-term prevention of bone loss. Ann Intern Med. 2000 Jul 4;133(1):72-3.

Meunier PJ. Calcium, vitamin D and vitamin K in the prevention of fractures due to osteoporosis. Osteoporos Int. 1999;9(Suppl 2):S48-52.

Outila TA, Lamberg-Allardt CJ. Ergocalciferol supplementation may positively affect lumbar spine bone mineral density of vegans. J Am Diet Assoc. 2000 Jun;100(6):629.

Pfeifer M, Begerow B, Minne HW, Abrams C, Nachtigall D, Hansen C. Effects of a short-term vitamin D and calcium supplementation on body sway and secondary hyperparathyroidism in elderly women. J Bone Miner Res. 2000 Jun;15(6):1113-8.

Recker RR, Davies KM, Dowd RM, Heaney RP. The effect of low-dose continuous estrogen and progesterone therapy with calcium and vitamin D on bone in elderly women. A randomized, controlled trial. Ann Intern Med. 1999 Jun 1;130(11):897-904.

Reid IR. The roles of calcium and vitamin D in the prevention of osteoporosis. Endocrinol Metab Clin North Am. 1998 Jun;27(2):389-98.

Stallings VA. Calcium and bone health in children: A review. Am J Ther. 1997 Jul-Aug;4(7-8):259-73.

Swaminathan R. Nutritional factors in osteoporosis. Int J Clin Pract. 1999 Oct-Nov;53(7):540-8.

Trombetti A, Gerbase MW, Spiliopoulos A, Slosman DO, Nicod LP, Rizzoli R. Bone mineral density in lung-transplant recipients before and after graft: Prevention of lumbar spine post-transplantation-accelerated bone loss by pamidronate. J Heart Lung Transplant. 2000 Aug;19(8):736-43.

Wical KE, Brussee P. Effects of a calcium and vitamin D supplement on alveolar ridge resorption in immediate denture patients. J Prosthet Dent. 1979 Jan;41(1):4-11.

Zamora SA, Rizzoli R, Belli DC, Slosman DO, Bonjour JP. Vitamin D supplementation during infancy is associated with higher bone mineral mass in prepubertal girls. J Clin Endocrinol Metab. 1999 Dec;84(12):4541-4.

VITAMIN K

What Is It?

Vitamin K (phylloquinone/menaquinone) is a fat-soluble vitamin required for blood clotting and bone formation. Good food sources include avocado, liver, and dark leafy greens (spinach, kale, broccoli). One cup of spinach provides almost twice the current RDA (about 120 mcg).

Claims

- Promotes blood clotting
- Improves bone density and bone strength

Theory

Vitamin K is involved in both blood clotting (via prothrombin synthesis) and bone metabolism (via carboxylation of osteocalcin). Although isolated vitamin K supplements are not available without a prescription, it is added in small amounts to most multivitamins and is frequently found as part of many bone formulas. As a dietary supplement for bone health, vitamin K promotes the adequate deposition of calcium, magnesium, and phosphorus within the bone matrix (through the action of a bone protein called osteocalcin). Vitamin K is required for full activity of the osteocalcin protein, and elderly subjects with low vitamin K intake have been shown to have suboptimal bone density and an increased risk of osteoporosis.

Scientific Support

Vitamin K's primary function is to regulate normal blood clotting (due to its role in the synthesis of prothrombin). The current RDA for vitamin K is 1 mcg per kilogram of body weight—so larger people require more vitamin K than smaller people (about 50 to 80 mcg for adults). The vitamin K content of most foods is very low (less than 10 mcg per 100 g). We get the majority of our vitamin K from a few leafy green vegetables (spinach, kale, lettuce, parsley, broccoli) and vegetable oils (soybean, cottonseed, canola, and olive) that contain high amounts (so if you don't eat these foods regularly, then you are unlikely to consume enough vitamin K). Of the two types of naturally occurring vitamin K, absorption of phylloquinone from plant foods is poor, and the small amounts of menaquinone produced by intestinal bacteria provide only a minor portion of daily requirements.

In bones, vitamin K mediates the gamma-carboxylation of glutamyl residues on several bone proteins, most notably the bone formation protein osteocalcin. High serum concentrations of undercarboxylated osteocalcin and low serum concentrations of vitamin K are associated with lower bone mineral density and increased risk of hip fracture. Women with higher vitamin K intakes have a significantly lower relative risk of hip fracture (about 30 percent lower) than women with lower vitamin K intake (less than 109 mcg per day). Risk of hip fracture is also reduced by almost half for women with the highest lettuce consumption (lettuce is high in vitamin K). Women who consumed one or more servings of lettuce per day were 45 percent less likely to have low bone density compared with women eating less than one serving of lettuce each week. These findings suggest that low dietary intake of vitamin K may increase the risk of hip fracture in women.

Studies in postmenopausal women have shown that an increased intake of vitamin K results in an increase in bone formation and a slowing of bone loss. Another study, conducted in female athletes, also showed that one month of vitamin K supplementation increased the body's ability to bind calcium in the bones and resulted in a 15 to 20 percent increase in bone formation and a 20 to 25 percent decrease in bone breakdown.

Safety

High intake of vitamin K, from either foods or supplements, is not recommended for individuals taking anticoagulant medications such as warfarin (Coumadin). It is widely assumed that a dietary vitamin K-warfarin interaction exists, and patients taking these medications are instructed to maintain a constant dietary intake of vitamin K (to avoid fluctuations in the activity of their blood-thinning medication). In most cases, a constant dietary intake of vitamin K from dietary supplements containing RDA levels (65 to 80 mcg) of vitamin K is the most acceptable practice for patients on these medications. As with any fat-soluble vitamin, chronic consumption of doses above RDA levels is not recommended due to concerns regarding buildup and toxicity.

Value

As an isolated dietary supplement, vitamin K is not available without a prescription. RDA levels of vitamin K are often included in many multivitamins and several complete bone formulas. For individuals who may not be consuming the recommended levels of vitamin K and for elderly individuals who may have a slightly higher dietary need for vitamin K, dietary supplements may be warranted to ensure optimal calcium deposition into bone tissue.

Dosage

The adult RDA ranges from 60 to 80 mcg per day. Natural forms of vitamin K found in foods are only about half as potent as synthetic versions, but both are used efficiently in the body. The levels of vitamin K found in most multivitamins and bone formulas (10 to 120 mcg) are considered safe.

WORKS CONSULTED

Booth SL, Tucker KL, Chen H, Hannan MT, Gagnon DR, Cupples LA, Wilson PW, Ordovas J, Schaefer EJ, Dawson-Hughes B, Kiel DP. Dietary vitamin K intakes are associated with hip fracture but not with bone mineral density in elderly men and women. Am J Clin Nutr. 2000 May;71(5):1201-8.

Craciun AM, Wolf J, Knapen MH, Brouns F, Vermeer C. Improved bone metabolism in female elite athletes after vitamin K supplementation. Int J Sports Med. 1998 Oct;19(7):479-84.

Meunier PJ. Calcium, vitamin D and vitamin K in the prevention of fractures due to osteoporosis. Osteoporos Int. 1999;9(Suppl 2):S48-52.

Reichel H. No effect of vitamin K1 supplementation on biochemical bone markers in haemodialysis patients. Nephrol Dial Transplant. 1999 Jan;14(1):249-50.

Chapter 8

Supplements for Joint Health

INTRODUCTION

Arthritis causes pain, disability, and restricted mobility in more than 40 million Americans. Until very recently, degenerative joint conditions were considered incurable side effects of old age to which we were all eventually bound to succumb. Dramatic breakthroughs in nutritional biochemistry, exercise physiology, and sports medicine, however, have begun to change the way health professionals, and the public at large, think about the treatment and prevention of bone and joint disease.

Right now, approximately 42 million Americans have arthritis. As the U.S. population ages, the total number of people with disability or functional impairment related to their bones and joints is expected to skyrocket. Over the next fifteen to twenty years, an estimated 100 to 110 million people will be affected enough to lose some degree of flexibility and mobility in their joints. Sobering statistics to be sure, but when considered in light of the dramatic increase in active lifestyles and sports participation among older Americans (up nearly 60 percent since 1990), it is clear that many people are not quite ready to accept these "inevitable consequences of aging" as part of their future.

CAUSES OF ARTHRITIS AND CONVENTIONAL TREATMENTS

In the most common form of arthritis, called osteoarthritis, joint cartilage becomes damaged—resulting in inflammation, pain, and reduced mobility and flexibility. The degeneration of joint cartilage is often referred to as a "wear and tear" condition in which the body's own restorative processes cannot keep up with the breakdown events, resulting in arthritis. Under normal conditions, connective tissues such as cartilage are undergoing a constant cycle of breakdown and repair referred to as "turnover"—a cycle which is normally balanced to maintain healthy cartilage.

As cartilage degradation outpaces restoration, pain and stiffness can result in reduced mobility. Conventional treatment typically involves analgesic and/or anti-inflammatory medications such as Tylenol, Advil, Aleve, or aspirin. A frequent side effect of many anti-inflammatory medications is gastrointestinal damage (ulcers) as well as the possibility of slowing cartilage repair processes even further (through an inhibition of certain enzymes).

PRACTICAL ADVICE

It makes little sense to talk about nutrition or dietary supplementation without trying to put it into the context of how it can help the entire body. For example, most people know that calcium is "good" for their bones, but you also need to consider your intake of other nutrients (such as vitamins D and K, and minerals such as magnesium, boron, and zinc).

The same goes for dietary supplements to support cartilage health. Virtually everybody who has even heard of nutraceuticals is aware of glucosamine and chondroitin as agents that may help nourish joint cartilage. Simply packing these supplements into a capsule, without considering essential cofactors required for the cartilage repair process, misses the entire point of using supplements to maintain health and well-being. Important cofactors for cartilage synthesis and maintenance, such as vitamins C and E, boron, copper, manganese, and zinc, must be present in the right amounts for the cartilage repair process to operate normally. In addition, a wide variety of nonnutrient factors such as boswellia, bromelain, papain, white willow bark, and curcumin may be able to enhance the process of connective tissue maintenance by reducing inflammation and improving circulation.

CONTRIBUTING FACTORS

It is important to note that because no two people are exactly the same, the overall effect of a given dietary supplement can vary from person to person. Some individuals may experience dramatic results in a short period of time, some may take longer to notice any benefits, and some may fail to achieve any noticeable benefits from a particular supplement (although it may be working just the same). A number of factors are known to influence the body's ability to undergo the normal process of connective tissue (cartilage) maintenance, including:

- *Aging* causes a number of biochemical and biomechanical changes in connective tissues such as cartilage and bones. For example, in joint cartilage, both the number of cartilage cells (chondrocytes) and their individual activity may decline with age. This means that the cartilage in older joints may be less able to repair damage and less resistant to injury than the cartilage in younger joints.
- *Obesity* is a known risk factor for joint pain and stiffness due to the increased chronic load delivered to joints. The primary weight-bearing joints of the body, the knees and hips, are particularly susceptible to damage from bearing excessive weight.
- *Genetic factors* are thought to play a role in connective tissue metabolism and may explain some of the variation in the overall risk for conditions such as arthritis and osteoporosis.
- *Physical activity* has the potential to significantly influence cartilage metabolism by enhancing transport of nutrients from the blood into the joint tissues where they can be used. Too little activity or too much mechanical stress may unbalance the cartilage repair process and impair function.
- *Medications,* including over-the-counter pain relievers such as aspirin, ibuprofen (Advil), and naproxen (Aleve), can interfere with the normal cartilage repair process. Although such medications are widely used for the temporary relief of pain and inflammation of arthritis and other injuries, their overall effect is to address the symptom of pain— not the underlying cause of tissue damage. Chronic use of such pain relievers may actually accelerate the very condition from which you are trying to get relief.

DIETARY SUPPLEMENTS

Glucosamine and Chondroitin

Perhaps the most widely used joint supplements, glucosamine and chondroitin have been used separately and in combination in several European countries as a first-line treatment for osteoarthritis for over twenty years. A number of studies have clearly shown that both glucosamine and chondroitin can reduce the pain and stiffness of arthritis and may even play a role in slowing the progression of the damage. In most cases, these supplements are significantly more effective than placebo and just as effective as common pain-relieving medications (with fewer side effects). Although they often take longer to start working, they may continue to work for a longer period of time. Most studies suggest that four to eight weeks of supplementation are needed at doses of 1,500 mg per day of glucosamine and/or 1,200 mg of chondroitin (the combination formula has not been shown to be any more effective than either supplement on its own).

Recent evidence published in top arthritis and medical journals such as the *Journal of Rheumatology* and *JAMA* suggests that chondroitin *does* indeed appear to be as effective as glucosamine in alleviating joint pain and stiffness. It is important to note, however, that the *combination* of glucosamine and chondroitin has yet to be shown to be any more effective than either ingredient on its own. In addition, chondroitin is approximately ten times more expensive than glucosamine, and the quality of the raw material has been the subject of recent controversy.

S-Adenosylmethionine (SAMe)

SAMe is the latest "darling" of the supplement world. A derivative of the amino acid methionine, SAMe (or "Sammy" as it is called) has been shown to alleviate pain and inflammation while improving flexibility and mobility in people suffering from arthritis. The overall effect of SAMe (200 to 1,200 mg per day) appears to be equivalent to common analgesic and anti-inflammatory medications (again, with fewer gastrointestinal side effects), but its cost relative to glucosamine and chondroitin is prohibitive for many people (although an added benefit for SAMe is its potential to also help combat mild depression—something that neither glucosamine nor chondroitin can do).

Methylsulfonylmethionine (MSM)

MSM is another of the newer entries into the joint supplement category. Although a lot of hype surrounds MSM as a beneficial supplement for treating arthritis and other degenerative joint conditions, the scientific evidence is quite meager. MSM is a methylated and sulfated version of the amino acid methionine, so as a dietary source of sulfur, it actually may have some benefits because sulfur is involved in a number of amino acid and protein metabolic pathways, including some related to cartilage synthesis and repair.

Hydrolyzed Collagen Protein (HCP)

HCP is also known as gelatin. Collagen is the chief structural protein that makes up connective tissues in the body (such as joint cartilage), and the hydrolyzed form is simply a modified form of the protein that has been broken down into smaller pieces by enzymes. By providing key amino acid building blocks for cartilage synthesis, HCP can help rebuild damaged cartilage.

A handful of small European studies have suggested that HCP can effectively reduce the joint pain and stiffness of arthritis—but the daily dose is high at about 7 to 10 g per day (good thing it's inexpensive).

Essential Fatty Acids (EFAs)

EFAs, such as those found in fish oil and some seed oils, may be effective in reducing inflammatory prostaglandins. For example, the omega-3 fatty acids EPA and DHA provide anti-inflammatory effects that may augment the overall joint benefits of primary joint supplements such as glucosamine. Dosage recommendations are typically in the 2 to 4 g per day range (for EPA and DHA)—or about 8 to 12 g of fish oil per day. As a vegetarian alternative to fish oils, essential fatty acids can be obtained from seed oils such as evening primrose, black currant and borage oils (about 5 to 10 g per day).

Antioxidants

Findings from the decade-long Framingham study have suggested that people with a high intake of antioxidants, particularly vitamins C and E, have a slower rate of cartilage degeneration and a better maintenance of overall joint function. Other studies have shown how bioflavonoids such as quercetin can help inhibit the synthesis of inflammatory prostaglandins to reduce swelling and pain.

Devil's Claw

This South American herb has been shown to provide pain relief in arthritic conditions (at doses of 1 to 3 g per day). Curiously, devil's claw appears to be most effective for joint pain originating in the lower back.

White Willow Bark

This natural source of salicin is sometimes called nature's aspirin because of its use as a mild anti-inflammatory. Raw white willow powders do not provide high enough concentrations of salicylates to provide much benefit, so be sure to look for an extract standardized to at least 20 percent total salicin content.

D,L-phenylalanine (DLPA)

A synthetic form of the amino acid phenylalanine, DLPA is typically used as a dietary supplement to reduce appetite, elevate mood, and reduce the sensation of pain. In the body, phenylalanine can be converted into another amino acid, tyrosine, and then into the neurotransmitters dopamine and norepinephrine (which have roles in transmitting pain signals). In addition, animal studies suggest that DLPA may increase brain levels of endorphins (the body's "feel-good" morphine-like compounds)—an effect that could potentially reduce pain.

Silicon

Like sulfur, the mineral silicon may help strengthen connective tissues such as cartilage by supporting the structural proteins that comprise the tissues. Horsetail extract is frequently used as a natural herbal source of silicon in some dietary supplements.

Boswellia serrata

Extract from the sap of boswellia is a traditional Indian herbal treatment for controlling inflammation, pain, and stiffness. Its effects in controlling inflammation have been compared to conventional nonsteroidal anti-inflammatory drugs (NSAIDs)—without the associated gastrointestinal side effects or progression of joint damage. Typical dosage recommendations are 600 to 1,200 mg per day of a 65 percent boswellic acid extract or 1,200 to 2,400 mg per day of a 35 percent extract (taken in divided doses two to four times per day).

Turmeric (Curcumin) and Ginger

Turmeric root extract is another traditional Indian remedy for controlling swelling and inflammation. Turmeric is a bright yellow spice used in Indian curry cooking and supplies curcumin, a powerful anti-inflammatory and antioxidant. Standardized turmeric root extracts can provide as much as 95 percent curcumin, which can be used two to four times per day in doses of 200 to 400 mg. Ginger also provides some mild anti-inflammatory effects in doses of 1 to 3 g per day (taken in two to three divided doses).

SUMMARY

There is little doubt in the minds of nutritionally oriented physicians and scientists that dietary supplements can indeed be helpful in supporting cartilage synthesis, repair, and maintenance (see Table 8.1). Glucosamine is among the most popular joint supplements—and at 1,500 mg per day appears to be quite safe and effective, but approximately four to eight weeks may be necessary before the joint benefits of glucosamine become evident. High levels of antioxidants in the diet, particularly vitamins C and E, have been reported to slow the rate of joint deterioration in the knees and reduce symptoms of pain and stiffness (compared to people who consume low levels of dietary antioxidants). Trace minerals such as boron, manganese, copper, selenium, silicon, sulfur, and zinc are known to influence connective tissue metabolism, and boron supplements have been associated with relief from joint pain and stiffness (at a dose of 3 to 6 mg per day for two months). *Boswellia serrata,* curcumin (from turmeric root), ginger, devil's claw, and white willow have anti-inflammatory actions similar to conventional nonsteroidal anti-inflammatory medications (NSAIDs)—but without the gastrointestinal side effects common to many NSAIDs.

TABLE 8.1. Primary Dietary Supplements for Joint Health

Ingredient	Dose (per day)	Primary claims
Boswellia	450-1,200 mg	Anti-inflammatory/pain reliever
Chondroitin	1,200 mg	Rebuilds joint cartilage
Collagen protein	7-10 g	Rebuilds joint cartilage
Devil's claw	750-6,000 mg	Reduces pain and inflammation
Glucosamine	1,500 mg	Rebuilds joint cartilage
Green-lipped mussel	500-3,000 mg	Reduces pain and inflammation
MSM	200-2,000 mg	Reduces pain
SAMe	200-1,200 mg	Reduces pain
Sea cucumber	500-2,000 mg	Reduces pain and inflammation

GLUCOSAMINE

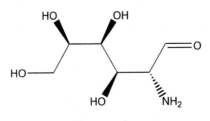

Glucosamine

What Is It?

Glucosamine is an aminopolysaccharide (a combination of an amino acid [glutamine] and a sugar [glucose]). Glucosamine is concentrated in joint cartilage, where it is incorporated into longer chains known as glyco-saminoglycans and finally into very large structures known as proteo-glycans. The proteoglycans function to attract water into the joint space for lubrication of the cartilage during movement.

Claims

- Reverses osteoarthritis
- Protects joints and tendons from injury
- Decreases inflammation

Theory

The major principle behind glucosamine supplementation is that the glucosamine is delivered to the joint space and incorporated into pro-teoglycans of joint cartilage to maintain structure and repair damage. Glucosamine may also stimulate chondrocytes (cartilage cells) to begin pro-ducing healthy new cartilage matrix (both collagen and proteoglycans).

Scientific Support

Numerous European studies and a handful of North American reports show a clear benefit of glucosamine supplements for relief of joint pain and stiffness associated with arthritis. Many of the studies have been criticized for lack of scientific control, short duration, and small size, but recent meta-analyses of the smaller studies have supported the beneficial role of glucosamine supplements as a safe and effective approach to treating osteoarthritis. In general, one to three months of glucosamine supplementation seems to be as effective as many analgesic and nonsteroidal anti-inflammatory drugs (NSAIDs), such as acetaminophen and ibuprofen, in reducing the joint pain of osteoarthritis. At least two very recent studies have shown that glucosamine may even be able to slow or stop the destruction of cartilage in the knee joints of people with osteoarthritis.

Safety

Occasional symptoms of gastrointestinal discomfort have been noted, but no significant adverse effects are associated with glucosamine supplementation. Although no long-term safety studies have been conducted in humans, animal studies on glucosamine have found it to be nontoxic. Diabetics may want to exercise a degree of caution when using glucosamine supplements, as several animal studies and one small human pilot study have suggested an increase in blood sugar levels during regular glucosamine consumption (although most of the animal studies have used injections of glucosamine).

Value

Glucosamine supplements tend to be among the more expensive products on the shelf. A one-month supply of capsules can range from $15 to well over $100. Because they have to be consumed for one to three months before any noticeable benefit is apparent, you may need to invest a significant amount of money before you realize any benefits. However, because arthritis pain is one of the most debilitating conditions, most people dealing with such pain would gladly invest a dollar or so per day in a supplement that relieved their discomfort and helped repair their damaged cartilage tissue. For people with existing chronic joint pain, glucosamine supplements are probably worth the significant dollar investment for the benefits that they deliver.

Dosage

No dose-response studies have been conducted with glucosamine supplements. Virtually all oral supplementation studies on glucosamine have used 1,500 mg per day, usually in three divided doses of 500 mg each. While this level appears to be effective, there is no information to suggest that a higher dose would work better or faster—or that a lower dose would be less effective. A common supplementation strategy, which can decrease the daily cost of supplements, is to consume 1,500 mg of glucosamine per day for the first sixty to ninety days, followed by a reduced intake of 250 to 750 mg per day as a "maintenance level." Following the initial sixty- to ninety-day period, dosage levels can be increased or decreased based on individual pain and stiffness levels.

WORKS CONSULTED

Barclay TS, Tsourounis C, McCart GM. Glucosamine. Ann Pharmacother. 1998 May;32(5):574-9.

da Camara CC, Dowless GV. Glucosamine sulfate for osteoarthritis. Ann Pharmacother. 1998 May;32(5):580-7.

Deal CL, Moskowitz RW. Nutraceuticals as therapeutic agents in osteoarthritis. The role of glucosamine, chondroitin sulfate, and collagen hydrolysate. Rheum Dis Clin North Am. 1999 May;25(2):379-95.

Delafuente JC. Glucosamine in the treatment of osteoarthritis. Rheum Dis Clin North Am. 2000 Feb;26(1):1-11.

Denham AC, Newton WP. Are glucosamine and chondroitin effective in treating osteoarthritis? J Fam Pract. 2000 Jun;49(6):571-2.

Donohoe M. Efficacy of glucosamine and chondroitin for treatment of osteoarthritis. JAMA. 2000 Sep 13;284(10):1241; discussion 1242.

Houpt JB, McMillan R, Wein C, Paget-Dellio SD. Effect of glucosamine hydrochloride in the treatment of pain of osteoarthritis of the knee. J Rheumatol. 1999 Nov;26(11):2423-30.

Leeb BF, Schweitzer H, Montag K, Smolen JS. A metaanalysis of chondroitin sulfate in the treatment of osteoarthritis. J Rheumatol. 2000 Jan;27(1):205-11.

Leffler CT, Philippi AF, Leffler SG, Mosure JC, Kim PD. Glucosamine, chondroitin, and manganese ascorbate for degenerative joint disease of the knee or low back: A randomized, double-blind, placebo-controlled pilot study. Mil Med. 1999 Feb;164(2):85-91.

Mautone G. Efficacy of glucosamine and chondroitin for treatment of osteoarthritis. JAMA. 2000 Sep 13;284(10):1241; discussion 1242.

McAlindon TE, LaValley MP, Felson DT. Efficacy of glucosamine and chondroitin for treatment of osteoarthritis. JAMA. 2000 Sep 13;284(10):1241.

McAlindon TE, LaValley MP, Gulin JP, Felson DT. Glucosamine and chondroitin for treatment of osteoarthritis: A systematic quality assessment and meta-analysis. JAMA. 2000 Mar 15;283(11):1469-75.

Rindone JP, Hiller D, Collacott E, Nordhaugen N, Arriola G. Randomized, controlled trial of glucosamine for treating osteoarthritis of the knee. West J Med. 2000 Feb;172(2):91-4.

Towheed TE, Anastassiades TP. Glucosamine and chondroitin for treating symptoms of osteoarthritis: Evidence is widely touted but incomplete. JAMA. 2000 Mar 15;283(11):1483-4.

CHONDROITIN SULFATE (CS)

What Is It?

Chondroitin sulfate (CS) falls into a category of compounds known as glycosaminoglycans—basically a long chain of specialized polysaccharides (or sugars). In the body, chondroitin is used as a building block for larger structures known as proteoglycans—which are in turn used to form connective tissues such as cartilage. Chondroitin is related in structure and function to another sugar derivative, glucosamine, both of which are widely used as dietary supplements to nourish joint cartilage. Chondroitin sulfate is not found in the diet in appreciable amounts—the primary source being animal cartilage (such as the trachea of cows).

Claims

- Alleviates joint pain associated with osteoarthritis
- Reduces inflammation

Theory

For many years, critics of CS's use for treating arthritis argued that the large size of the CS molecule would prevent it from being absorbed into the body. We now know, however, that as much as 10 to 20 percent of CS is absorbed intact (and perhaps substantially more for the newer low-molecular-weight chondroitin), while the remaining percentage is likely digested and absorbed as its component parts. The theory behind the use of CS to treat osteoarthritis involves two primary concepts. The first and most basic is that CS simply provides the raw material that cartilage needs to repair itself. The second theory is that CS may block the activity of enzymes that break down cartilage—an activity that may yield benefits in reducing inflammation and protecting cartilage from further damage.

Scientific Support

Until recently, the scientific evidence for the effectiveness of chondroitin sulfate in alleviating joint pain has been relatively week. Several small studies have shown some evidence for a reduction in joint pain—but several other studies have found no clear benefits. Very recently, however, separate groups of researchers have performed meta-analyses of all studies using CS to treat osteoarthritis. This type of statistical analysis gathers the evidence from the available research studies and looks at them together, allowing researchers to combine several small studies into one large analysis and obtain more "power" (a statistical term) to determine whether an actual beneficial effect exists for a treatment. Both research groups found that over the course of approximately four months of treatment, CS was significantly superior to placebo in relieving joint pain and that patients taking CS showed improvements of at least 50 percent in measurements such as pain level, joint stiffness, and walking speed. In other smaller studies, CS also appears to slow the progression of cartilage degradation in the knee joint—an effect measured by a stabilization of the medial femoro-tibial (knee) joint width.

Safety

Aside from some mild gastrointestinal complaints (heartburn and nausea), chondroitin sulfate has not been associated with any serious adverse side effects.

Value

Now that a bit more is known about the effectiveness of chondroitin sulfate, it appears that the supplement can indeed result in a reduction in the pain associated with osteoarthritis (following about two to four months of treatment). Because the scientific data are also quite strong for the effectiveness of glucosamine in alleviating joint pain, it may be wise to select chondroitin supplements that also include the effective dose of glucosamine (1,500 mg per day) as well. The key practical consideration for selecting a chondroitin supplement, however, is quality control—a problem that is widespread in the supplement industry. One study conducted at the University of Maryland found that at least half of the commercially available chondroitin supplements failed to supply the labeled amount of the ingredient—and some provided almost zero chondroitin.

Dosage

The typical recommendation for chondroitin supplementation is 1,200 mg per day. Although the daily dose is frequently supplied in divided doses of 400 mg (taken three times per day) or 600 mg (taken twice per day), taking the entire 1,200 mg in one dose appears to be just as effective in alleviating joint pain. A large number of dietary supplements combine chondroitin with glucosamine, but it is still not known whether this combination of ingredients is any better than either supplement on its own.

WORKS CONSULTED

Arthritis supplements. Do natural dietary supplements for arthritis really work? Johns Hopkins Med Lett Health After 50. 1999 Oct;11(8):8.

Klippel J. A "natural" approach to treating osteoarthritis. Health News. 2000 May;6(5):1-2.

McAlindon TE, LaValley MP, Gulin JP, Felson DT. Glucosamine and chondroitin for treatment of osteoarthritis: A systematic quality assessment and meta-analysis. JAMA. 2000 Mar 15;283(11):1469-75.

Towheed TE, Anastassiades TP. Glucosamine and chondroitin for treating symptoms of osteoarthritis: Evidence is widely touted but incomplete. JAMA. 2000 Mar 15;283(11):1483-4.

BOSWELLIA (BOSWELLIA SERRATA)

What Is It?

The boswellia tree produces a sap that has been used in traditional Indian medicine as a treatment for arthritis and inflammatory conditions.

Claims

- Anti-inflammatory
- Relieves pain associated with joint pain and sports injuries

Theory

The primary compounds thought to be responsible for the anti-inflammatory activity of boswellia are known as boswellic acids. These compounds are thought to interfere with enzymes that contribute to inflammation and pain.

Scientific Support

Only a handful of studies have been conducted on the effects of boswellia in treating sports injuries or arthritis, but at least a few have suggested that boswellic acids may possess anti-inflammatory activity at least as potent as that of common over-the-counter medications such as ibuprofen and aspirin. In one study of patients with rheumatoid arthritis, pain and swelling was reduced following three months of boswellia use.

Safety

In some cases, boswellia may be associated with mild gastrointestinal upset (heartburn, aftertaste, and nausea), but there are no reports of serious adverse side effects.

Value

Although further scientific studies need to be conducted to confirm the long-term safety and effectiveness of boswellia extracts, the plant has a long history of safe and effective use as a mild anti-inflammatory to reduce pain and stiffness and promote increased mobility (without many of the associated gastrointestinal side effects commonly reported for synthetic anti-inflammatory medications).

Dosage

The typical recommended dose of boswellia is 450 to 1,200 mg per day of an extract standardized to contain approximately 30 to 65 percent boswellic acids. The extract should be consumed in three divided doses of 150 to 400 mg each for approximately two to three months to achieve benefits in terms of reduced pain and improved mobility.

WORKS CONSULTED

Ammon HP. Salai Guggal—Boswellia serrata: From a herbal medicine to a non-redox inhibitor of leukotriene biosynthesis. Eur J Med Res. 1996 May 24; 1(8):369-70.

Boswellia serrata. Altern Med Rev. 1998 Aug;3(4):306-7.

Gupta I, Parihar A, Malhotra P, Singh GB, Ludtke R, Safayhi H, Ammon HP. Effects of Boswellia serrata gum resin in patients with ulcerative colitis. Eur J Med Res. 1997 Jan;2(1):37-43.

Kulkarni RR, Patki PS, Jog VP, Gandage SG, Patwardhan B. Treatment of osteoarthritis with a herbomineral formulation: A double-blind, placebo-controlled, cross-over study. J Ethnopharmacol. 1991 May-Jun;33(1-2):91-5.

Sander O, Herborn G, Rau R. Is H15 (resin extract of Boswellia serrata, "incense") a useful supplement to established drug therapy of chronic polyarthritis? Results of a double-blind pilot study. Z Rheumatol. 1998 Feb;57(1):11-6.

Singh GB, Atal CK. Pharmacology of an extract of salai guggal ex-Boswellia serrata, a new non-steroidal anti-inflammatory agent. Agents Actions. 1986 Jun;18(3-4):407-12.

METHYLSULFONYLMETHANE (MSM)

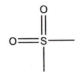

Methylsulfonylmethane

What Is It?

MSM is a metabolite of dimethylsulfoxide (DMSO). DMSO is a well-known solvent that is often used topically for its analgesic (pain-killing) and anti-inflammatory properties. The primary role of MSM as a dietary supplement is as a sulfur donor.

Claims

- Relieves arthritis pain and stiffness
- Increases growth hormone synthesis
- Stimulates immune function
- Supports connective tissue integrity (hair, nails, skin)

Theory

MSM, which is about one-third sulfur, acts as a dietary source of sulfur. Sulfur is involved in a wide variety of metabolic pathways and plays an important structural role in amino acid and protein metabolism. Sulfur is required for proper synthesis and maintenance of connective tissues such as skin, hair, nails, tendons, and cartilage. Many supplements claim MSM to be a dietary treatment for osteoarthritis based on the presence of sulfur in connective tissues such as collagen (collagen comprises nearly three-quarters of the solid portion of cartilage).

Scientific Support

Despite the wide range of anecdotal reports of MSM effectiveness, little compelling scientific evidence supports such claims—particularly for osteoarthritis. Several small-animal studies have suggested that MSM may play a role in resistance to stress and stimulation of immune system responses. Doses in the range of 1 to 5 mg/kg per day (approximately 70 to 350 mg for an average-sized man) over a period of two to four weeks appear to stimulate synthesis of immunoglobulins (in mice and chickens). In horses, larger doses (2.5 to 10 g per day) have been associated with improvements in hoof quality.

Safety

The best news about MSM is that it can be considered very safe (although not very effective) when used as a dietary supplement. In rats and dogs, toxic effects are reported only for extremely high doses that would correspond to well over 200 g per day for an average-sized man (about 8 oz of the stuff!).

Value

As a dietary sulfur source (its only valid benefit), MSM would appear to be an overpriced supplement option. There are a number of other less expensive yet equally effective dietary sources of sulfur, including eggs, meat, and fish—as well as sulfur-containing amino acids such as methionine and cystine or cysteine. Large doses of methionine, however, should also be accompanied by supplemental levels of key B vitamins such as folic acid, B_6, and B_{12}, which are known to reduce homocysteine levels (homocysteine is a metabolite of methionine, and high levels have been associated with an increased risk for cardiovascular disease).

Dosage

Typical dosage recommendations range from 2 to 5 g per day as a beginning or "loading" dose to about 50 to 200 mg per day for maintenance. Due to the lack of strong scientific evidence, however, MSM is not recommended as a particularly effective dietary supplement for joint health.

WORKS CONSULTED

Alam SS, Layman DL. Dimethyl sulfoxide inhibition of prostacyclin production in cultured aortic endothelial cells. Ann N Y Acad Sci. 1983;411:318-20.
Bertken R. "Crystalline DMSO": DMSO2. Arthritis Rheum. 1983 May;26(5):693-4.

Childs SJ. Dimethyl sulfone (DMSO2) in the treatment of interstitial cystitis. Urol Clin North Am. 1994 Feb;21(1):85-8.

Klandorf H, Chirra AR, DeGruccio A, Girman DJ. Dimethyl sulfoxide modulation of diabetes onset in NOD mice. Diabetes. 1989 Feb;38(2):194-7.

Layman DL. Growth inhibitory effects of dimethyl sulfoxide and dimethyl sulfone on vascular smooth muscle and endothelial cells in vitro. In Vitro Cell Dev Biol. 1987 Jun;23(6):422-8.

Layman DL, Jacob SW. The absorption, metabolism and excretion of dimethyl sulfoxide by rhesus monkeys. Life Sci. 1985 Dec 23;37(25):2431-7.

Morton JI, Siegel BV. Effects of oral dimethyl sulfoxide and dimethyl sulfone on murine autoimmune lymphoproliferative disease. Proc Soc Exp Biol Med. 1986 Nov;183(2):227-30.

Murav'ev IV, Venikova MS, Pleskovskaia GN, Riazantseva TA, Sigidin IA. Effect of dimethyl sulfoxide and dimethyl sulfone on a destructive process in the joints of mice with spontaneous arthritis. Patol Fiziol Eksp Ter. 1991 Mar-Apr;(2):37-9.

Pain. MSM: Does it work? Harv Health Lett. 2000 Aug;25(10):7.

Richmond VL. Incorporation of methylsulfonylmethane sulfur into guinea pig serum proteins. Life Sci. 1986 Jul 21;39(3):263-8.

HYDROLYZED COLLAGEN PROTEIN (HCP)/GELATIN

What Is It?

Hydrolyzed collagen protein (HCP) is also known as gelatin. Collagen is the chief structural protein that makes up connective tissues in the body (skin, bones, cartilage, tendons, and ligaments). *Hydrolyzed* collagen is simply a modified form of the protein that has been broken down into smaller pieces by enzymes. The hydrolysis process makes the protein easier to incorporate into dietary products and may ease the digestion and absorption of the amino acids by the intestine. HCP is often used as a general protein source in bodybuilding products because it is relatively inexpensive. HCP has most recently been used to promote joint health, nourish cartilage and bones, and help athletes recover from exercise and sports-related injuries.

Claims

- Rebuilds cartilage and bones
- Speeds injury repair
- Promotes tissue recovery following exercise
- Protects against overuse injuries (sprains, strains, tendonitis)

Theory

HCP is not generally considered a good source of high-quality protein such as you would find in meat, poultry, fish, and protein powders comprising soy, egg, or milk/whey proteins. On the one hand, HCP is a poor protein source because it is low in the sulfur-containing amino acids such as cystine (cysteine) and methionine. On the other hand, however, HCP is the richest dietary source of the primary amino acids that make up the collagen molecule—glycine, proline, hydroxyproline, lysine, and hydroxylysine. As a concentrated source of these collagen amino acids, HCP is thought to help nourish the collagen-containing tissues throughout the body such as cartilage, bones, tendons, ligaments, and skin.

Scientific Support

HCP has been used in Europe for decades as a dietary supplement and an alternative treatment for arthritis and osteoporosis. In several German and Czech studies, 7 to 10 g of HCP per day for one to three months has been shown to decrease the pain and stiffness associated with arthritis. In some studies, HCP was as effective as oral painkillers such as acetaminophen

(Tylenol), and in other studies, subjects were able to decrease or discontinue their use of analgesic medications while consuming HCP. Although proponents of HCP consumption claim that it "rebuilds" cartilage, this is merely speculation (although probably correct) based on the body of scientific data showing pain reduction. At least one small German study has shown a suppression of bone breakdown in osteoporotic women. In addition, athletes recovering from intense exercise training or sports injuries appear to be able to do so faster when consuming HCP.

Safety

No serious adverse side effects are known to exist for consumption of hydrolyzed collagen protein.

Value

As a joint support supplement, HCP is typically much less expensive than other popular joint supplements such as glucosamine and chondroitin, but the level and quality of the scientific evidence is also not nearly as strong. It may be possible, however, that because HCP and glucosamine/chondroitin products target different parts of the cartilage structure (collagen and proteoglycans, respectively), one ingredient or the other may work better for some individuals. Several products have recently been developed to include combinations of several ingredients designed to work on different parts of the connective tissue matrix simultaneously.

Dosage

Clinical studies suggest that at least 7 to 10 g per day over the course of thirty to ninety days is needed for reduction of pain in patients with moderate osteoarthritis. It is unknown whether lower doses would be as effective or if higher doses might even be more effective or work faster.

WORKS CONSULTED

Adam M, Hulejova H, Miterova S. The development of osteoarthrosis and the role of collagen in the pathophysiology of its development. Acta Chir Orthop Traumatol Cech. 1989 Oct;56(5):377-90.

Adam M, Krabcova M, Miterova L, von der Mark K, Kuhn K. The presence of collagen of type III in pathologically altered cartilage and bone. Cas Lek Cesk. 1980 Sep 26;119(39):1043-8.

Adam M, Krabcova M, Musilova J, Pesakova V, Brettschneider I, Deyl Z. Contribution to the mode of action of glycosaminoglycan-polysulphate (GAGPS) upon human osteoarthrotic cartilage. Biochemical study of the collagen and proteoglycan turnover. Arzneimittelforschung. 1980;30(10):1730-2.

Adam M, Musilova J. Cartilage and osteoarthrosis: Changes of collagen and proteoglycans. Czech Med. 1979;2(1-2):64-8.

Adam M, Musilova J, Deyl Z. Cartilage collagen in osteoarthrosis. Clin Chim Acta. 1976 May 17;69(1):53-9.

Adam M, Musilova J, Krabcova M, Brettschneider I, Pesakova V, Deyl Z. Effect of cartilage bone marrow extract on the metabolism of collagen in osteoarthrotic cartilage. Pharmacology. 1980;21(1):53-8.

Adam M, Novotna J, Deyl Z. Changes in collagen metabolism—another look at osteoarthrosis. Acta Biol Hung. 1984;35(2-4):181-7.

Adam M, Trnavsky K. Changes in the metabolism of collagen in progressive polyarthritis. Cas Lek Cesk. 1984 Jun 15;123(24):724-6.

Adam M, Vitasek R, Deyl Z, Felsch G, Musilova J, Olsovska Z. Collagen in rheumatoid arthritis. Clin Chim Acta. 1976 Jul 1;70(1):61-9.

Alleviating arthritis. Can gelatin promote joint health? Johns Hopkins Med Lett Health After 50. 1998 Aug;10(6):8.

Arborelius M Jr, Konttinen YT, Nordstrom DC, Solovieva SA. Gly-X-Y repeat sequences in the treatment of active rheumatoid arthritis. Rheumatol Int. 1999;18(4):129-35.

Becvar R, Myllyla R, Krbec M, Cech O, Adam M. Changes in collagen biosynthesis in patients with hip joint replacement surgery and reoperation. Acta Chir Orthop Traumatol Cech. 1991 May;58(3):178-84.

Brown KE, Leong K, Huang CH, Dalal R, Green GD, Haimes HB, Jimenez PA, Bathon J. Gelatin/chondroitin 6-sulfate microspheres for the delivery of therapeutic proteins to the joint. Arthritis Rheum. 1998 Dec;41(12):2185-95.

Krajickova J, Macek J, Medova N, Adam M. Excretion of proteoglycan degradation products in the urine in patients with rheumatoid arthritis and osteoarthrosis. Vnitr Lek. 1987 Feb;33(2):129-33.

Kuettner KE, Thonar EJ, Aydelotte MB. Modern aspects of articular cartilage biochemistry. Verh Dtsch Ges Inn Med. 1989;95:436-47.

Macek J, Adam M. Determination of collagen degradation products in human urine in osteoarthrosis. Z Rheumatol. 1987 Sep-Oct;46(5):237-40.

McDevitt CA. Biochemistry of articular cartilage. Nature of proteoglycans and collagen of articular cartilage and their role in ageing and in osteoarthrosis. Ann Rheum Dis. 1973 Jul;32(4):364-78.

Myllyla R, Becvar R, Adam M, Kivirikko KI. Markers of collagen metabolism in sera of patients with various rheumatic diseases. Clin Chim Acta. 1989 Aug 31;183(3):243-52.

Novotna J, Hulejova H, Svoboda T, Deyl Z, Adam M. The role of cartilage minor collagens in inducing arthritis. Z Rheumatol. 1991 Mar-Apr;50(2):93-8.

Novotna J, Hulejova H, Svoboda T, Trc T, Deyl Z, Adam M. Experimental models of arthritis induced by various cartilage collagen type. Cas Lek Cesk. 1989 Jan 27;128(5):139-45.

Schattenkirchner M. Treatment of arthrosis. Internist (Berl). 1990 Jan;31(1):82.

DEVIL'S CLAW

What Is It?

Devil's claw *(Harpagophytum procumbens),* also known as "grapple plant" or "grappling hook fruit" because of the look of the fruit, is a South African plant used medicinally to reduce pain and inflammation. Modern herbalists typically use devil's claw as a treatment for arthritis and low back pain.

Claims

- Relieves pain and inflammation
- Alleviates arthritis and low back pain

Theory

Devil's claw contains several iridoid glucoside compounds, such as harpagoside, which are thought to influence the synthesis of prostaglandins, eicosanoids, thromboxanes, and leukotrienes—all of which are involved in inflammation. By reducing the synthesis of these inflammatory prostaglandins, both pain and inflammation may be reduced.

Scientific Support

The German Commission E has approved the use of devil's claw for "degenerative disorders of the locomotor system"—making arthritis, tendonitis, and back pain common indications. Several double-blind studies have shown two to eight weeks of devil's claw treatment to reduce pain and improve mobility in cases of rheumatoid arthritis and osteoarthritis. In other studies, however, subjects with chronic back pain reported only a modest pain relief from devil's claw (if any). Animal studies have found anti-inflammatory and analgesic (pain-relieving) effects, and an in vitro (test-tube) study has shown reduced synthesis of inflammation mediators in human blood. Two other studies, however, have found no anti-inflammatory or analgesic effects for devil's claw. One study found high doses of devil's

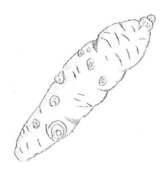

claw to be completely ineffective in reducing inflammation (in an animal model) and in inhibiting prostaglandin synthetase (in a test tube). These results suggest that devil's claw lacks the anti-inflammatory properties found in common anti-inflammatory medications. A more recent human study (1992) also found devil's claw (2 g per day containing 3 percent iridoid glucosides for three weeks) to lack anti-inflammatory activity (eicosanoid production—PGE2, PGF1, thromboxane, and leukotriene).

Overall, the results from test-tube, animal, and human studies on the benefits of devil's claw are conflicting—some studies show anti-inflammatory and pain-relieving effects and other studies show no benefit. It is possible that only certain types of inflammatory conditions respond sufficiently to devil's claw treatment. For example, in one study of back pain, twenty-five out of thirty subjects experienced significant reductions in pain levels and increases in mobility (by about 50 percent), whereas the remaining five subjects showed no change.

Safety

Devil's claw does not appear to be associated with adverse side effects or toxicity, aside from mild gastrointestinal distress. Because of its ability to stimulate secretion of gastric acids, individuals with gastric or duodenal ulcers should avoid devil's claw.

Value

At $15 to $20 for a one-month supply of devil's claw, a properly standardized extract (see Dosage) may be a useful and effective natural treatment for reducing pain and inflammation associated with arthritis and back pain. Since much of the research on devil's claw has been conducted on the extract from Lichtwer Pharma, it may be prudent to select products that include this particular extract.

Dosage

Typical dosage recommendations for devil's claw are 750 to 6,000 mg per day (taken in two to three divided doses) of a root extract standardized to contain 1 to 3 percent iridoid glycosides. The German Pharmacopoeia requires a minimum content of 1 percent harpagoside for devil's claw preparations. A total level of 24 to 60 mg of harpagoside would represent a clinically effective dose.

WORKS CONSULTED

Abou-Mandour A. Pharmaceutical-biological studies of the genus Harpagophytum. 2. Communication: Tissue cultures of Harpagophytum procumbens. Planta Med. 1977 May;31(3):238-44.

Baghdikian B, Lanhers MC, Fleurentin J, Ollivier E, Maillard C, Balansard G, Mortier F. An analytical study, anti-inflammatory and analgesic effects of Harpagophytum procumbens and Harpagophytum zeyheri. Planta Med. 1997 Apr;63(2):171-6.

Caprasse M. Description, identification and therapeutical uses of the "devil's claw": Harpagophytum procumbens DC. J Pharm Belg. 1980 Mar-Apr;35(2):143-9.

Erdos A, Fontaine R, Friehe H, Durand R, Poppinghaus T. Contribution to the pharmacology and toxicology of different extracts as well as the harpagoside from Harpagophytum procumbens DC. Planta Med. 1978 Aug;34(1):97-108.

Ficarra P, Ficarra R, Tommasini A, De Pasquale Costa R, Guarniera Fenech C, Ragusa S. HPLC analysis of a drug in traditional medicine: Harpagophytum procumbens DC. I. Boll Chim Farm. 1986 Jul;125(7):250-3.

Fontaine J, Elchami AA, Vanhaelen M, Vanhaelen-Fastre R. Biological analysis of Harpagophytum procumbens D.C. II. Pharmacological analysis of the effects of harpagoside, harpagide and harpagogenine on the isolated guinea-pig ileum. J Pharm Belg. 1981 Sep-Oct;36(5):321-4.

Grahame R, Robinson BV. Devils's claw (Harpagophytum procumbens): Pharmacological and clinical studies. Ann Rheum Dis. 1981 Dec;40(6):632.

McLeod DW, Revell P, Robinson BV. Investigations of Harpagophytum procumbens (Devil's Claw) in the treatment of experimental inflammation and arthritis in the rat. Br J Pharmacol. 1979 May;66(1):140P-1P.

Moussard C, Alber D, Toubin MM, Thevenon N, Henry JC. A drug used in traditional medicine, Harpagophytum procumbens: No evidence for NSAID-like effect on whole blood eicosanoid production in human. Prostaglandins Leukot Essent Fatty Acids. 1992 Aug;46(4):283-6.

Pourrat H, Texier O, Vennat B, Pourrat A, Gaillard J. Stability of iridoids of Harpagophytum procumbens DC. during the preparation of powders and atomized drugs. Ann Pharm Fr. 1985;43(6):601-6.

Tunmann P, Bauersfeld HJ. Further components from radix Harpagophytum procumbens DC. Arch Pharm (Weinheim). 1975 Aug;308(8):655-7.

Wegener T. Therapy of degenerative diseases of the musculoskeletal system with South African devil's claw. Wien Med Wochenschr. 1999;149(8-10):254-7.

Whitehouse LW, Znamirowska M, Paul CJ. Devil's Claw (Harpagophytum procumbens): No evidence for anti-inflammatory activity in the treatment of arthritic disease. Can Med Assoc J. 1983 Aug 1;129(3):249-51.

GREEN-LIPPED MUSSEL

What Is It?

Green-lipped mussel *(Perna canaliculus)* is sold as Seatone and Lyprinol—both of which are powdered forms of the mussel flesh (Seatone highlights its glycogen content, while Lyprinol highlights its lipid content). As a dietary supplement, green-lipped mussel can be considered a source of chondroitin and other glycosaminoglycans (as can sea cucumber and shark cartilage). The majority of green-lipped mussel comes from Australia or New Zealand. You'll know whether your supplement contains the right ingredient by its fishy smell.

Claims

- Relieves joint pain and stiffness (from arthritis)
- Reduces inflammation
- Enhances postexercise and injury recovery

Theory

Because green-lipped mussel contains a wide variety of glycosamino-glycans, it has been recommended as a natural therapy for maintaining and rebuilding connective tissues such as cartilage, tendons, and ligaments as well as for its anti-inflammatory properties.

Scientific Support

The anti-inflammatory effects of green-lipped mussel have been demonstrated in experimental animal models (usually mice with induced paw swelling). In these studies, green-lipped mussel appears to be effective in delaying or preventing inflammation (so mice with swollen feet should definitely take this supplement). The presence of anti-inflammatory fatty acids may provide an additive effect in controlling prostaglandin synthesis (potentially with pain-relieving effects). At least a few studies have shown an improvement of arthritic symptoms in dogs supplemented with 1 to 3 g of green-lipped mussel per day for two to four months (so dogs with stiff legs and hips are prime candidates for this supplement). Unfortunately, the scientific evidence for a beneficial effect in humans is quite weak. A couple of small studies conducted in the 1980s suggested that green-lipped mussel may be effective in relieving the joint pain and stiffness associated with arthritis (similar to effects seen for glucosamine and chondroitin), but follow-up studies found no beneficial effects.

Safety

No serious side effects are known, although individuals allergic to shell-fish should be especially cautious and avoid using supplements containing green-lipped mussel extract.

Value

At around $30 for a one-month supply of capsules (at a "low" dose), green-lipped mussel could be an effective anti-inflammatory for both mice and dogs—but human benefits are unclear. The purported health benefits of green-lipped mussel are likely due to various fatty acids and glucosamine-like compounds, which have both been shown to be effective in controlling inflammation and pain associated with arthritis and other conditions. On the downside, dosages that may be effective are high (making the product more expensive) and it stinks (like fish).

Dosage

Typical dosage recommendations are for 500 to 3,000 mg of green-lipped mussel extract per day, taken in two to three divided doses throughout the day.

WORKS CONSULTED

Caughey DE, Grigor RR, Caughey EB, Young P, Gow PJ, Stewart AW. Perna canaliculus in the treatment of rheumatoid arthritis. Eur J Rheumatol Inflamm. 1983;6(2):197-200.

Couch RA, Ormrod DJ, Miller TE, Watkins WB. Anti-inflammatory activity in fractionated extracts of the green-lipped mussel. N Z Med J. 1982 Nov 24;95(720):803-6.

Gibson RG, Gibson SL. Green-lipped mussel extract in arthritis. Lancet. 1981 Feb 21;1(8217):439.

Gibson RG, Gibson SL. New Zealand green-lipped mussel extract (Seatone) and rheumatoid arthritis. N Z Med J. 1981 May 27;93(684):343.

Gibson RG, Gibson SL. New Zealand green-lipped mussel extract (Seatone) in rheumatoid arthritis. N Z Med J. 1981 Jul 22;94(688):67-8.

Kosuge T, Tsuji K, Ishida H, Yamaguchi T. Isolation of an anti-histaminic substance from green-lipped mussel (Perna canaliculus). Chem Pharm Bull (Tokyo). 1986 Nov;34(11):4825-8.

Larkin JG, Capell HA, Sturrock RD. Seatone in rheumatoid arthritis: A six-month placebo-controlled study. Ann Rheum Dis. 1985 Mar;44(3):199-201.

Miller T, Wu H. In vivo evidence for prostaglandin inhibitory activity in New Zealand green-lipped mussel extract. N Z Med J. 1984 Jun 13;97(757):355-7.

Miller TE, Dodd J, Ormrod DJ, Geddes R. Anti-inflammatory activity of glycogen extracted from Perna canaliculus (NZ green-lipped mussel). Agents Actions. 1993;38(Spec No):C139-42.

Miller TE, Ormrod D. The anti-inflammatory activity of Perna canaliculus (NZ green lipped mussel). N Z Med J. 1980 Sep 10;92(667):187-93.

Rainsford KD, Whitehouse MW. Gastroprotective and anti-inflammatory properties of green lipped mussel (Perna canaliculus) preparation. Arzneimittelforschung. 1980;30(12):2128-32.

SEA CUCUMBER

What Is It?

Sea cucumbers *(bêche-de-mer)* are not cucumbers at all—or even members of the plant family, for that matter. Instead, sea cucumbers are swishy sea-dwelling animals related to the starfish. The sea cucumber's body wall is composed of five muscle strips running from front to back. At the front end of the animal, the mouth is ringed by feeding tentacles. They serve as "ocean filters" by sucking in sediments and recycling nutrients into the sea (feeding on microorganisms associated with sediment particles). For use as dietary supplements, the sea cucumbers are harvested from the sea, dried, and pulverized into powder for encapsulation. In many parts of Asia, sea cucumbers are considered a delicacy. The strong demand for them in Asian cuisine and in arthritis supplements has led to serious arguments about fisheries management and conservation issues in many parts of the world (because they grow very slowly, and it can take years to replenish populations that are overfished).

Claims

- Relieves joint pain and stiffness (from arthritis)

Theory

Because sea cucumber contains chondroitin and other mucupolysaccharides, it has been recommended as a treatment for arthritis to help rebuild joint cartilage.

Scientific Support

While several analytical reports denote the chondroitin and glycosaminoglycan content of various strains of sea cucumber, no published reports support its effectiveness in relieving arthritis pain and stiffness.

Safety

There are no known side effects, but potential anticoagulant (blood-thinning) effects at high doses.

Value

At about $7 to $20 for sixty 500 mg capsules (about a thirty-day supply), sea cucumber could be viewed as a cheap, but impure, source of chondroitin (as many people view shark cartilage). The likelihood of receiving significant benefit is slim and it may be prudent to select other supplements for alleviating joint pain such as glucosamine, HCP, SAMe, and boswellia.

Dosage

Typical dosage recommendations are 500 to 2,000 mg per day, usually taken in two divided doses (morning and evening).

WORKS CONSULTED

Imanari T, Washio Y, Huang Y, Toyoda H, Suzuki A, Toida T. Oral absorption and clearance of partially depolymerized fucosyl chondroitin sulfate from sea cucumber. Thromb Res. 1999 Feb 1;93(3):129-35.

Kariya Y, Watabe S, Hashimoto K, Yoshida K. Occurrence of chondroitin sulfate E in glycosaminoglycan isolated from the body wall of sea cucumber Stichopus japonicus. J Biol Chem. 1990 Mar 25;265(9):5081-5.

Mourao PA, Pereira MS, Pavao MS, Mulloy B, Tollefsen DM, Mowinckel MC, Abildgaard U. Structure and anticoagulant activity of a fucosylated chondroitin sulfate from echinoderm. Sulfated fucose branches on the polysaccharide account for its high anticoagulant action. J Biol Chem. 1996 Sep 27;271(39):23973-84.

Vieira RP, Mourao PA. Occurrence of a unique fucose-branched chondroitin sulfate in the body wall of a sea cucumber. J Biol Chem. 1988 Dec 5;263(34): 18176-83.

Vieira RP, Pedrosa C, Mourao PA. Extensive heterogeneity of proteoglycans bearing fucose-branched chondroitin sulfate extracted from the connective tissue of sea cucumber. Biochemistry. 1993 Mar 9;32(9):2254-62.

Chapter 9

Supplements for Mood and Brain Health

INTRODUCTION

When most people think about dietary supplements for brain function and mood elevation, they automatically think of the herbs ginkgo biloba for memory and St. John's wort for emotional balance. Although brain function and mood elevation are two distinct categories of health, there is consistent overlap between the two, so it is important to discuss them together. It is vitally important, however, for anybody with moderate to severe levels of depression to *immediately* consult his or her personal physician and not rely solely on dietary supplements to self-treat the condition. That said, it is important to note that mild depression, "the blues," and chronic unhappiness and lack of energy can oftentimes be a nonspecific response to a wide variety of stressors, hormone imbalances, or biochemical abnormalities.

It is no surprise that dietary supplements promoted for "brain health" (memory, concentration, and emotions) are among the top-selling products on the market. There are millions of tired and stressed-out people who can relate to promises of natural products that will enhance their brain function—and the number is continually growing as the worldwide population ages. With age, there is almost always some degree of memory loss, particularly in short-term memory and learning ability.

The slow progression of short-term memory loss is sometimes classified as age-related memory impairment or ARMI and may be due to subtle physiological and biochemical changes in the nervous system as we age (such as neuronal death and reduced neurotransmitter synthesis). The good news is that recent studies of cognitive function in older adults show quite clearly that individuals who "exercise" their brains on a regular basis show a significant slowing of mental impairment—sort of a "use it or lose it" situation.

An important part of maintaining optimal brain function is ensuring that the brain receives an adequate supply of oxygen. Cerebrovascular disease ("atherosclerosis of the brain") can affect blood circulation to the brain and lead to a progressive decline in memory and overall cognitive ability. Because the brain uses 20 to 30 percent of the body's total oxygen supply, it is quite sensitive to small changes in blood flow and oxygen delivery. Several dietary supplements, such as the wildly popular (and effective) ginkgo biloba, are thought to have benefits in treating or preventing age-related senility due to powerful effects on maintaining blood flow in the brain.

THE FIRST STEP—DIET AND EXERCISE

Physiologists and nutritionists regularly document the dramatic improvements in mood, emotions, confidence, and self-efficacy that are the result of some very simple lifestyle modifications. Regular exercise and adequate diet can result in profound changes in the body's own production of mood-elevating chemicals such as the endorphins that cause "runner's high" and neurotransmitters such as serotonin that contribute to emotional well-being. In general terms, *any* amount of exercise can help relieve mild to moderate depression and help elevate mood. Walking for 20 minutes on as many days of the week as possible (at least three times per week) might be a good place to start.

Now for the nutrition side of things. It will probably come as no surprise that diet is intimately tied to emotions. Just think about your feelings as you contemplate gorging yourself on that hot fudge sundae (guilty), followed by your feelings when you finally give in to the temptation (more guilt) and start eating (elation) until you get to the bottom of the bowl (disappointment). All kidding aside, the food that we eat directly influences our moods because the macronutrients (carbs, proteins, fats) and micronutrients (vitamins, minerals, and phytonutrients) ultimately act as potent neurochemicals in the body. For example, some people feel energized when following a low-fat, high-carbohydrate diet, while others are left feeling hungry, lethargic, and depressed.

For most people, the best advice for getting a handle on their emotional balance is to take a week or so to analyze how diet affects mood. Look at every speck of food that you eat and how it makes you feel. Once you feel that you know a bit about how certain foods influence your emotions, then you can decide where some of the dietary supplements outlined in this chapter may (or may not) fit into your lifestyle.

DIETARY SUPPLEMENTS

Vitamin B_6 is sort of the perennial "nerve supplement" as it has been recommended for dozens of conditions associated with nerve damage, maintenance, and repair (most often for carpal tunnel syndrome). Women taking birth control pills are sometimes at risk for having low vitamin B_6 levels (some oral contraceptives can accelerate B_6 destruction) and therefore may want to take a supplement (5 to 20 mg per day). Although the data are relatively weak, some forms of depression may be related to low or reduced levels of vitamin B_6 and iron and may respond to dietary supplements. In particular, the depressed emotions associated with premenstrual syndrome (PMS) may be related to low B_6 and/or iron levels. Doses of as much as 100 mg of B_6 and 10 to 20 mg of iron per day may be helpful in such situations (do not exceed 500 mg per day of B_6 or 30 mg of iron). In some children, low levels of B_6 and choline have been suggested as contributing factors in development of attention deficit hyperactivity disorder (ADHD or ADD).

Vitamin B_{12} is sometimes called the "senility vitamin" because levels are so often depressed in elderly individuals suffering from senile dementia. In many cases, high-dose vitamin B_{12} injections can improve many measures of mental function and help to elevate mood.

Vitamin E may, in some cases, slow the progression of Alzheimer's disease—probably due to the antioxidant effects of the vitamin in protecting brain cell membranes from oxidative free radical damage. Standard dosage recommendations of 400 to 800 international units (IU) for heart benefits may need to be increased to 1,000 IU or more to provide benefits for individuals suffering from dementia. Consult your personal physician before taking such high doses due to concerns about reduced blood clotting.

Several amino acids, such as phenylalanine, taurine, and tyrosine have been associated with improved mental function, particularly under conditions of chronic stress. In the case of tyrosine, conversion to the neurotransmitter norepinephrine may help elevate mood in mildly depressed individuals (although relatively high levels of 5 to 10 g are needed). During exercise, reduced levels of another group of amino acids, the branched chain amino acids (BCAA), have been linked to the onset of mental and physical fatigue. Supplementation with BCAAs before and during intense exercise can help delay the onset of fatigue and may help maintain mental performance.

A number of phospholipids (basically a fat with a phosphate group attached) can play a role in the production and metabolism of brain neurotransmitters. In particular, phosphatidylserine (PS) and phosphatidylcholine (PC) have shown promising results in reducing depression and promoting optimal brain function (200 to 800 mg of each per day). Lecithin, a mixture of several phospholipids extracted from soybeans, is often used as an inexpensive source of PC (about 25 percent) along with phosphatidylethanolamine (PE) and phosphatidylinositol (PI)—which make up an additional 40 percent or so of lecithin. Unfortunately, lecithin is a relatively poor source of PS unless it has been specifically enriched in this fraction. Phospholipids are both an important structural component of cell membranes, including those in nerves cells and the brain, and an important functional component for the synthesis of neurotransmitters such as acetylcholine needed for nerve transmission. Large doses of lecithin are typically needed to deliver the high levels of PS and PC that have been associated with improvements in cognitive function. For example, more than 10 g of lecithin are needed to provide about 2 to 3 g of PC. A single egg, on the other hand, contains 3 to 4 g of PC. Because PS is virtually nonexistent in lecithin, specialized (and expensive) supplements supplying 200 to 800 mg are needed for improvements in memory and cognitive performance. In patients suffering from the moderate to severe cognitive impairment common to Alzheimer's disease, three months of PS supplementation may improve memory and general mental function. Doses as high as 1,000 mg are well tolerated without significant side effects.

St. John's wort is probably the granddaddy of the "brain" herbs in terms of public popularity. Extracts of the herb are effective in treating mild to moderate depression (as effective as some of the older prescription antidepressants such as imipramine). Side effects for using standardized extracts (1 to 2 mg hypericin per day) are rare, but four to eight weeks may be needed before noticing results.

Ginkgo biloba is as popular as St. John's wort but with slightly different usage indications. Extracts of ginkgo leaves can improve circulation to the brain (and other parts of the body) and may boost memory and ability to concentrate. In individuals with cognitive dysfunction, ginkgo may have some benefits in slowing the loss of mental faculties. In people with normal brain function, ginkgo supplements are less likely to produce a noticeable effect on mental acuity, but the flavonoid compounds in ginkgo extracts may contribute to antioxidant protection of brain cells. Dosage recommendations for standardized extracts (at least 24 percent ginkgosides and 6 percent terpenes) are in the range of 120 to 250 mg per day, taken in two to three divided doses throughout the day.

A final herbal recommendation to support brain function and ability to focus is consumption of the adaptogenic herbs of the ginseng family. Both Asian and Siberian ginseng are frequently used to boost energy levels and maintain stamina. In some cases, these effects may also be perceived as an enhanced ability to concentrate. Depending on the standardized extract, 100 to 200 mg of Asian ginseng or 200 to 400 mg of Siberian ginseng (eleuthero) may be effective. For a summary of supplements discussed in this chapter, see Table 9.1.

TABLE 9.1. Dietary Supplements for Brain Function and Emotional Support

Ingredient	Dose (per day)	Primary claims
5-HTP	300-900 mg	Relieves mild depression
Choline	1-5 g	Improves memory
DLPA	75-200 mg	Elevates mood
Feverfew	25-125 mg	Prevents migraines
Ginkgo biloba	120-240 mg	Improves memory
Huperzine A	50 mcg	Improves memory
Kava-kava	50-150 mg	Antianxiety
Melatonin	1-10 mg	Antianxiety/sleep aid
Phosphatidylserine	100-1,000 mg	Improves memory
SAMe	200-600 mg	Relieves mild depression
St. John's wort	450-900 mg	Relieves mild depression
Valerian	250-500 mg	Antianxiety/sleep aid
Vinpocetine	10-30 mg	Improves memory

ST. JOHN'S WORT

What Is It?

St. John's wort *(Hypericum perforatum)*, also called Klamath weed, is a five-petaled yellow flower, which is especially plentiful in northern California and southern Oregon. The name "St. John's" comes from the red color of the extract (from squeezed buds and flowers), which was associated with the blood of St. John the Baptist and the fact that the herb typically flowers around the time of the feast of St. John. St. John's wort has been used for centuries for everything from "protection against evil spirits" (depression) and for wound healing to its most common present-day use as an antidepressant. The active ingredients in St. John's wort extract are unknown, but extracts standardized to contain napthodianthrone compounds such as hypericin and pseudohypericin along with phloroglucinols such as hyperforin and adhyperforin are known to be effective in alleviating mild to moderate depressive symptoms. St. John's wort also contains various flavonoids and proanthocyanidin polymers.

Claims

- Eases symptoms of mild to moderate depression
- Stabilizes mood, including seasonal mood changes
- Increases energy levels (in some people)
- Controls appetite and promotes weight loss (in some people)
- Improves tolerance to stress
- Improves sleep patterns in older people (caution: can interfere with sleep in some people)
- Aids in wound healing and in resistance to viral infection when applied topically

Theory

As an antidepressant, St. John's wort has been shown to inhibit an enzyme (catechol-*O*-methyltransferase) that degrades certain neurotransmitters such as dopamine. It has also been shown to inhibit serotonin re-uptake in the brain and to reduce expression of interleukin-6 and gamma-aminobutyric acid (GABA) uptake. Each of these actions can contribute to alleviating depression by slow-

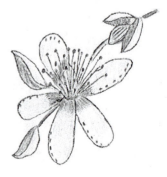

ing the recycling of neurotransmitters needed for maintaining emotional balance. As an antiviral agent, St. John's wort has been reputed to inhibit replication of several viruses, including herpes simplex, HIV, and the virus that causes mononucleosis.

Scientific Support

Several clinical studies have been conducted to determine the efficacy of St. John's wort for those with mild to moderate depression. In one review of twenty-three randomized trials (fifteen placebo-controlled and eight drug comparisons) including nearly 2,000 patients with mild or moderate depressive disorders, extracts of St. John's wort were nearly three times more effective than placebo, and were comparable to prescription antidepressants (with fewer side effects). Across the studies, fewer than 1 percent of those taking St. John's wort dropped out of the study, compared with a dropout rate of 3 percent of those taking a prescription antidepressant. Perhaps the most encouraging results were that in contrast to the high percentage of side effects in those taking prescription antidepressants (52.8 percent), only 19.8 percent of those taking St. John's wort experienced any adverse effects. Other well-controlled studies comparing the St. John's wort extract LI 160 (from Lichtwer Pharma) to prescription antidepressants such as Prozac (fluoxetine), sertraline (Zoloft), paroxetine (Paxil), imipramine, amitriptyline, and maprotiline have all found St. John's wort to be comparable in effectiveness, but superior to prescription drugs with regard to tolerability. Overall, more than a dozen double-blind placebo-controlled studies have been conducted (mostly small studies), with the majority supporting the case for the effectiveness of St. John's wort in alleviating mild to moderate depression.

In the one recent study in the literature that explored the use of St. John's wort as a retroviral agent for use in HIV-infected patients, over half of the patients discontinued treatment early because of severe cutaneous phototoxicity (skin sensitivity to sunlight exposure). Of those who remained in the study, there were no significant changes in virological markers. It should be noted that HIV-positive patients should *not* use St. John's wort without specific advice and consultation with their personal physicians, as the herb has been shown to almost completely inactivate the effects of certain antiviral medications (indinavir and other protease inhibitors).

Safety

St. John's wort is quite safe in terms of observed side effects, the most common of which are typically mild gastrointestinal upset, mild allergic reactions (skin rash), tiredness, and insomnia or restlessness. There have been no published reports of serious adverse side effects from taking the herb alone, and animal studies with large doses of St. John's wort have not shown any serious problems. The most commonly studied adverse effect of St. John's wort is its ability to cause photosensitivity, especially in fair-skinned individuals. This condition is reversible upon discontinuation of the herb. Thus, special care should be taken to avoid ultraviolet light, or to frequently apply sunscreen and wear sunglasses (due to an increased risk of cataracts) when it is necessary to be outside. Other side effects include gastrointestinal symptoms, dizziness, confusion and tiredness, and tend to be equivalent in incidence to placebo.

Scientific studies conducted in vitro (test-tube studies) have shown St. John's wort to be mutagenic and toxic to sperm, suggesting that it should not be taken when trying to become pregnant. On the flip side, St. John's wort has also been shown to interfere with the action of certain oral contraceptives (birth control pills). St. John's wort is not recommended for children or for women who are pregnant or lactating.

Although it is no longer believed that St. John's wort potentiates MAO inhibitors, consult your physician if you are taking MAO inhibitors or prescription antidepressants before you take St. John's wort.

Although direct side effects from consuming St. John's wort appear to be quite rare, several recent reports have raised the possibility that the herb may interact with and decrease the effectiveness of various medications, including HIV drugs (protease inhibitors), immunosuppressants (such as cyclosporin for organ transplants), digoxin (for congestive heart failure), blood thinners (Coumadin/warfarin), chemotherapy drugs (olanzapine/clozapine), and asthma medications (theophylline). If you are currently taking any of these or other prescription medications, *do not* begin taking *or* discontinue taking St. John's wort without first consulting your personal physician (abrupt withdrawal of the herb could increase blood levels of various medications, which could be dangerous in certain cases).

Value

St. John's wort appears to be helpful in about 50 to 60 percent of cases, but as with prescription antidepressants, the full effect takes about four to six weeks to develop. It is important to note that St. John's wort should *never* be used for the treatment of severe depression (feelings of suicide, extreme inability to cope with daily life, severe anxiety, or extreme fatigue)—physician-directed drug therapy may mean the difference between life and death.

That said, St. John's wort is sold in a variety of forms, including tea, drops, tablets, capsules, and even in a snack-chip form (not a joke). In tablet or capsule form, standardized St. John's wort (300 to 900 mg per day) typically costs between $20 and $30 per month—not a bad price for a relatively safe and effective dietary supplement for those with mild to moderate depression, anxiety, or seasonal affective disorder.

Dosage

The recommended dosage for St. John's wort is 900 mg per day (300 mg taken three times per day) of a 5:1 extract of the flowering tops and leaves standardized to contain 0.3 percent hypericin in a complex of other natural compounds, or 3 to 5 percent hyperforin (the main constituent that is thought to inhibit neurotransmitter reuptake). Minimal treatment time is four to six weeks. St. John's wort is sold in the United States only as an herbal supplement, although it is marketed as a drug in Germany for the treatment of mild depression and anxiety.

WORKS CONSULTED

Cott JM. In vitro receptor binding and enzyme inhibition by Hypericum perforatum extract. Pharmacopsychiatry. 1997 Sep;30(Suppl 2):108-12.

Cott JM, Fugh-Berman A. Is St. John's wort (Hypericum perforatum) an effective antidepressant? J Nerv Ment Dis. 1998 Aug;186(8):500-1.

Czekalla J, Gastpar M, Hubner WD, Jager D. The effect of hypericum extract on cardiac conduction as seen in the electrocardiogram compared to that of imipramine. Pharmacopsychiatry. 1997 Sep;30(Suppl 2):86-8.

De Vry J, Maurel S, Schreiber R, de Beun R, Jentzsch KR. Comparison of hypericum extracts with imipramine and fluoxetine in animal models of depression and alcoholism. Eur Neuropsychopharmacol. 1999 Dec;9(6):461-8.

Firenzuoli F, Luigi G. Safety of Hypericum perforatum. J Altern Complement Med. 1999 Oct;5(5):397-8.

Fugh-Berman A, Cott JM. Dietary supplements and natural products as psychotherapeutic agents. Psychosom Med. 1999 Sep-Oct;61(5):712-28.

Gaster B, Holroyd J. St John's wort for depression: A systematic review. Arch Intern Med. 2000 Jan 24;160(2):152-6.

Golsch S, Vocks E, Rakoski J, Brockow K, Ring J. Reversible increase in photosensitivity to UV-B caused by St. John's wort extract. Hautarzt. 1997 Apr;48(4):249-52.

Hansgen KD, Vesper J, Ploch M. Multicenter double-blind study examining the antidepressant effectiveness of the hypericum extract LI 160. J Geriatr Psychiatry Neurol. 1994 Oct;7(Suppl 1):S15-8.

Harrer G, Hubner WD, Podzuweit H. Effectiveness and tolerance of the hypericum extract LI 160 compared to maprotiline: A multicenter double-blind study. J Geriatr Psychiatry Neurol. 1994 Oct;7(Suppl 1):S24-8.

Holsboer-Trachsler E, Vanoni C. Clinical efficacy and tolerance of the hypericum special extract LI 160 in depressive disorders—a drug monitoring study. Schweiz Rundsch Med Prax. 1999 Sep 9;88(37):1475-80.

Hubner WD, Lande S, Podzuweit H. Hypericum treatment of mild depressions with somatic symptoms. J Geriatr Psychiatry Neurol. 1994 Oct;7(Suppl 1):S12-4.

Jobst KA, McIntyre M, St George D, Whitelegg M. Safety of St John's wort. Lancet. 2000 Feb 12;355(9203):575.

Johne A, Brockmoller J, Bauer S, Maurer A, Langheinrich M, Roots I. Pharmacokinetic interaction of digoxin with an herbal extract from St John's wort (Hypericum perforatum). Clin Pharmacol Ther. 1999 Oct;66(4):338-45.

Kasper S. Treatment of seasonal affective disorder (SAD) with hypericum extract. Pharmacopsychiatry. 1997 Sep;30(Suppl 2):89-93.

Laakmann G, Schule C, Baghai T, Kieser M. St. John's wort in mild to moderate depression: The relevance of hyperforin for the clinical efficacy. Pharmacopsychiatry. 1998 Jun;31(Suppl 1):54-9.

Linde K, Ramirez G, Mulrow CD, Pauls A, Weidenhammer W, Melchart D. St John's wort for depression—an overview and meta-analysis of randomised clinical trials. Br Med J. 1996 Aug 3;313(7052):253-8.

Martinez B, Kasper S, Ruhrmann S, Moller HJ. Hypericum in the treatment of seasonal affective disorders. J Geriatr Psychiatry Neurol. 1994 Oct;7(Suppl 1): S29-33.

Miller AL. St. John's Wort (Hypericum perforatum): Clinical effects on depression and other conditions. Altern Med Rev. 1998 Feb;3(1):18-26.

Miller JL. Study provides additional support for hypericum extract. Am J Health Syst Pharm. 2000 Feb 1;57(3):208, 213.

Muller WE, Rolli M, Schafer C, Hafner U. Effects of hypericum extract (LI 160) in biochemical models of antidepressant activity. Pharmacopsychiatry. 1997 Sep;30 (Suppl 2):102-7.

Myers J. Can an herb really help depression? Adv Nurse Pract. 1998 Mar;6(3):33-4.

Neary JT, Bu Y. Hypericum LI 160 inhibits uptake of serotonin and norepinephrine in astrocytes. Brain Res. 1999 Jan 23;816(2):358-63.

Nierenberg AA, Burt T, Matthews J, Weiss AP. Mania associated with St. John's wort. Biol Psychiatry. 1999 Dec 15;46(12):1707-8.

Pepping J. St. John's wort: Hypericum perforatum. Am J Health Syst Pharm. 1999 Feb 15;56(4):329-30.

Philipp M, Kohnen R, Hiller KO. Hypericum extract versus imipramine or placebo in patients with moderate depression: Randomised multicentre study of treatment for eight weeks. Br Med J. 1999 Dec 11;319(7224):1534-8.

Sommer H, Harrer G. Placebo-controlled double-blind study examining the effectiveness of an hypericum preparation in 105 mildly depressed patients. J Geriatr Psychiatry Neurol. 1994 Oct;7(Suppl 1):S9-11.

Stanga CY. Special dialogue: Herbal remedies for depression. Clin Cornerstone. 1999;1(4):55-7.

Stevinson C, Ernst E. Hypericum for depression. An update of the clinical evidence. Eur Neuropsychopharmacol. 1999 Dec;9(6):501-5.

Volz HP, Laux P. Potential treatment for subthreshold and mild depression: A comparison of St. John's wort extracts and fluoxetine. Compr Psychiatry. 2000 Mar-Apr;41(2 Suppl 1):133-7.

Vorbach EU, Arnoldt KH, Hubner WD. Efficacy and tolerability of St. John's wort extract LI 160 versus imipramine in patients with severe depressive episodes according to ICD-10. Pharmacopsychiatry. 1997 Sep;30(Suppl 2):81-5.

Vorbach EU, Hubner WD, Arnoldt KH. Effectiveness and tolerance of the hypericum extract LI 160 in comparison with imipramine: Randomized double-blind study with 135 outpatients. J Geriatr Psychiatry Neurol. 1994 Oct;7(Suppl 1):S19-23.

Wheatley D. LI 160, an extract of St. John's wort, versus amitriptyline in mildly to moderately depressed outpatients—a controlled 6-week clinical trial. Pharmacopsychiatry. 1997 Sep;30 (Suppl 2):77-80.

Wheatley D. Safety of St John's wort. Lancet. 2000 Feb 12;355(9203):576.

Williams JW Jr, Mulrow CD, Chiquette E, Noel PH, Aguilar C, Cornell J. A systematic review of newer pharmacotherapies for depression in adults: Evidence report summary. Ann Intern Med. 2000 May 2;132(9):743-56.

Woelk H, Burkard G, Grunwald J. Benefits and risks of the hypericum extract LI 160: Drug monitoring study with 3250 patients. J Geriatr Psychiatry Neurol. 1994 Oct;7(Suppl 1):S34-8.

Yu PH. Effect of the Hypericum perforatum extract on serotonin turnover in the mouse brain. Pharmacopsychiatry. 2000 Mar;33(2):60-5.

5-HYDROXYTRYPTOPHAN (5-HTP)

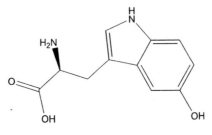

5-Hydroxytryptophan

What Is It?

5-HTP is a derivative of the amino acid tryptophan (via a hydroxyl group added to the 5 position). In the body, tryptophan is converted into 5-HTP, which then can be converted into serotonin (a potent neurotransmitter in the brain). Although 5-HTP is not found at any significant level in a normal diet, tryptophan is found in a wide variety of protein foods. The 5-HTP used in dietary supplements is derived from the seeds of an African plant *(Griffonia simplicifolia)*.

Claims

- Relieves mild to moderate depression
- Relieves insomnia and promotes restful sleep
- Promotes weight loss by suppressing appetite
- Reduces overall sensation of pain (migraine headaches, fibromyalgia, general muscle pain)

Theory

5-HTP is typically used to treat mild depression based on the theory that as a precursor to serotonin, supplements of 5-HTP can increase serotonin levels and influence mood, sleep patterns, and pain control. The amino acid tryptophan can also be broken down in the body to yield ribose and/or NAD—both of which have been associated with increased energy levels.

While these are certainly logical theories, the scientific evidence supporting them remains moderate at best.

Scientific Support

As just indicated, the overall scientific evidence for the effectiveness of 5-HTP is not very strong. In a few small studies, however, 5-HTP has been shown to be as effective as prescription antidepressant medications—and with fewer side effects—but there are just as many controlled clinical trials that have shown no effect of 5-HTP in alleviating mood disturbances. In other studies, doses of 5-HTP in the range of 300 to 900 mg per day have resulted in benefits by reducing pain (migraines and fibromyalgia), reducing appetite, and promoting sleep (possibly by increasing blood levels of melatonin). In some studies, it appears that there are "responders" (individuals who experience an elevation in 5-HTP levels in the blood) as well as "nonresponders" (who see no such increase).

Several studies have investigated 5-HTP supplementation in conjunction with SSRI medications (selective serotonin reuptake inhibitors such as fenfluramine and fluoxetine—Prozac). In this combination, 5-HTP could be expected to help increase serotonin synthesis, while the SSRIs would keep those levels elevated, but this hypothesis has not been particularly supported. In at least one study, 5-HTP actually appeared to cause an *increase* in depressive symptoms in healthy subjects—exactly the opposite effect that users of the supplement are looking for.

Safety

The most significant safety concern related to 5-HTP supplements is the remote possibility for contamination with a compound linked to a disorder known as eosinophilic myalgia syndrome (EMS). In 1989, an outbreak of EMS (which results in muscle pain and weakness, vomiting, headache, and, in rare cases, death) was linked to contaminated tryptophan supplements (not to the tryptophan per se, but to a contaminant in the tryptophan supplements). As a result, the FDA banned the sale of all tryptophan supplements (a move that has been widely criticized by people on both sides of the supplement debate). In some rare cases, 5-HTP supplements have been linked (anecdotally) to gastrointestinal distress, muscle pain, lethargy, and headaches.

The banned tryptophan supplements were manufactured from a bacterial source (fermentation process), while 5-HTP is extracted from the seeds of a plant—so it is less likely (although not impossible) that the contaminant associated with EMS (commonly known as "peak X") is present in 5-HTP supplements. However, the FDA issued a "talk paper" in 1998 that seemed to confirm the presence of peak X at low levels in several commercially available brands of 5-HTP—raising the possibility that EMS could strike those taking 5-HTP supplements. Although the FDA has not taken any action, such as removing 5-HTP from the market or issuing any precautions against it, anybody considering using this supplement should buy a brand from a reputable company. Some supplement manufacturers and raw material suppliers conduct quality control tests to confirm the absence of peak X in their 5-HTP supplements. If you decide to try 5-HTP, it is suggested that you contact the manufacturer of your supplement for confirmation that their products have undergone this type of analysis.

In addition to the safety considerations, 5-HTP supplements are not recommended for children or for women who are pregnant or lactating. Individuals currently taking prescription antidepressants, weight control medications, or herbal remedies for depression (such as St. John's wort) should not combine these treatments with 5-HTP supplements (except on the advice and guidance of a nutritionally oriented physician).

Value

Because commonly prescribed antidepressant medications are ineffective in about 30 percent of depressed patients, and because depression and anxiety disorders are associated with brain imbalances in serotonin, 5-HTP supplements would seem to be a logical approach to boosting serotonin levels and mood. Unfortunately, the scientific evidence for effectiveness is not strong—even though a few small studies have shown 5-HTP supplements to be beneficial in several serotonin-related conditions, many other studies have shown no benefits.

Dosage

The typical dose is 300 to 900 mg per day (usually in two to three doses throughout the day).

WORKS CONSULTED

5-hydroxytryptophan. Altern Med Rev. 1998 Jun;3(3):224-6.
Beckmann H, Kasper S. Serotonin precursors as antidepressive agents: A review. Fortschr Neurol Psychiatr. 1983 May;51(5):176-82.

Birdsall TC. 5-Hydroxytryptophan: A clinically-effective serotonin precursor. Altern Med Rev. 1998 Aug;3(4):271-80.

Byerley WF, Judd LL, Reimherr FW, Grosser BI. 5-Hydroxytryptophan: A review of its antidepressant efficacy and adverse effects. J Clin Psychopharmacol. 1987 Jun;7(3):127-37.

Cangiano C, Laviano A, Del Ben M, Preziosa I, Angelico F, Cascino A, Rossi-Fanelli F. Effects of oral 5-hydroxy-tryptophan on energy intake and macronutrient selection in non-insulin dependent diabetic patients. Int J Obes Relat Metab Disord. 1998 Jul;22(7):648-54.

Coppen AJ, Doogan DP. Serotonin and its place in the pathogenesis of depression. J Clin Psychiatry. 1988 Aug;49(Suppl):4-11.

De Benedittis G, Massei R. Serotonin precursors in chronic primary headache. A double-blind cross-over study with L-5-hydroxytryptophan vs. placebo. J Neurosurg Sci. 1985 Jul-Sep;29(3):239-48.

Fernstrom JD. Dietary effects on brain serotonin synthesis: Relationship to appetite regulation. Am J Clin Nutr. 1985 Nov;42(5 Suppl):1072-82.

Fernstrom JD. Effects on the diet on brain neurotransmitters. Metabolism. 1977 Feb;26(2):207-23.

Juhl JH. Fibromyalgia and the serotonin pathway. Altern Med Rev. 1998 Oct;3(5):367-75.

Meyers S. Use of neurotransmitter precursors for treatment of depression. Altern Med Rev. 2000 Feb;5(1):64-71.

van Praag HM. Management of depression with serotonin precursors. Biol Psychiatry. 1981 Mar;16(3):291-310.

van Praag HM. Serotonin precursors in the treatment of depression. Adv Biochem Psychopharmacol. 1982;34:259-86.

Yamada J, Sugimoto Y, Ujikawa M. The serotonin precursor 5-hydroxytryptophan elevates serum leptin levels in mice. Eur J Pharmacol. 1999 Oct 21;383(1):49-51.

Yamada J, Ujikawa M, Sugimoto Y. Serum leptin levels after central and systemic injection of a serotonin precursor, 5-hydroxytryptophan, in mice. Eur J Pharmacol. 2000 Oct 6;406(1):159-162.

PHENYLALANINE/D,L-PHENYLALANINE (DLPA)

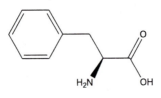

Phenylalanine

What Is It?

Phenylalanine is an essential amino acid—meaning that the body cannot synthesize it on its own and we must get it from the diet. The primary dietary sources of phenylalanine are high-protein foods such as meat, fish, eggs, and dairy products. Another significant dietary source for some people may be sugar-free products containing the artificial sweetener aspartame (Nutra-sweet), which is formed by a combination of phenylalanine with another amino acid, aspartic acid.

Amino acids exist in two forms, designated "L" and "D" forms. The L form is the naturally occurring form in foods, whereas the D form is the synthetic variety. When an amino acid is synthesized commercially, there is usually a mixture of the L and D forms. Sometimes the D form is removed, but in the case of phenylalanine, the combination of the two forms is used to take advantage of the unique characteristics of both forms. The combined form of the supplement is known as D,L-phenylalanine or DLPA.

Claims

- Maintains nervous system health
- Relieves depression
- Elevates mood
- Decreases pain
- Boosts memory
- Suppresses appetite

Theory

DLPA has two distinct fates in the body. The L form of phenylalanine can be converted in the body to another amino acid—tyrosine. Tyrosine, in turn, can be converted into one of several neurotransmitter molecules (L-dopa, norepinephrine, and epinephrine), each of which have important functions in brain metabolism. The D form of phenylalanine cannot be converted to tyrosine, but it can be converted to another compound called phenylethylamine (as can the L form), which may have effects in elevating mood, treating depression, and altering pain sensation.

Scientific Support

DLPA has been used to treat depression, Parkinson's disease, and painful conditions such as arthritis. In one study, phenylalanine supplements were able to elevate mood in thirty-one of forty subjects suffering from depression. Doses of DLPA from 75 to 200 mg per day over twenty days have been shown to be effective in treating depressed mood, agitation, and sleep disturbances. In some cases, depressed subjects were discharged without further treatment beyond continued use of the supplement. In another study, 150 to 200 mg of DLPA was compared to a prescription antidepressant (imipramine). Following thirty days of supplementation, DLPA was found to be as effective as the drug in treating depressive symptoms, indicating that DLPA has powerful antidepressant properties.

Safety

Megadose intakes of any amino acid are discouraged, and phenylalanine is no exception—nerve damage may result with intakes exceeding several grams per day. A condition known as phenylketonuria (PKU), in which phenylalanine cannot be broken down, requires individuals to follow a diet low in this amino acid. Do not take DLPA in conjunction with prescription antidepressants.

Value

Like 5-HTP, DLPA may have some benefits for people who may be concerned with possible drug/herb interactions reported for St. John's wort. Rarely used as a stand-alone supplement, DLPA may be better suited as an ingredient in a larger blend of nutrients or herbs targeting pain and depression or appetite and weight loss.

Dosage

The daily requirement of phenylalanine is probably about 1 g. Effective DLPA doses are in the 75 to 200 mg per day range.

WORKS CONSULTED

Anderson GH. Diet, neurotransmitters and brain function. Br Med Bull. 1981 Jan;37(1):95-100.

Anderson GH, Johnston JL. Nutrient control of brain neurotransmitter synthesis and function. Can J Physiol Pharmacol. 1983 Mar;61(3):271-81.

Ashley DV, Barclay DV, Chauffard FA, Moennoz D, Leathwood PD. Plasma amino acid responses in humans to evening meals of differing nutritional composition. Am J Clin Nutr. 1982 Jul;36(1):143-53.

Benevenga NJ, Steele RD. Adverse effects of excessive consumption of amino acids. Annu Rev Nutr. 1984;4:157-81.

Candito M, Aubin-Brunet V, Tonelli I, Feuillade P, Pringuey D, Chambon P, Darcourt G. Plasma tryptophan in a protein controlled diet in depressed patients. Encephale. 1994 May-Jun;20(3):327-32.

Contino MI, Bausano G. Nutritional approach to the therapy of pain: Recent findings. Recenti Prog Med. 1985 Sep;76(9):472-5.

Fernstrom JD. Can nutrient supplements modify brain function? Am J Clin Nutr. 2000 Jun;71(6 Suppl):1669S-75S.

Fernstrom JD. Dietary amino acids and brain function. J Am Diet Assoc. 1994 Jan;94(1):71-7.

Fernstrom JD. Dietary precursors and brain neurotransmitter formation. Annu Rev Med. 1981;32:413-25.

Fernstrom JD. Effects of precursors on brain neurotransmitter synthesis and brain functions. Diabetologia. 1981 Mar;20 (Suppl):281-9. Review.

Fernstrom JD, Fernstrom MH. Dietary effects on tyrosine availability and catecholamine synthesis in the central nervous system: Possible relevance to the control of protein intake. Proc Nutr Soc. 1994 Jul;53(2):419-29.

Growdon JH, Cohen EL, Wurtman RJ. Treatment of brain disease with dietary precursors of neurotransmitters. Ann Intern Med. 1977 Mar;86(3):337-9.

Growdon JH, Wurtman RJ. Nutrients and neurotransmitters. N Y State J Med. 1980 Sep;80(10):1638-9.

Haze JJ. Toward an understanding of the rationale for the use of dietary supplementation for chronic pain management: The serotonin model. Cranio. 1991 Oct;9(4):339-43.

Hommes FA, Lee JS. The control of 5-hydroxytryptamine and dopamine synthesis in the brain: A theoretical approach. J Inherit Metab Dis. 1990;13(1):37-57.

King RB. Pain and tryptophan. J Neurosurg. 1980 Jul;53(1):44-52.

Lehnert H, Reinstein DK, Strowbridge BW, Wurtman RJ. Neurochemical and behavioral consequences of acute, uncontrollable stress: Effects of dietary tyrosine. Brain Res. 1984 Jun 15;303(2):215-23.

Lieberman HR. Behavioral changes caused by nutrients. Bibl Nutr Dieta. 1986; (38):219-24.

Lieberman HR, Corkin S, Spring BJ, Growdon JH, Wurtman RJ. Mood, performance, and pain sensitivity: Changes induced by food constituents. J Psychiatr Res. 1982-83;17(2):135-45.

Lucca A, Lucini V, Catalano M, Smeraldi E. Neutral amino acid availability in two major psychiatric disorders. Prog Neuropsychopharmacol Biol Psychiatry. 1995 Jul;19(4):615-26.

Melamed E, Glaeser B, Growdon JH, Wurtman RJ. Plasma tyrosine in normal humans: Effects of oral tyrosine and protein-containing meals. J Neural Transm. 1980;47(4):299-306.

Nurmikko T, Pertovaara A, Pontinen PJ, Marnela KM, Oja SS. Effect of L-tryptophan supplementation on ischemic pain. Acupunct Electrother Res. 1984;9(1):45-55.

Pogson CI, Knowles RG, Salter M. The control of aromatic amino acid catabolism and its relationship to neurotransmitter amine synthesis. Crit Rev Neurobiol. 1989;5(1):29-64.

Previc FH. Dopamine and the origins of human intelligence. Brain Cogn. 1999 Dec;41(3):299-350.

Seltzer S. Dietary control of chronic maxillofacial pain. Endod Dent Traumatol. 1985 Jun;1(3):89-95.

Seltzer S, Dewart D, Pollack RL, Jackson E. The effects of dietary tryptophan on chronic maxillofacial pain and experimental pain tolerance. J Psychiatr Res. 1982-83;17(2):181-6.

Seltzer S, Marcus R, Stoch R. Perspectives in the control of chronic pain by nutritional manipulation. Pain. 1981 Oct;11(2):141-8.

Seltzer S, Stoch R, Marcus R, Jackson E. Alteration of human pain thresholds by nutritional manipulation and L-tryptophan supplementation. Pain. 1982 Aug; 13(4):385-93.

Spring B. Recent research on the behavioral effects of tryptophan and carbohydrate. Nutr Health. 1984;3(1-2):55-67.

Strain GW. Nutrition, brain function and behavior. Psychiatr Clin North Am. 1981 Aug;4(2):253-68.

Thurmond JB, Brown JW. Effect of brain monoamine precursors on stress-induced behavioral and neurochemical changes in aged mice. Brain Res. 1984 Mar 26;296(1):93-102.

Warfield CA, Stein JM. The nutritional treatment of pain. Hosp Pract (Off Ed). 1983 Jul;18(7):100N-100P.

Wurtman RJ. Food consumption, neurotransmitter synthesis, and human behaviour. Experientia Suppl. 1983;44:356-69.

Wurtman RJ. Nutrients that modify brain function. Sci Am. 1982 Apr;246(4):50-9.

Zeisel SH. Dietary influences on neurotransmission. Adv Pediatr. 1986;33:23-47.

PHOSPHATIDYLSERINE (PS)

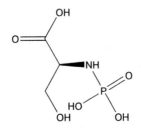

Phosphatidylserine

What Is It?

Phosphatidylserine (PS) is a phospholipid—a molecule made up of two fatty acids and a phosphate group attached to a glycerol backbone. PS is concentrated in cells of the brain, where it may be related to brain cell function and neurotransmitter metabolism. PS is also found in other cell membranes, such as muscle tissue and cells of the immune system, where it may play both structural and functional roles in muscle metabolism and immune system function.

Claims

- Prevents muscle breakdown
- Stimulates immune function
- Maintains brain function, memory, and cognitive ability

Theory

PS has been shown to reduce blood levels of cortisol, a hormone produced in response to stress. One of the effects of elevated cortisol production is accelerated amino acid catabolism, which could lead to muscle breakdown. Suppression of cortisol levels could theoretically maintain muscle mass during periods of increased stress and intense training.

Scientific Support

PS, like other phospholipids, is a major constituent of cellular membranes. Maintenance of membrane integrity is a crucial component of proper function, but there is little direct evidence that PS supplements improve membrane integrity or cellular function. PS has, however, been linked to a suppression of cortisol secretion during periods of intense training (20 to 30 percent)—an effect that may help enhance recovery and repair, particularly following intense exercise or injury.

As a brain-support nutrient, PS has been validated through double-blind trials for improving memory, learning, concentration, word recall, and mood in middle-aged and elderly subjects with dementia or age-related cognitive decline. In animal studies, long-term phosphatidylserine treatment has been shown to maintain the integrity of neuronal structures in the brain that have been altered by the aging process. These are logical findings, as PS is particularly enriched in the brain and has an excellent benefit-to-risk profile compared to traditional treatments for memory loss.

It is interesting to note that PS could also be considered a "general stress" nutrient—providing benefits for athletes subjected to the physical stress of exercise as well as for individuals who are under chronic emotional stress from hectic lifestyles, job deadlines, and many of the other stresses of modern life.

Safety

It appears that no significant side effects are associated with dietary supplements containing phosphatidylserine, but due to concerns about "mad cow disease," it is generally recommended to select PS supplements derived from soybeans versus those forms extracted from cow brains.

Value

PS may be recommended for individuals under increased physical or emotional stress or for athletes recovering from a particularly strenuous bout of exercise (e.g., after running a marathon).

Dosage

Concentrated PS supplements are available in doses of 50 to 100 mg per day, but they are very expensive. For brain and mental support, 500 to 1,000 mg per day of PS are recommended for a month or so, followed by a lower maintenance dose of approximately 500 mg per day. Athletes may need as much as 1 to 2 g (1,000 to 2,000 mg) immediately before or following intense training to help suppress cortisol secretion and promote muscle recovery (but this level of PS would cost over $100 per month, making these levels far from commercially viable).

WORKS CONSULTED

Bell JM, Lundberg PK. Effects of a commercial soy lecithin preparation on development of sensorimotor behavior and brain biochemistry in the rat. Dev Psychobiol. 1985 Jan;18(1):59-66.

Diboune M, Ferard G, Ingenbleek Y, Bourguignat A, Spielmann D, Scheppler-Roupert C, Tulasne PA, Calon B, Hasselmann M, Sauder P, et al. Soybean oil, blackcurrant seed oil, medium-chain triglycerides, and plasma phospholipid fatty acids of stressed patients. Nutrition. 1993 Jul-Aug;9(4):344-9.

DiPalma JR. Nutritional pharmacology. Am Fam Physician. 1985 Aug;32(2):171-3.

Farquharson J, Jamieson EC, Abbasi KA, Patrick WJ, Logan RW, Cockburn F. Effect of diet on the fatty acid composition of the major phospholipids of infant cerebral cortex. Arch Dis Child. 1995 Mar;72(3):198-203.

Fenton WS, Hibbeln J, Knable M. Essential fatty acids, lipid membrane abnormalities, and the diagnosis and treatment of schizophrenia. Biol Psychiatry. 2000 Jan 1;47(1):8-21.

Growdon JH, Wurtman RJ. Dietary influences on the synthesis of neurotransmitters in the brain. Nutr Rev. 1979 May;37(5):129-36.

Hals J, Bjerve KS, Nilsen H, Svalastog AG, Ek J. Essential fatty acids in the nutrition of severely neurologically disabled children. Br J Nutr. 2000 Mar; 83(3):219-25.

Jamieson EC, Abbasi KA, Cockburn F, Farquharson J, Logan RW, Patrick WA. Effect of diet on term infant cerebral cortex fatty acid composition. World Rev Nutr Diet. 1994;75:139-41.

Jumpsen JA, Lien EL, Goh YK, Clandinin MT. During neuronal and glial cell development diet n-6 to n-3 fatty acid ratio alters the fatty acid composition of phosphatidylinositol and phosphatidylserine. Biochim Biophys Acta. 1997 Jul 12;1347(1):40-50.

Kelly GS. Nutritional and botanical interventions to assist with the adaptation to stress. Altern Med Rev. 1999 Aug;4(4):249-65.

Khalsa DS. Integrated medicine and the prevention and reversal of memory loss. Altern Ther Health Med. 1998 Nov;4(6):38-43.

Kohn G, Sawatzki G, van Biervliet JP, Rosseneu M. Diet and the essential fatty acid status of term infants. Acta Paediatr Suppl. 1994 Sep;402:69-74.

Leathwood PD. Neurotransmitter precursors and brain function. Bibl Nutr Dieta. 1986;(38):54-71.

Lutz M. Diet as a determinant of central nervous system development: Role of essential fatty acids. Arch Latinoam Nutr. 1998 Mar;48(1):29-34.

Mahadik SP, Mukherjee S, Horrobin DF, Jenkins K, Correnti EE, Scheffer RE. Plasma membrane phospholipid fatty acid Composition of cultured skin fibroblasts from schizophrenic patients: Comparison with bipolar patients and normal subjects. Psychiatry Res. 1996 Jul 31;63(2-3):133-42.

Monteleone P, Beinat L, Tanzillo C, Maj M, Kemali D. Effects of phosphatidylserine on the neuroendocrine response to physical stress in humans. Neuroendocrinology. 1990 Sep;52(3):243-8.

Monteleone P, Maj M, Beinat L, Natale M, Kemali D. Blunting by chronic phosphatidylserine administration of the stress-induced activation of the hypothalamo-pituitary-adrenal axis in healthy men. Eur J Clin Pharmacol. 1992;42(4):385-8.

Newman PE. Could diet be one of the causal factors of Alzheimer's disease? Med Hypotheses. 1992 Oct;39(2):123-6.

Rosenberg GS, Davis KL. Precursors of acetylcholine: Considerations underlying their use in Tourette syndrome. Adv Neurol. 1982;35:407-12.

Sato N, Murakami Y, Nakano T, Sugawara M, Kawakami H, Idota T, Nakajima I. Effects of dietary nucleotides on lipid metabolism and learning ability of rats. Biosci Biotechnol Biochem. 1995 Jul;59(7):1267-71.

Wurtman RJ. Nutrients that modify brain function. Sci Am. 1982 Apr;246(4):50-9.

CHOLINE

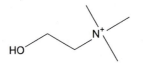

Choline

What Is It?

Choline is an essential nutrient, a B vitamin. It can be manufactured in the body (from the amino acid methionine), although there is some debate whether it can be made in sufficient amounts for optimal health. Folic acid and vitamin B_{12} are also needed to process choline. Choline plays a role in liver function, cardiovascular health, and brain development (as an amine precursor for the neurotransmitter acetylcholine). The recommended amount of choline is 425 mg per day for women and 550 mg per day for men. Food sources of choline include egg yolks (the major dietary source), organ meats, and legumes. Choline is available in supplemental form as lecithin (or phosphatidylcholine) as well as purified choline capsules and as an ingredient in sports bars and drinks.

Claims

- Memory aid/brain development
- Cardiovascular protection
- Cancer prevention
- Boosts energy levels and delays fatigue

Theory

Because choline is an important constituent of cell membranes, it has functions in virtually every bodily system. Choline participates in lipid (fat) transport in the body and may reduce accumulation of fat in the liver. As a dietary supplement and ergogenic aid, however, claims surrounding choline are due mostly to its role as a component of acetylcholine (the neurotransmitter needed for conduction of nerve signals and brain function). Claims for it typically involve mental performance, memory, and reaction time.

Scientific Support

During pregnancy, choline intake of the mother may influence memory and brain development in the growing infant. Studies on choline and lecithin supplementation clearly show an increase in blood choline levels following supplementation with 1 to 5 g of choline (or 5 to 15 g of lecithin). Choline supplements have also been shown to improve marathon performance and endurance cycling ability (time to exhaustion), but they have failed to demonstrate a beneficial effect on shorter duration high-intensity exercise such as sprinting.

Safety

No adverse effects of choline supplements are noted at levels of 1 to 2 g, whereas doses closer to 5 g may be associated with side effects such as diarrhea, nausea, and abdominal discomfort. There have also been anecdotal reports of "fishy body odor" in people consuming high daily doses of choline or lecithin.

Value

Although adequate maternal choline intake has been shown to be important for fetal brain development during pregnancy, dietary sources of choline (eggs and peanuts) are the preferred method of increasing choline intake for pregnant women. Among endurance athletes, choline supplements may be warranted due to a presumed low intake of choline (due to reliance on a high-carbohydrate diet for energy) and an increased loss of choline following exercise.

Dosage

The average diet supplies about 400 to 900 mg of choline daily, which is presumed to be adequate. Choline was designated as an essential nutrient by the Food and Nutrition Board of the National Academy of Sciences in April 1998. The recommended amount of choline is 425 mg per day for women and 550 mg per day for men. Supplemental levels of 1 to 5 g of choline may help improve exercise performance and promote adequate mental function.

WORKS CONSULTED

Bell JM, Lundberg PK. Effects of a commercial soy lecithin preparation on development of sensorimotor behavior and brain biochemistry in the rat. Dev Psychobiol. 1985 Jan;18(1):59-66.

Diboune M, Ferard G, Ingenbleek Y, Bourguignat A, Spielmann D, Scheppler-Roupert C, Tulasne PA, Calon B, Hasselmann M, Sauder P, et al. Soybean oil, blackcurrant seed oil, medium-chain triglycerides, and plasma phospholipid fatty acids of stressed patients. Nutrition. 1993 Jul-Aug;9(4):344-9.

Farquharson J, Jamieson EC, Abbasi KA, Patrick WJ, Logan RW, Cockburn F. Effect of diet on the fatty acid composition of the major phospholipids of infant cerebral cortex. Arch Dis Child. 1995 Mar;72(3):198-203.

Fenton WS, Hibbeln J, Knable M. Essential fatty acids, lipid membrane abnormalities, and the diagnosis and treatment of schizophrenia. Biol Psychiatry. 2000 Jan 1;47(1):8-21.

Growdon JH, Wurtman RJ. Dietary influences on the synthesis of neurotransmitters in the brain. Nutr Rev. 1979 May;37(5):129-36.

Hals J, Bjerve KS, Nilsen H, Svalastog AG, Ek J. Essential fatty acids in the nutrition of severely neurologically disabled children. Br J Nutr. 2000 Mar;83(3):219-25.

Jamieson EC, Abbasi KA, Cockburn F, Farquharson J, Logan RW, Patrick WA. Effect of diet on term infant cerebral cortex fatty acid composition. World Rev Nutr Diet. 1994;75:139-41.

Jumpsen J, Lien EL, Goh YK, Clandinin MT. Small changes of dietary (n-6) and (n-3)/fatty acid content ration alter phosphatidylethanolamine and phosphatidylcholine fatty acid composition during development of neuronal and glial cells in rats. J Nutr. 1997 May;127(5):724-31.

Kelly GS. Nutritional and botanical interventions to assist with the adaptation to stress. Altern Med Rev. 1999 Aug;4(4):249-65.

Khalsa DS. Integrated medicine and the prevention and reversal of memory loss. Altern Ther Health Med. 1998 Nov;4(6):38-43.

Kohn G, Sawatzki G, van Biervliet JP, Rosseneu M. Diet and the essential fatty acid status of term infants. Acta Paediatr Suppl. 1994 Sep;402:69-74.

Leathwood PD. Neurotransmitter precursors and brain function. Bibl Nutr Dieta. 1986;(38):54-71.

Leathwood PD, Schlosser B. Phosphatidylcholine, choline and cholinergic function. Int J Vitam Nutr Res Suppl. 1986;29:49-67.

Lutz M. Diet as a determinant of central nervous system development: Role of essential fatty acids. Arch Latinoam Nutr. 1998 Mar;48(1):29-34.

Mahadik SP, Mukherjee S, Horrobin DF, Jenkins K, Correnti EE, Scheffer RE. Plasma membrane phospholipid fatty acid composition of cultured skin fibroblasts from schizophrenic patients: Comparison with bipolar patients and normal subjects. Psychiatry Res. 1996 Jul 31;63(2-3):133-42.

Newman PE. Could diet be one of the causal factors of Alzheimer's disease? Med Hypotheses. 1992 Oct;39(2):123-6.

Rosenberg GS, Davis KL. Precursors of acetylcholine: Considerations underlying their use in Tourette syndrome. Adv Neurol. 1982;35:407-12.

Wurtman RJ. Nutrients that modify brain function. Sci Am. 1982 Apr;246(4):50-9.

Zeisel SH. Choline: An important nutrient in brain development, liver function and carcinogenesis. J Am Coll Nutr. 1992 Oct;11(5):473-81.

Zeisel SH, Blusztajn JK. Choline and human nutrition. Annu Rev Nutr. 1994;14:269-96.

Zeisel SH, Growdon JH, Wurtman RJ, Magil SG, Logue M. Normal plasma choline responses to ingested lecithin. Neurology. 1980 Nov;30(11):1226-9.

GINKGO BILOBA

What Is It?

Ginkgo biloba is often referred to as a "living fossil" because it is believed to be the world's oldest living tree species at about 200 million years old. Various parts of the ginkgo tree have been used in traditional Chinese medicine for over 4,000 years, reportedly in the treatment of respiratory ailments, to improve circulation, as a digestive aid, as a tonic for memory loss in the elderly, and as a longevity elixir. In Germany, ginkgo is a top-selling over-the-counter and prescription drug. Modern ginkgo extracts are produced from the leaves of cultivated trees and still enjoy great popularity for the treatment of various disorders. High quality ginkgo biloba extract is normally standardized to 24 percent ginkgo flavone glycosides and 6 percent terpene lactones.

Claims

- Improves memory and mental sharpness
- Alleviates symptoms of Alzheimer's disease
- Antidepressant
- Improves circulation, thins blood, and promotes cardiovascular health
- Antioxidant

Theory

The two groups of phytochemicals to which ginkgo is normally standardized, ginkgo flavone glycosides and terpene lactones, are considered to be the primary active constituents. The flavone glycosides, which include quercetin, kaempherol, and isorhamnetin, are responsible for the antioxidant properties of ginkgo extract. The terpene lactones, which include ginkgolides A, B, and C, as well as bilobalide, possess several activities. These activities include neuroprotection, improvement of choline uptake in brain synapses, and inhibition of platelet activating factor (which reduces the tendency of the blood to clot).

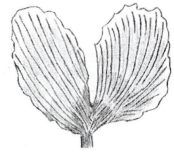

Scientific Support

Laboratory and clinical studies have found a great deal of support for the majority of claims made for the therapeutic use of ginkgo biloba extract. The German Commission E approves ginkgo for effective therapy in cases of memory deficits, impaired concentration, depression, dizziness, tinnitus (ringing in the ears), or headache. The primary groups of dementias targeted for treatment with ginkgo are primary degenerative dementia, vascular dementia, and mixed forms of both. Ginkgo is also approved for use in the improvement of pain-free walking in patients diagnosed with intermittent claudication or peripheral arterial occlusive disease (both are conditions in which improved circulation helps relieve symptoms). Lastly, Commission E recommends ginkgo for vertigo and tinnitus, which also may be caused by inadequate circulation.

A wide variety of clinical studies have been conducted on the benefits of ginkgo biloba extract, many in Germany, but several in the United States. Major findings include:

- Enhanced oxygen use and improvement of tolerance to hypoxia (lack of oxygen)
- Increased brain circulation and inhibition or prevention of brain damage due to trauma and/or toxicity
- Promotion of eye health and protection of retina
- Neurotransmitter support, inhibition of age-related loss of choline receptors, and stimulation of choline uptake in the hippocampus region of the brain
- Memory support (increased memory performance and learning capacity)
- Improved systemic circulation (improvement of blood flow, particularly in microcirculation of capillaries)
- Cardiovascular risk factor reduction (antioxidant effects, reduces activity of platelet-activating factor, which reduces tendency of blood to clot)
- General neuroprotective effects

One meta-analysis analyzed over forty clinical studies investigating ginkgo biloba extract for the treatment of cerebral insufficiency (which is associated with age-related mental decline or dementia). The resulting analysis concluded that ginkgo is effective in reducing all symptoms of cerebral insufficiency and impaired mental function.

In a placebo-controlled, double-blind, randomized study, seventy-two patients with cerebral insufficiency (lack of blood flow to the brain) were subjected to a computerized test of short-term memory. At the end of six weeks, the group receiving ginkgo biloba extract exhibited a statistically significant improvement in short-term memory capacity, while the placebo group showed no significant increase.

Clinical evidence indicates that ginkgo may be useful in the treatment of certain types of depression, notably "resistant" depression. At least one study demonstrated a reduction of cerebral blood flow in depressed patients. In one placebo-controlled study, patients who continued to exhibit symptoms of depression after the use of antidepressants were given 240 mg per day of ginkgo biloba extract. The patients receiving ginkgo experienced a significant reduction in depressive symptoms as well as an improvement in cognitive function. In an open clinical trial of sixty patients having erectile dysfunction, 50 percent of the patients regained potency and 25 percent showed improved arterial blood flow following six months of supplementation with 60 mg per day of ginkgo biloba.

There has been some question as to the ability of ginkgo to improve cognitive function in healthy subjects (which is very difficult to measure). However, two recent studies of healthy volunteers measured brain activity using sensitive electroencephalography (EEG) and found that dosages of 120 to 240 mg of ginkgo biloba extract increase cognitive function (measured as alpha wave activity) within 30 minutes (peak measures were recorded two to three hours after consuming the supplements). The enhancement in alpha wave activity was similar to that achieved through the use of drugs that improve cognitive function. Both studies concluded that ginkgo biloba extract improves cognitive function in healthy subjects.

Safety

Ginkgo is, very rarely, associated with gastrointestinal upset, allergic skin reaction, and headache. There are no known contraindications or interactions with other drugs. Ginkgo is not known to be toxic at high dosages, although its inhibition of platelet-activating factor could pose a concern to individuals with blood clotting problems or taking anticoagulant medications (so check with your doctor before taking ginkgo).

Value

Ginkgo is valuable for a broad array of health concerns related to problems with microcirculation—whether in the brain, legs, or sex organs. Ginkgo's neuroprotective effects are also well established, and its benefits in improving mental function and memory in healthy subjects look promising.

Dosage

The general consensus is that for the treatment of microcirculation problems in the extremities, including vertigo, tinnitus, and intermittent claudication, a dosage of 120 to 160 mg per day is suitable. For treatment of dementia, mild depression, and improvement of cognitive abilities, higher doses (about 240 mg per day) are recommended. For best results, daily dosage is typically split into two to three divided doses. Be sure to look for an extract standardized to at least 24 percent ginkgo flavone glycosides and 6 percent terpene lactones—this is the type of extract that has been shown to be effective in virtually every clinical trial.

WORKS CONSULTED

Agnoli A, Fiorani P, Pistolese GR. Preliminary results in the modifications of cerebral blood flow using xenon-133 during administration of ginkgo-biloba. Minerva Med. 1973 Nov 7;64(79 Suppl):4166-73.

Allard M. Treatment of the disorders of aging with Ginkgo biloba extract. From pharmacology to clinical medicine. Presse Med. 1986 Sep 25;15(31):1540-5.

al-Zuhair H, Abd el-Fattah A, el-Sayed MI. The effect of meclofenoxate with ginkgo biloba extract or zinc on lipid peroxide, some free radical scavengers and the cardiovascular system of aged rats. Pharmacol Res. 1998 Jul;38(1):65-72.

Christen Y. Oxidative stress and Alzheimer disease. Am J Clin Nutr. 2000 Feb; 71(2):621S-9S.

Deberdt W. Interaction between psychological and pharmacological treatment in cognitive impairment. Life Sci. 1994;55(25-26):2057-66.

Diamond BJ, Shiflett SC, Feiwel N, Matheis RJ, Noskin O, Richards JA, Schoenberger NE. Ginkgo biloba extract: Mechanisms and clinical indications. Arch Phys Med Rehabil. 2000 May;81(5):668-78.

Fowler JS, Wang GJ, Volkow ND, Logan J, Franceschi D, Franceschi M, MacGregor R, Shea C, Garza V, Liu N, Ding YS. Evidence that gingko biloba extract does not inhibit MAO A and B in living human brain. Life Sci. 2000 Jan 21;66(9):PL141-6.

Garg RK, Nag D, Agrawal A. A double blind placebo controlled trial of ginkgo biloba extract in acute cerebral ischaemia. J Assoc Physicians India. 1995 Nov;43(11):760-3.

Gsell W, Reichert N, Youdim MB, Riederer P. Interaction of neuroprotective substances with human brain superoxide dismutase. An in vitro study. J Neural Transm Suppl. 1995;45:271-9.

Hannequin D, Thibert A, Vaschalde Y. Development of a model to study the anti-edema properties of Ginkgo biloba extract. Presse Med. 1986 Sep 25;15(31):1575-6.

Heiss WD. Pharmacologic modification of the circulation in the brain. Bull Schweiz Akad Med Wiss. 1980 Apr;36(1-3):183-207.

Heiss WD. Therapy of cerebral ischemia. Z Kardiol. 1987;76(Suppl 4):87-98.

Hemmer R, Tzavellas O. On cerebral effect of plant preparation from Ginkgo biloba. Arzneimittelforschung. 1967 Apr;17(4):491-3.

Hofferberth B. The effect of Ginkgo biloba extract on neurophysiological and psychometric measurement results in patients with psychotic organic brain syndrome. A double-blind study against placebo. Arzneimittelforschung. 1989 Aug;39(8):918-22.

Hoyer S. Possibilities and limits of therapy of cognition disorders in the elderly. Z Gerontol Geriatr. 1995 Nov-Dec;28(6):457-62.

Itil TM, Eralp E, Ahmed I, Kunitz A, Itil KZ. The pharmacological effects of ginkgo biloba, a plant extract, on the brain of dementia patients in comparison with tacrine. Psychopharmacol Bull. 1998;34(3):391-7.

Ivaniv OP. The results of using different forms of a Ginkgo biloba extract (EGb 761) in the combined treatment of patients with circulatory encephalopathy. Lik Sprava. 1998 Dec;(8):123-8.

Khalsa DS. Integrated medicine and the prevention and reversal of memory loss. Altern Ther Health Med. 1998 Nov;4(6):38-43.

Kidd PM. A review of nutrients and botanicals in the integrative management of cognitive dysfunction. Altern Med Rev. 1999 Jun;4(3):144-61.

Kleijnen J, Knipschild P. Ginkgo biloba. Lancet. 1992 Nov 7;340(8828):1136-9.

Koltringer P, Eber O, Klima G, Rothlauer W, Wakonig P, Langsteger W, Lind P. Microcirculation in parenteral Ginkgo biloba extract therapy. Wien Klin Wochenschr. 1989 Mar 17;101(6):198-200.

Kunkel H. EEG profile of three different extractions of Ginkgo biloba. Neuropsychobiology. 1993;27(1):40-5.

Massoni G, Piovella C, Fratti L. Effects on microcirculation of Ginkgo-biloba in elderly people. G Gerontol. 1972 May;20(5):444-50.

Perry EK, Pickering AT, Wang WW, Houghton P, Perry NS. Medicinal plants and Alzheimer's disease: Integrating ethnobotanical and contemporary scientific evidence. J Altern Complement Med. 1998 Winter;4(4):419-28.

Perry EK, Pickering AT, Wang WW, Houghton PJ, Perry NS. Medicinal plants and Alzheimer's disease: From ethnobotany to phytotherapy. J Pharm Pharmacol. 1999 May;51(5):527-34.

Pidoux B. Effects of Ginkgo biloba extract on functional brain activity. An assessment of clinical and experimental studies. Presse Med. 1986 Sep 25;15(31):1588-91.

Pitchumoni SS, Doraiswamy PM. Current status of antioxidant therapy for Alzheimer's disease. J Am Geriatr Soc. 1998 Dec;46(12):1566-72.

Pospelova ML, Barnaulov OD. The antihypoxic and antioxidant action of medicinal plants as the basis for their use in destructive brain diseases. Fiziol Cheloveka. 2000 Jan-Feb;26(1):100-6.

Raabe A, Raabe M, Ihm P. Therapeutic follow-up using automatic perimetry in chronic cerebroretinal ischemia in elderly patients. Prospective double-blind study with graduated dose ginkgo biloba treatment. Klin Monatsbl Augenheilkd. 1991 Dec;199(6):432-8.

Racagni G, Brunello N, Paoletti R. Neuromediator changes during cerebral aging. The effect of Ginkgo biloba extract. Presse Med. 1986 Sep 25;15(31):1488-90.

Ramassamy C, Averill D, Beffert U, Bastianetto S, Theroux L, Lussier-Cacan S, Cohn JS, Christen Y, Davignon J, Quirion R, Poirier J. Oxidative damage and protection by antioxidants in the frontal cortex of Alzheimer's disease is related to the apolipoprotein E genotype. Free Radic Biol Med. 1999 Sep;27(5-6):544-53.

Reisecker F. Therapy approaches in cerebral cognitive deficits—neuropsychiatric aspects. Wien Med Wochenschr. 1996;146(21-22):546-8.

Saponaro A. Modifications of the rheogram of cranial retinal vessels following administration of ginkgo-biloba. Minerva Med. 1973 Nov 7;64(79 Suppl):4194-8.

Sastre J, Pallardo FV, Garcia de la Asuncion J, Vina J. Mitochondria, oxidative stress and aging. Free Radic Res. 2000 Mar;32(3):189-98.

Semlitsch HV, Anderer P, Saletu B, Binder GA, Decker KA. Cognitive psychophysiology in nootropic drug research: Effects of Ginkgo biloba on event-related potentials (P300) in age-associated memory impairment. Pharmacopsychiatry. 1995 Jul;28(4):134-42.

Spinnewyn B, Blavet N, Clostre F. Effects of Ginkgo biloba extract on a cerebral ischemia model in gerbils. Presse Med. 1986 Sep 25;15(31):1511-5.

Taillandier J, Ammar A, Rabourdin JP, Ribeyre JP, Pichon J, Niddam S, Pierart H. Treatment of cerebral aging disorders with Ginkgo biloba extract. A longitudinal multicenter double-blind drug vs. placebo study. Presse Med. 1986 Sep 25;15(31):1583-7.

Warburton DM. Clinical psychopharmacology of Ginkgo biloba extract. Presse Med. 1986 Sep 25;15(31):1595-604.

Winter JC. The effects of an extract of Ginkgo biloba, EGb 761, on cognitive behavior and longevity in the rat. Physiol Behav. 1998 Feb 1;63(3):425-33.

HUPERZINE A (HupA)

What Is It?

Huperzine A is a purified alkaloid extract from a Chinese moss, *Huperzia serrata* (as such, it is really more of a naturally derived drug than a true herbal remedy). The moss has been used in traditional Chinese medicine for treating fever, inflammation, schizophrenia, and memory loss. As a modern herbal supplement, huperzine A (HupA) is used therapeutically to treat Alzheimer's disease and other age-associated memory impairments.

Claims

- Improves memory
- Enhances learning ability
- Treats senile dementia and Alzheimer's disease

Theory

The theory of how HupA may work has to do with a specific neurotransmitter called acetylcholine. Acetylcholine is released into the space between two nerve cells (the synapse), where it stimulates a transfer of the nerve impulse from one nerve cell to the next. After the nerve impulse has been transmitted, an enzyme called acetylcholine esterase breaks down acetylcholine and the nervous signal is ended. In some memory disorders, such as Alzheimer's disease and senile dementia, acetylcholine may be destroyed too quickly, so the nerve impulse is either too weak to be received or it is incompletely transmitted between nerve cells. HupA seems to inhibit the activity of acetylcholine esterase, so the breakdown of acetylcholine is slowed and the strength and duration of the nerve impulse is improved. This inhibition of acetylcholine breakdown may be the reason for the effect of HupA on improving memory and overall cognitive processes.

Scientific Support

The effects of HupA have been investigated in laboratory and clinical settings—with the overall findings that HupA is a potent, reversible, and selective inhibitor of acetylcholine esterase, with a rapid absorption and penetration into the brain in animal tests. It exhibits memory-enhancing activities in animal and clinical trials. Compared to existing medications for the treatment of Alzheimer's disease, such as tacrine, physostigmine, and donepezil, HupA possesses a longer duration of action and higher therapeutic index, and the peripheral cholinergic side effects are minimal at therapeutic doses. HupA may also reduce neuronal cell death caused by glutamate, an action that further enhances the potential value of HupA as a therapeutic agent for Alzheimer's disease.

In animal studies, daily oral administration of huperzine A has been shown to produce a significant improvement in learning ability (maze tasks) that is strongly correlated with promotion of blood flow and inhibition of acetylcholinesterase activity in various regions of the brain (cortex and hippocampus).

In humans, the effects of HupA are considered a promising therapeutic agent for Alzheimer's disease and memory deficit. In one study of 103 patients with Alzheimer's disease (multicenter, prospective, double-blind, parallel, placebo controlled, and randomized), fifty received 200 mcg of HupA and fifty-three received a placebo for eight weeks. Study results showed that about 58 percent (twenty-nine out of fifty) of patients treated with HupA showed significant improvements in their memory, cognitive, and behavioral functions versus only 36 percent of those receiving the placebo. No adverse side effects were reported. In another study of teenage Chinese students, the effect of HupA on memory and learning performance was studied using a double-blind, matched-pair, placebo-controlled design in which thirty-four pairs of students complaining of memory inadequacy were given HupA (100 mcg HupA, taken twice per day) or a look-alike placebo for four weeks. At the end of the trial, the students receiving HupA had significantly higher scores on tests of memory (memory quotient) compared to the placebo group.

Safety

The reported side effects for HupA are generally quite mild, such as dizziness and headaches. However, because no long-term safety studies have been conducted, children and women who are pregnant or nursing should avoid HupA except on the specific advice and guidance of a physician (animal studies have shown that HupA can pass from mother to fetus). There have also been isolated reports of possible liver and kidney toxicity associated with raw preparations of the huperzine moss, so a purified extract is recommended. Huperzine occurs in two forms, "A" and "B," as well as two enantiomers (–) and (+). The most biologically active form of huperzine appears to be (–) Huperzine A. It should be noted that because the safety window between an effective dose of HupA (50 to 200 mcg) and a potentially toxic dose (above 500 mcg) is small, users of Huperzine A should exercise extreme caution.

Value

As a treatment for Alzheimer's disease, dementia, age-associated memory impairment, and senile memory disorders, HupA has shown some impressive results with virtually no side effects. The popularity of other memory and brain herbals, such as ginkgo, ginseng, and 5-HTP, attests to the fact that this is an area of great concern to many people—and the typical price for HupA preparations is quite reasonable at less than $1 per day.

Dosage

Typical dosage recommendations for purified and standardized HupA extracts are 50 mcg, taken twice per day, although doses of 30 to 200 mcg per day have been used in clinical studies to treat Alzheimer's disease, dementia, age-associated memory impairment, and senile memory disorders.

WORKS CONSULTED

Ashani Y, Grunwald J, Kronman C, Velan B, Shafferman A. Role of tyrosine 337 in the binding of huperzine A to the active site of human acetylcholinesterase. Mol Pharmacol. 1994 Mar;45(3):555-60.

Ashani Y, Peggins JO 3rd, Doctor BP. Mechanism of inhibition of cholinesterases by huperzine A. Biochem Biophys Res Commun. 1992 Apr 30;184(2):719-26.

Bai DL, Tang XC, He XC. Huperzine A, a potential therapeutic agent for treatment of Alzheimer's disease. Curr Med Chem. 2000 Mar;7(3):355-74.

Geib SJ, Tuckmantel W, Kozikowski AP. Huperzine A—a potent acetylcholinesterase inhibitor of use in the treatment of Alzheimer's disease. Acta Crystallogr C. 1991 Apr 15;47(Pt 4):824-7.

Patocka J. Huperzine A—an interesting anticholinesterase compound from the Chinese herbal medicine. Acta Medica (Hradec Kralove). 1998;41(4):155-7.

Pepping J. Huperzine A. Am J Health Syst Pharm. 2000 Mar 15;57(6):530, 533-4.

Pilotaz F, Masson P. Huperzine A: An acetylcholinesterase inhibitor with high pharmacological potential. Ann Pharm Fr. 1999 Sep;57(5):363-73.

Saxena A, Qian N, Kovach IM, Kozikowski AP, Pang YP, Vellom DC, Radic Z, Quinn D, Taylor P, Doctor BP. Identification of amino acid residues involved in the binding of Huperzine A to cholinesterases. Protein Sci. 1994 Oct;3(10):1770-78.

Sun QQ, Xu SS, Pan JL, Guo HM, Cao WQ. Huperzine-A capsules enhance memory and learning performance in 34 pairs of matched adolescent students. Chung Kuo Yao Li Hsueh Pao. 1999 Jul;20(7):601-3.

Tang XC. Huperzine A (shuangyiping): A promising drug for Alzheimer's disease. Chung Kuo Yao Li Hsueh Pao. 1996 Nov;17(6):481-4.

Wang LM, Han YF, Tang XC. Huperzine A improves cognitive deficits caused by chronic cerebral hypoperfusion in rats. Eur J Pharmacol. 2000 Jun 9;398(1):65-72.

Xiao XQ, Wang R, Han YF, Tang XC. Protective effects of huperzine A on beta-amyloid(25-35) induced oxidative injury in rat pheochromocytoma cells. Neurosci Lett. 2000 Jun 9;286(3):155-8.

Xu SS, Cai ZY, Qu ZW, Yang RM, Cai YL, Wang GQ, Su XQ, Zhong XS, Cheng RY, Xu WA, Li JX, Feng B. Huperzine-A in capsules and tablets for treating patients with Alzheimer disease. Chung Kuo Yao Li Hsueh Pao. 1999 Jun;20(6):486-90.

Xu SS, Gao ZX, Weng Z, Du ZM, Xu WA, Yang JS, Zhang ML, Tong ZH, Fang YS, Chai XS, et al. Efficacy of tablet huperzine-A on memory, cognition, and behavior in Alzheimer's disease. Chung Kuo Yao Li Hsueh Pao. 1995 Sep; 16(5):391-5.

Zhang RW, Tang XC, Han YY, Sang GW, Zhang YD, Ma YX, Zhang CL, Yang RM. Drug evaluation of huperzine A in the treatment of senile memory disorders. Chung Kuo Yao Li Hsueh Pao. 1991 May;12(3):250-2.

Zhu XZ. Development of natural products as drugs acting on central nervous system. Mem Inst Oswaldo Cruz. 1991;86(Suppl 2):173-5.

VINPOCETINE

What Is It?

Vinpocetine is an extract of *Vinca minor,* also known as the periwinkle plant. A derivative of the alkaloid vincamine, vinpocetine is used around the world (in about thirty-five countries) in the treatment of stroke and vascular dementia to enhance blood flow to specific regions of the brain as well as to reduce damage from free radicals. In Europe, a Hungarian company (Gedeon Richter) markets vinpocetine as a drug (Cavinton) for the treatment of various cerebral insufficiency conditions and as the "only drug" that improves cerebral metabolism (glucose and oxygen uptake), increases ATP concentration, and selectively increases blood flow to the brain (without lowering blood flow to other parts of the body).

Claims

- Memory enhancer
- Treatment for Alzheimer's disease
- Treatment for stroke
- Improves circulation (especially to the brain)
- Antioxidant

Theory

Vinpocetine is known to have effects in dilating blood vessels, enhancing circulation to the brain, improving oxygen utilization, and reducing blood clotting by making red blood cells more pliable and inhibiting platelet aggregation. It is also thought to possess various actions as an antioxidant.

Scientific Support

A number of studies on vinpocetine have shown significant improvements in cognitive function in patients suffering from mild to moderate dementia (10 mg, taken three times per day for four months). In general, scientific studies support the claims that vinpocetine enhances overall brain function and cognitive ability (memory) in those recovering from stroke, Alzheimer's disease, and age-related declines in memory (typically measured using standard memory tests). In one study, the effect of vinpocetine (Cavinton) on cerebral glucose metabolism was studied in chronic stroke patients (using positron emission tomography, PET scans), showing that vinpocetine significantly improved the transport of glucose (both uptake and release) in the brain and especially in the brain tissue around the area damaged by the stroke. These changes appeared to be related to increased blood in the entire region in and around the area of damage. Over the ten- to twenty-year history of clinical vinpocetine (Cavinton) use in Europe, thousands of patients with different cerebrovascular diseases have shown improvement (75 to 85 percent of patients) on measures of cognitive function.

Safety

Overall, side effects of vinpocetine are quite rare, typically minor, and disappear with discontinuance of consumption. Rarely, side effects such as gastrointestinal upset, low blood pressure (hypotension), dry mouth, insomnia, headaches, and heart palpitations (rapid heartbeat) have been reported. Because it can reduce the ability of blood to clot, vinpocetine should be avoided by individuals with a tendency to bleed and by anybody taking anticoagulant therapy (Coumadin/warfarin). Also, the safety of vinpocetine has not been adequately documented for pregnant or lactating women or for children.

Value

At about $25 to $30 for a one-month supply, vinpocetine may represent a significant value for individuals suffering from Alzheimer's disease or stroke as well as for the individual seeking a boost in mental power. In the case of Alzheimer's disease or other severe cognitive impairment, vinpocetine may need to be used for several weeks before seeing any improvement, whereas memory enhancement benefits may be noticeable within a week or so in otherwise healthy individuals. It may also be possible for vinpocetine to potentiate or increase the effect of other supplements (such as ginkgo, huperzine, and phosphatidylserine) and either enhance the effect or allow dosing at a lower level of each compound.

Dosage

Typical dosage recommendations for vinpocetine are 5 to 10 mg, taken two to three times per day with meals (to increase absorption and reduce gastrointestinal discomfort).

WORKS CONSULTED

Balestreri R, Fontana L, Astengo F. A double-blind placebo controlled evaluation of the safety and efficacy of vinpocetine in the treatment of patients with chronic vascular senile cerebral dysfunction. J Am Geriatr Soc. 1987;35:425-30.

Burtsev EM, Savkov VS, Shprakh VV, Burtsev ME. 10-year experience with using Cavinton in cerebrovascular disorders. Zh Nevropatol Psikhiatr Im S S Korsakova. 1992;92(1):56-60.

Hindmarch I, Fuchs HH, Erzigkeit H. Efficacy and tolerance of vinpocetine in ambulant patients suffering from mild to moderate organic psychosyndromes. Int Clin Psychopharmacol. 1991;6:31-43.

Hitzenberger G, Sommer W, Grandt R. Influence of vinpocetine on warfarin-induced inhibition of coagulation. Int J Clin Pharmacol Ther Toxicol. 1990; 28:323-8.

Itil TM, Eralp E, Ahmed I, Kunitz A, Itil KZ. The pharmacological effects of ginkgo biloba, a plant extract, on the brain of dementia patients in comparison with tacrine. Psychopharmacol Bull. 1998;34(3):391-7.

Kiss B, Karpati E. Mechanism of action of vinpocetine. Acta Pharm Hung. 1996 Sep;66(5):213-24.

Lohmann A, Dingler E, Sommer W, Schaffler K, Wober W, Schmidt W. Bioavailability of vinpocetine and interference of the time of application with food intake. Arzneimittelforschung. 1992;42:914-7.

Olah VA, Balla G, Balla J, Szabolcs A, Karmazsin L. An in vitro study of the hydroxyl scavenger effect of Caviton. Acta Paediatr Hung. 1990;30:309-16.

Osawa M, Maruyama S. Effects of TCV-3B (Vinpocetine) on blood viscosity in ischemic cerebrovascular disease. Ther Hung. 1985;33:7-12.

Otomo E, Atarashi J, Araki G. Comparison of Vinpocetine with ifenprodil tartrate and dihydroergotoxine mesylate treatment and results of long-term treatment with Vinpocetine. Curr Ther Res. 1985;37:811-21.

Sauer D, Rischke R, Beck T, Rossberg C, Mennel HD, Bielenberg GW, Krieglstein J. Vinpocetine prevents ischaemic cell damage in rat hippocampus. Life Sci. 1988;43:1733-9.

Szakall S, Boros I, Balkay L, Emri M, Fekete I, Kerenyi L, Lehel S, Marian T, Molnar T, Varga J, Galuska L, Tron L, Bereczki D, Csiba L, Gulyas B. Cerebral effects of a single dose of intravenous vinpocetine in chronic stroke patients: A PET study. J Neuroimaging 1998 Oct;8(4):197-204.

Tamaki N, Kusunoki T, Matsumoto S. The effect of Vinpocetine on cerebral blood flow in patients with cerebrovascular disease. Ther Hung. 1985;33:13-21.

Thal LJ, Salmon DP, Lasker B, Bower D, Klauber MR. The safety and lack of efficacy of vinpocetine in Alzheimer's disease. J Am Geriatr Soc. 1989;37:515-20.

Vamosi B, Molnar L, Demeter J, Tury F. Comparative study of the effect of Ethyl Apovincaminate and Xanthinol Nicotinate in cerebrovascular diseases. Arzneimittel Forschung 1976;28:1980-4.

KAVA-KAVA

What Is It?

Kava *(Piper methysticum)* is the root of a pepper plant used by Pacific islanders (e.g., from Fiji, Hawaii) for centuries as a ceremonial intoxicant to help people relax and socialize. More recent uses suggest a role for kava in relieving anxiety and tension. Kava is reported to create a feeling of calmness without dulling the mind or causing hangovers as alcohol does. Heavy consumption may be associated with effects similar to alcohol intoxication (do not use kava in conjunction with alcohol) and may lead to a condition of itchy, scaly skin when used at high levels for prolonged periods of time.

Traditional preparation of the kava root involves cutting up freshly dug roots, chewing them up, and spitting them into a large communal bowl containing water or coconut milk. This unappetizing mixture is then mixed around, strained to remove any remaining large pieces, and passed around for everyone to share. It all sounds pretty disgusting, but early Christian missionaries to the islands actually tried to ban kava parties because people were having such a good time preparing and passing the kava drinks. If you can't stomach the chewing and spitting part of kava preparation, the roots can be pounded until soft, then soaked in fluid before drinking. If you've ever tried the brew, it has a somewhat bitter taste reminiscent of dirt and a slightly numbing or tingling sensation on the tongue.

No doubt, kava is not prepared or consumed very often by the traditional route by average supplement users in the United States. Instead, the kava roots are dried and ground into a powder by machines. The powder can then be packed into capsules or tablets, blended into drinks, or dissolved in an alcohol-based extract. Americans spend about $30 to $50 million annually on kava-containing products. Due to increasing demand for kava root in dietary supplements, the wholesale price for a pound of dried root has almost doubled in the last couple of years to about $10 per pound.

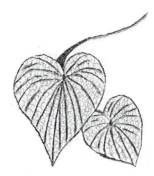

Claims

- Alleviates anxiety and promotes relaxation
- Aids sleep
- Balances mood and relieves depression

- Eases symptoms of menopause (hot flashes)
- Analgesic/headache remedy

Theory

The active ingredients, chemicals called kavalactones, act as a mild central nervous system depressant. The kavalactone content in kava roots can vary significantly from plant to plant (3 to 20 percent) depending on the growing, harvesting, and processing conditions.

Scientific Support

Although no well-designed studies have been conducted on kava in humans in the United States, several projects have been carried out in Europe. These overseas trials of kava have largely been conducted in Germany, and have found kava to be helpful in alleviating anxiety and other emotional problems related to stress. No side effects or withdrawal symptoms have been noted during kava supplementation studies or when people stopped taking the supplement. One study assessed various interpersonal problems and psychological stressors, finding that after four weeks, the group taking kava supplements showed statistically significant decreases in stress in every category measured, in contrast to the placebo group, which showed little variation in any area.

Safety

No side effects or withdrawal symptoms have been noted during kava supplementation studies or when people stopped taking kava. It is presently unknown whether prolonged use of kava is safe or whether any risks are associated with combining kava with other drugs or natural products. In rare instances, kava abuse can result in temporary skin and liver problems, which clear up when kava consumption is discontinued. On March 25, 2002, the United States Food and Drug Administration (FDA) issued a consumer advisory of the potential risk of liver injury associated with the use of kava. Although the FDA has not made a final determination about the risks associated with kava, more than twenty case studies suggesting kava-related liver damage have prompted regulatory agencies in Germany, Canada, and the United Kingdom to warn consumers about the potential risks of kava use. Although liver damage appears to be exceedingly rare, and may not be related to kava at all, the FDA believes that consumers should be informed of this potential risk.

Because kava depresses the nervous system, it should not be taken with alcohol or in conjunction with antianxiety drugs such as Valium. In addition, although kava appears helpful for alleviating cases of mild to moderate anxiety, self-medication with kava is probably not appropriate for individuals with major anxiety conditions. Additionally, it is advisable to refrain from using kava before driving. There was an interesting case in Maryland in 1999, when a police officer pulled over a man for driving erratically. The man slurred his speech and had difficulty walking, so the officer assumed he was intoxicated, despite the man's insistence that he had not been drinking. Blood alcohol measures indicated no alcohol in the man's system. After further questioning, it was discovered that the man had recently consumed several cups of kava tea.

Value

For temporary relief of mild anxiety and alleviation of feelings of stress, kava may be an effective dietary supplement for many people.

Dosage

Supplements should provide an extract standardized for kavalactone content and delivering the equivalent of 50 to 150 mg of kavalactones. A 100 mg dose of a 70 percent kavalactone standardized extract, consumed one to three times per day, is an effective dose for alleviating mild anxiety.

WORKS CONSULTED

Almeida JC, Grimsley EW. Coma from the health food store: Interaction between kava and alprazolam. Ann Intern Med. 1996 Dec 1;125(11):940-1.

Burton-Bradley BG. Kava kava. Mental health in Papua New Guinea. Med J Aust. 1974 Aug 17;2(2 Suppl):17-9.

Cantor C. Kava and alcohol. Med J Aust. 1997 Nov 17;167(10):560.

Cauffield JS, Forbes HJ. Dietary supplements used in the treatment of depression, anxiety, and sleep disorders. Lippincotts Prim Care Pract. 1999 May-Jun;3(3):290-304.

Cawte J. Psychoactive substances of the South Seas: Betel, kava and pituri. Aust N Z J Psychiatry. 1985 Mar;19(1):83-7.

Cerrato PL. Natural tranquilizers? RN. 1998 Dec;61(12):61-2.

Duffield AM, Jamieson DD, Lidgard RO, Duffield PH, Bourne DJ. Identification of some human urinary metabolites of the intoxicating beverage kava. J Chromatogr. 1989 Jul 28;475:273-81.

Ford CS. Ethnographical aspects of kava. Psychopharmacol Bull. 1967 Dec;4(3):12.

Fugh-Berman A, Cott JM. Dietary supplements and natural products as psychotherapeutic agents. Psychosom Med. 1999 Sep-Oct;61(5):712-28.

Garner LF, Klinger JD. Some visual effects caused by the beverage kava. J Ethnopharmacol. 1985 Jul;13(3):307-11.

Gleitz J, Beile A, Wilkens P, Ameri A, Peters T. Antithrombotic action of the kava pyrone (+)-kavain prepared from Piper methysticum on human platelets. Planta Med. 1997 Feb;63(1):27-30.

Heiligenstein E, Guenther G. Over-the-counter psychotropics: A review of melatonin, St John's wort, valerian, and kava-kava. J Am Coll Health. 1998 May;46(6):271-6.

Heinze HJ, Munthe TF, Steitz J, Matzke M. Pharmacopsychological effects of oxazepam and kava-extract in a visual search paradigm assessed with event-related potentials. Pharmacopsychiatry. 1994 Nov;27(6):224-30.

Herberg KW. Effect of Kava-Special Extract WS 1490 combined with ethyl alcohol on safety-relevant performance parameters. Blutalkohol. 1993 Mar;30(2):96-105.

Holmes LD. Piper methysticum (kava). The function of kava in modern Samoan culture. Psychopharmacol Bull. 1967 Dec;4(3):9.

Jappe U, Franke I, Reinhold D, Gollnick HP. Sebotropic drug reaction resulting from kava-kava extract therapy: A new entity? J Am Acad Dermatol. 1998 Jan;38(1):104-6.

Kava. Lancet. 1988 Jul 30;2(8605):258-9.

Kinder C, Cupp MJ. Kava: An herbal sedative. Nurse Pract. 1998 Jun;23(6):14, 156.

Kinzler E, Kromer J, Lehmann E. Effect of a special kava extract in patients with anxiety-, tension-, and excitation-states of non-psychotic genesis. Double blind study with placebos over 4 weeks. Arzneimittelforschung. 1991 Jun;41(6):584-8.

Mack RB. A less than Pacific odyssey: The use of kava. N C Med J. 1999 Mar-Apr;60(2):91-3.

Mathews JD, Riley MD, Fejo L, Munoz E, Milns NR, Gardner ID, Powers JR, Ganygulpa E, Gununuwawuy BJ. Effects of the heavy usage of kava on physical health: Summary of a pilot survey in an aboriginal community. Med J Aust. 1988 Jun 6;148(11):548-55.

Muller B, Komorek R. Treatment with Kava—the root to combat stress. Wien Med Wochenschr. 1999;149(8-10):197-201.

Munte TF, Heinze HJ, Matzke M, Steitz J. Effects of oxazepam and an extract of kava roots (Piper methysticum) on event-related potentials in a word recognition task. Neuropsychobiology. 1993;27(1):46-53.

Norton SA, Ruze P. Kava dermopathy. J Am Acad Dermatol. 1994 Jul;31(1):89-97.

Nowakowska E, Ostrowicz A, Chodera A. Kava-kava preparations—alternative anxiolytics. Pol Merkuriusz Lek. 1998 Mar;4(21):179-180a.

Pepping J. Kava: Piper methysticum. Am J Health Syst Pharm. 1999 May 15;56(10):957-8, 960.

Pfeiffer CC, Murphree HB, Goldstein L. Effect of kava in normal subjects and patients. Psychopharmacol Bull. 1967 Dec;4(3):12.

Piper methysticum (kava kava). Altern Med Rev. 1998 Dec;3(6):458-60.

Pittler MH, Ernst E. Efficacy of kava extract for treating anxiety: Systematic review and meta-analysis. J Clin Psychopharmacol. 2000 Feb;20(1):84-9.

Riesenberg SH. Ancient kava ceremony re-enacted on Pahn Kedira, Ponape. Psychopharmacol Bull. 1967 Dec;4(3):5-8.

Rotblatt MD. Cranberry, feverfew, horse chestnut, and kava. West J Med. 1999 Sep;171(3):195-8.

Ruze P. Kava-induced dermopathy: A niacin deficiency? Lancet. 1990 Jun 16;335(8703):1442-5.

Schelosky L, Raffauf C, Jendroska K, Poewe W. Kava and dopamine antagonism. J Neurol Neurosurg Psychiatry. 1995 May;58(5):639-40.

Scherer J. Kava-kava extract in anxiety disorders: An outpatient observational study. Adv Ther. 1998 Jul-Aug;15(4):261-9.

Singh YN. Kava: An overview. J Ethnopharmacol. 1992 Aug;37(1):13-45.

Spillane PK, Fisher DA, Currie BJ. Neurological manifestations of kava intoxication. Med J Aust. 1997 Aug 4;167(3):172-3.

Tinsley JA. The hazards of psychotropic herbs. Minn Med. 1999 May;82(5):29-31.

Uebelhack R, Franke L, Schewe HJ. Inhibition of platelet MAO-B by kava pyrone-enriched extract from Piper methysticum Forster (kava-kava). Pharmacopsychiatry. 1998 Sep;31(5):187-92.

Volz HP, Kieser M. Kava-kava extract WS 1490 versus placebo in anxiety disorders—a randomized placebo-controlled 25-week outpatient trial. Pharmacopsychiatry. 1997 Jan;30(1):1-5.

Warnecke G. Psychosomatic dysfunctions in the female climacteric. Clinical effectiveness and tolerance of Kava Extract WS 1490. Fortschr Med. 1991 Feb 10;109(4):119-22.

Wong AH, Smith M, Boon HS. Herbal remedies in psychiatric practice. Arch Gen Psychiatry. 1998 Nov;55(11):1033-44.

S-ADENOSYLMETHIONINE (SAMe)

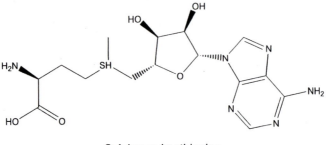

S-Adenosylmethionine

What Is It?

S-adenosylmethionine (SAMe) is a form of the sulfur-containing amino acid methionine, combined with adenosine (part of the energy compound ATP). Like methionine, SAMe is involved in numerous metabolic processes in the body that require sulfur, such as the methylation reactions. The body typically manufactures all the SAMe that it requires (from methionine consumed in protein foods), but a defect in methylation or a deficiency in any of the cofactors required for SAMe production (methionine, choline, B vitamins) is theorized to reduce the body's ability to produce SAMe.

Claims

- Relieves depression/elevates mood
- Reduces arthritis pain
- Maintains antioxidant status (via glutathione)

Theory

It has been hypothesized that a defect in the body's methylation process is central to the biochemical basis of certain neuropsychiatric disorders. For example, folic acid, which is involved in methylation reactions in the body, has been linked to depression when consumed at deficient levels (probably due to a lowering of brain serotonin levels). There is a high incidence of folate deficiency in depression, and there are indications in the literature that some depressed patients who are folate deficient respond to folate supplementation. Folate deficiency is also known to lower levels of SAMe, while supplemental levels are an effective antidepressant that raise brain serotonin levels. It is suggested that low levels of serotonin in some depressed patients may be a secondary consequence of low levels of SAMe.

Scientific Support

Tissue levels of SAMe have been found to be low in the elderly and in patients suffering from depression. SAMe has performed as well as conventional antidepressant drugs in studies of depression, where it has been demonstrated that SAMe can alter mood states. The mechanism for the effectiveness of SAMe is unclear, but is likely to be related to increasing levels of brain neurotransmitters such as serotonin and dopamine.

Safety

SAMe has been shown to be effective in elevating mood and treating depression—without some of the more commonly reported side effects found with prescription antidepressants (impotence, nervousness, trouble sleeping, and headaches).

High dietary intake of methionine, however, is associated with the potential for significant adverse side effects. High levels of methionine can lead to high levels of a particular metabolite, homocysteine, which has been associated with an increased risk for cardiovascular disease. In the presence of inadequate levels of B-complex vitamins (folic acid and vitamins B_6 and B_{12}), homocysteine levels may increase and may damage the inner lining of blood vessels, leading to cardiovascular complications.

Value

SAMe has the distinct advantage of being a naturally occurring compound in the body, which suggests that supplementation with SAMe is simply providing an additional dietary source of this nutrient. Other antidepressant compounds that are available as dietary supplements, such as St. John's wort, could be viewed as more of a pharmacological approach to relieving depression because they are not found in the body. This is more a matter of semantics, however, as both compounds have been shown to be effective in elevating mood and relieving mild depression.

Dosage

It is important to note that dietary supplements of methionine do not appear to elevate SAMe levels or have the same effect on mood states found with SAMe. Doses of 200 to 600 mg per day may be effective in elevating mood and treating mild depression.

WORKS CONSULTED

Baldessarini RJ. Biological transmethylation involving S-adenosylmethionine: Development of assay methods and implications for neuropsychiatry. Int Rev Neurobiol. 1975;18:41-67.

Baldessarini RJ. Neuropharmacology of S-adenosyl-L-methionine. Am J Med. 1987 Nov 20;83(5A):95-103.

Bottiglieri T, Godfrey P, Flynn T, Carney MW, Toone BK, Reynolds EH. Cerebrospinal fluid S-adenosylmethionine in depression and dementia: Effects of treatment with parenteral and oral S-adenosylmethionine. J Neurol Neurosurg Psychiatry. 1990 Dec;53(12):1096-8.

Bottiglieri T, Hyland K. S-adenosylmethionine levels in psychiatric and neurological disorders: A review. Acta Neurol Scand Suppl. 1994;154:19-26.

Bottiglieri T, Hyland K, Reynolds EH. The clinical potential of ademetionine (S-adenosylmethionine) in neurological disorders. Drugs. 1994 Aug; 48(2): 137-52.

Bressa GM. S-adenosyl-l-methionine (SAMe) as antidepressant: Meta-analysis of clinical studies. Acta Neurol Scand Suppl. 1994;154:7-14.

Cantoni GL, Mudd SH, Andreoli V. Affective disorders and S-adenosylmethionine: A new hypothesis. Trends Neurosci. 1989 Sep;12(9):319-24.

Carney MW. Neuropharmacology of S-adenosyl methionine. Clin Neuropharmacol. 1986;9(3):235-43.

Carney MW, Edeh J, Bottiglieri T, Reynolds EM, Toone BK. Affective illness and S-adenosyl methionine: A preliminary report. Clin Neuropharmacol. 1986;9(4): 379-85.

Carney MW, Toone BK, Reynolds EH. S-adenosylmethionine and affective disorder. Am J Med. 1987 Nov 20;83(5A):104-6.

Del Vecchio M, Amati A, Vacca L, Zizolfi S. Monitoring S-adenosyl-methionine blood levels and antidepressant effect. Acta Neurol (Napoli). 1980 Dec;2(6):488-95.

Fava M, Rosenbaum JF, MacLaughlin R, Falk WE, Pollack MH, Cohen LS, Jones L, Pill L. Neuroendocrine effects of S-adenosyl-L-methionine, a novel putative antidepressant. J Psychiatr Res. 1990;24(2):177-84.

Goodnick PJ, Sandoval R. Psychotropic treatment of chronic fatigue syndrome and related disorders. J Clin Psychiatry. 1993 Jan;54(1):13-20.

Masturzo P, Gianrossi R, Carolei A, Barreca T, Murialdo G. Effect of S-adenosyl-methionine (SAMe) on some endocrine parameters in normal adult subjects. Minerva Med. 1976 Sep 19;67(43):2801-4.

Morrison LD, Becker L, Kish SJ. S-adenosylmethionine decarboxylase in human brain. Regional distribution and influence of aging. Brain Res Dev Brain Res. 1993 Jun 8;73(2):237-41.

Morrison LD, Bergeron C, Kish SJ. Brain S-adenosylmethionine decarboxylase activity is increased in Alzheimer's disease. Neurosci Lett. 1993 May 14;154(1-2): 141-4.

Morrison LD, Sherwin AL, Carmant L, Kish SJ. Activity of S-adenosylmethionine decarboxylase, a key regulatory enzyme in polyamine biosynthesis, is increased in epileptogenic human cortex. Arch Neurol. 1994 Jun;51(6):581-4.

Morrison LD, Smith DD, Kish SJ. Brain S-adenosylmethionine levels are severely decreased in Alzheimer's disease. J Neurochem. 1996 Sep;67(3):1328-31.

Newman PE. Alzheimer's disease revisited. Med Hypotheses. 2000 May;54(5):774-6.

Otero Losada ME, Rubio MC. The importance of methylation reactions in the biochemistry of catecholaminergic and serotoninergic neurons. Medicina (B Aires). 1991;51(3):267-72.

Passeri M, Ceccato S. Significance of transmethylation and S-adenosylmethionine (SAM) in the management of Parkinson's disease with L-dopa. Minerva Med. 1972 Apr 21;63(30):1722-59.

Piccinin GL, Gerardi AU, Piccirilli M, Araco M. The neurochemical bases of the use of SAM in psychiatry. Clin Ter. 1980 Jul 15;94(1):113-6.

Reynolds EH, Carney MW, Toone BK. Methylation and mood. Lancet. 1984 Jul 28;2(8396):196-8.

Reynolds EH, Stramentinoli G. Folic acid, S-adenosylmethionine and affective disorder. Psychol Med. 1983 Nov;13(4):705-10.

Rosenbaum JF, Fava M, Falk WE, Pollack MH, Cohen LS, Cohen BM, Zubenko GS. The antidepressant potential of oral S-adenosyl-l-methionine. Acta Psychiatr Scand. 1990 May;81(5):432-6.

Salmaggi P, Bressa GM, Nicchia G, Coniglio M, La Greca P, Le Grazie C. Double-blind, placebo-controlled study of S-adenosyl-L-methionine in depressed postmenopausal women. Psychother Psychosom. 1993;59(1):34-40.

Tramoni AV, Azorin JM. Therapeutic indications of S-adenosyl methionine in neuropsychiatry. Encephale. 1988 May-Jun;14(3):113-8.

Trolin CG, Lofberg C, Trolin G, Oreland L. Brain ATP: L-methionine S-adenosyltransferase (MAT), S-adenosylmethionine (SAM) and S-adenosylhomocysteine (SAH): Regional distribution and age-related changes. Eur Neuropsychopharmacol. 1994 Dec;4(4):469-77.

VALERIAN

What Is It?

Valerian *(Valeriana officinalis* or *Valeriana radix)* has been used as a medicinal antianxiety herb and sleep aid since the days of the Romans. The dried roots of the plant are used in teas, tinctures, and capsule or tablet forms.

Claims

- Promotes relaxation and induces sleep
- Calms nerves and reduces anxiety

Theory

It is unclear which of the numerous compounds is the true active ingredient, but the combination of compounds appears to work together in the brain in a manner similar to the action of prescription tranquilizers such as Valium and Halcion.

Scientific Support

Valerian taken before bedtime appears to reduce the amount of time that it takes to fall asleep. It is unknown, however, whether the quality of the sleep is affected by valerian consumption. Valerian is generally regarded as a mild tranquilizer and has been deemed safe by the German Commission E for treating "restlessness and sleeping disorders brought on by nervous conditions."

Safety

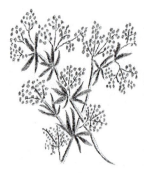

Occasional reports of headaches and mild nausea are documented, but habituation or dependency is unlikely when used as directed. Valerian should be avoided by pregnant and lactating women and should not be consumed by children. Individuals currently taking sedative drugs or antidepressant medications should be advised by their personal physician before taking valerian. Do not take valerian in conjunction with alcohol or other tranquilizers and do not consume for more than two weeks.

Value

As a mild tranquilizer and sleep aid, valerian may be an effective herb for dealing with temporary feelings of anxiety, nervousness, or insomnia. The effects of valerian are generally quite mild when compared to prescription products and synthetic OTC products.

Dosage

Because the activity and strength of valerian preparations can vary significantly from one product to the next, it is recommended to select a standardized product (0.5 to 1.0 percent valerenic acids) whenever possible and to follow the directions on the particular product. As a general guideline, approximately 250 to 500 mg of a 5-6:1 extract can be taken before bed (as a sleep aid) or as needed as a mild tranquilizer.

WORKS CONSULTED

Balderer G, Borbely AA. Effect of valerian on human sleep. Psychopharmacology (Berl). 1985;87(4):406-9.

Cauffield JS, Forbes HJ. Dietary supplements used in the treatment of depression, anxiety, and sleep disorders. Lippincotts Prim Care Pract. 1999 May-Jun;3(3):290-304.

Cerrato PL. Natural tranquilizers? RN. 1998 Dec;61(12):61-2.

Dominguez RA, Bravo-Valverde RL, Kaplowitz BR, Cott JM. Valerian as a hypnotic for Hispanic patients. Cultur Divers Ethni Minor Psychol. 2000 Feb;6(1):84-92.

Donath F, Quispe S, Diefenbach K, Maurer A, Fietze I, Roots I. Critical evaluation of the effect of valerian extract on sleep structure and sleep quality. Pharmacopsychiatry. 2000 Mar;33(2):47-53.

Dorn M. Efficacy and tolerability of Baldrian versus oxazepam in non-organic and non-psychiatric insomniacs: A randomised, double-blind, clinical, comparative study. Forsch Komplementarmed Klass Naturheilkd. 2000 Apr;7(2):79-84.

Fugh-Berman A, Cott JM. Dietary supplements and natural products as psychotherapeutic agents. Psychosom Med. 1999 Sep-Oct;61(5):712-28.

Garges HP, Varia I, Doraiswamy PM. Cardiac complications and delirium associated with valerian root withdrawal. JAMA. 1998 Nov 11;280(18):1566-7.

Gerhard U, Hobi V, Kocher R, Konig C. Acute sedative effect of a herbal relaxation tablet as compared to that of bromazepam. Schweiz Rundsch Med Prax. 1991 Dec 27;80(52):1481-6.

Haas LF. Neurological stamp. Valeriana officinalis (garden heliotrope). J Neurol Neurosurg Psychiatry. 1996 Mar;60(3):255.

Heiligenstein E, Guenther G. Over-the-counter psychotropics: A review of melatonin, St John's wort, valerian, and kava-kava. J Am Coll Health. 1998 May;46(6):271-6.

Houghton PJ. The biological activity of Valerian and related plants. J Ethnopharmacol. 1988 Feb-Mar;22(2):121-42.

Houghton PJ. The scientific basis for the reputed activity of Valerian. J Pharm Pharmacol. 1999 May;51(5):505-12.

Kammerer E. Phytogenic sedatives-hypnotics—does a combination of valerian and hops have a value in the modern drug repertoire? Z Arztl Fortbild (Jena). 1993 Apr 12;87(5):401-6.

Khawaja IS, Marotta RF, Lippmann S. Herbal medicines as a factor in delirium. Psychiatr Serv. 1999 Jul;50(7):969-70.

Kirkwood CK. Management of insomnia. J Am Pharm Assoc (Wash). 1999 Sep-Oct;39(5):688-96.

Kohnen R, Oswald WD. The effects of valerian, propranolol, and their combination on activation, performance, and mood of healthy volunteers under social stress conditions. Pharmacopsychiatry. 1988 Nov;21(6):447-8.

Kuhlmann J, Berger W, Podzuweit H, Schmidt U. The influence of valerian treatment on "reaction time, alertness and concentration" in volunteers. Pharmacopsychiatry. 1999 Nov;32(6):235-41.

Last G. On the treatment of insomnia. Hippokrates. 1969 Jan 15;40(1):28-33.

Leathwood PD, Chauffard F. Aqueous extract of valerian reduces latency to fall asleep in man. Planta Med. 1985 Apr;(2):144-8.

Leathwood PD, Chauffard F. Quantifying the effects of mild sedatives. J Psychiatr Res. 1982-83;17(2):115-22.

Leathwood PD, Chauffard F, Heck E, Munoz-Box R. Aqueous extract of valerian root (Valeriana officinalis L.) improves sleep quality in man. Pharmacol Biochem Behav. 1982 Jul;17(1):65-71.

Lindahl O, Lindwall L. Double blind study of a valerian preparation. Pharmacol Biochem Behav. 1989 Apr;32(4):1065-6.

Molodozhnikova LM. Medicinal valerian. Feldsher Akush. 1988 Jan;53(1):44-6.

Plushner SL. Valerian: Valeriana officinalis. Am J Health Syst Pharm. 2000 Feb 15;57(4):328, 333, 335.

Schmitz M, Jackel M. Comparative study for assessing quality of life of patients with exogenous sleep disorders (temporary sleep onset and sleep interruption disorders) treated with a hops-valerian preparation and a benzodiazepine drug. Wien Med Wochenschr. 1998;148(13):291-8.

Schulz H, Stolz C, Muller J. The effect of valerian extract on sleep polygraphy in poor sleepers: A pilot study. Pharmacopsychiatry. 1994 Jul;27(4):147-51.

Straube G. The importance of valerian roots in therapy. Ther Ggw. 1968 Apr;107(4):555-62.

Thierolf H. Contribution on the treatment of nervous manifestations. Landarzt. 1964 Sep 10;40(25):1086-7.

Tucakov J. Comparative ethnomedical study of Valeriana officinalis L. Glas Srp Akad Nauka [Med]. 1965;(18):131-50.

Vonderheid-Guth B, Todorova A, Brattstrom A, Dimpfel W. Pharmacodynamic effects of valerian and hops extract combination (Ze 91019) on the quantitative-topographical EEG in healthy volunteers. Eur J Med Res. 2000 Apr 19;5(4):139-44.

Wagner J, Wagner ML, Hening WA. Beyond benzodiazepines: Alternative pharmacologic agents for the treatment of insomnia. Ann Pharmacother. 1998 Jun;32(6):680-91.

Willey LB, Mady SP, Cobaugh DJ, Wax PM. Valerian overdose: A case report. Vet Hum Toxicol. 1995 Aug;37(4):364-5.

Wong AH, Smith M, Boon HS. Herbal remedies in psychiatric practice. Arch Gen Psychiatry. 1998 Nov;55(11):1033-44.

MELATONIN

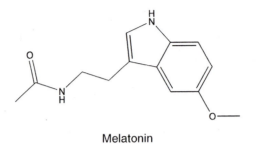

Melatonin

What Is It?

Melatonin is a hormone produced by the pineal gland in the brain. It is synthesized from the amino acid tryptophan. In humans, melatonin appears to have an inhibitory effect on early maturation.

Claims

- Promotes sleep
- Reduces symptoms of jet lag
- Slows the aging process
- Acts as an antioxidant

Theory

In animals, melatonin seems to help regulate seasonal behaviors (mating, molting, hibernation), which are related to daily light/dark cycles. In humans, melatonin helps regulate our "internal clock." The onset of darkness results in an increased production of melatonin in the brain, while the light of morning tells the brain to stop producing melatonin. Melatonin levels are ten times higher at night than during the day.

Scientific Support

Melatonin supplementation has been shown to lower core body temperature, produce acute hypnotic effects, and induce the onset of sleep in a variety of subjects including military pilots, jet-lagged travelers, elderly patients, and individuals with delayed sleep disorder. Melatonin has also shown some benefit in helping to reset the biological clock of shift workers, who tend to have peak melatonin levels during the day.

As an antioxidant, melatonin has shown benefits in protecting cells against oxidative stress by scavenging hydroxyl radicals and preventing oxidative damage to DNA, lipids, and cellular proteins. Melatonin is also thought to play a role in the regulation of the human menstrual cycle, as evidenced by the finding that women with hypothalamic amenorrhea (lack of menstrual periods) have melatonin levels three times higher than normal. High-dose melatonin supplements have been used pharmacologically in studies to suppress ovulation for birth control purposes.

Safety

The interaction of melatonin with other supplements or drugs is unknown, but some studies suggest that melatonin can induce or deepen depression in susceptible individuals. Melatonin supplements may also be dangerous for people with cardiovascular risks, due to the possibility of vasoconstriction and increased blood pressure. The National Institutes of Health has warned about possible dangers of melatonin supplementation, including infertility, reduced sex drive in males, hypothermia, retinal damage, and interference with hormone replacement therapy. Information regarding the long-term effects of melatonin supplements is unavailable.

Value

Melatonin can be viewed as a relatively inexpensive and nonaddictive alternative to over-the-counter chemical sleep aids. It may be particularly useful as a short-term regulator of sleep/wake cycles in cases such as recovering from jet lag.

Dosage

Studies of melatonin as a sleep aid or for relief of symptoms associated with jet lag have shown 1 to 10 mg to be effective, depending on the degree of sleep disturbance. High-dose melatonin supplements (around 50 mg) may disrupt female fertility and menstrual patterns and should be avoided except under the supervision of a reproductive physician.

WORKS CONSULTED

Arendt J, Deacon S. Treatment of circadian rhythm disorders—melatonin. Chronobiol Int. 1997 Mar;14(2):185-204.

Avery D, Lenz M, Landis C. Guidelines for prescribing melatonin. Ann Med. 1998 Feb;30(1):122-30.

Chase JE, Gidal BE. Melatonin: Therapeutic use in sleep disorders. Ann Pharmacother. 1997 Oct;31(10):1218-26.

Defrance R, Quera-Salva MA. Therapeutic applications of melatonin and related compounds. Horm Res. 1998;49(3-4):142-6.

Jan JE, Espezel H. Melatonin treatment of chronic sleep disorders. Dev Med Child Neurol. 1995 Mar;37(3):279-80.

Jan JE, Espezel H, Freeman RD, Fast DK. Melatonin treatment of chronic sleep disorders. J Child Neurol. 1998 Feb;13(2):98.

Kato M, Kajimura N, Sekimoto M, Watanabe T, Takahashi K. Melatonin treatment for rhythm disorder. Psychiatry Clin Neurosci. 1998 Apr;52(2):262-3.

Kendler BS. Melatonin: Media hype or therapeutic breakthrough? Nurse Pract. 1997 Feb;22(2):66-7, 71-2, 77.

Kryger MH. Controversies in sleep medicine: Melatonin. Sleep. 1997 Oct;20(10):898.

Kuhn WF, Wellman A. The use of melatonin as a potential treatment for shiftwork sleep disorder. Acad Emerg Med. 1998 Aug;5(8):842-3.

Lewy AJ, Ahmed S, Jackson JM, Sack RL. Melatonin shifts human circadian rhythms according to a phase-response curve. Chronobiol Int. 1992 Oct;9(5):380-92.

McArthur AJ, Lewy AJ, Sack RL. Non-24-hour sleep-wake syndrome in a sighted man: Circadian rhythm studies and efficacy of melatonin treatment. Sleep. 1996 Sep;19(7):544-53.

Okawa M, Uchiyama M, Ozaki S, Shibui K, Kamei Y, Hayakawa T, Urata J. Melatonin treatment for circadian rhythm sleep disorders. Psychiatry Clin Neurosci. 1998 Apr;52(2):259-60.

Sack RL, Hughes RJ, Edgar DM, Lewy AJ. Sleep-promoting effects of melatonin: At what dose, in whom, under what conditions, and by what mechanisms? Sleep. 1997 Oct;20(10):908-15.

Sack RL, Lewy AJ, Hughes RJ. Use of melatonin for sleep and circadian rhythm disorders. Ann Med. 1998 Feb;30(1):115-21.

Skene DJ, Deacon S, Arendt J. Use of melatonin in circadian rhythm disorders and following phase shifts. Acta Neurobiol Exp (Warsz). 1996;56(1):359-62.

Skene DJ, Lockley SW, Arendt J. Melatonin in circadian sleep disorders in the blind. Biol Signals Recept. 1999 Jan-Apr;8(1-2):90-5.

Skene DJ, Lockley SW, Arendt J. Use of melatonin in the treatment of phase shift and sleep disorders. Adv Exp Med Biol. 1999;467:79-84.

Tzischinsky O, Pal I, Epstein R, Dagan Y, Lavie P. The importance of timing in melatonin administration in a blind man. J Pineal Res. 1992 Apr;12(3):105-8.

Zhdanova IV, Lynch HJ, Wurtman RJ. Melatonin: A sleep-promoting hormone. Sleep. 1997 Oct;20(10):899-907.

FEVERFEW

What Is It?

Feverfew *(Tanacetum parthenium)* is a member of the daisy family. It has been used in traditional medicine as far back as the first century for inflammatory conditions and to prevent the occurrence of migraine headaches. Traditionally consumed as whole or dried leaves, or as a tea, feverfew is available in supplemental form as an encapsulated powder standardized for the potential active ingredient, known as parthenolide.

Claims

- Prevents migraine headaches
- Reduces severity of migraine episodes
- Anti-inflammatory activity (may help arthritis)

Theory

The dried leaves of feverfew contain compounds known as sesquiterpene lactones, of which parthenolide is the most prevalent (85 percent) and is thought to be the primary active constituent.

Scientific Support

Laboratory and clinical studies have shown an effect of feverfew leaves and extracts on inflammatory processes including arachidonate metabolism and platelet functions. Feverfew extracts produce a clear inhibition of histamine release and reduced production of prostaglandins, which may explain some of the anti-inflammatory activities of feverfew. Parthenolide and related sesquiterpenes may interfere with serotonin release from platelets (excess serotonin release from platelets has been suggested as a primary cause of migraines), suggesting a possible mechanism by which feverfew functions to inhibit smooth muscle cell contraction and prevent migraines from occurring.

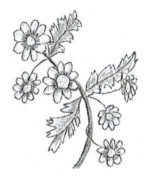

In subjects consuming 80 mg of feverfew per day for one month, 25 percent experienced a reduction in the number of migraine attacks and a clear reduction in the occurrence of the nausea and vomiting that often accompany migraine attacks. In another study, in which subjects consumed 100 mg per day of dried feverfew leaves (standardized to contain 0.2 mg parthenolide), migraine intensity was reduced following sixty days.

Safety

A number of side effects have been noted in clinical studies, including mouth ulcers, gastrointestinal discomfort, and dry mouth. Women who are pregnant or lactating should avoid consuming feverfew, as should any individuals with a known sensitivity to other members of the same plant family, such as ragweed and chamomile. Long-term use may be associated with an anticoagulant (blood-thinning) effect, so feverfew should probably not be used in conjunction with other blood-thinning agents.

Value

Migraines can cause excruciating pain and often completely incapacitate the sufferer. Feverfew is relatively inexpensive, safe, and has shown clear effects in reducing the number of migraine attacks in some people. It is important to look for a supplement that is standardized to at least 0.2 percent parthenolide, thus ensuring that you are actually consuming what is thought to be the primary active constituent of the whole plant.

Dosage

Most studies have used dosages ranging from 25 to 125 mg of feverfew leaf per day, with a parthenolide content of at least 0.2 mg (0.2 to 0.9 percent). Supplements should be taken prophylactically to prevent the occurrence of migraines, rather than in an attempt to relieve a migraine attack once it occurs. A month or two may pass before the therapeutic effect is achieved. Some alternative practitioners recommend an occasional break from treatment, but be aware that a "rebound" syndrome has been reported in which tension and headaches follow the discontinuance of feverfew consumption.

WORKS CONSULTED

Abourashed EA, Khan IA. Determination of parthenolide in selected feverfew products by liquid chromatography. J AOAC Int. 2000 Jul-Aug; 83(4):789-92.
Awang DV. Feverfew products. CMAJ. 1997 Sep 1;157(5):510-1.

Barsby RW, Knight DW, McFadzean I. A chloroform extract of the herb feverfew blocks voltage-dependent potassium currents recorded from single smooth muscle cells. J Pharm Pharmacol. 1993 Jul;45(7):641-5.

Barsby RW, Salan U, Knight DW, Hoult JR. Feverfew and vascular smooth muscle: Extracts from fresh and dried plants show opposing pharmacological profiles, dependent upon sesquiterpene lactone content. Planta Med. 1993 Feb;59(1):20-5.

Barsby RW, Salan U, Knight DW, Hoult JR. Feverfew extracts and parthenolide irreversibly inhibit vascular responses of the rabbit aorta. J Pharm Pharmacol. 1992 Sep;44(9):737-40.

Barsby R, Salan U, Knight DW, Hoult JR. Irreversible inhibition of vascular reactivity by feverfew. Lancet. 1991 Oct 19;338(8773):1015.

Groenewegen WA, Heptinstall S. A comparison of the effects of an extract of feverfew and parthenolide, a component of feverfew, on human platelet activity in-vitro. J Pharm Pharmacol. 1990 Aug;42(8):553-7.

Groenewegen WA, Knight DW, Heptinstall S. Progress in the medicinal chemistry of the herb feverfew. Prog Med Chem. 1992;29:217-38.

Hayes NA, Foreman JC. The activity of compounds extracted from feverfew on histamine release from rat mast cells. J Pharm Pharmacol. 1987 Jun;39(6):466-70.

Heptinstall S. Feverfew—an ancient remedy for modern times? J R Soc Med. 1988 Jul;81(7):373-4.

Heptinstall S, Awang DV, Dawson BA, Kindack D, Knight DW, May J. Parthenolide content and bioactivity of feverfew (Tanacetum parthenium (L.) Schultz-Bip.). Estimation of commercial and authenticated feverfew products. J Pharm Pharmacol. 1992 May;44(5):391-5.

Heptinstall S, Groenewegen WA, Spangenberg P, Losche W. Inhibition of platelet behaviour by feverfew: A mechanism of action involving sulphydryl groups. Folia Haematol Int Mag Klin Morphol Blutforsch. 1988;115(4):447-9.

Knight DW. Feverfew: Chemistry and biological activity. Nat Prod Rep. 1995 Jun;12(3):271-6.

Loesche W, Groenewegen WA, Krause S, Spangenberg P, Heptinstall S. Effects of an extract of feverfew (Tanacetum parthenium) on arachidonic acid metabolism in human blood platelets. Biomed Biochim Acta. 1988;47(10-11):S241-3.

Loesche W, Mazurov AV, Voyno-Yasenetskaya TA, Groenewegen WA, Heptinstall S, Repin VS. Feverfew—an antithrombotic drug? Folia Haematol Int Mag Klin Morphol Blutforsch. 1988;115(1-2):181-4.

Murphy JJ, Heptinstall S, Mitchell JR. Randomised double-blind placebo-controlled trial of feverfew in migraine prevention. Lancet. 1988 Jul 23;2(8604):189-92.

Pattrick M, Heptinstall S, Doherty M. Feverfew in rheumatoid arthritis: A double blind, placebo controlled study. Ann Rheum Dis. 1989 Jul;48(7):547-9.

Pittler MH, Vogler BK, Ernst E. Feverfew for preventing migraine. Cochrane Database Syst Rev. 2000;(3):CD002286.

Prusinski A, Durko A, Niczyporuk-Turek A. Feverfew as a prophylactic treatment of migraine. Neurol Neurochir Pol. 1999;33(Suppl 5):89-95.

Pugh WJ, Sambo K. Prostaglandin synthetase inhibitors in feverfew. J Pharm Pharmacol. 1988 Oct;40(10):743-5.

Rotblatt MD. Cranberry, feverfew, horse chestnut, and kava. West J Med. 1999 Sep;171(3):195-8.

Sriramarao P, Rao PV. Allergenic cross-reactivity between Parthenium and ragweed pollen allergens. Int Arch Allergy Immunol. 1993;100(1):79-85.

Sumner H, Salan U, Knight DW, Hoult JR. Inhibition of 5-lipoxygenase and cyclooxygenase in leukocytes by feverfew. Involvement of sesquiterpene lactones and other components. Biochem Pharmacol. 1992 Jun 9;43(11):2313-20.

Vogler BK, Pittler MH, Ernst E. Feverfew as a preventive treatment for migraine: A systematic review. Cephalalgia. 1998 Dec;18(10):704-8.

Williams CA, Harborne JB, Geiger H, Hoult JR. The flavonoids of Tanacetum parthenium and T. vulgare and their anti-inflammatory properties. Phytochemistry. 1999 Jun;51(3):417-23.

Wong HC. Is feverfew a pharmacologic agent? CMAJ. 1999 Jan 12;160(1):21-2.

Zhou JZ, Kou X, Stevenson D. Rapid extraction and high-performance liquid chromatographic determination of parthenolide in feverfew (Tanacetum parthenium). J Agric Food Chem. 1999 Mar;47(3):1018-22.

Chapter 10

Supplements for Heart Health

INTRODUCTION

According to the American Heart Association, nearly 60 million Americans suffer from one or more forms of cardiovascular disease. When we add in individuals with elevated levels of blood cholesterol, the number approaches 100 million Americans who may be in need of specific diet and lifestyle recommendations for achieving and maintaining heart health.

When it comes to dietary supplements, the vast majority of products are overwhelmingly focused on lowering cholesterol levels, or in DSHEA parlance, "maintaining healthy cholesterol levels"—but there is a great deal more to heart health than a simple cholesterol level. For example, about 50 million Americans have hypertension (high blood pressure), 12 million have coronary artery disease, and more than 7 million heart attacks and 5 million strokes are reported each year. Although deaths from cardiovascular disease (CVD) have dropped more than 20 percent over the last twenty years, CVD still claims almost 1 million American lives each year (about 2,500 deaths each *day*)—making it the leading killer (ahead of deaths from cancer, accidents, and AIDS).

Aside from the generalized recommendations that we typically hear for heart health (lose weight, exercise more, and eat less fat and more fruits and vegetables), there are a number of potentially beneficial dietary supplements that may help to lower cholesterol (chromium, red yeast rice, alfalfa, plant stanols or sterols, soy protein) reduce blood pressure (omega-3 fatty acids, garlic), increase heart muscle function (hawthorn, carnitine, coenzyme Q10), and have other generally positive effects on heart health (such as control of blood levels of homocysteine, glucose, and insulin). It is important to keep in mind, however, that no supplement regimen will counteract a poor diet or sedentary lifestyle, but it *may* provide an added measure of support to genuine nutrition and fitness programs.

Because heart disease results not from a single cause, but from a number of related risk factors, it must be addressed from several different perspectives. For example, heart disease risk can be increased by smoking, diabetes, obesity, high blood pressure, high cholesterol, elevated homocysteine, high stress levels, lack of exercise, and hereditary factors (family history). That's the bad news. The *good* news is that, aside from your genetic makeup, you have a great deal of control over each of these risk factors.

In developing a personal heart health strategy, it might help to think of three main goals and to progress toward each one via the combination of diet, exercise, and dietary supplements that works best for you. The primary goals for attaining improved heart health are:

- Opening blood vessels
- Strengthening the heart muscle
- Controlling free radical damage

OPENING BLOOD VESSELS

Diet

Dietary intake of fat and cholesterol are strongly associated with heart health, but while important, they are far from being the only factors to consider in terms of cardiovascular disease risk. Most people are aware of the differences between low-density lipoproteins (LDL—the "bad" cholesterol) and high-density lipoproteins (HDL—the "good" cholesterol). Many are not aware, however, of the complex chain of events that actually leads to the development of plaque buildup and narrowing of the blood vessels—a process that involves cholesterol, saturated and *trans* fats, triglycerides, homocysteine, glucose, insulin, free radicals, and a host of contributing factors.

If you have your cholesterol level checked and your doctor tells you that it is elevated (above 240 mg/dl), he or she may suggest a popular form of prescription medication designed to reduce cholesterol levels. These drugs, known as "statins," are among the best-selling pharmaceuticals of all time—often generating over $1 billion per drug per year for pharmaceutical companies. Some of the top statins, such as lovastatin (Mevacor) and simvastatin (Zocor) from Merck, atorvastatin (Lipitor) from Warner-Lambert, and pravastatin (Pravachol) from Bristol Myers-Squibb, may be able to reduce serum cholesterol levels by nearly 40 percent (a *huge* amount).

Because many of the statin medications are associated with adverse side effects, however, it may be wise to try diet and exercise alterations before opting for drug therapy (especially if your cholesterol levels are between 200 and 240 mg/dl). Dietary changes such as reducing saturated fat and *trans* fat intake can help lower LDL levels, while regular exercise can help raise HDL levels. In addition, pay attention to daily intake of refined carbohydrates, which can cause rapid elevations in triglycerides, blood sugar, and insulin—each of which can damage blood vessels and promote plaque buildup above and beyond the direct effects of cholesterol-related factors.

Exercise

There is no doubt that regular exercise is associated with a lower risk of heart disease compared to a sedentary lifestyle. One reason may be due to the close association between obesity, hypertension, elevated cholesterol levels, and elevated blood glucose and insulin levels. Health experts estimate that almost three-quarters of the American population is overweight and that obesity is a direct cause of about 25 percent of health care expenditures related to heart disease.

Again, despite the bad news about obesity and heart disease, the good news is that a great deal can be done about the situation—and that means exercise. Until recently, exercise recommendations consisted of working yourself half to death—the "no pain, no gain" philosophy of exercise. The most recent exercise recommendations for heart health, however, encourage people to do something—*anything*—so long as they get up and get active. Although it would be terrific for everybody to strive for at least 30 minutes of moderate aerobic activity three or more times a week to help elevate their HDL levels, *something* is a whole lot better than *nothing,* and even a walk around the block can help improve blood sugar regulation, blood lipid profiles, blood pressure, and help control body weight.

Supplements

Essential fatty acids (EFAs) are associated with many aspects of cardiovascular health. One of the best sources of EFAs is flaxseed oil (also known as linseed oil) because of the unique balance of omega-3 (linolenic acid) and omega-6 (linoleic acid) fatty acids. Most Americans consume an imbalanced diet providing mostly omega-6 fats (from vegetable oils) and very few omega-3s—a situation that can lead to constricted blood vessels, elevated blood pressure, and an increased tendency of the blood to clot. Because flaxseed oil is about 60 percent omega-3 and 20 percent omega-6 fatty acids, it already provides a healthy balance of these fatty acids in the right ratio to promote heart health. Fish oil and other marine oils can be a much more concentrated source of omega-3 fatty acids, providing as much as 180 mg of DHA and 120 mg of EPA per gram of high-quality oil.

B-complex vitamins such as folic acid, B_6, and B_{12} are needed for the proper metabolism of homocysteine (a metabolite of the amino acid methionine). Homocysteine has been linked to blood vessel damage and a heightened risk of heart disease. Many people think of folic acid only as a "pregnancy" vitamin because of its role in preventing neural tube defects—but postmenopausal women can benefit from folate supplements because they often have higher blood levels of homocysteine than premenopausal women. Supplements providing as little as 400 to 800 mcg of folic acid alone or in combination with vitamins B_6 (2 to 10 mg) and B_{12} (2 to 30 mcg) have been shown to effectively lower elevated homocysteine levels.

Niacin, another B vitamin, can help lower cholesterol and triglyceride levels, but only at very high doses of 1 to 3 g per day. High doses of niacin, however, often cause the skin to flush, an unpleasant side effect that causes many people to stop taking the supplement. The same cholesterol-lowering benefits of niacin (and a lower risk of side effects) may be obtained by combining a smaller dose of the vitamin with other supplements such as red yeast rice or chromium.

Chromium is typically recommended for controlling blood sugar levels, but it also plays a role in helping to manage cholesterol levels and heart health. In diabetics, chromium can help improve blood sugar control—an effect that has direct heart benefits in preventing blood vessel damage and formation of atherosclerotic plaques.

Garlic is a frequent addition to supplement formulas intended to promote heart health—and with good reason. Garlic intake has been associated with reduced cholesterol and triglyceride levels as well as an inhibition of blood clotting (a blood-thinning effect) and a modest lowering of blood pressure.

Ginkgo biloba may help to improve blood circulation to all parts of the body, including the heart. Although ginkgo has no direct impact on lowering cholesterol or homocysteine levels, its effects on dilating blood vessels and reducing blood clotting may help promote heart health by improving heart muscle efficiency. Ginkgo also appears to be effective in reducing the leg pain associated with intermittent claudication—where lack of blood flow to the legs causes pain when walking.

Red yeast rice is a traditional Chinese food used to spice dishes such as Peking duck. Because it naturally contains several compounds that can reduce cholesterol production in the liver (via inhibition of an enzyme called HMG-CoA reductase)—red yeast rice may be an effective alternative to statin drugs for people who have borderline elevated cholesterol (200 to 240 mg/dl).

Plant compounds known as *stanols* and *sterols* are being formulated into margarine and other food products for their benefits in blocking the absorption of cholesterol from foods (because of similarities in chemical structure). These types of margarine have been shown in several studies to be capable of lowering LDL cholesterol levels by 10 to 15 percent without affecting HDL levels.

Alfalfa supplements are theorized to help lower cholesterol due to a combination of fiber and saponins, which can bind to cholesterol in the diet and bile acids in the intestines—both of which would increase the amount of cholesterol lost from the body in feces.

Arginine is an amino acid that serves as a precursor to nitric oxide, a compound needed for proper dilation of blood vessels. The popularity of this supplement as a circulation enhancer is evident from arginine's inclusion in supplements for everything from sexual fitness to bodybuilding. Medical foods targeted directly at heart disease patients may provide as much as 3 to 6 g of arginine per day as a way to help open blood vessels and promote blood flow.

Soluble fiber (upward of 7 to 10 g per day) can reduce total cholesterol and LDL levels by 5 to 10 percent via directly binding to cholesterol and bile acids in the intestines and flushing them out of the body in the feces.

Soy protein can help lower LDL cholesterol by about 10 percent, a fact that spurred the FDA to approve a health claim for foods that "25 grams of soy protein a day, as part of a diet low in saturated fat and cholesterol, may help reduce the risk of heart disease" (FDA Talk Paper, T99-48. October 20, 1999).

STRENGTHENING THE HEART MUSCLE

Diet

Although there are no direct dietary strategies for increasing the strength of the heart muscles, several dietary approaches can help minimize damage to blood vessels and the associated strain on the heart. Aside from dietary recommendations centered on fat and cholesterol intake, a word about sodium and alcohol is appropriate. Public concern about salt intake waxes and wanes with media reports supporting or refuting the theory that salt intake is linked to high blood pressure. The most current scientific opinion is that about 50 to 60 percent of people with elevated blood pressure are salt sensitive—meaning that excessive salt (sodium) intake can raise their blood pressure, while salt restriction can help lower it. This does not mean that salt consumption *causes* hypertension in "normal" people who do not exhibit a salt sensitivity.

Regarding alcohol, moderate consumption (one to two drinks per day) has been associated with reduced risk for heart disease (most notably for red wine—the so-called French paradox). The reasons for this interesting finding may be due partly to the alcohol (which can open blood vessels) and partly to a high level of antioxidants (flavonoids), which can help protect blood vessel linings and prevent the oxidation of LDL cholesterol.

Exercise

Regular exercise should be "taken" just as you take your supplements, as a daily dose—because consistency is the key to delivering the benefits in terms of helping you lose weight, reduce cholesterol, control blood sugar, lower blood pressure, strengthen the heart muscle, and alleviate stress. It is well established that people who are less fit are five to ten times more likely to die from cardiovascular disease than those who are highly fit.

Supplements

Magnesium is one of the top "strengthening" nutrients when it comes to heart health. Not only does magnesium play a vital role in controlling muscle contraction and relaxation, it is involved in regulating blood pressure (by relaxing blood vessels) and can help reduce the tendency of blood to clot.

Coenzyme Q10 plays an important role in the "energetics" of the heart, where it participates in the production of energy used for muscle contractions. CoQ10 supplementation has been linked to improvements in heart muscle contraction strength—so much so that patients with congestive heart failure (CHF) show clinically important improvements on measures such as fluid accumulation (edema) and incidence of chest pain (angina). Individuals currently taking statin medications or red yeast rice supplements, both of which operate as inhibitors of the HMG CoA reductase enzyme, should be aware that these agents may suppress the body's own production of CoQ10—making supplements even more important.

Potassium, one of several electrolytes that are important for muscle contractions, has been associated with beneficial effects in preventing hypertension. Several studies have shown that increasing potassium intake can help reduce blood pressure in patients with hypertension and that strokes may be linked with reduced potassium levels in the blood. In most cases, however, the amount of potassium associated with these cardiovascular benefits can be easily obtained from common foods (bananas, citrus fruit, and orange juice), so supplemental levels may not be necessary.

Hawthorn berry is frequently recommended as a "tonic" supplement for the heart. It has been used to help control abnormal heart beat (arrhythmia) and has been a traditional remedy for both high and low blood pressure. Because hawthorn has a relatively high concentration of bioflavonoids, it also possesses strong antioxidant benefits.

Carnitine is an amino acid that is involved in the transport of fatty acids into the mitochondria for oxidation. As such, it is directly involved in the metabolism of the heart's major fuel source—fat. An increase in the energy efficiency of the heart muscle would allow greater energy production, a more forceful muscle contraction, and greater delivery of blood and oxygen to the rest of the body. In patients recovering from heart attacks and bypass surgery, carnitine has been shown to improve exercise tolerance and allow patients to perform greater amounts of work at higher intensities.

CONTROLLING FREE RADICAL DAMAGE

Diet

Antioxidant nutrients such as vitamins C and E, and minerals such as selenium and zinc, are potent scavengers of reactive molecules called free radicals. Free radicals have been implicated in diseases such as cancer, heart disease, and even the aging process itself. Other nonnutrient antioxidants such as the flavonoids and carotenoids can provide added cellular protection against free radical damage. The *best* source of phytonutrient antioxidants such as carotenoids and flavonoids is a frequent and varied intake of brightly colored fruits and vegetables. These phytonutrients are pigments that give fruits and veggies their characteristic colors (the brighter the better) and provide protection from free radical damage.

Exercise

Intense physical activity is frequently cited as a cause of oxidative damage from an increased production of free radicals (and it is). Exercise also induces the body to increase its production of specialized antioxidant enzymes to help counteract the increase in free radical production and protect the tissues most susceptible to damage (lungs, muscles, and heart tissue). Both exercise and dietary supplementation of cysteine and alpha lipoic acid can enhance the body's own production of glutathione, one of the most potent endogenous antioxidants.

Supplements

Among nutritional antioxidants, *vitamin E* is almost certainly "king of the hill" (although vitamin C is a close second—perhaps the "queen"?). Vitamin E has been studied more than any other nutrient for its antioxidant properties and for its specific role in helping to prevent heart attacks (by reducing oxidation of LDL cholesterol and by reducing the tendency of the blood to clot). The majority of studies suggest that 400 to 800 IU of vitamin E per day (levels almost impossible to achieve in the diet) can reduce the risk of death from cardiovascular disease by 30 to 60 percent when compared to a placebo. More recent studies, however, have found that 400 IU of vitamin E does not reduce the incidence of heart attacks or stroke in patients with *established* heart disease, and still other studies suggest that vitamin E from *foods* may be more effective in controlling heart disease risk than vitamin E from supplements. Does this mean that vitamin E supplements are useless? No—but it does mean that vitamin E should not be viewed as the panacea or cure for heart disease that some people make it out to be. Although vitamin E supplements appear to be beneficial for many people, they are clearly no magic bullet.

Vitamin C, or ascorbic acid, also performs as an antioxidant—but unlike vitamin E (a fat-soluble vitamin), vitamin C acts as a water-soluble antioxidant within the watery environment inside and between cells. Thus, the antioxidant benefits of vitamins C and E complement each other very nicely to deliver a one-two punch to free radicals (and prevent them from damaging blood vessel linings and fragile heart tissue). One of the key benefits of supplemental vitamin C is its ability to help regenerate vitamin E after it has come in contact with a free radical—thus recharging vitamin E to fight again.

Grape seed extract is an excellent source of flavonoid compounds (oligomeric proanthocyanidins, or OPCs) that perform as powerful antioxidants and as blood vessel strengtheners. *Green tea extract* is a rich source of another class of polyphenols, the catechins, which also perform antioxidant functions to protect LDL cholesterol and blood vessel linings from oxidative damage. The "antioxidant network" is a term frequently used to denote the interrelated nature of antioxidant and free radical metabolism. The network involves a complex interplay between vitamin and mineral antioxidants (C, E, selenium, zinc), phytonutrients (flavonoids, carotenoids), and other nonnutrient compounds such as alpha lipoic acid to create a multidimensional protection from cellular oxidation.

SUMMARY

In general, a wide variety of dietary supplements may be effective in promoting heart health from a number of different angles (see Table 10.1). It is very important, however, to view such supplements as just that—*supplements*—to an otherwise sound regimen of diet and exercise. Part of this regi-

TABLE 10.1. Primary Dietary Supplements for Heart Health

Ingredient	Dose (per day)	Primary claim
Alfalfa	250-1,000 mg	Lowers cholesterol
Coenzyme Q10	100-200 mg	Heart tonic
Folic acid	200-600 mcg	Reduces homocysteine
Garlic	2-4 g	Lowers blood pressure
Hawthorn	100-300 mg	Heart tonic
Niacin	250-2,000 mg	Lowers cholesterol
Omega-3 fatty acids	2-6 g	Reduces blood clotting
Red yeast rice	1-3 g	Lowers cholesterol
Soy protein	25-50 g	Lowers cholesterol
Vitamin B_{12}	6-12 mcg	Reduces homocysteine
Vitamin B_6	2-4 mg	Reduces homocysteine

men includes regular checkups to monitor blood pressure and blood levels of lipids, glucose, homocysteine, and (if possible) insulin. Review the dietary checklist for some tips to help you achieve heart health:

- Exercise.
- Eat more fruits and veggies—the brighter the color, the better—and include members of the "cruciferous" family such as cabbage, broccoli, and Brussels sprouts.
- Eat fewer fried foods and cut down on saturated fat and partially hydrogenated *trans* fat whenever possible.
- Eat fewer fatty acids of the omega-6 variety (found in corn oil, safflower oil, and sunflower oil) and eat more of the omega-3 variety (found in flaxseed oil, fish oil, and cold-water fish such as salmon, mackerel, tuna, and sardines).
- Eat more soluble fiber.
- Consume more OPCs (found in red wine, purple grape juice, and grape seed or green tea extract).
- Eat more garlic.
- Take a balanced multivitamin supplement that provides the key B-complex nutrients for heart health (niacin, folic acid, B_6, and B_{12}).

RED YEAST RICE (RYR)

What Is It?

Red yeast rice (RYR) is a traditional Chinese spice used to flavor and color food such as Peking duck. The red yeast *(Monascus purpureus)* is grown on white rice and then fermented, creating the product known as red yeast rice. The yeast is then inactivated and the rice/yeast mixture is powdered. In traditional Chinese medicine, red yeast rice is used for "healthy blood" and to "strengthen the heart," while modern dietary supplements use RYR to lower cholesterol levels. In many Asian countries, total daily RYR consumption from foods ranges from 10 to 50 g per day, while Western use as a dietary supplement is often in the range of 1 to 3 g per day.

Claims

- Lowers cholesterol and triglyceride levels
- Heart disease protection

Theory

Red yeast rice contains a number of naturally occurring compounds known as monacolins. Monacolins are known to inhibit the activity of an enzyme in the liver (HMG-CoA reductase) that is needed to produce cholesterol. RYR also contains a mix of sterols (sitosterol, campesterol, and stigmasterol), isoflavones, and unsaturated fatty acids, which are thought to contribute to the cholesterol and lipid-lowering effects of the monacolins. Of the dozen or so monacolins found in RYR, one of them, monacolin K, is also known as lovastatin and is synthesized and marketed by the pharmaceutical giant Merck as Mevacor for reducing elevated cholesterol and triglyceride levels. Although the precise mechanism of action for RYR is not completely understood, the activity of the monacolins on reducing cholesterol synthesis does not appear to be sufficient to account for the entire effect observed in studies of RYR supplementation. For example, the dose of total monacolins reported in clinical trials is 9.6 to 13.5 mg per day, while the recommended dose of lovastatin is 20 mg—suggesting that the cholesterol-lowering effects of RYR may be due to the combined actions of monacolins and other constituents such as sterols and fatty acids (possibly by simultaneously reducing cholesterol synthesis and absorption while also promoting cholesterol excretion).

Scientific Support

Animal studies (mostly in rabbits) have clearly shown that consumption of red yeast rice reduces total and LDL cholesterol levels by 40 to 60 percent and triglyceride levels by 50 to 60 percent. The animal studies have also shown that RYR can inhibit the formation of atherosclerotic plaques. Several human studies have also shown the benefits of RYR in reducing elevated cholesterol and correcting dyslipidemia. In one study of subjects with elevated cholesterol levels (230 mg/dl), 1.2 g of RYR per day (13.5 mg total monacolins) reduced total cholesterol by 23 percent, LDL by 31 percent, and triglycerides by 34 percent, while HDL was elevated by 20 percent, following eight weeks of supplementation. In another study, subjects with elevated cholesterol were given RYR (10 to 13 mg total monacolins) and showed a 20 to 36 percent reduction in cholesterol and triglyceride levels. A recent study used a combination of diet (American Heart Association Step 1 Diet) with RYR supplements and found that a two-month course of RYR supplements (2.4 g per day, containing 9.6 mg total monacolins) reduced total cholesterol by 16 percent, LDL by 21 percent, and total triglyceride levels by 25 percent, while HDL levels increased by 15 percent. Discontinuation of RYR supplements following the treatment led to a rapid return of serum lipids to prestudy levels—despite adherence of the subjects to the American Heart Association Step 1 diet.

Safety

In both animal and human studies, red yeast rice appears to be quite safe as a dietary supplement. No serious side effects have been reported in human trials, although mild gastrointestinal symptoms are possible. It is important to note that some potentially serious adverse side effects have been noted for prescription statin medications such as lovastatin (muscle pain and damage with flulike symptoms). Although such side effects have not been noted in published studies on RYR, some supplement manufacturers err on the side of caution and post a warning label on their products to alert consumers to the possibility. Because of the likely mechanism of action of monacolins in the liver, you should not exceed the recommended amount (see Dosage), nor should RYR be taken by pregnant or lactating women or individuals with liver disease.

Value

As a natural approach to controlling moderately elevated cholesterol levels (between 200 to 240 mg/dl), red yeast rice supplements appear to be a safe and effective addition to a prudent diet and exercise regimen. For individuals with cholesterol levels well below 200 mg/dl, RYR supplements probably do not justify the cost ($1 to $1.50 per day), while individuals with cholesterol levels above 240 mg/dl should consult with their personal physician to discuss the appropriateness of prescription medications for lowering cholesterol levels.

Dosage

Doses of 1.2 to 2.4 g per day of red yeast rice (9.6 to 13.5 mg of total monacolins) have been used to effectively reduce elevated cholesterol and triglyceride levels in several clinical trials.

WORKS CONSULTED

Havel R. Dietary supplement or drug? The case of cholestin. Am J Clin Nutr. 1999;69:175-6.

Heber D. Dietary supplement or drug? The case for cholestin. Am J Clin Nutr. 1999;70:106-8.

Heber D. Reply to EG Bliznakov. Am J Clin Nutr. 2000;71:153-4.

Heber D, Yip I, Ashley JM, Elashoff DA, Elashoff RM, Go VL. Cholesterol-lowering effects of a proprietary Chinese red-yeast-rice dietary supplement. Am J Clin Nutr. 1999;69:231-6.

Li C, Zhu Y, Wang Y. Monascus purpureus-fermented rice (red yeast rice): A natural food product that lowers blood cholesterol in animal models of hypercholesterolemia. Nutr Res. 1998;18:71-81.

Qin S, Zhang W, Qi P. Elderly patients with primary hyperlipidemia benefited from treatment with a Monascus purpureus rice preparation: A placebo-control, double-blind clinical trial. 39th Annual Conference on Cardiovascular Disease Epidemiology and Prevention. Orlando, Florida. March 25, 1999.

Rippe J, Bonovich K, Colfer H. A multicenter, self-controlled study of cholestin in subjects with elevated cholesterol. 39th Annual Conference on Cardiovascular Disease Epidemiology and Prevention. Orlando, Florida. March 25, 1999.

Wang J, Lu Z, Chi J. Multicenter clinical trial of the serum lipid-lowering effects of a Monascus purpureus (red yeast) rice preparation from traditional Chinese medicine. Cur Ther Res. 1997;58:964-97.

SOY

What Is It?

"Soy" refers to many products derived from the soybean. In terms of health and wellness, the two most important dietary supplements derived from soybeans are isolated and concentrated soy proteins and soy extracts, which contain a large amount of compounds called isoflavones. The isoflavones have been associated with a wide variety of beneficial health effects ranging from protection from cancer and osteoporosis to a reduction in hot flashes and other symptoms of menopause. Soy protein, which may or may not contain a high level of isoflavones (depending on how it is processed) has been associated with a reduction in serum cholesterol and triglyceride levels and may protect against the development of coronary heart disease.

Claims

- Reduces cholesterol and triglyceride levels
- Reduces risk of heart disease
- Suppresses menopausal symptoms (hot flashes)
- Slows bone breakdown (osteoporosis)

Theory

Depending on the method of processing, many soy foods contain a relatively high content of chemical compounds called isoflavones, which possess weak estrogen-like effects and relatively powerful antioxidant properties. Under conditions of high estrogen exposure, which may promote certain cancers, the isoflavone compounds tend to block the adverse effects of estrogen and may prevent growth of cancer cells. Under conditions of low estrogen exposure, such as during menopause, the isoflavones tend to act as weak estrogens, which may be just enough to help alleviate some of the symptoms associated with menopause, such as hot flashes, headaches, and mood swings. In terms of heart disease risk, both isoflavones and concentrated soy proteins provide benefits via anti-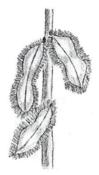

oxidant effects (from the isoflavones) and cholesterol lowering (from the protein).

Scientific Support

In general, soybeans, like most legumes, have a high protein content (35 to 40 percent for whole soybeans). After processing, protein powders composed of soy *concentrate* provide about 70 percent protein, while the even more purified protein source soy *isolate* may contain close to 90 percent protein. As a protein source, soy tends to be somewhat low in the sulfur-containing amino acids such as cysteine and methionine. This has led to the perception that soy protein is a less desirable source of dietary protein than foods with higher sulfur content, such as meat, milk, and eggs. When the digestibility of the protein is taken into account, however, isolated soy protein scores on par with egg white and milk proteins. Consumption of soy foods and soy proteins has been associated with beneficial health effects for heart disease, osteoporosis, cancer, and menopausal symptoms. It is still unclear, however, whether these effects are due to the displacement of animal protein with vegetable protein or the combination of soy protein with the phytonutrients known as isoflavones.

Isoflavones

Soy is the richest dietary source of isoflavones. Typical soy foods such as tofu might contain about 40 to 100 mg of isoflavones per ounce. Soy milk provides about 100 to 150 mg of isoflavones per 8 oz glass. The isoflavones function as phytoestrogens in the body, where they possess weak estrogen-like effects. The two primary isoflavones found in soy are daidzein and genistein, both of which have been associated with the health benefits mentioned previously. The chemical structure of isoflavones is similar enough to that of estrogen that they can bind to the estrogen receptor on cells, yet different enough that they have only very weak estrogen effects. Among the different soy-based protein powders on the market, the isoflavone content can vary significantly, from almost zero for products extracted using alcohol to certified levels of 2 to 5 mg per gram of protein. In many Asian countries where the incidence of heart disease, cancer, and menopausal symptoms is low, the daily isoflavone intake is estimated at 25 to 50 mg per day. In contrast, the average Western intake is less than 5 mg per day.

Heart Protection

Results from a number of studies show the cholesterol-lowering benefits of including soy protein in the diet. Drops in total cholesterol, LDL, and triglycerides, with no lowering of HDL (good) cholesterol levels, has been shown with soy protein intakes of 25 to 50 g per day, typically taken in two to four divided doses throughout the day. Such intakes have also been shown to reduce the susceptibility of the LDL particles to oxidation, which is thought to be a crucial step that promotes cholesterol buildup on artery walls.

Cancer Risk

Epidemiological studies have suggested that Asian diets may provide protection from several cancers, including those of the breast, prostate gland, and colon. As mentioned, the action of isoflavones as weak estrogens allows them to bind to estrogen receptors and block some of the detrimental effects of estrogen such as promotion of cancer cell growth. Tamoxifen, a prescription drug for treating breast cancer, is thought to act as an anti-estrogen by binding to the estrogen receptor and blocking the growth-promoting effects of estrogen in cancer cells. Women using tamoxifen have a lower incidence of breast cancer and a 30 to 40 percent reduction in breast cancer cell growth rate. The isoflavones in soy are chemically similar to tamoxifen and, therefore, may also reduce the risk of hormone-dependent cancers via the same estrogen-blocking mechanism.

Bone Health

Soy protein consumption has been shown to reduce bone breakdown and slow calcium loss in an animal model of osteoporosis, suggesting a possible beneficial role in preventing osteoporosis in humans. A diet high in soy protein has been shown to improve bone density after six months. In addition, soybeans have a relatively high calcium content, a large portion of which may be retained in soy protein powders. It is also interesting to note that soy protein seems to cause less loss of calcium from the body than other dietary sources of protein, which may promote calcium loss and bone breakdown at high levels. Ipriflavone, a synthetic isoflavone drug prescribed in Europe, is metabolized in the body into daidzein, and has potent effects on reducing bone resorption in postmenopausal women.

Safety

Dietary consumption of soy-based protein concentrate or soy isolate is not associated with any significant side effects, aside from the mild gastrointestinal issues (bloating, flatulence) associated with any high-protein diet.

High doses of concentrated isoflavone extracts are probably safe at levels up to about 200 mg per day (the estimated amount contained in the average Japanese diet). Since the long-term effects of isolated isoflavone supplements are unknown and the potential for proestrogenic effects may exist for megadose isoflavone consumption, it is prudent to keep total isoflavone intake close to the levels found in dietary amounts.

Value

As a high-quality protein source, soy-based protein powders provide an excellent amino acid profile along with the added benefits for heart health, cancer protection, bone maintenance, and, in postmenopausal women, relief from postmenopausal symptoms. For women who cannot or choose not to select hormone replacement therapy following menopause, isoflavone supplements may provide an effective alternative way to treat some of the symptoms associated with menopause, including hot flashes, night sweats, headaches, vaginal dryness, and mood swings.

Dosage

- As a protein supplement, as needed (typical protein recommendations are 1 to 2 g of protein per kilogram of body weight).
- For heart health, 25 to 50 g of soy protein isolate per day is effective in reducing cholesterol and triglyceride levels.
- For menopausal symptoms, 25 to 50 mg of isoflavones per day is effective in alleviating some symptoms (e.g., hot flashes). Do not exceed more than 200 mg per day.

WORKS CONSULTED

Adlercreutz H. Epidemiology of phytoestrogens. Baillieres Clin Endocrinol Metab. 1998 Dec;12(4):605-23.

Clarkson TB, Anthony MS. Phytoestrogens and coronary heart disease. Baillieres Clin Endocrinol Metab. 1998 Dec;12(4):589-604.

Dwyer J. Overview: Dietary approaches for reducing cardiovascular disease risks. J Nutr. 1995 Mar;125(3 Suppl):656S-65S.

Figtree GA, Griffiths H, Lu YQ, Webb CM, MacLeod K, Collins P. Plant-derived estrogens relax coronary arteries in vitro by a calcium antagonistic mechanism. J Am Coll Cardiol. 2000 Jun;35(7):1977-85.

Gooderham MH, Adlercreutz H, Ojala ST, Wahala K, Holub BJ. A soy protein isolate rich in genistein and daidzein and its effects on plasma isoflavones concentrations, platelet aggregation, blood lipids and fatty acid composition of plasma phospholipid in normal men. J Nutr. 1996 Aug;126(8):2000-6.

Jacques H, Laurin D, Moorjani S, Steinke FH, Gagne C, Brun D, Lupien PJ. Influence of diets containing cow's milk or soy protein beverage on plasma lipids in children with familial hypercholesterolemia. J Am Coll Nutr. 1992 Jun;11 (Suppl):69S-73S.

Knight DC, Eden JA. A review of the clinical effects of phytoestrogens. Obstet Gynecol. 1996 May;87(5 Pt 2):897-904.

Krauss RM, Chait A, Stone NJ. Soy protein and serum lipids. N Engl J Med. 1995 Dec 21;333(25):1715-6.

Merz-Demlow BE, Duncan AM, Wangen KE, Xu X, Carr TP, Phipps WR, Kurzer MS. Soy isoflavones improve plasma lipids in normocholesterolemic, premenopausal women. Am J Clin Nutr. 2000 Jun;71(6):1462-9.

Messina M. Diet-heart statement. Circulation. 1994 Nov;90(5):2564-5.

Messina M. Modern applications for an ancient bean: Soybeans and the prevention and treatment of chronic disease. J Nutr. 1995 Mar;125(3 Suppl):567S-9S.

Mitchell JH, Collins AR. Effects of a soy milk supplement on plasma cholesterol levels and oxidative DNA damage in men—a pilot study. Eur J Nutr. 1999 Jun;38(3):143-8.

Samsonov MA, Vasil'ev AV, Pogozheva AV, Pokrovskaia GR, Mal'tsev GI, Biiasheva IR, Orlova LA. The effect of a soy protein isolate and sources of polyunsaturated omega-3 fatty acids in an anti-atherosclerotic diet on the lipid spectrum of blood serum and immunological indicators in patients with ischemic heart disease and hypertension. Vopr Med Khim. 1992 Sep-Oct;38(5):47-50.

Tham DM, Gardner CD, Haskell WL. Clinical review 97: Potential health benefits of dietary phytoestrogens: A review of the clinical, epidemiological, and mechanistic evidence. J Clin Endocrinol Metab. 1998 Jul;83(7):2223-35.

Tikkanen MJ, Adlercreutz H. Dietary soy-derived isoflavone phytoestrogens. Could they have a role in coronary heart disease prevention? Biochem Pharmacol. 2000 Jul 1;60(1):1-5.

Wilson TA, Behr SR, Nicolosi RJ. Addition of guar gum and soy protein increases the efficacy of the American Heart Association (AHA) step I cholesterol-lowering diet without reducing high density lipoprotein cholesterol levels in non-human primates. J Nutr. 1998 Sep;128(9):1429-33.

Wong WW, Smith EO, Stuff JE, Hachey DL, Heird WC, Pownell HJ. Cholesterol-lowering effect of soy protein in normocholesterolemic and hypercholesterolemic men. Am J Clin Nutr. 1998 Dec;68(6 Suppl):1385S-9S.

Yetley EA, Park YK. Diet and heart disease: Health claims. J Nutr. 1995 Mar; 125(3 Suppl):679S-85S.

ESSENTIAL FATTY ACIDS
AND OMEGA-3 FATTY ACIDS

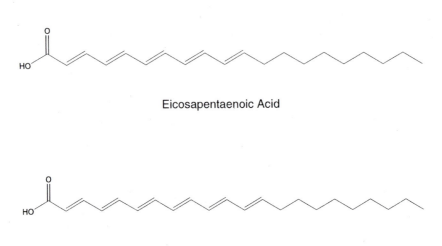

Eicosapentaenoic Acid

Docosahexaenoic Acid

What Is It?

"Essential fatty acids" refers to two fatty acids (linoleic acid and lino-lenic acid) that our bodies cannot synthesize and thus must be consumed in the diet (vitamins and minerals are also termed "essential" because we cannot make them and therefore must consume them). These essential fatty acids are needed for the production of compounds known as eicosanoids, which help regulate blood clotting, blood pressure, heart rate, immune response, and a wide variety of other biological processes.

Linoleic acid is a polyunsaturated fatty acid with eighteen carbon atoms and two double bonds. Linoleic acid is considered an omega-6 or n-6 fatty acid because the first of its double bonds occurs at the sixth carbon from the omega end. It is also referred to as C18:2n6 (meaning it has eighteen carbons, two double bonds, first double bond at n-6 position). It is found in vegetable and nut oils such as sunflower, safflower, corn, soy, and peanut oil. Most Americans get adequate levels of these omega-6 oils in their diets due to a high consumption of vegetable oil–based margarine, salad dressings, and mayonnaise.

Linolenic acid, or alpha-linolenic acid, is also an eighteen-carbon poly-unsaturated fatty acid, but it is classified as an omega-3 or n-3 fatty acid because its first double bond (of three) is at the third carbon from the omega end. It is also known as C18:3n3 (eighteen carbons, three double bonds, first double bond at the n-3 position). Good dietary sources are flaxseed oil (51 percent linolenic acid), canola oil (9 percent), and walnuts (7 percent) as well as margarine derived from canola oil. For example, a tablespoon of canola oil or canola oil margarine provides about 1 g of linolenic acid.

Claims

- Promotes brain development
- Treatment for attention-deficit hyperactivity disorder (ADHD)
- Supports cardiovascular health/reduces blood clotting
- Anti-inflammatory (rheumatoid arthritis, ulcerative colitis, Crohn's disease)
- Reduces blood pressure/dilates blood vessels

Theory

If you think back to the type of diet humans evolved to eat (the "caveman diet"), it provided a much more balanced mix of n-3 and n-6 fatty acids. Over the last century, modern diets have come to rely heavily on fats derived from vegetable oils (n-6), bringing the ratio of n-6 to n-3 fatty acids from the caveman's ratio of 1:1 to the modern-day range of 20-30:1—yikes! The unbalanced intake of high n-6 fatty acids and low n-3 fatty acids sets the stage for increases in blood viscosity (and the tendency of blood to clot), vasoconstriction (with elevated blood pressure), and inflammatory processes (involved in everything from heart health to pain levels).

Fatty acids of the n-3 variety, however, have opposing biological effects to the n-6 fatty acids—meaning that a higher intake of n-3 oils can deliver anti-inflammatory, antithrombotic, and vasodilatory effects that can lead to benefits in terms of heart disease, hypertension, diabetes, and a wide variety of inflammatory conditions such as rheumatoid arthritis and ulcerative colitis.

In the body, linoleic acid (n-6) is metabolized to arachidonic acid—a precursor to specific "bad" eicosanoids that can promote vasoconstriction and elevated blood pressure. Linolenic acid (n-3), however, is metabolized in the body to EPA (eicosapentaenoic acid) and DHA (docosahexaenoic acid). EPA serves as the precursor to prostaglandin E3, which may have vasodilatory properties on blood vessels—effects that can counteract the vasoconstriction caused by n-6 fatty acids. DHA has been associated with optimal brain development in infants.

Scientific Support

Recent studies have shown consumption of linolenic acid and other n-3 fatty acids to offer protection against heart disease and heart attacks. This effect is thought to be mediated through the synthesis of EPA and DHA. Fish oils contain large amounts of both EPA and DHA, and the majority of studies in this area have used various concentrations of fish oil supplements to demonstrate the health benefits of these essential fatty acids. For example, 1 g of menhaden oil (a common fish source) provides about 300 mg of these fatty acids. EPA is known to induce an antithrombotic (clot-preventing) effect through its inhibition of platelet cyclooxygenase (which converts arachidonic acid to thromboxane A2) and the "less sticky" platelets that result. Fish oil, and its high content of EPA and DHA, may also protect against heart disease through an anti-inflammatory effect (via reduced cytokine production and/or increased nitric oxide production in the endothelium).

Consumption of broiled or baked fish, two or more times per week, is associated with a 40 percent reduction in risk of rheumatoid arthritis. In one study, eight weeks of omega-3 supplementation (9 to 10 g per day) resulted in significant improvements in joint pain and stiffness among arthritis sufferers.

Flaxseed, a rich plant source of omega-3 fatty acids, has been shown to lower both systolic and diastolic blood pressure (1 to 2 tablespoons daily). Epidemiological studies have shown that subjects with high intakes of linolenic acid (n-3) have been shown to have a 50 percent reduced risk of heart disease, which may be partly due to beneficial effects on blood pressure, cholesterol levels, blood clotting, and heart rhythm. Indeed, omega-3 fatty acids are known to reduce thromboxane activity, which could explain the benefits of omega-3s in reducing platelet aggregation (blood clotting) and blood vessel constriction.

There is also some evidence that omega-3 fatty acids from fish oil and flaxseed may help improve insulin sensitivity, modulate lipid metabolism, and combat both mild depression and ADHD. Although the data are far from clear, it is known that omega-3 fatty acids are concentrated in the brain and that children and adults suffering from depression and/or ADHD typically show suboptimal blood levels of essential fatty acids. In addition, population studies suggest that high consumption of fish (rich in omega-3s) may be related to a lower risk of depression, including postpartum depression. Mothers pass large amounts of essential fatty acids to their babies during the last three months of fetal brain development and via breast milk—so much that new mothers have only half the normal blood levels of omega-3 fatty acids, and nursing mothers may have even lower levels.

A recent expert scientific advisory board at the National Institutes of Health highlighted the importance of a balanced intake of n-6 and n-3 fatty acids to reduce the adverse effects of elevated arachidonic acid (a metabolic product of n-6 metabolism). The committee recommended a reduction in the intake of n-6 fatty acids (linoleic acid) and an increase in n-3 (linolenic acid, DHA, EPA) intake. Adequate intake recommendations were established for the first time for the support of cardiovascular health in adults and brain development in infants (see Dosage).

A number of scientific studies suggest that diets high in omega-3 oils may protect against the development of diseases such as heart disease, attention deficit disorder, arthritis, colitis, and other inflammatory diseases. It has been convincingly shown that omega-3 fatty acids can reduce triglyceride levels in the blood. The effects of omega-3s on cholesterol levels, however, are inconsistent and may require excessive doses of fish oil to be effective. In rare instances, high-dose fish oil supplements may even increase serum cholesterol levels in genetically predisposed individuals.

A major heart-protective effect of omega-3 oil is its effect in reducing the "stickiness" of platelets in the blood—thus reducing the likelihood of formation of blood clots. Regular consumption of fish is clearly linked to a reduced incidence of heart attacks. In some studies, it even appears that the real importance isn't how much fish you eat, but that you eat it at all. In other words, eating fish once a week appears to be just as effective as eating it three or four times each week.

A recent study in the *Archives of General Psychiatry* suggests that 10 g of fish oil per day is effective in preventing the dramatic mood swings commonly observed in depressive states. Such results hold promise for treating other disorders such as ADHD.

Safety

No serious adverse side effects should be expected from regular consumption of essential fatty acid supplements or omega-3 oils—whether from fish oil or other common oil supplements (see Value). Due to the tendency of n-3 fatty acids to reduce platelet aggregation ("thin" the blood), increased bleeding times can occur in some individuals.

Value

The most common supplemental sources of essential fatty acids are fish oil, a good source of the omega-3 fatty acids. Other oils, such as flaxseed, borage seed, and evening primrose are rich sources of essential fatty acids but typically do not provide the high levels of concentrated EPA and DHA found in many fish oil supplements. The highest quality fish oil supplements should provide 18 to 30 percent EPA and 12 to 20 percent DHA. The higher the EPA and DHA content, the better (but also more expensive).

Dosage

The best dietary sources of omega-3 fatty acids are fish such as trout, tuna, salmon, mackerel, herring, and sardines, which all contain about 1 to 2 g of n-3 oils per 3 to 4 oz serving (for nonfish sources, see Table 10.2). A minimum of 4 to 5 g of linoleic acid (but no more than 6 to 7 g) and 2 to 3 g of linolenic acid are recommended per day. Supplements of linoleic acid (n-6) are typically not needed, whereas linolenic acid (n-3) supplements (4 to 10 g per day) and/or concentrated EPA/DHA supplements (400 to 1000 mg per day) are recommended to support cardiovascular health. Total DHA and EPA intake should approach about 1g per day—about evenly split between the two. Pregnant and lactating women are advised to increase their DHA intake somewhat so that they consume least 300 mg of DHA daily to ensure adequate brain development in their growing babies. When using flax as a concentrated source of essential fatty acids, a typical dose is 1 to 2 tablespoons per day.

TABLE 10.2. Vegetarian Sources of Essential Fatty Acids

Source	Alpha-linolenic (C18:3w3) Omega-3	Linoleic acid (C18:2w6) Omega-6	Gamma-linoleic (C18:3w6) Omega-6	Oleic acid (C18:1w9) Omega-9
Linseed (flax)	45	15	0	39
Hemp seed	20	60	3	13
Black currant	13	52	17	10
Borage	1	37	23	16
Olive	0	10	0	71
Evening primrose	0	68	9	8

WORKS CONSULTED

Adams PB, Lawson S, Sanigorski A, Sinclair AJ. Arachadonic acid to eicosapentaenoic acid ratio in blood correlates positively with clinical symptoms of depression. Lipids.1996;31(Suppl): S157-61.

Angerer P, von Schacky C. N-3 polyunsaturated fatty acids and the cardiovascular system. Curr Opin Lipidol. 2000 Feb;11(1):57-63.

Appel LJ, Miller ER 3rd, Seidler AJ, Whelton PK. Does supplementation of diet with fish oil reduce blood pressure? A meta-analysis of controlled clinical trials. Arch Intern Med. 1993;153:1429-38.

Cerrato PL. Omega-3 fatty acids: Nothing fishy here! RN. 1999 Aug;62(8):59-60.

Charnock JS. Omega-3 polyunsaturated fatty acids and ventricular fibrillation: The possible involvement of eicosanoids. Prostaglandins Leukot Essent Fatty Acids. 1999 Oct;61(4):243-7.

Christensen JH, Christensen MS, Dyerberg J, Schmidt EB. Heart rate variability and fatty acid content of blood cell membranes: A dose-response study with n-3 fatty acids. Am J Clin Nutr. 1999 Sep;70(3):331-7.

Connor WE. Importance of n-3 fatty acids in health and disease. Am J Clin Nutr. 2000 Jan;71(1 Suppl):171S-5S.

de Deckere EA, Korver O, Verschuren PM, Katan MB. Health aspects of fish and n-3 polyunsaturated fatty acids from plant and marine origin. Eur J Clin Nutr. 1998;52(10):749-53.

de Lorgeril M, Renaud S, Mamelle N, Salen P, Martin JL, Monjaud I, Guidollet J, Touboul P, Delaye J. Mediterranean alpha-linolenic acid-rich diet in secondary prevention of coronary heart disease. Lancet. 1994;343:1454-9.

Edwards R, Peet M, Shay J, Horrobin D. Omega-3 polyunsaturated fatty acids in the diet and in the red blood cell membranes of depressed patients. J Affect Disord. 1998;48:149-55.

Ferretti A, Flanagan VP. Antithromboxane activity of dietary alpha-linolenic acid: A pilot study. Prostaglandins Leukot Essent Fatty Acids. 1996;54:451-5.

Hamazaki T, Sawazaki S, Itomura M, Asaoka E, Nagao Y, Nishimura N, Yazawa K, Kuwamori T, Kobayashi M. The effect of docosahexaenoic acid on aggression in young adults. J Clin Invest. 1996;97(4):1129-34.

Holman RT, Johnson SB, Ogburn PL. Deficiency of essential fatty acids and membrane fluidity during pregnancy and lactation. Proc Natl Acad Sci. 1991;88:4835-9.

Horrocks LA, Yeo YK. Health benefits of docosahexaenoic acid. Pharmacol Res. 1999 Sep;40(3):211-25.

Hu FB, Stampfer MJ, Manson JE, Rimm EB, Wolk A, Colditz GA, Hennekens CH, Willett WC. Dietary intake of alpha-linolenic acid and risk of fatal ischemic heart disease among women. Am J Clin Nutr. 1999;69(5):890-7.

Kremer JM, Lawrence DA, Petrillo GF, Litts LL, Mullaly PM, Rynes RI, Stocker RP, Parhami N, Greenstein NS, Fuchs BR. Effects of high-dose fish oil on rheumatoid arthritis after stopping nonsteroidal anti-inflammatory drugs. Clinical and immune correlates. Arthritis Rheumatism. 1995 Aug;38(8):1107-14.

Leaf A, Kang JX, Xiao YF, Billman GE. Dietary n-3 fatty acids in the prevention of cardiac arrhythmias. Curr Opin Clin Nutr Metab Care. 1998 Mar;1(2):225-8.

Maes M, Smith R, Christophe A, Cosyns P, Desnyder R, Meltzer H. Fatty acid composition in major depression: Decreased omega-3 fractions in cholesteryl esters and increased C20:4 omega 6/C20:5 omega 3 ratio in cholesteryl esters and phospholipids. J Affect Disord. 1996;38:35-46.

Marckmann P, Gronbaek M. Fish consumption and coronary heart disease mortality. A systematic review of prospective cohort studies. Eur J Clin Nutr. 1999 Aug;53(8):585-90.

Meydani M. Omega-3 fatty acids alter soluble markers of endothelial function in coronary heart disease patients. Nutr Rev. 2000 Feb;58(2 Pt 1):56-9.

Miller M. Current perspectives on the management of hypertriglyceridemia. Am Heart J. 2000 Aug;140(2):232-40.

O'Keefe JH Jr, Harris WS. From Inuit to implementation: Omega-3 fatty acids come of age. Mayo Clin Proc. 2000 Jun;75(6):607-14.

Oomen CM, Feskens EJ, Rasanen L, Fidanza F, Nissinen AM, Menotti A, Kok FJ, Kromhout D. Fish consumption and coronary heart disease mortality in Finland, Italy, and The Netherlands. Am J Epidemiol. 2000 May 15;151(10):999-1006.

Roche HM, Gibney MJ. Effect of long-chain n-3 polyunsaturated fatty acids on fasting and postprandial triacylglycerol metabolism. Am J Clin Nutr. 2000 Jan;71(1 Suppl):232S-7S.

Schmidt EB, Dyerberg J. n-3 fatty acids and coronary heart disease—the urgent need of clinical trials. Lipids. 1999;34(Suppl):S303-5.

Shapiro JA, Koepsell TD, Voigt LF, Dugowson CE, Kestin M, Nelson JL. Diet and rheumatoid arthritis in women: A possible protective effect of fish consumption. Epidemiology. 1996 May;7(3):256-63.

Simopoulos AP. Essential fatty acids in health and chronic disease. Am J Clin Nutr. 1999 Sep;70(3 Suppl):560S-9S.

Simopoulos AP. Evolutionary aspects of omega-3 fatty acids in the food supply. Prostaglandins Leukot Essent Fatty Acids. 1999 May-Jun;60(5-6):421-9.

Singer P. Effects of dietary oleic, linoleic and alpha-linolenic acids on blood pressure, serum lipids, lipoproteins and the formation of eicosanoid precursors in patients with mild essential hypertension. J Human Hypertension. 1990;4:227-33.

Singleton CB, Walker BD, Campbell TJ. N-3 polyunsaturated fatty acids and cardiac mortality. Aust N Z J Med. 2000 Apr;30(2):246-51.

Siscovick DS, Raghunathan T, King I, Weinmann S, Bovbjerg VE, Kushi L, Cobb LA, Copass MK, Psaty BM, Lemaitre R, Retzlaff B, Knopp RH. Dietary intake of long-chain n-3 polyunsaturated fatty acids and the risk of primary cardiac arrest. Am J Clin Nutr. 2000 Jan;71(1 Suppl):208S-12S.

Stark KD, Park EJ, Maines VA, Holub BJ. Effect of a fish-oil concentrate on serum lipids in postmenopausal women receiving and not receiving hormone replacement therapy in a placebo-controlled, double-blind trial. Am J Clin Nutr. 2000 Aug;72(2):389-94.

Stevens LJ, Zentall SS, Abate ML, Kuczek T, Burgess JR. Omega-3 fatty acids in boys with behavior, learning, and health problems. Physiol Behav. 1996 Apr-May;59(4-5):915-20.

Torjesen PA, Birkeland KI, Anderssen SA, Hjermann I, Holme I, Urdal P. Lifestyle changes may reverse development of the insulin resistance syndrome. Diabetes Care. 1997;30:26-31.

Virkkunen ME, Horrobin DF, Jenkins DK, Manku MS. Plasma phospholipid essential fatty acids and prostaglandins in alcoholic, habitually violent, and impulsive offenders. Biol Psychiatry. 1987;22:1087-96.

von Schacky C. n-3 fatty acids and the prevention of coronary atherosclerosis. Am J Clin Nutr. 2000 Jan;71(1 Suppl):224S-7S.

GARLIC

What Is It?

It's not just for warding off vampires anymore—garlic (the stinking rose) has been used for centuries for its reported benefits in promoting heart health and preventing infection.

Claims

- Reduces serum cholesterol and triglycerides
- Inhibits platelet aggregation (thins blood)
- Lowers blood pressure

Theory

The cardioprotective benefits associated with garlic are generally attributed to the various sulfur compounds that can be isolated from the raw clove. These compounds, which include alliin, allicin, S-allylcysteine, S-methylcysteine, and many others are found in varying concentrations in garlic, chives, leeks, shallots, and onions, but the chemical composition may vary considerably depending on processing methods. The chemical responsible for the pungent smell of garlic, allicin, is produced from alliin via the action of alliinase and is thought to contribute to many of the health effects associated with garlic supplements.

Scientific Support

The health benefits of garlic supplements are controversial. Although quite a large number of studies seem to indicate a beneficial cardiovascular effect of garlic supplements, the most well-controlled studies generally suggest a lack of any beneficial effects. For example, in a study of children with elevated blood cholesterol and triglycerides, eight weeks of garlic supplementation (900 mg per day) produced no significant effect on total cholesterol, triglycerides, LDL, or HDL. It is possible that these children, who had severe cases of familial hyperlipidemia, did not respond to the garlic supplements be-

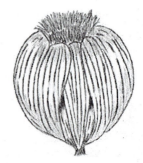

cause their medical condition was too advanced for treatment with a mild approach such as dietary supplementation. However, a multicenter study carried out over twelve weeks (also using 900 mg per day) also found no significant lipid or lipoprotein changes following garlic supplementation. The Food and Drug Administration has gone so far as to issue a ruling to prohibit the use of a claim for a relationship between garlic, decreased serum cholesterol, and the risk of cardiovascular disease in adults.

The lack of effect in these studies may have been due to the dose used— 900 mg per day. Larger doses of garlic (4 to 10 g per day) have been more consistently associated with beneficial effects. For example, in a study of thirty patients with coronary artery disease, garlic supplements (four capsules per day, equivalent to 4 g of raw garlic) showed a significant reduction in serum cholesterol and triglyceride levels as well as an inhibition of platelet aggregation (reduced blood clotting). Further supporting the cardiovascular benefits in humans is a well-controlled study that compared the effect of aged garlic extract on blood lipids in a group of forty-one men with moderately elevated cholesterol levels. Each subject received about 7 g of garlic extract per day over the course of six months. The major findings were a reduction in total serum cholesterol of approximately 7 percent and a drop in LDL of 4 to 5 percent. In addition, there was a 5.5 percent decrease in systolic blood pressure and a modest reduction of diastolic blood pressure in response to aged garlic extract. The overall conclusion of the study was that "dietary supplementation with aged garlic extract has beneficial effects on the lipid profile and blood pressure of moderately hypercholesterolemic subjects" (Steiner et al., 1996).

Safety

Adverse side effects associated with garlic supplements are rare. Occasionally, mild gastrointestinal symptoms such as heartburn and nausea may occur with high intakes. In some cases, high doses of garlic may potentiate the antithrombotic (blood-thinning) effects of anti-inflammatory medications such as aspirin and dietary supplements such as vitamin E and fish oil.

Value

A major concern with all garlic supplements is the total level of sulfur-containing compounds or total allicin potential of commercial products. Raw garlic is more potent than cooked garlic, and fresh garlic is more potent than old garlic. Deodorized garlic supplements contain alliin, which is converted to active allicin (the smelly form) in the body. Because the precise mechanism by which garlic helps lower cholesterol is unknown, it is prudent to select a product with high allicin potential.

Dosage

The German Commission E monographs recommend a dose of 4 g of fresh garlic per day to lower blood lipids. This amount of garlic would be equivalent to approximately 18,000 mcg (18 mg) of alliin (9 mg of allicin) and 500 mcg of S-allylcysteine.

WORKS CONSULTED

Arora RC, Arora S. Comparative effect of clofibrate, garlic and onion on alimentary hyperlipemia. Atherosclerosis. 1981 Jul;39(4):447-52.

Arora RC, Arora S, Gupta RK. The long-term use of garlic in ischemic heart disease—an appraisal. Atherosclerosis. 1981 Oct;40(2):175-9.

Arora RC, Arora S, Nigam P. Rationale of garlic use in ischemic heart disease? Mater Med Pol. 1985 Jan-Mar;17(1):48-50.

Breithaupt-Grogler K, Belz GG. Epidemiology of the arterial stiffness. Pathol Biol (Paris). 1999 Jun;47(6):604-13.

Breithaupt-Grogler K, Ling M, Boudoulas H, Belz GG. Protective effect of chronic garlic intake on elastic properties of aorta in the elderly. Circulation. 1997 Oct 21;96(8):2649-55.

Buck C, Donner AP, Simpson H. Garlic oil and ischaemic heart disease. Int J Epidemiol. 1982 Sep;11(3):294-5.

Buck C, Simpson H, Willan A. Ischaemic heart-disease and garlic. Lancet. 1979 Jul 14;2(8133):104-5.

Chutani SK, Bordia A. The effect of fried versus raw garlic on fibrinolytic activity in man. Atherosclerosis. 1981 Feb-Mar;38(3-4):417-21.

Craig WJ. Phytochemicals: Guardians of our health. J Am Diet Assoc. 1997 Oct;97(10 Suppl 2):S199-204.

Fogarty M. Garlic's potential role in reducing heart disease. Br J Clin Pract. 1993 Mar-Apr;47(2):64-5.

Herbal insurance. Does an allium a day keep the doctor away? Harv Health Lett. 1998 Jun;23(8):7.

Holzgartner H, Schmidt U, Kuhn U. Comparison of the efficacy and tolerance of a garlic preparation vs. bezafibrate. Arzneimittelforschung. 1992 Dec;42(12):1473-7.

Jepson RG, Kleijnen J, Leng GC. Garlic for peripheral arterial occlusive disease. Cochrane Database Syst Rev. 2000;(2):CD000095.

Morcos NC. Modulation of lipid profile by fish oil and garlic combination. J Natl Med Assoc. 1997 Oct;89(10):673-8.

Mostafa MG, Mima T, Ohnishi ST, Mori K. S-allylcysteine ameliorates doxorubicin toxicity in the heart and liver in mice. Planta Med. 2000 Mar;66(2):148-51.

Munday R, Munday CM. Low doses of diallyl disulfide, a compound derived from garlic, increase tissue activities of quinone reductase and glutathione transferase in the gastrointestinal tract of the rat. Nutr Cancer. 1999;34(1):42-8.

Randerson K. Cardiology update. Garlic and the healthy heart. Nurs Stand. 1993 Apr 14-20;7(30):51.

Simons LA, Balasubramaniam S, von Konigsmark M, Parfitt A, Simons J, Peters W. On the effect of garlic on plasma lipids and lipoproteins in mild hyper-cholesterolaemia. Atherosclerosis. 1995 Mar;113(2):219-25.

Slepko GI, Lobareva LS, Mikhalenko LI, Shatniuk LN. Biologically active garlic compounds and perspectives of their use in the therapeutic and prophylactic diet. Vopr Pitan. 1994;(5):28-32.

Steiner M, Khan AH, Holbert D, Lin RI. A double-blind crossover study in moderately hypercholesterolemic men that compared the effect of aged garlic extract and placebo administration on blood lipids. Am J Clin Nutr. 1996 Dec;64(6): 866-70.

Vialettes B. Mediterranean nutrition: A model for the world? Arch Mal Coeur Vaiss. 1992 Sep;85(Spec No 2):135-8.

HAWTHORN

What Is It?

Hawthorn, or *Crataegus oxyacantha,* grows as a thorny shrub with white or pink flowers and berries that resemble miniature apples. This shrub is native to northern temperate climates in Asia, Europe, and eastern North America. As far back as the Renaissance, Europeans used this supplement for digestive ailments; beginning in the late 1800s, doctors in Europe began to use hawthorn to treat heart disease as well. More recently, hawthorn has been used mostly as a cardiotonic to strengthen the heart muscle and promote more forceful contractions.

Claims

- Prevents plaque buildup on arteries (atherosclerosis)
- Lowers blood pressure
- Improves oxygen use by the heart to aid in congestive heart failure

Theory

Hawthorn contains a group of chemicals known as flavonoids that are the main active group of components and are thought to work together to aid the heart in several ways. First, hawthorn extract can dilate vessels to the heart, thus improving blood flow to this vital organ. By dilating these vessels, hawthorn decreases vessel resistance and therefore lowers blood pressure. In addition, with improved oxygen utilization, the heart is more efficient and functions better in individuals suffering from ailments such as congestive heart failure. Finally, as an antioxidant, hawthorn is claimed to maintain healthy collagen matrices of arterial walls so that the vessels remain elastic.

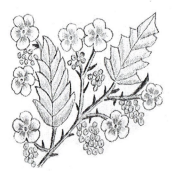

Scientific Support

Because heart disease is such a prevalent and lethal condition, compounds thought to aid those with coronary ailments generate a great deal of interest. In a controlled study using patients with heart disease caused by high blood pressure or decreased oxygen to the heart, those receiving hawthorn had significant, although subjective, improvements in problems associated with their condition. In a study of people with chronic chest pain, hawthorn was 85 percent effective compared to only 37 percent for those receiving placebo on measures of chest pain and cardiac performance.

Safety

Although no serious side effects have been documented following treatment with hawthorn, those with cardiovascular problems should not take hawthorn without first consulting a physician. Because heart ailments tend to occur in people beyond childbearing age, studies testing hawthorn's safety in pregnant or lactating women have not been conducted. It is therefore not recommended that such women take hawthorn unless a physician prescribes the supplement.

Value

Hawthorn typically costs approximately $10 for a thirty-day supply. The level of scientific support, coupled with the low cost, makes hawthorn a viable alternative for promoting general heart health.

Dosage

Hawthorn is sold in capsule, liquid, and tea form, although general recommendations are for 100 to 300 mg per day, taken in two to three divided doses.

WORKS CONSULTED

Leuchtgens H. Crataegus Special Extract WS 1442 in NYHA II heart failure. A placebo controlled randomized double-blind study. Fortschr Med. 1993 Jul 20;111(20-21):352-4.

Loew D. Phytogenic drugs in heart diseases exemplified by Crataegus. Wien Med Wochenschr. 1999;149(8-10):226-8.

Tauchert M, Gildor A, Lipinski J. High-dose Crataegus extract WS 1442 in the treatment of NYHA stage II heart failure. Herz. 1999 Oct;24(6):465-74.

Weikl A, Assmus KD, Neukum-Schmidt A, Schmitz J, Zapfe G, Noh HS, Siegrist J. Crataegus Special Extract WS 1442. Assessment of objective effectiveness in patients with heart failure. Fortschr Med. 1996 Aug 30;114(24):291-6.

COENZYME Q10 (CoQ10)/UBIQUINONE

What Is It?

Coenzyme Q10, or CoQ10, is found in the mitochondria of all cells. CoQ10 functions as part of the cellular system that generates energy from oxygen (in the form of ATP) for bodily processes. CoQ10 can also act as an antioxidant to help prevent cellular damage from free radicals created during exercise and during the generation of energy.

Claims

- Slows the aging process
- Increases energy
- Strengthens the heart
- Enhances endurance and aerobic performance
- Lowers blood pressure

Theory

Coenzyme Q10 is part of the respiratory chain as an electron/proton carrier. It functions in the production of ATP in the mitochondria of the cell. CoQ10 is synthesized in the cell—probably in the endoplasmic reticulum—and is found in highest concentration in cells of the heart, muscles, liver, kidney, and pancreas. CoQ10 has also been shown to exhibit activity as a free radical scavenger and antioxidant. The theory of CoQ10 supplementation posits that consumption of CoQ10 increases tissue and mitochondrial CoQ10 levels and supports ATP production as well as serving an antioxidant function.

Scientific Support

Since CoQ10 levels peak around age twenty and decline with age, it seems logical that supplemental CoQ10 might be beneficial in older adults. Animal studies, however, have not demonstrated any increase in life span following CoQ10 supplementation.

The antioxidant effects of CoQ10 are well established. A number of studies have shown that CoQ10 reduces the initiation and propagation of lipid peroxidation (free radical damage) in cell membranes and in lipoprotein fractions. Additionally, combined supplementation of CoQ10 plus vitamin

E produces a synergistic antioxidant effect on lipoproteins and "spares" the vitamin E.

In heart disease, CoQ10 has shown benefits in patients with heart failure—with 50 mg daily for four weeks resulting in improvements in dyspnea, heart rate, blood pressure, and ankle edema. Cardiac patients supplemented with CoQ10 prior to heart surgery tend to recover sooner and maintain blood and tissue levels of CoQ10 better than patients not receiving supplements. In addition, individuals taking cholesterol-lowering medications (HMG-CoA reductase inhibitors such as pravastatin) may benefit from CoQ10 supplements because these medications can reduce blood levels of CoQ10.

Data are most conflicting for CoQ10 as an ergogenic aid for athletic performance. Because of its role in ATP synthesis, it is logical that supplemental CoQ10 may support the process of cellular energy production. Research in this area has been inconclusive, however, with some studies showing a benefit and others showing no effect.

Safety

CoQ10 has a good safety profile, and daily doses of 50 to 100 mg are well tolerated. Reported side effects are rare, but tend to be various forms of epigastric distress (heartburn, nausea, stomachache), which can be prevented by consuming the supplement with a meal.

Value

For athletes, the data do not consistently support the use of supplemental CoQ10 as an ergogenic performance aid. As an antioxidant, especially in combination with other antioxidants such as vitamins C and E, CoQ10 appears to be beneficial. For heart patients, CoQ10 appears to be especially indicated, particularly in those patients who may be taking cholesterol-lowering medications (HMG-CoA reductase inhibitors such as pravastatin).

Dosage

Intakes of 100 to 200 mg per day have been studied with no apparent adverse side effects, but muscle damage has been noted in at least one study of 120 mg per day over twenty days (perhaps due to a pro-oxidant effect and free radical damage in the muscle).

WORKS CONSULTED

Giugliano D. Dietary antioxidants for cardiovascular prevention. Nutr Metab Cardiovasc Dis. 2000 Feb;10(1):38-44.

Greenberg S, Frishman WH. Co-enzyme Q10: A new drug for cardiovascular disease. J Clin Pharmacol. 1990 Jul;30(7):596-608.

Gvozdjakova A, Kucharska J, Mizera S, Braunova Z, Schreinerova Z, Schramekova E, Pechan I, Fabian J. Coenzyme Q10 depletion and mitochondrial energy disturbances in rejection development in patients after heart transplantation. Biofactors. 1999;9(2-4):301-6.

Harker-Murray AK, Tajik AJ, Ishikura F, Meyer D, Burnett JC, Redfield MM. The role of coenzyme Q10 in the pathophysiology and therapy of experimental congestive heart failure in the dog. J Card Fail. 2000 Sep;6(3):233-42.

Hofman-Bang C, Rehnqvist N, Swedberg K, Wiklund I, Astrom H. Coenzyme Q10 as an adjunctive in the treatment of chronic congestive heart failure. The Q10 Study Group. J Card Fail. 1995 Mar;1(2):101-7.

Khatta M, Alexander BS, Krichten CM, Fisher ML, Freudenberger R, Robinson SW, Gottlieb SS. The effect of coenzyme Q10 in patients with congestive heart failure. Ann Intern Med. 2000 Apr 18;132(8):636-40.

Kim Y, Sawada Y, Fujiwara G, Chiba H, Nishimura T. Therapeutic effect of coenzyme Q10 on idiopathic dilated cardiomyopathy: Assessment by iodine-123 labelled 15-(p-iodophenyl)-3(R,S)-methylpentadecanoic acid myocardial single-photon emission tomography. Eur J Nucl Med. 1997 Jun;24(6):629-34.

Kogan AK, Syrkin AL, Drinitsina SV, Kokanova IV. The antioxidant protection of the heart by coenzyme Q10 in stable stenocardia of effort. Patol Fiziol Eksp Ter. 1999 Oct-Dec;(4):16-9.

Kontush A, Reich A, Baum K, Spranger T, Finckh B, Kohlschutter A, Beisiegel U. Plasma ubiquinol-10 is decreased in patients with hyperlipidaemia. Atherosclerosis. 1997 Feb 28;129(1):119-26.

Kucharska J, Gvozdjakova A, Mizera S, Braunova Z, Schreinerova Z, Schramekova E, Pechan I, Fabian J. Participation of coenzyme Q10 in the rejection development of the transplanted heart: A clinical study. Physiol Res. 1998;47(6):399-404.

Kucharska J, Gvozdjakova A, Mizera S, Margitfalvi P, Schreinerova Z, Schramekova E, Solcanska K, Notova P, Pechan I, Fabian J. Coenzyme Q10 and alpha-tocopherol in patients after heart transplantation. Bratisl Lek Listy. 1996 Oct;97(10):603-6.

Langsjoen PH, Langsjoen AM. Overview of the use of CoQ10 in cardiovascular disease. Biofactors. 1999;9(2-4):273-84.

Langsjoen PH, Langsjoen A, Willis R, Folkers K. Treatment of hypertrophic cardiomyopathy with coenzyme Q10. Mol Aspects Med. 1997;18 (Suppl):S145-51.

Miyake Y, Shouzu A, Nishikawa M, Yonemoto T, Shimizu H, Omoto S, Hayakawa T, Inada M. Effect of treatment with 3-hydroxy-3-methylglutaryl coenzyme A reductase inhibitors on serum coenzyme Q10 in diabetic patients. Arzneimittelforschung. 1999 Apr;49(4):324-9.

Mortensen SA. Coenzyme Q10 as an adjunctive therapy in patients with congestive heart failure. J Am Coll Cardiol. 2000 Jul;36(1):304-5.

Munkholm H, Hansen HH, Rasmussen K. Coenzyme Q10 treatment in serious heart failure. Biofactors. 1999;9(2-4):285-9.

Naito T. Abnormal cardiac index measured by means of systolic time intervals and the effect of co-enzyme Q10 in thyroid disorders. Nippon Naibunpi Gakkai Zasshi. 1986 May 20;62(5):619-30.

Oda T. Recovery of the systolic time intervals by coenzyme Q10 in patients with a load-induced cardiac dysfunction. Mol Aspects Med. 1997;18 (Suppl):S153-8.

Overvad K, Diamant B, Holm L, Holmer G, Mortensen SA, Stender S. Coenzyme Q10 in health and disease. Eur J Clin Nutr. 1999 Oct;53(10):764-70.

Sacher HL, Sacher ML, Landau SW, Kersten R, Dooley F, Sacher A, Sacher M, Dietrick K, Ichkhan K. The clinical and hemodynamic effects of coenzyme Q10 in congestive cardiomyopathy. Am J Ther. 1997 Feb-Mar;4(2-3):66-72.

Sinatra ST. Coenzyme Q10: A vital therapeutic nutrient for the heart with special application in congestive heart failure. Conn Med. 1997 Nov;61(11):707-11.

Sinatra ST. Refractory congestive heart failure successfully managed with high dose coenzyme Q10 administration. Mol Aspects Med. 1997;18 (Suppl):S299-305.

Singh RB, Wander GS, Rastogi A, Shukla PK, Mittal A, Sharma JP, Mehrotra SK, Kapoor R, Chopra RK. Randomized, double-blind placebo-controlled trial of coenzyme Q10 in patients with acute myocardial infarction. Cardiovasc Drugs Ther. 1998 Sep;12(4):347-53.

Soja AM, Mortensen SA. Treatment of chronic cardiac insufficiency with coenzyme Q10, results of meta-analysis in controlled clinical trials. Ugeskr Laeger. 1997 Dec 1;159(49):7302-8.

Soja AM, Mortensen SA. Treatment of congestive heart failure with coenzyme Q10 illuminated by meta-analyses of clinical trials. Mol Aspects Med. 1997;18 (Suppl):S159-68.

Syrkin AL, Kogan AK, Drinitsina SV, Kuznetsov AB, Pechorina EA, Frenkel EE, Kuleshova NN, Golovnia LD. The use of the antioxidant coenzyme Q10 as a cytoprotection variant in ischemic heart disease. Klin Med (Mosk). 1998;76(7):24-8.

Taggart DP, Jenkins M, Hooper J, Hadjinikolas L, Kemp M, Hue D, Bennett G. Effects of short-term supplementation with coenzyme Q10 on myocardial protection during cardiac operations. Ann Thorac Surg. 1996 Mar;61(3):829-33.

Weston SB, Zhou S, Weatherby RP, Robson SJ. Does exogenous coenzyme Q10 affect aerobic capacity in endurance athletes? Int J Sport Nutr. 1997 Sep;7(3):197-206.

Willis R, Anthony M, Sun L, Honse Y, Qiao G. Clinical implications of the correlation between coenzyme Q10 and vitamin B6 status. Biofactors. 1999;9(2-4):359-63.

Yamamoto Y, Yamashita S. Plasma ratio of ubiquinol and ubiquinone as a marker of oxidative stress. Mol Aspects Med. 1997;18 (Suppl):S79-84.

Zhou M, Zhi Q, Tang Y, Yu D, Han J. Effects of coenzyme Q10 on myocardial protection during cardiac valve replacement and scavenging free radical activity in vitro. J Cardiovasc Surg (Torino). 1999 Jun;40(3):355-61.

VITAMIN B₆

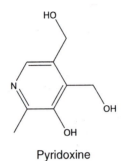

Pyridoxine

What Is It?

Vitamin B₆ (pyridoxine) is a water-soluble vitamin. It is also known by the names pyridoxine, pyridoxamine, and pyridoxal. Vitamin B₆ performs functions as a cofactor for about seventy different enzyme systems—most of which have something to do with amino acid and protein metabolism. Because vitamin B₆ is also involved in the synthesis of neurotransmitters in the brain and nerve cells, it is frequently recommended as a nutrient to support mental function (mood) and nerve conduction. Some athletic supplements include vitamin B₆ because of its role in the conversion of glycogen to glucose for energy in muscle tissue. Food sources include poultry, fish, whole grains, and bananas.

Claims

- Reduces blood levels of homocysteine
- Supports optimal nervous system function
- May improve emotional outlook/mood (serotonin synthesis)
- Needed for hemoglobin synthesis and red blood cell growth
- Immune support (white blood cell development)
- Relieves pain and inflammation of arthritis and carpal tunnel syndrome

Theory

Vitamin B₆, like most of the B vitamins, is involved as a cofactor in a wide variety of enzyme systems. As such, structure/function claims can be made for virtually any health condition. For example, because B_6 is needed in the conversion of the amino acid tryptophan into niacin, a common B_6 claim relates to "healthy cholesterol levels" (because niacin can help lower cholesterol in some people). Because B_6 also plays a role in prostaglandin synthesis, claims are often made for B_6 in regulating blood pressure, heart function, and pain levels (each of which is partially regulated by prostaglandins). Vitamin B_6 needs are increased in individuals consuming a high-protein diet as well as in women taking oral contraceptives (birth control pills).

Scientific Support

Vitamin B_6 supplements (in conjunction with folic acid) have been shown to have a significant effect in reducing plasma levels of homocysteine (an amino acid metabolite linked to increased risk of atherosclerosis). When combined with magnesium (300 mg per day as magnesium oxide), vitamin B_6 (10 mg per day) appears to reduce oxalate excretion and decrease the occurrence of kidney stones.

Vitamin B_6 is often recommended as a treatment for carpal tunnel syndrome (CTS). In the vast majority of cases, CTS is caused by repetitive hand or wrist motions (such as typing), which causes inflammation and nerve compression in a region of the wrist known as the carpal tunnel. CTS is also known to occur in some women during pregnancy, in which case the nerve compression may be related to water retention and swelling rather than to repetitive motion. B_6 is the most frequently recommended dietary supplement in cases of CTS (traditional treatments often include rest, splints, anti-inflammatory medications, and surgery). In some cases of CTS, approximately 100 to 300 mg of vitamin B_6 in divided doses has been shown to alleviate symptoms—although these results are not consistent, and several studies have found no benefit of vitamin B_6 in treating CTS.

Safety

As a water-soluble B vitamin, B_6 is generally very safe as a dietary supplement. Excessive intakes (2 to 6 g acutely or 500 mg chronically) are associated with sensory neuropathy (loss of feeling in the extremities)—which may or may not be reversible. The RDA for vitamin B_6 is only 2 mg per day, an amount contained in virtually all multivitamin supplements. Pregnant and lactating women should not take more than 100 mg of vitamin B_6 per day.

Value

Vitamin B_6 is rarely needed as an isolated supplement. Since B_6 deficiency rarely occurs by itself, it makes sense to get your B_6 as part of a more complete B complex or multivitamin supplement.

Dosage

The daily value for vitamin B_6 is 2 mg.

WORKS CONSULTED

Aybak M, Sermet A, Ayyildiz MO, Karakilcik AZ. Effect of oral pyridoxine hydrochloride supplementation on arterial blood pressure in patients with essential hypertension. Arzneimittelforschung. 1995 Dec;45(12):1271-3.

B vitamins and heart disease. Harv Health Lett. 1998 Oct;23(12):8.

B vitamins may cut heart disease risk. Harv Health Lett. 1998 Apr;23(6):8.

Baldewicz T, Goodkin K, Feaster DJ, Blaney NT, Kumar M, Kumar A, Shor-Posner G, Baum M. Plasma pyridoxine deficiency is related to increased psychological distress in recently bereaved homosexual men. Psychosom Med. 1998 May-Jun;60(3):297-308.

Bender DA. Non-nutritional uses of vitamin B6. Br J Nutr. 1999 Jan;81(1):7-20.

Bendich A. The potential for dietary supplements to reduce premenstrual syndrome (PMS) symptoms. J Am Coll Nutr. 2000 Feb;19(1):3-12.

Bigazzi M, Ferraro S, Ronga R, Scarselli G, Bruni V, Olivotti AL. Effect of vitamin B6 on the serum concentration of pituitary hormones in normal humans and under pathologic conditions. J Endocrinol Invest. 1979 Apr-Jun;2(2):117-24.

Blackburn G. Getting enough folate and B6? Health News. 1998 Mar 10;4(3):3, 5.

Bonke D. Influence of vitamin B1, B6, and B12 on the control of fine motoric movements. Bibl Nutr Dieta. 1986;(38):104-9.

Bostom AG, Shemin D, Verhoef P, Nadeau MR, Jacques PF, Selhub J, Dworkin L, Rosenberg IH. Elevated fasting total plasma homocysteine levels and cardiovascular disease outcomes in maintenance dialysis patients. A prospective study. Arterioscler Thromb Vasc Biol. 1997 Nov;17(11):2554-8.

Collier J. Vitamin B-6: Food or medicine? The rules—and the politics—are different. Br Med J. 1998 Jul 11;317(7151):92-3.

Donner MG, Schwandt P, Richter WO. Homocysteine and coronary heart disease. Is slight or moderate homocysteinemia related to increased risk of coronary heart disease? Fortschr Med. 1997 Jul 20;115(20-21):24-30.

Ellis JM, McCully KS. Prevention of myocardial infarction by vitamin B6. Res Commun Mol Pathol Pharmacol. 1995 Aug;89(2):208-20.

Fanapour PC, Yug B, Kochar MS. Hyperhomocysteinemia: An additional cardio-vascular risk factor. WMJ. 1999 Dec;98(8):51-4.

Fillmore CM, Bartoli L, Bach R, Park Y. Nutrition and dietary supplements. Phys Med Rehabil Clin N Am. 1999 Aug;10(3):673-703.

Folsom AR, Nieto FJ, McGovern PG, Tsai MY, Malinow MR, Eckfeldt JH, Hess DL, Davis CE. Prospective study of coronary heart disease incidence in relation to fasting total homocysteine, related genetic polymorphisms, and B vitamins: The Atherosclerosis Risk in Communities (ARIC) study. Circulation. 1998 Jul 21;98(3):204-10.

Guilarte TR. Vitamin B6 and cognitive development: Recent research findings from human and animal studies. Nutr Rev. 1993 Jul;51(7):193-8.

Gupta A, Moustapha A, Jacobsen DW, Goormastic M, Tuzcu EM, Hobbs R, Young J, James K, McCarthy P, van Lente F, Green R, Robinson K. High homo-cysteine, low folate, and low vitamin B6 concentrations: Prevalent risk factors for vascular disease in heart transplant recipients. Transplantation. 1998 Feb 27;65(4):544-50.

Heap LC, Peters TJ, Wessely S. Vitamin B status in patients with chronic fatigue syndrome. J R Soc Med. 1999 Apr;92(4):183-5.

Kirksey A, Wasynczuk AZ. Morphological, biochemical, and functional conse-quences of vitamin B6 deficits during central nervous system development. Ann N Y Acad Sci. 1993 Mar 15;678:62-80.

Kodentsova VM, Vrzhesinskaia OA, Kharitonchik LA, Spirichev VB. B group vi-tamin metabolism in duodenal ulcer disease, hypertension, and ischemic heart disease. Vopr Med Khim. 1994 Mar-Apr;40(2):41-5.

Lalouschek W, Aull S, Deecke L, Schnider P, Uhl F, Zeiler K. Hyperhomo-cyst(e)inemia—an independent risk factor of stroke. Fortschr Neurol Psychiatr. 1996 Jul;64(7):271-7.

Leowattana W, Mahanonda N, Bhuripunyo K, Pokum S. Association between se-rum homocysteine, vitamin B12, folate and Thai coronary artery disease pa-tients. J Med Assoc Thai. 2000 May;83(5):536-42.

Littell JT. Relationship of dietary folate and vitamin B6 with coronary heart disease in women. JAMA. 1998 Aug 5;280(5):418-9.

Liu S, Stampfer MJ, Hu FB, Giovannucci E, Rimm E, Manson JE, Hennekens CH, Willett WC. Whole-grain consumption and risk of coronary heart disease: Re-sults from the Nurses' Health Study. Am J Clin Nutr. 1999 Sep;70(3):412-9.

Mikati MA, Trevathan E, Krishnamoorthy KS, Lombroso CT. Pyridoxine-depend-ent epilepsy: EEG investigations and long-term follow-up. Electroencephalogr Clin Neurophysiol. 1991 Mar;78(3):215-21.

Molimard R, Marillaud A, Paille A, Le Devehat C, Lemoine A, Dougny M. Impair-ment of memorization by high doses of pyridoxine in man. Biomedicine. 1980 May;32(2):88-92.

Newman PE. Can reduced folic acid and vitamin B12 levels cause deficient DNA methylation producing mutations which initiate atherosclerosis? Med Hypothe-ses. 1999 Nov;53(5):421-4.

Omenn GS, Beresford SA, Motulsky AG. Preventing coronary heart disease: B vi-tamins and homocysteine. Circulation. 1998 Feb 10;97(5):421-4.

Ramakrishna T. Vitamins and brain development. Physiol Res. 1999;48(3):175-87.

Rimm EB, Willett WC, Hu FB, Sampson L, Colditz GA, Manson JE, Hennekens C, Stampfer MJ. Folate and vitamin B6 from diet and supplements in relation to risk of coronary heart disease among women. JAMA. 1998 Feb 4;279(5):359-64.

Saw SM. Homocysteine and atherosclerotic disease: The epidemiologic evidence. Ann Acad Med Singapore. 1999 Jul;28(4):565-8.

Selhub J, Jacques PF, Bostom AG, D'Agostino RB, Wilson PW, Belanger AJ, O'Leary DH, Wolf PA, Rush D, Schaefer EJ, Rosenberg IH. Relationship between plasma homocysteine, vitamin status and extracranial carotid-artery stenosis in the Framingham Study population. J Nutr. 1996 Apr;126(4 Suppl): 1258S-65S.

Selhub J, Jacques PF, Bostom AG, D'Agostino RB, Wilson PW, Belanger AJ, O'Leary DH, Wolf PA, Schaefer EJ, Rosenberg IH. Association between plasma homocysteine concentrations and extracranial carotid-artery stenosis. N Engl J Med. 1995 Feb 2;332(5):286-91.

Selhub J, Jacques PF, Wilson PW, Rush D, Rosenberg IH. Vitamin status and intake as primary determinants of homocysteinemia in an elderly population. JAMA. 1993 Dec 8;270(22):2693-8.

Simon J, Racek J, Rosolova H. Homocysteine, a less well-known risk factor in cardiac and vascular diseases. Cas Lek Cesk. 1996 May 2;135(9):263-5.

Sunder-Plassmann G, Floth A, Fodinger M. Hyperhomocysteinemia in organ transplantation. Curr Opin Urol. 2000 Mar;10(2):87-94.

Turner SL, Bechtel GA. Homocysteine and the heart. Adv Nurse Pract. 1999 Mar;7(3):71-3.

Ubbink JB. Vitamin nutrition status and homocysteine: An atherogenic risk factor. Nutr Rev. 1994 Nov;52(11):383-7.

Vermaak WJ, Barnard HC, Potgieter GM, Theron HD. Vitamin B6 and coronary artery disease. Epidemiological observations and case studies. Atherosclerosis. 1987 Feb;63(2-3):235-8.

Warren CJ. What is homocysteine? Am J Nurs. 1999 Oct;99(10):39-41.

Willis R, Anthony M, Sun L, Honse Y, Qiao G. Clinical implications of the correlation between coenzyme Q10 and vitamin B6 status. Biofactors. 1999;9(2-4): 359-63.

VITAMIN B_{12}

What Is It?

Vitamin B_{12} (cobalamin) is a water-soluble B vitamin. B_{12} is also known as cobalamin because it contains cobalt. The form of B_{12} most commonly used in dietary supplements is called cyanocobalamin. B_{12} is only produced by bacteria, so it is only found in food products of animal origin and in some fermented vegetable products such as tempeh and miso (fermented soybeans). B_{12} functions in a wide variety of metabolic processes, many of which are involved in transferring methyl groups between amino acids. B_{12} works closely with another B vitamin, folic acid, in reactions involved with DNA synthesis, blood cell formation, nervous system maintenance, and heart health. If that weren't enough, B_{12} is also involved in the metabolism of proteins, fats, and carbohydrates, as it is needed to produce succinyl CoA, an intermediary in the Krebs cycle, which generates ATP for cellular energy.

Claims

- Reduces blood levels of homocysteine
- Improves memory/promotes concentration
- Increases energy
- Reduces heart disease risk

Theory

Vitamin B_{12} absorption begins in the stomach, where it must combine with intrinsic factor, a compound synthesized by the stomach and required for proper absorption of B_{12} in the small intestine. Inadequate production of intrinsic factor and hydrochloric acid (stomach acid) in the elderly is a common cause of vitamin B_{12} deficiency. Because B_{12} is stored in the liver, the symptoms of deficiency develop very slowly, typically not showing up for five to ten years. Strict vegetarians (vegans), who consume only plant foods, are at the highest risk for developing B_{12} deficiency and should consider supplements.

Scientific Support

Mental Parameters

Vitamin B_{12} levels decrease with age and various measures of cognitive impairment are associated with reduced B_{12} status. In one study of subjects suffering from senile dementia, 78 percent of the subjects had metabolic cobalamin deficiency. Among those subjects supplemented with vitamin B_{12}, significant improvements in IQ, motor function, and mental state were noted.

Heart Disease Risk

Elevated plasma homocysteine concentrations are considered to be a risk factor for vascular disease and birth defects such as neural tube defects. Recent studies have shown that plasma homocysteine can be lowered by folic acid (400 to 800 mcg) combined with vitamin B_{12} (6 mcg). The combination of B_{12} with folic acid is significantly more effective in reducing homocysteine levels than is folic acid alone.

Safety

There are no confirmed reports of toxic side effects associated with vitamin B_{12} supplements—even at the very high injected doses commonly used to restore cognitive function in elderly subjects suffering from B_{12} deficiency. Oral intakes as high as 3,000 mcg are considered nontoxic.

Value

For individuals at highest risk for vitamin B_{12} deficiency, strict vegetarians and elderly persons with reduced B_{12} absorption, supplements are highly recommended. Most complete multivitamin supplements contain vitamin B_{12} at RDA or higher levels. Higher intakes from specific B_{12} or B-complex products may be warranted for high-risk individuals.

Dosage

The daily value for vitamin B_{12} is 6 mcg.

WORKS CONSULTED

Adachi S, Kawamoto T, Otsuka M, Todoroki T, Fukao K. Enteral vitamin B12 supplements reverse postgastrectomy B12 deficiency. Ann Surg. 2000 Aug; 232(2):199-201.

Baik HW, Russell RM. Vitamin B12 deficiency in the elderly. Annu Rev Nutr. 1999;19:357-77.

Booth GL, Wang EE. Preventive health care, 2000 update: Screening and management of hyperhomocysteinemia for the prevention of coronary artery disease events. The Canadian Task Force on Preventive Health Care. CMAJ. 2000 Jul 11;163(1):21-9.

Carmel R, Green R, Jacobsen DW, Rasmussen K, Florea M, Azen C. Serum cobalamin, homocysteine, and methylmalonic acid concentrations in a multiethnic elderly population: Ethnic and sex differences in cobalamin and metabolite abnormalities. Am J Clin Nutr. 1999 Nov;70(5):904-10.

Chandna SM, Tattersall JE, Nevett G, Tew CJ, O'Sullivan J, Greenwood RN, Farrington K. Low serum vitamin B12 levels in chronic high-flux haemodialysis patients. Nephron. 1997;75(3):259-63.

Cheliout-Heraut F, Durand MC, Desterbecq E, Dizien O, de Lattre J. Visual, auditory and somatosensory potentials in the diagnosis of vitamin B12 deficiency. Neurophysiol Clin. 1997;27(1):59-65.

Favier M, Hininger I. Vitamins: B1, B6, B12. Consequences of a deficiency, of excessive vitamins and value of systematic supplementation. J Gynecol Obstet Biol Reprod (Paris). 1997;26 (Suppl 3):100-8.

Fenech M, Aitken C, Rinaldi J. Folate, vitamin B12, homocysteine status and DNA damage in young Australian adults. Carcinogenesis. 1998 Jul;19(7):1163-71.

Gomes-Trolin C, Gottfries CG, Regland B, Oreland L. Influence of vitamin B12 on brain methionine adenosyltransferase activity in senile dementia of the Alzheimer's type. J Neural Transm Gen Sect. 1996;103(7):861-72.

Grange DK, Finlay JL. Nutritional vitamin B12 deficiency in a breastfed infant following maternal gastric bypass. Pediatr Hematol Oncol. 1994 May-Jun; 11(3):311-8.

Guyonnet S, Nourhashemi F, Ousset PJ, de Glisezinski I, Riviere D, Albarede JL, Vellas B. Alzheimer's disease and nutrition. Rev Neurol (Paris). 1999 May;155(5):343-9.

Hassing L, Wahlin A, Winblad B, Backman L. Further evidence on the effects of vitamin B12 and folate levels on episodic memory functioning: A population-based study of healthy very old adults. Biol Psychiatry. 1999 Jun 1;45(11):1472-80.

Hokin BD, Butler T. Cyanocobalamin (vitamin B-12) status in Seventh-day Adventist ministers in Australia. Am J Clin Nutr. 1999 Sep;70(3 Suppl):576S-8S.

Houston DK, Johnson MA, Nozza RJ, Gunter EW, Shea KJ, Cutler GM, Edmonds JT. Age-related hearing loss, vitamin B-12, and folate in elderly women. Am J Clin Nutr. 1999 Mar;69(3):564-71.

Howard JM, Azen C, Jacobsen DW, Green R, Carmel R. Dietary intake of cobalamin in elderly people who have abnormal serum cobalamin, methylmalonic acid and homocysteine levels. Eur J Clin Nutr. 1998 Aug;52(8):582-7.

La Rue A, Koehler KM, Wayne SJ, Chiulli SJ, Haaland KY, Garry PJ. Nutritional status and cognitive functioning in a normally aging sample: A 6-y reassessment. Am J Clin Nutr. 1997 Jan;65(1):20-9.

Lobo A, Naso A, Arheart K, Kruger WD, Abou-Ghazala T, Alsous F, Nahlawi M, Gupta A, Moustapha A, van Lente F, Jacobsen DW, Robinson K. Reduction of homocysteine levels in coronary artery disease by low-dose folic acid combined with vitamins B6 and B12. Am J Cardiol. 1999 Mar 15;83(6):821-5.

Loew D, Wanitschke R, Schroedter A. Studies on vitamin B12 status in the elderly—prophylactic and therapeutic consequences. Int J Vitam Nutr Res. 1999 May;69(3):228-33.

Lovblad K, Ramelli G, Remonda L, Nirkko AC, Ozdoba C, Schroth G. Retardation of myelination due to dietary vitamin B12 deficiency: Cranial MRI findings. Pediatr Radiol. 1997 Feb;27(2):155-8.

Mano Y. Aging of brain and the maintenance of the function. Hokkaido Igaku Zasshi. 1996 May;71(3):321-4.

Nilsson-Ehle H. Age-related changes in cobalamin (vitamin B12) handling. Implications for therapy. Drugs Aging. 1998 Apr;12(4):277-92.

Novy MA. Are strict vegetarians at risk of vitamin B12 deficiency? Cleve Clin J Med. 2000 Feb;67(2):87-8.

Quinn K, Basu TK. Folate and vitamin B12 status of the elderly. Eur J Clin Nutr. 1996 Jun;50(6):340-2.

Ramakrishna T. Vitamins and brain development. Physiol Res. 1999;48(3):175-87.

Riedel WJ, Jorissen BL. Nutrients, age and cognitive function. Curr Opin Clin Nutr Metab Care. 1998 Nov;1(6):579-85.

Robinson M, White FJ, Cleary MA, Wraith E, Lam WK, Walter JH. Increased risk of vitamin B12 deficiency in patients with phenylketonuria on an unrestricted or relaxed diet. J Pediatr. 2000 Apr;136(4):545-7.

Romero-Blanco M, Sanchez-Caballero F, Jimenez-Hernandez MD. Epilepsy and coma as the presentation of vitamin B12 deficiency. Rev Neurol. 1999 Sep 1-15;29(5):492.

Stojsavljevic N, Levic Z, Drulovic J, Dragutinovic G. A 44-month clinical-brain MRI follow-up in a patient with B12 deficiency. Neurology. 1997 Sep;49(3):878-81.

Sudo K, Tashiro K. Cerebral white matter lesions associated with vitamin B12 deficiency. Neurology. 1998 Jul;51(1):325-6.

Swain R. An update of vitamin B12 metabolism and deficiency states. J Fam Pract. 1995 Dec;41(6):595-600.

Tan SV, Guiloff RJ. Hypothesis on the pathogenesis of vacuolar myelopathy, dementia, and peripheral neuropathy in AIDS. J Neurol Neurosurg Psychiatry. 1998 Jul;65(1):23-8.

Tucker KL, Rich S, Rosenberg I, Jacques P, Dallal G, Wilson PW, Selhub J. Plasma vitamin B-12 concentrations relate to intake source in the Framingham Offspring study. Am J Clin Nutr. 2000 Feb;71(2):514-22.

van Asselt DZ, de Groot LC, van Staveren WA, Blom HJ, Wevers RA, Biemond I, Hoefnagels WH. Role of cobalamin intake and atrophic gastritis in mild cobalamin deficiency in older Dutch subjects. Am J Clin Nutr. 1998 Aug;68(2):328-34.

Wahlin A, Hill RD, Winblad B, Backman L. Effects of serum vitamin B12 and folate status on episodic memory performance in very old age: A population-based study. Psychol Aging. 1996 Sep;11(3):487-96.

Weir DG, Scott JM. Brain function in the elderly: Role of vitamin B12 and folate. Br Med Bull. 1999;55(3):669-82.

Wynn M, Wynn A. The danger of B12 deficiency in the elderly. Nutr Health. 1998;12(4):215-26.

Zeitlin A, Frishman WH, Chang CJ. The association of vitamin B 12 and folate blood levels with mortality and cardiovascular morbidity incidence in the old old: The Bronx aging study. Am J Ther. 1997 Jul-Aug;4(7-8):275-81.

FOLIC ACID

What Is It?

Folic acid is a B vitamin that plays an important role in DNA and RNA synthesis, production of red blood cells, and maintenance of the nervous system. Fruits and veggies are the best dietary source (for folic think—"foliage"), with dark leafy greens, oranges and orange juice, beans and peas leading the way. Brewer's yeast is also a good source of folic acid and other B vitamins.

Claims

- Prevents neural tube birth defects
- Promotes heart health (reduced plasma homocysteine levels)

Theory

Because folic acid has functions in DNA synthesis and nervous system maintenance, it has been linked to growth and development of the fetus during pregnancy. Clinical evidence clearly shows that adequate folic acid intake reduces the risk of brain and spinal cord birth defects. Due to its role in red blood cell formation and homocysteine metabolism and the fact that folic acid deficiency results in megaloblastic anemia, supplemental levels are often associated with maintenance of energy levels and heart health.

Scientific Support

It is abundantly clear that an adequate intake of folic acid is essential during pregnancy. Overwhelming evidence shows that women given folic acid supplements during pregnancy are less likely to deliver babies with neural tube birth defects such as spina bifida. Oral contraceptives ("the pill") have been associated with lower folate levels in women who conceive soon after they stop taking the pill. In some cases, former contraceptive users and women who have delivered babies with neural tube defects may especially benefit from supplemental levels of folate in their diets.

The U.S. Department of Health recommends that pregnant women (and those trying to conceive) should take a daily folic acid supplement of 400 mcg (0.4 mg). The U.S. Public Health Service recommends that all women of childbearing age consume the same amount of folic acid each day to decrease the risk of having a pregnancy affected by a neural tube defect (just in case). Three strategies are available to women to achieve this goal: eat more foods with naturally occurring folate (fruits and veggies); eat foods fortified with folic acid; or use dietary supplements.

Despite the wide-ranging benefits of adequate folic acid intake and the widespread public awareness of these benefits, as many as 68 to 87 percent of American women of childbearing age still have folic acid intakes below the recommended 400 mcg per day. Elderly populations are also thought to be at increased risk for folate deficiencies, which may exacerbate their already high risk of heart disease, cancer, and neurological impairments. Several recent studies have suggested that folate supplementation should be considered in elderly people, especially those with elevated plasma total homocysteine levels and cardiovascular disease, as well as in individuals who experience neuropsychiatric disorders. Because of the possibility that high-dose folate supplements will mask the symptoms of vitamin B_{12} (cyanocobalamin) deficiencies (which are also common in the elderly), folic acid supplements should be given in conjunction with B_{12}.

Safety

Extremely high intakes (1 to 5 mg per day) have been associated with masking the signs and symptoms of pernicious anemia (vitamin B_{12} deficiency) and should be avoided.

Value

Because folic acid is destroyed during cooking, levels are typically highest in raw or lightly steamed vegetables. The chemical form of folic acid found in foods, monoglutamic acid (conjugated), however, is less well absorbed than the synthetic form, polyglutamic acid (unconjugated), which is found in dietary supplements. This suggests that supplemental forms of folic acid may even be warranted in high-risk individuals in addition to a well-balanced intake of fruits and vegetables.

Dosage

The daily value for folic acid is 400 mcg—an amount that *all* women of childbearing age should consume each day. Like the other B vitamins, dietary needs may be somewhat elevated during times of stress and during pregnancy and lactation. In the elderly, a daily folate supplement of 500 mcg may be warranted, although it should not replace a diet rich in fruit and vegetables.

WORKS CONSULTED

Bailey LB. New standard for dietary folate intake in pregnant women. Am J Clin Nutr. 2000 May;71(5 Suppl):1304S-7S.

Boddie AM, Dedlow ER, Nackashi JA, Opalko FJ, Kauwell GP, Gregory JF 3rd, Bailey LB. Folate absorption in women with a history of neural tube defect-affected pregnancy. Am J Clin Nutr. 2000 Jul;72(1):154-8.

Brouwer IA, van Dusseldorp M, Thomas CM, Duran M, Hautvast JG, Eskes TK, Steegers-Theunissen RP. Low-dose folic acid supplementation decreases plasma homocysteine concentrations: A randomized trial. Am J Clin Nutr. 1999 Jan;69(1):99-104.

Bunout D, Garrido A, Suazo M, Kauffman R, Venegas P, de la Maza P, Petermann M, Hirsch S. Effects of supplementation with folic acid and antioxidant vitamins on homocysteine levels and LDL oxidation in coronary patients. Nutrition. 2000 Feb;16(2):107-10.

Carmody BJ, Arora S, Avena R, Cosby K, Sidawy AN. Folic acid inhibits homocysteine-induced proliferation of human arterial smooth muscle cells. J Vasc Surg. 1999 Dec;30(6):1121-8.

Cortes F, Hirsch S, de la Maza MP. The importance of folic acid in current medicine. Rev Med Chil. 2000 Feb;128(2):213-20.

Czeizel AE, Timar L, Sarkozi A. Dose-dependent effect of folic acid on the prevention of orofacial clefts. Pediatrics. 1999 Dec;104(6):e66.

de Walle HE, Cornel MC, de Smit DJ, de Jong-Van Den Berg LT. Preconceptional use of folic acid amongst women of advanced maternal age. Prenat Diagn. 1999 Oct;19(10):996-7.

Einarson A, Parshuram C, Koren G. Periconceptional use of folic acid to reduce the rates of neural tube defects: Is it working? Reprod Toxicol. 2000 Jul-Aug;14(4):291-2.

Elkin AC, Higham J. Folic acid supplements are more effective than increased dietary folate intake in elevating serum folate levels. BJOG. 2000 Feb;107(2):285-9.

Fiatarone Singh MA, Bernstein MA, Ryan AD, O'Neill EF, Clements KM, Evans WJ. The effect of oral nutritional supplements on habitual dietary quality and quantity in frail elders. J Nutr Health Aging. 2000;4(1):5-12.

Folic acid for the prevention of neural tube defects. American Academy of Pediatrics. Committee on Genetics. Pediatrics. 1999 Aug;104(2 Pt 1):325-7.

Ford ES, Ballew C. Dietary folate intake in US adults: Findings from the third National Health and Nutrition Examination Survey. Ethn Dis. 1998 Autumn;8(3):299-305.

Henry A, Crowther CA. Universal periconceptional folate supplementation: Chasing a dream? Med J Aust. 2000 Apr 17;172(8):407-8.

Kim YI. Folate and cancer prevention: A new medical application of folate beyond hyperhomocysteinemia and neural tube defects. Nutr Rev. 1999 Oct;57(10):314-21.

Ladipo OA. Nutrition in pregnancy: Mineral and vitamin supplements. Am J Clin Nutr. 2000 Jul;72(1 Suppl):280S-90S.

Lee EY, Kim JS, Lee HJ, Yoon DS, Han BG, Shim YH, Choi SO. Do dialysis patients need extra folate supplementation? Adv Perit Dial. 1999;15:247-50.

Lewis CJ, Crane NT, Wilson DB, Yetley EA. Estimated folate intakes: Data updated to reflect food fortification, increased bioavailability, and dietary supplement use. Am J Clin Nutr. 1999 Aug;70(2):198-207.

Lumley J, Watson L, Watson M, Bower C. Periconceptional supplementation with folate and/or multivitamins for preventing neural tube defects. Cochrane Database Syst Rev. 2000;(2):CD001056.

Mackey AD, Picciano MF. Maternal folate status during extended lactation and the effect of supplemental folic acid. Am J Clin Nutr. 1999 Feb;69(2):285-92.

Mahomed K. Folate supplementation in pregnancy. Cochrane Database Syst Rev. 2000;(2):CD000183.

Mahomed K. Iron and folate supplementation in pregnancy. Cochrane Database Syst Rev. 2000;(2):CD001135.

McNulty H, Cuskelly GJ, Ward M. Response of red blood cell folate to intervention: Implications for folate recommendations for the prevention of neural tube defects. Am J Clin Nutr. 2000 May;71(5 Suppl):1308S-11S.

Molloy AM, Mills JL, Kirke PN, Weir DG, Scott JM. Folate status and neural tube defects. Biofactors. 1999;10(2-3):291-4.

Rolschau J, Kristoffersen K, Ulrich M, Grinsted P, Schaumburg E, Foged N. The influence of folic acid supplement on the outcome of pregnancies in the county of Funen in Denmark. Eur J Obstet Gynecol Reprod Biol. 1999 Dec;87(2):105-10; discussion 103-4.

Rothenberg SP. Increasing the dietary intake of folate: Pros and cons. Semin Hematol. 1999 Jan;36(1):65-74.

Scholl TO, Johnson WG. Folic acid: Influence on the outcome of pregnancy. Am J Clin Nutr. 2000 May;71(5 Suppl):1295S-303S.

Suitor CW, Bailey LB. Food folate vs synthetic folic acid: A comparison. J Am Diet Assoc. 1999 Mar;99(3):285.

Werler MM, Hayes C, Louik C, Shapiro S, Mitchell AA. Multivitamin supplementation and risk of birth defects. Am J Epidemiol. 1999 Oct 1;150(7):675-82.

Werler MM, Louik C, Mitchell AA. Achieving a public health recommendation for preventing neural tube defects with folic acid. Am J Public Health. 1999 Nov; 89(11):1637-40.

Williams CN. Should folic acid supplementation be used to reduce the risk of cancer in ulcerative colitis? Can J Gastroenterol. 1999 Nov;13(9):715-6.

Zhang S, Hunter DJ, Hankinson SE, Giovannucci EL, Rosner BA, Colditz GA, Speizer FE, Willett WC. A prospective study of folate intake and the risk of breast cancer. JAMA. 1999 May 5;281(17):1632-7.

NIACIN

What Is It?

Niacin is a water-soluble B vitamin—and the common name for two very different compounds: nicotinic acid and niacinamide. Like all B vitamins, niacin plays a role in many aspects of energy metabolism and nervous system function. One of the most common uses for supplemental niacin is cholesterol regulation (used at very high doses—see Dosage). Rich dietary sources of niacin include many high-protein foods such as meat, chicken, tuna and other fatty fish, peanuts, pork, and milk.

Claims

- Lowers cholesterol and triglyceride levels (nicotinic acid)
- Prevents/treats diabetes (niacinamide)
- Improves circulation (inositol hexaniacinate)
- Relieves arthritis (niacinamide)

Theory

Because niacin is involved in the proper functioning of more than 200 metabolic enzymes, it plays a role in a wide range of bodily processes, including synthesis of hormones and blood cells and the release of energy from fats, carbohydrates, and proteins. As a nutrient (vitamin B_3) consumed at low doses (20 to 40 mg), there is virtually no difference between the chemical forms of niacin. In the mid-1950s, however, it was shown that high doses of niacin (as nicotinic acid) could lower cholesterol levels (although the exact mechanism of action is still not known). The other form of niacin (nicotinamide or niacinamide) does not provide a cholesterol-lowering effect, but there is some evidence that it may be helpful in preventing the development of childhood diabetes (Type I) in high-risk children. It should be cautioned that there is a strong possibility of liver inflammation with large doses of any form of niacin (see Safety).

Scientific Support

Niacin has been studied for its cardiovascular benefits in numerous clinical trials. The primary cardiovascular measures such as cholesterol and triglyceride levels, heart attacks, and strokes are all significantly reduced with niacin therapy (sometimes used alone and sometimes used along with other drug therapy). Overall, the use of niacin (nicotinic acid, but not niacinamide) to prevent or treat elevated blood lipids and reduce cardiovascular disease risk is well substantiated. In a large number of clinical trials, nicotinic acid has been shown to consistently lower total and LDL ("bad") cholesterol (by about 15 to 20 percent) and triglycerides (by 10 to 25 percent), while increasing levels of HDL ("good") cholesterol (by 15 to 25 percent). The down side is that the amount of niacin needed to lower cholesterol levels also tends to result in "niacin intolerance" in 15 to 40 percent of people who try it, as well as the unpleasant side effect of skin flushing (similar to hot flashes) and the serious risk of liver damage (see Safety).

Niacin supplements are available in regular and slow-release forms. The slow-release forms of nicotinic acid are intended for prolonged release of niacin during its six- to eight-hour transit time in the intestines, but they are also associated with greater toxicity, and safe doses are only about half of normal-release forms of niacin.

There have also been some reports that niacinamide (but not nicotinic acid) may be effective in controlling blood sugar and possibly preventing the development of diabetes in certain high-risk children. Although niacinamide is being used in trials to prevent or delay the development of insulin-dependent diabetes, the nicotinic acid form of niacin has been shown to cause insulin resistance and increased insulin secretion in normal subjects—so the jury is still out on the benefits of using high-dose niacin supplements to treat or control diabetes.

Safety

In the high doses used for controlling cholesterol levels (anything above 100 mg per day), nicotinic acid can cause skin flushing and itching as well as headaches and hypotension (lightheadedness and low blood pressure). The niacinamide form of niacin does not cause these side effects, but it is not effective in reducing cholesterol levels, so it is seldom taken in such high doses. The slow-release versions of niacin supplements for controlling blood lipids have the potential for causing liver damage (even at "lower" doses of 500 mg per day)—so blood tests to monitor for liver damage are recommended, and high-dose niacin supplementation should only be undertaken on the advice and guidance of a physician. The inositol hexaniacinate (niacinol) form of niacin may be less likely to cause liver damage than time-release forms. Anybody with liver disease, including those who consume more than two drinks of alcohol daily, should not take high-dose niacin except on specific medical advice.

Value

Because niacin is cheap, its effectiveness in reducing cholesterol levels may be an inexpensive way to reduce a known risk factor for cardiovascular disease. When monitored properly, niacin therapy can be almost as effective as the popular (and expensive) "statin" drugs for lowering cholesterol and triglyceride levels. It is important to note that, despite the fact that niacin is a B vitamin, high-dose niacin therapy should really be considered drug therapy and not nutritional therapy.

Dosage

Although the daily value for niacin is only 20 mg, and the body can convert tryptophan (an amino acid) into niacin, a cholesterol-lowering dose of niacin (as nicotinic acid, *not* niacinamide or nicotinamide) is typically in the range of 250 to 2,000 mg per day. Dosing is usually started at the low end (250 mg per day), increasing the dose by 250 mg each week or two until blood lipid levels start to normalize (or side effects develop). Side effects are usually minimized by increasing the dosage slowly to the common therapeutic range of 1,000 to 2,000 mg per day. Niacin should be divided into two to three separate doses of no more than 500 to 750 mg per dose. In some cases, the skin flushing and itching side effects can be reduced somewhat by combining niacin with aspirin (which also has a beneficial cardiovascular effect via reduced blood clotting). All niacin therapy (at doses exceeding 100 mg per day) should be supervised and monitored by a physician.

WORKS CONSULTED

Capuzzi DM, Guyton JR, Morgan JM, Goldberg AC, Kreisberg RA, Brusco OA, Brody J. Efficacy and safety of an extended-release niacin (Niaspan): A long-term study. Am J Cardiol. 1998 Dec 17;82(12A):74U-81U.

Cunningham JJ. Micronutrients as nutriceutical interventions in diabetes mellitus. J Am Coll Nutr. 1998 Feb;17(1):7-10.

Gardner SF, Marx MA, White LM, Granberry MC, Skelton DR, Fonseca VA. Combination of low-dose niacin and pravastatin improves the lipid profile in diabetic patients without compromising glycemic control. Ann Pharmacother. 1997 Jun;31(6):677-82.

Goldberg AC. Clinical trial experience with extended-release niacin (Niaspan): Dose-escalation study. Am J Cardiol. 1998 Dec 17;82(12A):35U-38U.

Greenbaum CJ, Kahn SE, Palmer JP. Nicotinamide's effects on glucose metabolism in subjects at risk for IDDM. Diabetes. 1996 Nov;45(11):1631-4.

Guyton JR, Blazing MA, Hagar J, Kashyap ML, Knopp RH, McKenney JM, Nash DT, Nash SD. Extended-release niacin vs gemfibrozil for the treatment of low levels of high-density lipoprotein cholesterol. Niaspan-Gemfibrozil Study Group. Arch Intern Med. 2000 Apr 24;160(8):1177-84.

Guyton JR, Capuzzi DM. Treatment of hyperlipidemia with combined niacin-statin regimens. Am J Cardiol. 1998 Dec 17;82(12A):82U-4U.

Guyton JR, Goldberg AC, Kreisberg RA, Sprecher DL, Superko HR, O'Connor CM. Effectiveness of once-nightly dosing of extended-release niacin alone and in combination for hypercholesterolemia. Am J Cardiol. 1998 Sep 15;82(6):737-43.

Hale PJ, Nattrass M. The short-term effect of nicotinic acid on intermediary metabolism in insulin-dependent diabetes mellitus. Ann Clin Biochem. 1991 Jan;28(Pt 1):39-43.

Jin FY, Kamanna VS, Kashyap ML. Niacin accelerates intracellular ApoB degradation by inhibiting triacylglycerol synthesis in human hepatoblastoma (HepG2) cells. Arterioscler Thromb Vasc Biol. 1999 Apr;19(4):1051-9.

Kashyap ML. Mechanistic studies of high-density lipoproteins. Am J Cardiol. 1998 Dec 17;82(12A):42U-8U.

Knopp RH. Clinical profiles of plain versus sustained-release niacin (Niaspan) and the physiologic rationale for nighttime dosing. Am J Cardiol. 1998 Dec 17; 82(12A):24U-8U.

Knopp RH, Alagona P, Davidson M, Goldberg AC, Kafonek SD, Kashyap M, Sprecher D, Superko HR, Jenkins S, Marcovina S. Equivalent efficacy of a time-release form of niacin (Niaspan) given once-a-night versus plain niacin in the management of hyperlipidemia. Metabolism. 1998 Sep;47(9):1097-104.

McCulloch DK, Kahn SE, Schwartz MW, Koerker DJ, Palmer JP. Effect of nicotinic acid-induced insulin resistance on pancreatic B cell function in normal and streptozocin-treated baboons. J Clin Invest. 1991 Apr;87(4):1395-401.

Morgan JM, Capuzzi DM, Guyton JR. A new extended-release niacin (Niaspan): Efficacy, tolerability, and safety in hypercholesterolemic patients. Am J Cardiol. 1998 Dec 17;82(12A):29U-34U.

O'Connor PJ, Rush WA, Trence DL. Relative effectiveness of niacin and lovastatin for treatment of dyslipidemias in a health maintenance organization. J Fam Pract. 1997 May;44(5):462-7.

Philipp CS, Cisar LA, Saidi P, Kostis JB. Effect of niacin supplementation on fibrinogen levels in patients with peripheral vascular disease. Am J Cardiol. 1998 Sep 1;82(5):697-9, A9.

Schuna AA. Safe use of niacin. Am J Health Syst Pharm. 1997 Dec 15;54(24):2803.

Sikand G, Kashyap ML, Yang I. Medical nutrition therapy lowers serum cholesterol and saves medication costs in men with hypercholesterolemia. J Am Diet Assoc. 1998 Aug;98(8):889-94.

Singh GR, Menon PS, Shah P, Virmani A. Early onset juvenile diabetes mellitus controlled with nicotinic acid therapy. Indian J Pediatr. 1994 Jul-Aug;61(4):441-2.

Thomas VL, Gropper SS. Effect of chromium nicotinic acid supplementation on selected cardiovascular disease risk factors. Biol Trace Elem Res. 1996 Dec; 55(3):297-305.

Virtanen SM, Aro A. Dietary factors in the aetiology of diabetes. Ann Med. 1994 Dec;26(6):469-78.

Ziajka PE, Wehmeier T. Peripheral neuropathy and lipid-lowering therapy. South Med J. 1998 Jul;91(7):667-8.

ARGININE

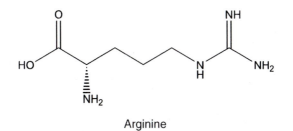

Arginine

What Is It?

Arginine is an amino acid that functions as a precursor to nitric oxide (NO), which is needed for optimal dilation of blood vessels and control of blood pressure and blood flow.

Claims

- Protection from heart disease
- Reduces cholesterol
- Lowers blood pressure
- Improves poor circulation

Theory

Arginine is a key component of the nitric oxide pathway, an important cascade of reactions involved in vasodilation and related to cardiovascular function. Arginine supplements have been associated with reduced symptoms associated with coronary artery disease and may be capable of slowing the progression of atherosclerosis. In the body, arginine serves as the substrate for the nitric oxide synthase enzyme, which catalyzes the oxidation of arginine to produce citrulline and NO. In the cells that line the blood vessels (endothelium cells), nitric oxide production causes vasodilatation (opening of the vessels). NO is involved in the overall regulation of systemic vascular resistance, where it inhibits the adherence of cells and foreign substances to the blood vessel walls and helps suppress the overgrowth of smooth muscle cells in the lining of the vessels. Because humans can synthesize arginine, it has been classified as a nonessential amino acid. Recent evidence suggests, however, that the synthesis rate of arginine in the body is insufficient for op-timal health—which would reclassify arginine as a semiessential or condi-tionally essential amino acid.

Scientific Support

In people with elevated cholesterol levels, it is common to see a reduced ability of the endothelium to produce NO and, therefore, to dilate effec-tively. In addition, because NO production may be limited, blood cells such as monocytes and platelets are more likely to attach themselves to the inner vessel wall and lead to blockages. Arginine supplements (8 to 21 g per day) have been shown to restore endothelial vasodilation in the coronary arteries of people (and rabbits) with high cholesterol and reduce the ability of blood cells to adhere to the vessel walls. Improvements in coronary artery blood flow and reductions in myocardial ischemia and walking pain due to clau-dication have been noted with arginine supplements (9 to 14 g per day).

Safety

Arginine supplements have been used safely in patients with heart dis-ease in doses up to more than 20 g per day.

Value

For individuals at risk for coronary artery disease, including those who experience ischemia due to reduced blood flow and oxygen delivery, arginine supplements may be an effective strategy for improving circulation to the heart and other affected areas (such as vessels in the calves).

Dosage

The daily arginine requirement has been calculated to be approximately 9 to 12 g per day (based on calculations for a 70 kg person). Since the aver-age American diet contains only about 3 to 5 g of arginine per day, there would appear to be a deficit between intake and requirements. Importantly, the primary dietary sources of arginine, like all amino acids, are meats and other high-protein foods (nuts, eggs).

WORKS CONSULTED

Alexander JW, Levy A, Custer D, Valente JF, Babcock G, Ogle CK, Schroeder TJ. Arginine, fish oil, and donor-specific transfusions independently improve cardiac allograft survival in rats given subtherapeutic doses of cyclosporin. J Parenter Enteral Nutr. 1998 May-Jun;22(3):152-5.

Brown SA, Langford K, Tarver S. Effects of certain vasoactive agents on the long-term pattern of blood pressure, heart rate, and motor activity in cats. Am J Vet Res. 1997 Jun;58(6):647-52.

Chaloupecky V, Hucin B, Tlaskal T, Kostelka M, Kucera V, Janousek J, Skovranek J, Sprongl L. Nitrogen balance, 3-methylhistidine excretion, and plasma amino acid profile in infants after cardiac operations for congenital heart defects: The effect of early nutritional support. J Thorac Cardiovasc Surg. 1997 Dec;114(6): 1053-60.

Chin-Dusting JP, Kaye DM, Lefkovits J, Wong J, Bergin P, Jennings GL. Dietary supplementation with L-arginine fails to restore endothelial function in forearm resistance arteries of patients with severe heart failure. J Am Coll Cardiol. 1996 Apr;27(5):1207-13.

Dadmarz M, van der Burg C, Milakofsky L, Hofford JM, Vogel WH. Effects of stress on amino acids and related compounds in various tissues of fasted rats. Life Sci. 1998;63(16):1485-91.

de Lorgeril M, Salen P, Monjaud I, Delaye J. The "diet heart" hypothesis in secondary prevention of coronary heart disease. Eur Heart J. 1997 Jan;18(1):13-8.

Fraser GE. Diet and coronary heart disease: Beyond dietary fats and low-density-lipoprotein cholesterol. Am J Clin Nutr. 1994 May;59(5 Suppl):1117S-23S.

Fraser GE. Nut consumption, lipids, and risk of a coronary event. Clin Cardiol. 1999 Jul;22(7 Suppl):III11-5.

Gnadinger MP, Weidmann P, Rascher W, Lang RE, Hellmuller B, Uehlinger DE. Plasma arginine-vasopressin levels during infusion of synthetic atrial natriuretic peptide on different sodium intakes in man. J Hypertens. 1986 Oct;4(5):623-9.

Hayakawa H, Raij L. Nitric oxide synthase activity and renal injury in genetic hypertension. Hypertension. 1998 Jan;31(1 Pt 2):266-70.

Hayashi T, Fukuto JM, Ignarro LJ, Chaudhuri G. Gender differences in atherosclerosis: Possible role of nitric oxide. J Cardiovasc Pharmacol. 1995 Nov;26(5):792-802.

He H, Kimura S, Fujisawa Y, Tomohiro A, Kiyomoto K, Aki Y, Abe Y. Dietary L-arginine supplementation normalizes regional blood flow in Dahl-Iwai salt-sensitive rats. Am J Hypertens. 1997 May;10(5 Pt 2):89S-93S.

Ikeda K, Nara Y, Tagami M, Yamori Y. Nitric oxide deficiency induces myocardial infarction in hypercholesterolaemic stroke-prone spontaneously hypertensive rats. Clin Exp Pharmacol Physiol. 1997 May;24(5):344-8.

Laurant P, Demolombe B, Berthelot A. Dietary L-arginine attenuates blood pressure in mineralocorticoid-salt hypertensive rats. Clin Exp Hypertens. 1995 Oct;17(7):1009-24.

Lou H, Kodama T, Wang YN, Katz N, Ramwell P, Foegh ML. L-arginine prevents heart transplant arteriosclerosis by modulating the vascular cell proliferative response to insulin-like growth factor-I and interleukin-6. J Heart Lung Transplant. 1996 Dec;15(12):1248-57.

Manning RD Jr, Hu L, Reckelhoff JF. Role of nitric oxide in the arterial pressure and renal adaptations to long-term changes in sodium intake. Am J Physiol. 1997 Apr;272(4 Pt 2):R1162-9.

Rajamohan T, Kurup PA. Lysine: Arginine ratio of a protein influences cholesterol metabolism. Part 1—Studies on sesame protein having low lysine:arginine ratio. Indian J Exp Biol. 1997 Nov;35(11):1218-23.

Siani A, Pagano E, Iacone R, Iacoviello L, Scopacasa F, Strazzullo P. Blood pressure and metabolic changes during dietary L-arginine supplementation in humans. Am J Hypertens. 2000 May;13(5 Pt 1):547-51.

Stechenko LO, Sahach VF, Tkachenko MM, Skybins'ka TR, Andriienko TV. The effect of L-arginine on the ultrastructure of atrial cardiomyocytes in experimental hypercholesterolemia. Fiziol Zh. 1999;45(1-2):72-9.

Wu G, Flynn NE, Flynn SP, Jolly CA, Davis PK. Dietary protein or arginine deficiency impairs constitutive and inducible nitric oxide synthesis by young rats. J Nutr. 1999 Jul;129(7):1347-54.

ALFALFA

What Is It?

Alfalfa *(Medicago sativa)* is a plant with a long history of use around the world as a livestock feed. Middle Eastern cultures have long used alfalfa as fodder for horses, claiming it increased speed and strength of the animals, which led to the name "Al-fal-fa," meaning "father of all foods." The fiber-rich alfalfa plant, like beans and peas, is a member of the legume family and can be found in modern dietary supplements as an ingredient intended to lower cholesterol, increase energy levels, and "detoxify." the blood.

Claims

- Reduces cholesterol and blood sugar levels
- Promotes general liver health and "detoxifies" the body
- Relieves pain and stiffness of arthritis and bursitis
- Alleviates menopausal side effects (hot flashes)
- Increases energy levels and reduces fatigue

Theory

Like other members of the legume family, alfalfa is a fairly good source of protein (up to 50 percent), B-complex vitamins, and several minerals (calcium, magnesium, phosphorus, iron, and potassium). Due to its generally high nutritive value, alfalfa could possibly help to prevent fatigue associated with vitamin or mineral deficiency or protein energy malnutrition in disadvantaged parts of the world. In addition, alfalfa also contains saponins, which, like those found in various ginseng roots, may have adaptogenic or stimulatory actions on the cardiovascular and nervous systems. Alfalfa is also promoted as a "detoxifier" for the liver and bloodstream, possibly due to its alkalizing nature. Finally, the isoflavone/phytoestrogen content of alfalfa may explain claims of anticancer activity and benefits in relieving menopausal symptoms.

Scientific Support

Scientific or clinical evidence in support of the claimed benefits of alfalfa is either scanty or totally lacking. Laboratory evidence (animal and test-tube studies) shows that saponins and other compounds in alfalfa are capable of binding to cholesterol and bile salts. In the GI tract, cholesterol and bile salt binding may prevent or slow dietary absorption of cholesterol and therefore help lower cholesterol levels in the blood. In one small study, fifteen patients with elevated cholesterol levels were given alfalfa (40 g, three times per day for eight weeks). Results showed an average 17 to 18 percent reduction in total and LDL cholesterol levels, with some patients exhibiting decreases in the range of 26 to 30 percent. The authors of the study concluded that alfalfa can be helpful in normalizing serum cholesterol concentrations—although the convenience of adding 120 g of alfalfa (almost 4 oz) to a supplement regimen is debatable.

Safety

At the typical dosages found in commercially available alfalfa supplements (less than a few grams per day), there are no reported or expected adverse side effects, aside from a potential mild blood-thinning effect associated with coumestrol and other phytonutrients. There are reports in the medical literature, however, which suggest that large doses of alfalfa seeds may induce or aggravate lupus or a related inflammatory connective tissue disease. Potential aggravating substances may include a particular amino acid (canavanine) found in alfalfa seeds. As such, it may be advisable for individuals with systemic lupus erythematosus to exercise caution when using alfalfa-based supplements (or avoid them altogether).

Value

Due to the lack of strong clinical evidence of benefits for alfalfa-based supplements, it appears to have little or no therapeutic value at this time other than possible cholesterol-lowering benefits at very high doses (and there are better choices such as red yeast rice, fiber, and soy).

Dosage

Typical dosage recommendations for alfalfa for lowering cholesterol levels range from 250 to 1,000 mg, taken two to three times daily with meals. Doses of several hundred grams per day may be needed to result in appreciable changes in serum cholesterol levels.

WORKS CONSULTED

Brown AC. Lupus erythematosus and nutrition: A review of the literature. J Ren Nutr. 2000 Oct;10(4):170-83.

Casanova M, You L, Gaido KW, Archibeque-Engle S, Janszen DB, Heck HA. Developmental effects of dietary phytoestrogens in Sprague-Dawley rats and interactions of genistein and daidzein with rat estrogen receptors alpha and beta in vitro. Toxicol Sci. 1999 Oct;51(2):236-44.

Cowgill UM. The distribution of selenium and mortality owing to acquired immune deficiency syndrome in the continental United States. Biol Trace Elem Res. 1997 Jan;56(1):43-61.

Elakovich SD, Hampton JM. Analysis of coumestrol, a phytoestrogen, in alfalfa tablets sold for human consumption. J Agric Food Chem. 1984 Jan-Feb;32(1):173-5.

Kurzer MS, Xu X. Dietary phytoestrogens. Annu Rev Nutr. 1997;17:353-81.

Malinow MR, Bardana EJ Jr, Pirofsky B, Craig S, McLaughlin P. Systemic lupus erythematosus-like syndrome in monkeys fed alfalfa sprouts: Role of a nonprotein amino acid. Science. 1982 Apr 23;216(4544):415-7.

Molgaard J, von Schenck H, Olsson AG. Alfalfa seeds lower low density lipoprotein cholesterol and apolipoprotein B concentrations in patients with type II hyperlipoproteinemia. Atherosclerosis. 1987 May;65(1-2):173-9.

Montanaro A, Bardana EJ Jr. Dietary amino acid-induced systemic lupus erythematosus. Rheum Dis Clin North Am. 1991 May;17(2):323-32.

Whittam J, Jensen C, Hudson T. Alfalfa, vitamin E, and autoimmune disorders. Am J Clin Nutr. 1995 Nov;62(5):1025-6.

Chapter 11

Supplements for Immune System Support

INTRODUCTION

The first thing to keep in mind about dietary supplements to support the immune system is that there is a huge difference between chronic supplementation (to support the immune system on a regular basis) and acute supplementation (to battle an existing infection). For example, the popular immunostimulant herb echinacea appears to be quite effective (when standardized for the right compounds) in stimulating immune system activity to battle a *new* infection—but it is not recommended for prolonged or continuous use due to concerns about cellular toxicity. Likewise, vitamin C and zinc would be appropriate at low doses for chronic protection, whereas higher levels are effective on a short-term basis for direct activity against invading pathogens.

Bolstering immunity is, of course, the primary key to preventing infection in the first place. When it comes to prevention, it is always a good idea to keep your immune system humming throughout the year (not just when cold and flu season comes rumbling into town). The following section provides a number of points to consider for supporting immune system function, including nutrition, exercise, rest, fluid intake, and exposure to pathogens.

SUPPORTING IMMUNE SYSTEM FUNCTION

Exposure to Pathogens

Viruses cause colds and flu, and bacteria can cause all sorts of unpleasant effects (gastrointestinal cramps, fever, diarrhea, etc.). Probably the most effective way to reduce your exposure to any pathogen is to wash your hands as frequently as possible. One of the primary ways that viruses and bacteria are transferred between people is through secondary contact—someone with the "bug" touches something, like a handrail or doorknob, and then you touch the same object and pick it up there. Frequent hand washing can reduce the chance that you'll transfer those pathogens from your hand to your eyes or nose—where they'll enter your body and begin the infection process.

Fluid Intake

Why is it that our mothers and grandmothers always made us drink more fluids when a cold came on? Mostly, it's because your body needs that extra fluid to "flush out" the infection via several routes including increased mucus production. In the more severe influenza infections, dehydration can result from fluid lost in vomit and diarrhea—so be sure to replace all losses plus some extra for good measure.

Exercise

Regular physical activity is a vital part of maintaining optimal immune function—those who exercise at a *moderate* level at least a couple of times each week are far less likely to get sick than sedentary individuals. On the other hand, be aware that *extreme* exercise—whether extremely intense or extremely long in duration (such as marathons or triathlons)—has been associated with reduced immune protection and an increased risk of infection (primarily upper respiratory tract infections in competitive athletes).

Nutrition

Any significant nutrient deficiency can impair functioning of the immune system. Thus, it is always a wise idea to include a complete multivitamin supplement as part of your total immune system support. Be sure to look for a multivitamin that supplies at least RDA levels for selenium and zinc. Many popular products contain some of them, so check the labels and add additional amounts as needed to reach the suggested intake. To round out your nutrient armory, consider adding key amino acids such as N-acetyl-cysteine (1 to 2 g per day) or glutamine (1 to 5 g per day)—both of which have been linked to elevated immune system responses. Finally, a number of immune-stimulating herbs and herbal blends are available—the most effective of which seem to be echinacea, goldenseal, and astragalus.

SUPPLEMENTS

Echinacea is the king of the immune function herbs (with over 300 scientific studies on its immune-enhancing effects). It is important to note that the primary use of echinacea is in the acute (short-term) treatment of the common cold—*not* for prolonged use (past a few weeks) as general immune system support. Also, echinacea is generally not recommended for use by individuals with autoimmune disorders (such as multiple sclerosis or rheumatoid arthritis) due to its immune-stimulating properties. The best use of echinacea is immediate consumption following acute exposure to an infected individual (meaning that as soon as Aunt Mary coughs on you, you should reach for the echinacea).

Goldenseal is a popular herb for immune system stimulation due to its high content of berberine. Because of the endangered status of goldenseal, however, many consumers (and supplement manufacturers) are turning to other berberine-containing herbs such as barberry and Oregon grape, which also appear to be quite effective alternatives for immune system support. Berberine has been shown to block the adherence of various infectious bacteria (such as streptococci) to the body's respiratory linings—but berberine-containing herbs are known to cause uterine contractions, so they should be avoided during pregnancy.

Astragalus has been used as an herbal tonic for centuries in traditional Chinese medicine (TCM) and in Native American folk medicine. Astragalus is used primarily for prevention throughout the cold and flu season—a different usage than the more popular echinacea, which is best used for early-stage treatment as soon as you feel a cold or flu coming on. Most of what we know about astragalus, however, comes from test-tube and animal experiments, which show that astragalus can help fight bacteria and viruses by enhancing various aspects of the body's normal immune response (the function of specific immune system cells such as T cells, lymphocytes, and neutrophils). In TCM, astragalus is often combined with other tonic herbs such as ginseng, cordyceps, or ashwagandha to keep the immune system humming during periods of high stress.

A number of *mushrooms* are used in TCM to support immune system strength. Among the more popular are shiitake, maitake, and reishi—all of which contain various polysaccharide and amino acid fractions that may help stimulate immune cell activity and get the immune system ready to do battle with invading pathogens. Although they are not completely understood, current theory suggests that the complex polysaccharides and small protein structures present in herbs such as astragalus and mushrooms act as immunomodulators because of similarities between these compounds and the cellular surfaces of pathogenic bacteria (although the herbs lack the infectivity that pathogens have).

Nettle leaf is an herbal treatment for the symptoms of hay fever and other mild allergic conditions. It may act as a gentle antihistamine to help alleviate the sneezing, nasal congestion, and itchy, watery eyes without many of the common side effects of synthetic antihistamines (nervousness, insomnia, drowsiness). Common dosage recommendations are in the range of 300 to 500 mg of nettle leaf, taken two to three times per day.

Probiotics, which are also called "beneficial bacteria," are quite effective for supporting immune function. The most popular variety used in dietary supplements, *Lactobacillus acidophilus* and *Bifidobacteria bifidum,* have been shown in hundreds of studies to boost immune function via their effects on increasing white blood cell numbers, activity, and effectiveness. Used in conjunction with prebiotics (indigestible carbohydrates that feed the growth of friendly bacteria in the intestines) such as fructooligosaccharides (FOS), probiotic organisms can displace certain pathogenic microbes in the intestines to prevent disease. Typical dosage recommendations are in the range of 2 to 4 billion organisms per day—but be careful to select a product that is fresh and has been transported and stored under proper conditions (refrigeration is best).

Vitamin C is the perennial immune booster and cold fighter. Despite the exaggerated tale that vitamin C *prevents* the common cold, it is clear that regular consumption of amounts of vitamin C above the RDA (500 mg to 2 g daily) can help reduce the duration and severity of colds. In fact, clinical studies now suggest that about 1 g of vitamin C consumed on a regular basis throughout the cold and flu season can reduce cold incidence by about 20 percent and cold duration by almost 40 percent. Vitamin C can also act as a natural antihistamine to help open up congested airways. In some people, however, high doses (500 mg or more) can produce mild diarrhea or gas, so you may need to experiment to find the most effective dose for you (reduce intake until symptoms disappear).

Often used in conjunction with vitamin C are a wide variety of *bioflavonoids,* such as quercetin, rutin, hesperidin, and a number of catechins and polyphenols found in green tea, grape seed, and pine bark extracts. All possess powerful antioxidant functions that can both strengthen immune system cells and protect healthy body tissues from damage, while some, such as quercetin, may also work as an antihistamine. Taken separately or in combination in mixed bioflavonoid complexes, these phytochemical compounds can be taken at dosages of several hundred milligrams per day to help prevent infections and alleviate mild symptoms of colds, flu, and allergies such as hay fever.

Vitamin A is an effective immune system nutrient because it helps keep bacteria and viruses from penetrating the protective mucous membranes (mouth, nose, stomach, lungs) and gaining a foothold in the body. Since vitamin A is fat-soluble, people on low-fat diets may be limiting their consumption of foods rich in vitamin A (liver and dairy) and should consider a supplement. For men and postmenopausal women, vitamin A is considered relatively safe up to 25,000 IU (7,500 mcg retinol equivalents [RE]) per day. In pregnant women, or in those who could become pregnant, less than

10,000 IU (3,000 mcg RE) per day is more prudent—as high-dose vitamin A is linked to birth defects and other damaging effects in the developing fetus. *All women considering becoming pregnant should discuss vitamin A supplementation with a personal physician.* A safer alternative may be to consider a mixed carotenoid supplement, because beta-carotene can be converted into vitamin A in the body—but only at levels that the body requires.

Selenium is a building block of the body's key antioxidant enzyme, glutathione peroxidase (GPx). GPx is also thought to play a key role in helping immune system cells protect us from invading viruses and bacteria. Selenium has shown positive results as an important immune system nutrient in studies of AIDS, chronic fatigue syndrome, and cancer (some forms of which may be caused by viruses). When combined with zinc, these two nutrients provide a boost to general immunity. Since few Americans get the recommended amounts of either selenium or zinc from their diets, a dietary supplement may be needed—especially during the cold and flu season. To achieve intake levels associated with enhanced immunity, consider a supplement providing selenium (200 mcg per day) and zinc (15 to 30 mg per day) together.

Zinc lozenges have become one of the most popular natural approaches to treating the common cold, and there is actually some good scientific evidence to support their use. Zinc lozenges appear to reduce cold symptoms such as sore throats, hoarseness, and coughing—and may even be able to shorten the duration of colds by a full day or so. Like vitamin C, zinc is an essential nutrient for optimal functioning of the immune system—and they both possess significant antiviral activity when consumed at elevated levels for a short period of time. It also appears, however, that some forms of zinc lozenges may be more effective than others (due to the total amount of ionized zinc that the lozenge actually releases into the mouth and throat). At least one study has shown that lozenges containing zinc gluconate plus citric acid, sorbitol, or mannitol may not deliver high enough levels of ionized zinc—whereas lozenges that contained glycine (an amino acid) appeared to deliver a greater quantity of ionized zinc. For a list of supplements and dosages, see Table 11.1.

TABLE 11.1. Dietary Supplements for General Immune System Support

Supplement	Dose (per day)
Astragalus	250-500 mg
Beta-glucans	10-200 mg
Cat's claw	20-60 mg
Colostrum	1-10 g
Echinacea	250-500 mg
Glutamine	1-10 g
Goldenseal	250-500 mg
Iron	3-18 mg
Mixed carotenoids	5-50 mg
Perilla seed oil	3-6 g
Selenium	100-200 mcg
Vitamin A	5,000-10,000 IU*
Vitamin C	250-1,000 mg
Vitamin E	200-800 IU
Zinc	15-45 mg

*Women who are pregnant or who may become pregnant should *not* exceed the RDA for preformed vitamin A unless directed to do so by their personal physician.

ECHINACEA

What Is It?

Echinacea is a flower native to North America, which has been used as a common herbal remedy by Native American tribes for treating and preventing colds, flu, and other infections. In Europe, echinacea preparations are primarily used to stimulate the immune system and help the body resist common cold infections affecting the throat and nasal passages. There are three different echinacea species *(purpurea, angustifolia,* and *pallida)*— each of which possess various concentrations of active compounds in different parts of each plant (roots, stems, leaves, flowers).

Claims

* Stimulates immune system function
* Reduces duration and intensity of upper respiratory tract infections (colds and flu)

Theory

Various polysaccharide compounds (long sugar molecules) found in echinacea extracts have been shown to stimulate the growth and activity of cells of the immune system (macrophages, natural killer cells, T-cells). Such activation of protective mechanisms is thought to increase the body's defenses against infection by bacteria and viruses. Of the compounds with potential immune-stimulating activity, various derivatives of caffeic acid such as echinoside, flavonoids, and polysaccharides have been implicated as the primary immunostimulatory constituents in the various echinacea species. Mechanistically, the polysaccharide fraction of echinacea is known to inhibit hyaluronidase, an enzyme secreted by bacteria. Bacteria produce hyaluronidase in order to break down host cell membranes and penetrate the cells. Inhibition of this enzyme by echinacea fractions may be one of the mechanisms by which echinacea supplements help prevent infection.

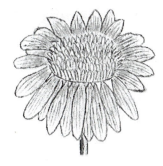

Scientific Support

. Owing to the widespread popularity of echinacea supplements for treating and preventing the symptoms associated with colds and flu, a number of clinical studies have been done, which show a clear benefit of echinacea extracts in reducing the duration and severity of flulike symptoms. Another handful of studies show no measurable benefits associated with echinacea supplements, but most of these studies can be criticized based on methodological or biochemical criteria such as using a nonstandardized herbal extract. It is important to note that many differences exist between various echinacea formulations, so the different commercially available echinacea preparations may have widely variable results.

In rats, echinacea treatment results in a significant increase in immune response to infection (assessed by immunoglobulin levels). In test-tube studies, macrophages are stimulated by echinacea to produce significantly higher levels of interleukins (IL-1, TNF-alpha, IL-6, and IL-10)—suggesting a possible activation of the immune system. Stimulation of T-cell replication, natural killer cell activity, and numbers of macrophages and neutrophils have been noted in a number of studies of cellular immunity.

Overall, across the hundreds of echinacea studies from the lab to the clinic, evidence from at least a dozen clinical trials shows that echinacea is effective in either treating or preventing upper respiratory tract infections (URTIs)—otherwise known as colds and flu (about a half-dozen clinical trials show no effect). Aside from the dozens of clinical trials in humans with colds, the majority of other echinacea studies (showing various active compounds in the herb) are analytical chemistry studies and test-tube studies of immune cell function. Among the clinical studies showing a beneficial effect of echinacea extracts in promoting immune function in human subjects, supplements have been shown to accelerate recovery from cold symptoms and reduce the incidence of cold-related infections. In most cases, cold and flu symptoms resolve one to four days earlier in subjects taking echinacea than in those taking a placebo.

Safety

When taken as directed, no toxicity or serious side effects are associated with acute echinacea use, although typical recommendations caution against long-term use.

Value

As a treatment for cold and flu symptoms, echinacea may be beneficial in reducing the severity and duration of symptoms. Echinacea preparations should not, however, be viewed as a cure for the common cold.

Dosage

Approximately 250 to 500 mg per day of a concentrated extract (5-6:1) is a typical dosage recommendation. Five to six parts of the raw herb is concentrated down to provide one part of the extract. Due to the significant differences between various echinacea preparations available on the market, however, it is important to select a standardized product. For example, 500 mg per day of one echinacea extract may be effective (based on the presence of active compounds), whereas 1,000 mg of another extract may be ineffective (if the level of active constituents is too low). Consumers are strongly urged to select a product standardized for the presence of active immune-stimulating compounds—either liquid products composed of the "fresh pressed juice" from echinacea or encapsulated extracts standardized for total content of alkamides and polysaccharides. For treatment of cold or flulike symptoms, it is generally recommended that echinacea supplements be taken as soon as symptoms are noticed and continued two to four times per day for one to two weeks.

WORKS CONSULTED

Abdullah T. A strategic call to utilize Echinacea-garlic in flu-cold seasons. J Natl Med Assoc. 2000 Jan;92(1):48-51.

Binns SE, Purgina B, Bergeron C, Smith ML, Ball L, Baum BR, Arnason JT. Light-mediated antifungal activity of Echinacea extracts. Planta Med. 2000 Apr;66(3): 241-4.

Borchers AT, Keen CL, Stern JS, Gershwin ME. Inflammation and Native American medicine: The role of botanicals. Am J Clin Nutr. 2000 Aug;72(2):339-47.

Currier NL, Miller SC. Natural killer cells from aging mice treated with extracts from echinacea purpurea are quantitatively and functionally rejuvenated. Exp Gerontol. 2000 Aug;35(5):627-39.

Ertel G, Manley H, McQueen C, Bryant P. Information on additional Echinacea trials. J Fam Pract. 1999 Dec;48(12):1001-2.

Giles JT, Palat CT 3rd, Chien SH, Chang ZG, Kennedy DT. Evaluation of echinacea for treatment of the common cold. Pharmacotherapy. 2000 Jun;20(6):690-7.

Gunning K. Echinacea in the treatment and prevention of upper respiratory tract infections. West J Med. 1999 Sep;171(3):198-200.

Henneicke-von Zepelin H, Hentschel C, Schnitker J, Kohnen R, Kohler G, Wustenberg P. Efficacy and safety of a fixed combination phytomedicine in the treatment of the common cold (acute viral respiratory tract infection): Results of a random-ised, double blind, placebo controlled, multicentre study. Curr Med Res Opin. 1999;15(3):214-27.

Hu C, Kitts DD. Studies on the antioxidant activity of Echinacea root extract. J Agric Food Chem. 2000 May;48(5):1466-72.

Kim HO, Durance TD, Scaman CH, Kitts DD. Retention of alkamides in dried echinacea purpurea. J Agric Food Chem. 2000 Sep;48(9):4187-92.

Kim HO, Durance TD, Scaman CH, Kitts DD. Retention of caffeic acid derivatives in dried echinacea purpurea. J Agric Food Chem. 2000 Sep;48(9):4182-6.

Lindenmuth GF, Lindenmuth EB. The efficacy of echinacea compound herbal tea preparation on the severity and duration of upper respiratory and flu symptoms: A randomized, double-blind placebo-controlled study. J Altern Complement Med. 2000 Aug;6(4):327-34.

Lord RW Jr. Echinacea for upper respiratory infections. J Fam Pract. 1999 Dec;48(12):939-40.

Mazza G, Cottrell T. Volatile components of roots, stems, leaves, and flowers of Echinacea species. J Agric Food Chem. 1999 Aug;47(8):3081-5.

Melchart D, Linde K, Fischer P, Kaesmayr J. Echinacea for preventing and treating the common cold. Cochrane Database Syst Rev. 2000;(2):CD000530.

Percival SS. Use of echinacea in medicine. Biochem Pharmacol. 2000 Jul 15;60(2):155-8.

Perry NB, van Klink JW, Burgess EJ, Parmenter GA. Alkamide levels in Echinacea purpurea: Effects of processing, drying and storage. Planta Med. 2000 Feb; 66(1):54-6.

Rininger JA, Kickner S, Chigurupati P, McLean A, Franck Z. Immunopharmaco-logical activity of Echinacea preparations following simulated digestion on murine macrophages and human peripheral blood mononuclear cells. J Leukoc Biol. 2000 Oct;68(4):503-10.

Turner RB, Riker DK, Gangemi JD. Ineffectiveness of echinacea for prevention of experimental rhinovirus colds. Antimicrob Agents Chemother. 2000 Jun;44(6): 1708-9.

Wustenberg P, Henneicke-von Zepelin HH, Kohler G, Stammwitz U. Efficacy and mode of action of an immunomodulator herbal preparation containing echinacea, wild indigo, and white cedar. Adv Ther. 1999 Jan-Feb;16(1):51-70.

GOLDENSEAL

What Is It?

Goldenseal *(Hydrastis canadensis)* is a common perennial plant that grows in the wild from Georgia to Canada. In the nineteenth century, the expansion of farming lands and the popularity of its medicinal properties among the early settlers and Native Americans caused goldenseal to become an endangered species. It is now cultivated, and its high price and demand may result in adulterated products. As a result of the endangered status of goldenseal, a handful of environmentally conscious supplement companies are substituting other berberine-containing herbs for goldenseal in their immune-support formulas. Other plants that contain relatively high concentrations of berberine (the alkaloid thought to contribute to the immune-stimulating effect of goldenseal) include goldenthread *(Coptis chinensis),* Oregon grape *(Berberis aquifolium),* barberry *(Berberis vulgaris),* and tree turmeric *(Berberis aristata).*

Claims

- Immune system support (immunostimulant/antimicrobial)
- Anticancer effects (colon cancer)
- Antioxidant
- Treats/prevents urinary tract infections

Theory

Goldenseal contains several alkaloids in its roots, stems, and leaves that are believed to be the active components: hydrastin (4 percent), berberine (6 percent), and canadine. Berberine possesses some antibacterial activity by either directly killing bacteria or preventing bacterial attachment to the cell walls of the host, as well as some antioxidant properties and smooth muscle relaxation effects.

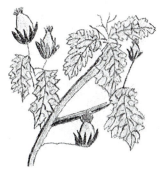

Scientific Support

No scientific studies evaluating the effect of goldenseal on humans have been reported at this point. Only animal, animal tissue, and in vitro testing have been done, and there is a long history of folk medicine use of goldenseal. A recent animal study tested the effectiveness of goldenseal as an immunostimulant. The study measured the formation of specific antibodies in rats injected with an antigen (a compound that stimulates an immune response). An extract of goldenseal root was consumed in the rats' drinking water for six weeks. Results of the study indicated that goldenseal caused a significant increase in antibodies (IgM) from day one to day fifteen compared to the control group, but that this benefit disappeared after day fifteen. A similar experiment was done using an echinacea extract, showing that the animals receiving echinacea had increased antibodies (IgG) from day one to day twenty-five, but this benefit also disappeared by day twenty-five.

Berberine, one of the alkaloids found in goldenseal, was found to decrease the activity of an enzyme involved in tumor growth (arylamine N-acetyltransferase) in a colon cancer cell culture. Whether goldenseal supplements would have any effect on colon cancer in humans remains to be tested.

Safety

Goldenseal is generally considered safe, but it should not be used during pregnancy or lactation and should be avoided by individuals with high blood pressure or other cardiovascular diseases.

Value

Goldenseal is often found in combination with echinacea and is claimed to help in the treatment of upper respiratory infections. No well-designed studies back this claim. The immunomodulation benefits of goldenseal root extract have been shown in a recent study on laboratory animals, but the results may not be applicable to a human population exposed to different antigens or microorganisms.

Dosage

Recommended doses of the powdered root range from 4 to 6 g per day, while dosage of the root extract ranges from 250 to 500 mg, taken three times per day. Products are typically standardized to berberine or total alkaloid levels (approximately 5 percent) and, as for echinacea, use should not exceed three weeks.

WORKS CONSULTED

Berberine. Altern Med Rev. 2000 Apr;5(2):175-7.

Blecher MB, Douglass K. Gold in goldenseal. Hosp Health Netw. 1997 Oct 20;71(20):50-2.

Budzinski JW, Foster BC, Vandenhoek S, Arnason JT. An in vitro evaluation of human cytochrome P450 3A4 inhibition by selected commercial herbal extracts and tinctures. Phytomedicine. 2000 Jul;7(4):273-82.

Iwasa K, Moriyasu M, Nader B. Fungicidal and herbicidal activities of berberine related alkaloids. Biosci Biotechnol Biochem. 2000 Sep;64(9):1998-2000.

Marinova EK, Nikolova DB, Popova DN, Gallacher GB, Ivanovska ND. Suppression of experimental autoimmune tubulointerstitial nephritis in BALB/c mice by berberine. Immunopharmacology. 2000 Jun;48(1):9-16.

Rehman J, Dillow JM, Carter SM, Chou J, Le B, Maisel AS. Increased production of antigen-specific immunoglobulins G and M following in vivo treatment with the medicinal plants Echinacea angustifolia and Hydrastis canadensis. Immunol Lett. 1999 Jun 1;68(2-3):391-5.

ASTRAGALUS

What Is It?

Astragalus is an herb from traditional Chinese medicine (TCM) that is traditionally used for its immune-enhancing properties but is also recommended for "deficiency of Qi" (life force)—which might include symptoms such as lack of energy and fatigue. The plant is native to Northern China and Mongolia, and there are over 2,000 types of astragalus worldwide.

Claims

- Stimulates immune system
- Provides cancer protection
- Acts as an adaptogen (nonspecific resistance to stress)
- Boosts energy levels

Theory

Several chemical constituents of astragalus have been identified as potential active compounds, including saponins, flavonoids, polysaccharides, and glycosides. Astragalus is often combined with other adaptogenic herbs, such as ginseng, and promoted as a guard against various internal and external stressors. Combination of astragalus with echinacea is common for protection against common infections of the mucous membranes (cold and flu).

Scientific Support

Most of the scientific data on astragalus comes from Chinese clinical evidence, in which astragalus appears to stimulate the immune system in patients with infections. At least one clinical trial in the United States has shown astragalus to boost T-cell levels close to normal in some cancer patients, suggesting the possibility of a synergistic effect of astragalus with chemotherapy. In animal studies, astragalus extracts have been effective in preventing infection of mice by an influenza virus, possibly by increasing the phagocytotic activity of the white blood cells of the immune system.

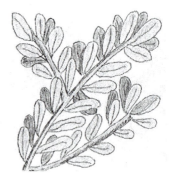

Safety

When used as recommended, astragalus has no known side effects, but gastrointestinal distress and diarrhea are possible at high intakes.

Value

Astragalus is available as a single-ingredient supplement, but it may be even more effective in lower doses (100 to 200 mg per day) when combined with other immune-stimulating herbs and nutrients.

Dosage

Approximately 500 mg per day is recommended for stimulation of the immune system and to provide resistance to the effects of stress. Divided doses of 250 mg per day of a standardized root extract are preferred.

WORKS CONSULTED

Chu DT, Lepe-Zuniga J, Wong WL, LaPushin R, Mavligit GM. Fractionated extract of Astragalus membranaceus, a Chinese medicinal herb, potentiates LAK cell cytotoxicity generated by a low dose of recombinant interleukin-2. J Clin Lab Immunol. 1988 Aug;26(4):183-7.

Chu DT, Sun Y, Lin JR. Immune restoration of local xenogeneic graft-versus-host reaction in cancer patients in vitro and reversal of cyclophosphamide-induced immune suppression in the rat in vivo by fractionated Astragalus membranaceus. Chung Hsi I Chieh Ho Tsa Chih. 1989 Jun;9(6):351-4, 326.

Chu DT, Wong WL, Mavligit GM. Immunotherapy with Chinese medicinal herbs. I. Immune restoration of local xenogeneic graft-versus-host reaction in cancer patients by fractionated Astragalus membranaceus in vitro. J Clin Lab Immunol. 1988 Mar;25(3):119-23.

Chu DT, Wong WL, Mavligit GM. Immunotherapy with Chinese medicinal herbs. II. Reversal of cyclophosphamide-induced immune suppression by administration of fractionated Astragalus membranaceus in vivo. J Clin Lab Immunol. 1988 Mar;25(3):125-9.

Fang JY. Effect of fu-zheng qu-xie on gastric disease infected with Campylobacter pyloridis. Chung Hsi I Chieh Ho Tsa Chih. 1991 Mar;11(3):150-2, 133.

He J, Li Y, Wei S, Guo M, Fu W. Effects of mixture of Astragalus membranaceus, Fructus Ligustri lucidi and Eclipta prostrata on immune function in mice. Hua Hsi I Ko Ta Hsueh Hsueh Pao. 1992 Sep;23(4):408-11.

Lau BH, Ruckle HC, Botolazzo T, Lui PD. Chinese medicinal herbs inhibit growth of murine renal cell carcinoma. Cancer Biother. 1994 Summer;9(2):153-61.

Pang SF. The effect of vitamin A and Astragalus on the splenic T lymphocyte-CFU of burned mice. Chung Hua Cheng Hsing Shao Shang Wai Ko Tsa Chih. 1989 Jun;5(2):122-4, 159.

Rittenhouse JR, Lui PD, Lau BH. Chinese medicinal herbs reverse macrophage suppression induced by urological tumors. J Urol. 1991 Aug;146(2):486-90.

Sinclair S. Chinese herbs: A clinical review of Astragalus, Ligusticum, and Schizandrae. Altern Med Rev. 1998 Oct;3(5):338-44.

Sugiura H, Nishida H, Inaba R, Iwata H. Effects of exercise in the growing stage in mice and of Astragalus membranaceus on immune functions. Nippon Eiseigaku Zasshi. 1993 Feb;47(6):1021-31.

Sun Y, Hersh EM, Talpaz M, Lee SL, Wong W, Loo TL, Mavligit GM. Immune restoration and/or augmentation of local graft versus host reaction by traditional Chinese medicinal herbs. Cancer. 1983 Jul 1;52(1):70-3.

Wang Y, Qian XJ, Hadley HR, Lau BH. Phytochemicals potentiate interleukin-2 generated lymphokine-activated killer cell cytotoxicity against murine renal cell carcinoma. Mol Biother. 1992 Sep;4(3):143-6.

Yoshida Y, Wang MQ, Liu JN, Shan BE, Yamashita U. Immunomodulating activity of Chinese medicinal herbs and Oldenlandia diffusa in particular. Int J Immunopharmacol. 1997 Jul;19(7):359-70.

Zhao KS, Mancini C, Doria G. Enhancement of the immune response in mice by Astragalus membranaceus extracts. Immunopharmacology. 1990 Nov-Dec; 20(3):225-33.

Zhou Y, Yan XZ. Experimental study of qi deficiency syndrome and Codonopsis pillosulae and Astragalus injection on the immune response in mice. Chung Hsi I Chieh Ho Tsa Chih. 1989 May;9(5):286-8, 262.

VITAMIN A

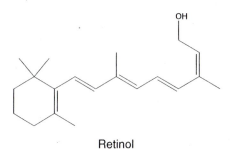

Retinol

What Is It?

Vitamin A is a fat-soluble vitamin that is part of a family of compounds including retinol, retinal, and beta-carotene. Beta-carotene is also known as "pro-vitamin A" because it can be converted into vitamin A when additional levels are required. Food sources of vitamin A include organ meats such as liver and kidney, egg yolks, butter, fortified dairy products such as milk, some margarines, and cod liver oil.

Claims

- Skin health (as both a topical cosmetic and an oral dietary supplement)
- Treats acne or other skin ailments
- Promotes eyesight and vision
- Prevents infection
- Antiaging
- Anticancer

Theory

Vitamin A is needed by all of the body's tissues for general growth and repair processes and is especially important for bone formation, healthy skin and hair, night vision, and function of the immune system. Because of these myriad functions, the health claims associated with vitamin A are numerous.

Scientific Support

Vitamin A may help boost immune system function and resistance to infection. The clinical and laboratory evidence to support such supplement claims is quite extensive. Vitamin A derivatives are also widely used in cosmetics and dermatological treatments designed to combat skin aging and treat acne. In addition, Vitamin A has been used for decades as a treatment for various vision-related conditions, including night blindness, cataracts, conjunctivitis, retinopathy, and macular degeneration.

Safety

Be aware that because it is fat soluble, vitamin A can be stored in the body, and levels can build up over time. Possible toxicity can result with high-dose supplementation (50,000 IU per day) leading to vomiting, headaches, joint pain, skin irritation, gastrointestinal distress, and hair loss. Extreme caution should be exercised during pregnancy, as high-dose vitamin A has been associated with teratogenic effects (birth defects). A maximum intake of 5,000 IU of vitamin A is suggested during pregnancy.

Value

High-dose supplementation of any isolated nutrient is generally not recommended. Virtually all standard multivitamin supplements contain either preformed vitamin A and/or beta-carotene as an ingredient.

Dosage

The daily value for vitamin A is 5,000 IU for adults. Children should consume no more than 3,500 IU daily. Although there is no established DV for beta-carotene, a daily intake of 5 to 20 mg would roughly approach the levels achieved by a diet high in fruits and vegetables.

WORKS CONSULTED

Allende LM, Corell A, Madrono A, Gongora R, Rodriguez-Gallego C, Lopez-Goyanes A, Rosal M, Arnaiz-Villena A. Retinol (vitamin A) is a cofactor in CD3-induced human T-lymphocyte activation. Immunology. 1997 Mar;90(3):388-96.

Chandra RK. Nutrition and immunoregulation. Significance for host resistance to tumors and infectious diseases in humans and rodents. J Nutr. 1992 Mar; 122(3 Suppl):754-7.

Daudu PA, Kelley DS, Taylor PC, Burri BJ, Wu MM. Effect of a low beta-carotene diet on the immune functions of adult women. Am J Clin Nutr. 1994
Dec;60(6):969-72.

Elitsur Y, Neace C, Liu X, Dosescu J, Moshier JA. Vitamin A and retinoic acids
immunomodulation on human gut lymphocytes. Immunopharmacology. 1997
Jan;35(3):247-53.

Fortes C, Forastiere F, Agabiti N, Fano V, Pacifici R, Virgili F, Piras G, Guidi L,
Bartoloni C, Tricerri A, Zuccaro P, Ebrahim S, Perucci CA. The effect of zinc
and vitamin A supplementation on immune response in an older population.
J Am Geriatr Soc. 1998 Jan;46(1):19-26.

Kutukculer N, Akil T, Egemen A, Kurugol Z, Aksit S, Ozmen D, Turgan N,
Bayindir O, Caglayan S. Adequate immune response to tetanus toxoid and failure of vitamin A and E supplementation to enhance antibody response in healthy
children. Vaccine. 2000 Jul 1;18(26):2979-84.

Molina EL, Patel JA. A to Z: Vitamin A and zinc, the miracle duo. Indian J Pediatr.
1996 Jul-Aug;63(4):427-31.

Penn ND, Purkins L, Kelleher J, Heatley RV, Mascie-Taylor BH, Belfield PW. The
effect of dietary supplementation with vitamins A, C and E on cell-mediated immune function in elderly long-stay patients: A randomized controlled trial. Age
Ageing. 1991 May;20(3):169-74.

Quadro L, Gamble MV, Vogel S, Lima AA, Piantedosi R, Moore SR, Colantuoni V,
Gottesman ME, Guerrant RL, Blaner WS. Retinol and retinol-binding protein:
Gut integrity and circulating immunoglobulins. J Infect Dis. 2000 Sep;182
(Suppl 1):S97-102.

Ravaglia G, Forti P, Maioli F, Bastagli L, Facchini A, Mariani E, Savarino L, Sassi
S, Cucinotta D, Lenaz G. Effect of micronutrient status on natural killer cell immune function in healthy free-living subjects aged >/=90 y. Am J Clin Nutr.
2000 Feb;71(2):590-8.

Rosales FJ, Kjolhede C. A single 210-mumol oral dose of retinol does not enhance
the immune response in children with measles. J Nutr. 1994 Sep;124(9):1604-14.

Rumore MM. Vitamin A as an immunomodulating agent. Clin Pharm. 1993 Jul;
12(7):506-14.

Schmidt K. Antioxidant vitamins and beta-carotene: Effects on immunocompe-
tence. Am J Clin Nutr. 1991 Jan;53(1 Suppl):383S-5S.

Semba RD. Vitamin A, immunity, and infection. Clin Infect Dis. 1994 Sep;19(3):489-99.

Semba RD. The role of vitamin A and related retinoids in immune function. Nutr
Rev. 1998 Jan;56(1 Pt 2):S38-48.

Semba RD. Vitamin A and immunity to viral, bacterial and protozoan infections.
Proc Nutr Soc. 1999 Aug;58(3):719-27.

Semba RD, Muhilal, Scott AL, Natadisastra G, Wirasasmita S, Mele L, Ridwan E,
West KP Jr, Sommer A. Depressed immune response to tetanus in children with
vitamin A deficiency. J Nutr. 1992 Jan;122(1):101-7.

Thurnham DI. Micronutrients and immune function: Some recent developments.
J Clin Pathol. 1997 Nov;50(11):887-91.

van Poppel G, Spanhaak S, Ockhuizen T. Effect of beta-carotene on immunological indexes in healthy male smokers. Am J Clin Nutr. 1993 Mar;57(3):402-7.

West CE, Rombout JH, van der Zijpp AJ, Sijtsma SR. Vitamin A and immune function. Proc Nutr Soc. 1991 Aug;50(2):251-62.

GLUTAMINE

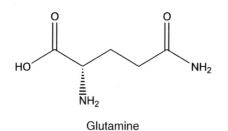

Glutamine

What Is It?

Glutamine is the most abundant amino acid in the body, making up approximately half of the free amino acids in the blood and muscle. As a nonessential amino acid, glutamine can be produced in the body by conversion from another amino acid, glutamic acid (primarily by the skeletal muscle and liver). Glutamine's main functions in the body include serving as a precursor in the synthesis of other amino acids and for conversion into glucose for energy. Cells of the immune system, the small intestine, and the kidney are the major consumers of glutamine.

Claims

- Boosts immune system function
- Maintains muscle mass/prevents muscle catabolism (breakdown)
- Enhances glycogen storage
- Aids recovery from exercise

Theory

Intense exercise training results in a well-described drop in plasma glutamine levels. Chronically low glutamine levels have been implicated as a possible contributing factor in athletic overtraining syndrome as well as the transient immunosuppression and increased risk of infections that typically affects competitive athletes during intense training and competition. Under conditions of metabolic stress, the body's need for glutamine may exceed its ability to produce adequate levels—meaning that a dietary source is required to prevent catabolism of skeletal muscle, the primary source of stored glutamine in the body.

Scientific Support

A significant body of scientific literature exists to support the beneficial effects of glutamine supplementation in maintaining muscle mass and immune system function in critically ill patients and in those recovering from extensive burns and major surgery. When plasma glutamine levels fall, skeletal muscles may enter a state of catabolism in which muscle protein is degraded to provide free glutamine for the rest of the body. Since skeletal muscle is the major source of glutamine (other than the diet), prolonged deficits in plasma glutamine can lead to a significant loss of skeletal muscle protein and muscle mass.

In recent years, at least a half-dozen studies have been conducted on glutamine supplementation in athletes, and a strong rationale exists for the efficacy of glutamine supplements in athletic populations. For example, glutamine's role in immune system support has been shown to prevent infections following intense bouts of physical activity (which tend to reduce plasma glutamine levels). Glutamine supplements have also been shown to play a role in counteracting the catabolic (muscle-wasting) effects of stress hormones such as cortisol, which are typically elevated by strenuous exercise. The function of glutamine in stimulating glycogen synthase, the enzyme that controls the synthesis and storage of glycogen fuel storage in muscles and liver, may provide a mechanism by which glutamine supplements promote enhanced fuel stores. Glutamine is also thought to increase cell volume, where it may stimulate the activity of enzymes in the liver and muscles involved in glycogen storage as well as those involved in anabolic activities such as protein synthesis. Glutamine supplements have also been hypothesized to increase levels of growth hormone, which may be expected to help stimulate protein synthesis and encourage gains in muscle mass and strength, but reliable evidence for this effect of glutamine supplements has not been demonstrated by clinical studies.

Safety

Glutamine supplements are well tolerated at levels up to at least 20 g per day, and intakes of as much as 40 g per day should induce no significant adverse effects outside of mild gastrointestinal discomfort. As with any isolated amino acid supplement, consumption in two to four divided doses throughout the day should increase total body stores without posing significant absorption issues.

Value

Glutamine supplements are relatively inexpensive compared to other amino acid supplements. For anybody exposed to heightened levels of stress, such as those recovering from injury, surgery, or intense exercise, glutamine supplements represent an economical way to promote tissue repair, reduce muscle catabolism, and help prevent infections.

Dosage

For the immune system support and anticatabolic actions that are of interest to most athletes, recommended doses range from 1 to 10 g.

WORKS CONSULTED

Alvestrand A, Bergstrom J, Furst P, Germanis G, Widstam U. Effect of essential amino acid supplementation on muscle and plasma free amino acids in chronic uremia. Kidney Int. 1978 Oct;14(4):323-9.

Aoki TT. Metabolic adaptations to starvation, semistarvation, and carbohydrate restriction. Prog Clin Biol Res. 1981;67:161-77.

Aoki TT, Brennan MF, Fitzpatrick GF, Knight DC. Leucine meal increases glutamine and total nitrogen release from forearm muscle. J Clin Invest. 1981 Dec;68(6):1522-8.

Bonau RA, Jeevanandam M, Moldawer L, Blackburn GL, Daly JM. Muscle amino acid flux in patients receiving branched-chain amino acid solutions after surgery. Surgery. 1987 Apr;101(4):400-7.

Calder PC, Yaqoob P. Glutamine and the immune system. Amino Acids. 1999; 17(3):227-41.

Carli F, Webster J, Ramachandra V, Pearson M, Read M, Ford GC, McArthur S, Preedy VR, Halliday D. Aspects of protein metabolism after elective surgery in patients receiving constant nutritional support. Clin Sci (Colch). 1990 Jun; 78(6):621-8.

Castell LM, Newsholme EA. The effects of oral glutamine supplementation on athletes after prolonged, exhaustive exercise. Nutrition. 1997 Jul-Aug;13(7-8): 738-42.

Elia M, Folmer P, Schlatmann A, Goren A, Austin S. Amino acid metabolism in muscle and in the whole body of man before and after ingestion of a single mixed meal. Am J Clin Nutr. 1989 Jun;49(6):1203-10.

Giesecke K, Magnusson I, Ahlberg M, Hagenfeldt L, Wahren J. Protein and amino acid metabolism during early starvation as reflected by excretion of urea and methylhistidines. Metabolism. 1989 Dec;38(12):1196-200.

Gleeson M, Bishop NC. Elite athlete immunology: Importance of nutrition. Int J Sports Med. 2000 May;21 (Suppl 1):S44-50.

Greenhaff PL, Gleeson M, Maughan RJ. The effects of diet on muscle pH and metabolism during high intensity exercise. Eur J Appl Physiol Occup Physiol. 1988;57(5):531-9.

Haymond MW, Strobel KE, DeVivo DC. Muscle wasting and carbohydrate homeostasis in Duchenne muscular dystrophy. Neurology. 1978 Dec;28(12):1224-31.

Lundeberg S, Belfrage M, Wernerman J, von der Decken A, Thunell S, Vinnars E. Growth hormone improves muscle protein metabolism and whole body nitrogen economy in man during a hyponitrogenous diet. Metabolism. 1991 Mar;40(3):315-22.

McKenzie DC. Markers of excessive exercise. Can J Appl Physiol. 1999 Feb;24(1):66-73.

Newsholme EA, Calder PC. The proposed role of glutamine in some cells of the immune system and speculative consequences for the whole animal. Nutrition. 1997 Jul-Aug;13(7-8):728-30.

Nieman DC. Exercise immunology: Future directions for research related to athletes, nutrition, and the elderly. Int J Sports Med. 2000 May;21(Suppl 1):S61-8.

Ruderman NB. Muscle amino acid metabolism and gluconeogenesis. Annu Rev Med. 1975;26:245-58.

Ruderman NB, Berger M. The formation of glutamine and alanine in skeletal muscle. J Biol Chem. 1974 Sep 10;249(17):5500-6.

Russell DM, Walker PM, Leiter LA, Sima AA, Tanner WK, Mickle DA, Whitwell J, Marliss EB, Jeejeebhoy KN. Metabolic and structural changes in skeletal muscle during hypocaloric dieting. Am J Clin Nutr. 1984 Apr;39(4):503-13.

Schedl HP, Maughan RJ, Gisolfi CV. Intestinal absorption during rest and exercise: Implications for formulating an oral rehydration solution (ORS). Proceedings of a roundtable discussion. April 21-22, 1993. Med Sci Sports Exerc. 1994 Mar;26(3):267-80.

Shephard RJ, Shek PN. Heavy exercise, nutrition and immune function: Is there a connection? Int J Sports Med. 1995 Nov;16(8):491-7.

Shephard RJ, Shek PN. Immunological hazards from nutritional imbalance in athletes. Exerc Immunol Rev. 1998;4:22-48.

Smith DJ, Norris SR. Changes in glutamine and glutamate concentrations for tracking training tolerance. Med Sci Sports Exerc. 2000 Mar;32(3):684-9.

Walsh NP, Blannin AK, Robson PJ, Gleeson M. Glutamine, exercise and immune function. Links and possible mechanisms. Sports Med. 1998 Sep;26(3):177-91.

Young LS, Bye R, Scheltinga M, Ziegler TR, Jacobs DO, Wilmore DW. Patients receiving glutamine-supplemented intravenous feedings report an improvement in mood. J Parenter Enteral Nutr. 1993 Sep-Oct;17(5):422-7.

Zanker CL, Swaine IL, Castell LM, Newsholme EA. Responses of plasma glutamine, free tryptophan and branched-chain amino acids to prolonged exercise after a regime designed to reduce muscle glycogen. Eur J Appl Physiol Occup Physiol. 1997;75(6):543-8.

ZINC

What Is It?

Zinc is an essential trace mineral that has functions as part of about 300 different enzymes. As such, zinc plays a role in virtually all biochemical pathways and physiological processes. More than 90 percent of the body's zinc is stored in the bones (30 percent) and muscles (60 percent), but zinc is also found in virtually all body tissues. The richest dietary sources of zinc are seafood (especially oysters), meat, fish, eggs, and poultry.

Claims

- Wound healing
- Immune system support
- Reduces length and severity of colds (in lozenge form)
- Supports a healthy prostate gland (prevents benign prostatic hyperplasia [BPH])
- Increases fertility (sperm production)

Theory

Because zinc is an essential part of nearly 300 different biochemical pathways, structure/function claims can be made for the nutrient's role in a wide variety of processes including digestion, wound healing, energy production, growth, cellular repair, collagen synthesis, bone strength, cognitive function, carbohydrate metabolism (glucose utilization and insulin production), and reproductive function. Even mild zinc deficiency has been associated with depressed immunity, decreased sperm count, and impaired memory. Perhaps the most popular claim for zinc is for its role in immunity, where zinc delivered in lozenge form may interfere with the replication of the cold virus (rhinovirus).

Scientific Support

There is certainly sufficient evidence supporting the use of zinc lozenges in reducing the duration and severity of colds. Although concentrated zinc lozenges can help kill cold viruses in the mouth and throat, it is important to begin using them as soon as possible following the onset of cold symptoms (ideally within the first twenty-four to forty-eight hours). Test-tube studies have shown that zinc can block the cold virus from replicating—an effect that could help the body's natural immune defenses get a jump on killing the viruses. Most studies of the effect of zinc lozenges (typically zinc gluconate or zinc acetate) on the common cold have shown that subjects in the supplement group tend to have fewer symptomatic days (on average two to three fewer sick days) than subjects receiving a placebo (measured in terms of coughing, sore throat, nasal congestion, and headache).

Occasionally, high-dose zinc supplements are recommended to diabetic patients. Such patients commonly suffer from increased loss of zinc and reduced body stores of zinc. High doses of zinc have been shown to mimic the effects of insulin in reducing blood sugar and promoting wound healing. These effects, however, should be considered preliminary, and high-dose zinc supplements are not recommended for diabetics except on the advice of their personal physician.

Exercise performance has also been associated with adequate zinc status—especially in athletes who avoid red meat, concentrate their diets too much on carbohydrates, or follow an overly restricted dietary regime. Low zinc intake (below 3 mg per day) has been linked to reduced activity of a zinc-containing enzyme in red blood cells called carbonic anhydrase (which helps red blood cells transport carbon dioxide from tissues to the lungs to be exhaled). Mild to moderate zinc deficiency can lead to significant reductions in the body's ability to take up and use oxygen, remove carbon dioxide, and generate energy during high-intensity exercise.

Zinc has also been linked to enhanced bone formation and reduction of bone loss, both alone and in combination with plant isoflavones such as genistein. When used together with isoflavones, it appears that the isoflavonoid effect on bone is enhanced by zinc and may have a potent role in prevention of bone loss.

Safety

The short-term use of zinc at therapeutic doses for cold relief (see Dosage) is assumed to be safe, and chronic supplementation with zinc at levels two to three times the current RDA should not be expected to pose any significant adverse side effects. However, high doses of zinc are not recommended for periods of more than two weeks due to concerns of immune system depression, interference with copper absorption, and other long-term health effects such as increased risk for heart disease. High doses of zinc (gram levels) can cause nausea, diarrhea, and vomiting.

Value

If you've never tried some of the zinc lozenges on the market, get ready for the distinct (bad) flavor of zinc—which is notoriously difficult to cover with any level of flavorings and sweeteners. For many people, however, the slightly metallic taste that zinc lozenges can leave in your mouth is a small price to pay for the quicker relief from cold symptoms.

Dosage

The daily value for zinc is 15 mg—a level that should be adequate for support of bone metabolism and optimal physical performance. As therapy for colds, however, higher levels are required—in the range of 13 to 23 mg (in lozenge form) taken every two hours for no more than two weeks. These levels appear to be quite effective for reducing the duration and severity of cold symptoms compared to not taking zinc lozenges. Try to select lozenges that are free from excipients such as sorbitol (a sweetener), citric acid (a flavoring), and mannitol (a sweetener), as these ingredients may bind zinc in the mouth and reduce its bioavailability and effectiveness. It is also important to note that other supplements, particularly high levels of calcium and iron, can decrease zinc absorption, while complexation (chelation) with various amino acids (such as glycine, histidine, and aspartate) or other organic compounds (such as gluconate or picolinate) may increase zinc bioavailability.

WORKS CONSULTED

Abbasi AA, Prasad AS, Rabbani P, DuMouchelle E. Experimental zinc deficiency in man. Effect on testicular function. J Lab Clin Med. 1980 Sep;96(3):544-50.

Brun JF, Dieu-Cambrezy C, Charpiat A, Fons C, Fedou C, Micallef JP, Fussellier M, Bardet L, Orsetti A. Serum zinc in highly trained adolescent gymnasts. Biol Trace Elem Res. 1995 Jan-Mar;47(1-3):273-8.

Couzy F, Lafargue P, Guezennec CY. Zinc metabolism in the athlete: Influence of training, nutrition and other factors. Int J Sports Med. 1990 Aug;11(4):263-6.

Gleeson M, Bishop NC. Elite athlete immunology: Importance of nutrition. Int J Sports Med. 2000 May;21(Suppl 1):S44-50.

Hunt CD, Johnson PE, Herbel J, Mullen LK. Effects of dietary zinc depletion on seminal volume and zinc loss, serum testosterone concentrations, and sperm morphology in young men. Am J Clin Nutr. 1992 Jul;56(1):148-57.

Krotkiewski M, Gudmundsson M, Backstrom P, Mandroukas K. Zinc and muscle strength and endurance. Acta Physiol Scand. 1982 Nov;116(3):309-11.

Lukaski HC. Magnesium, zinc, and chromium nutriture and physical activity. Am J Clin Nutr. 2000 Aug;72(2 Suppl):585S-93S.

McDonald R, Keen CL. Iron, zinc and magnesium nutrition and athletic performance. Sports Med. 1988 Mar;5(3):171-84.

Nishi Y. Anemia and zinc deficiency in the athlete. J Am Coll Nutr. 1996 Aug; 15(4):323-4.

Prasad AS. Zinc deficiency in human subjects. Prog Clin Biol Res. 1983;129:1-33.

Prasad AS, Cossack ZT. Neutrophil zinc: An indicator of zinc status in man. Trans Assoc Am Physicians. 1982;95:165-76.

Shephard RJ, Shek PN. Immunological hazards from nutritional imbalance in athletes. Exerc Immunol Rev. 1998;4:22-48.

Suboticanec K, Stavljenic A, Bilic-Pesic L, Gorajscan M, Gorajscan D, Brubacher G, Buzina R. Nutritional status, grip strength, and immune function in institutionalized elderly. Int J Vitam Nutr Res. 1989;59(1):20-8.

COLOSTRUM

What Is It?

Colostrum is the clear or cloudy "premilk" that female mammals secrete after giving birth and prior to producing milk. Colostrum for dietary supplements is usually derived from bovine sources (cows) and contains various immunoglobulins (also called antibodies) and antimicrobial factors (i.e., lactoferrin, lactoperoxidase, lysozyme, and growth factors).

Claims

- Immune support
- Reduction of diarrhea
- Gastrointestinal support
- Improved exercise performance and recovery

Theory

Bovine colostrum contains the same disease resistance factors (immunoglobins) that are found in human breast milk and unpasteurized cow's milk. Among the wide variety of immune factors that may be effective against various viruses, bacteria, yeast, and other invaders are immunoglobins, antibodies, lactoferrin, lactalbumin, glycoproteins, cytokines (such as IL-1, IL-6, and interferon Y), and various polypeptides, growth factors, vitamins, and minerals. The antibodies present in colostrum are thought to combine with disease-causing microorganisms in the GI tract. By adhering to pathogens, colostrum antibodies may be able to reduce the adhesive properties of bacteria and decrease their ability to attach to the intestinal wall (which could prevent their entrance into the body). It is unlikely that the full antimicrobial benefits of colostrum can be realized unless you happen to be a calf, because the immunoglobulins are largely digested in the gut and cannot be absorbed intact. It may be possible, however, for *partially* digested immunoglobulin fragments to retain a small portion of their functional properties.

Scientific Support

It is no secret that in response to a disease (or vaccination), the body produces specialized antibodies and general defense components to fight invading infections. It is also no secret that infants fed baby formula (instead of breast milk) are more prone to a variety of infections because pasteurized infant formula contains none of the active antibodies and other immune components that are naturally present in human breast milk.

In infants, it has been shown that intact immunoglobulin molecules and active fragments are still capable of delivering some immune activity after traveling through the digestive tract (based on test-tube studies). Whether the same is true for adults is largely unknown. It is known, however, that active antibodies can be recovered in the intestines and feces following colostrum consumption (about half of the ingested dose is still present after six hours).

Several small clinical studies of colostrum consumption have been conducted, although many are only published as abstracts. In one study, the administration of bovine immunoglobulins (in a mouth rinse) reduced yeast infections in bone marrow transplant patients. At least a few studies have shown the benefits of ingesting colostrum in neutralizing the activity of several strains of bacteria and parasites that cause diarrhea. In another study of children and adults with chronic gastritis, symptoms were improved and inflammation was reduced, suggesting that colostrum may be effective against *H. pylori* (the bacteria that causes ulcers).

In terms of sports performance, one study looked at thirty-nine males during an eight-week running program (three runs of 45 minutes per week) while consuming colostrum (60 g per day) or whey protein. The study found no differences in plasma IGF-1 concentrations in either group during the study period, but the colostrum group ran further and did more work than the placebo group (equal to a 2 percent increase in performance). Another study examined rowing performance in a group of elite female rowers. Eight rowers completed a nine-week training program while consuming either colostrum (60 g per day) or whey protein. By week nine, rowers consuming colostrum had greater increases in the distance covered and work done compared to the whey protein group.

One of the only published references on bovine colostrum consumption suggests that it can help prevent and treat the gastric injury associated with nonsteroidal anti-inflammatory drugs (NSAIDs) and may also be of value for the treatment of other ulcerative conditions of the bowel. The study, which examined rats and mice, found a 30 to 60 percent reduction in gastric injury following colostrum treatment.

Taken together, the available evidence for bovine colostrum is adequate to support its benefits as a mild immune-supporting supplement—particularly when interactions with pathogens in the intestinal tract are possible. It is unlikely, however, that colostrum would provide immune benefits against *airborne* pathogens and upper respiratory tract infections such as colds and influenza.

Safety

No adverse side effects are expected up to doses of 60 g per day—but individuals with milk allergies should avoid bovine colostrum.

Value

The price range for colostrum products is quite large—between $15 and $40 for a one-month supply of capsules or powder. Of special note is the fact that most capsule-form products provide no more than 1 g of colostrum per serving, while powder forms may go up to about 5 to 10 g. These amounts are well below the levels shown to be effective in the studies mentioned (as much as 60 g per day)—meaning that a clinically effective dose might cost you $30 per *day* and mean that you're swallowing as many as sixty capsules. Whether or not lower levels of colostrum are effective in boosting immune system function is unknown.

Dosage

Typical dosage recommendations for commercial products range from 1 to 6 g per day, but the majority of available research has used doses of about ten times as much (60 g in some studies). It is unknown whether these small (1 to 6 g) doses will provide the benefits demonstrated in clinical studies.

WORKS CONSULTED

Buckley J, Abbott M, Martin D, Brinkworth G, Whyte P. Effect of an oral bovine colostrum supplement (intact TM) on running performance. Abstract from: 1998 Australian Conference of Science and Medicine in Sport, Adelaide, South Australia, October 1998.

Greenberg PD, Cello JP. Treatment of severe diarrhea caused by Cryptosporidium parvum with oral bovine immunoglobulins concentrate in patients with AIDS. J AIDS Hum Retrovirol. 1996;13:348-54.

Kelly CP, Chetham S, Keates S, Bostwick EF, Roush AM, Castagliuolo I, LaMont JT, Pothoulakis C. Survival of anti-Clostridium difficile bovine immunoglobulin concentrate in the human gastrointestinal tract. Antimicrobial Agents Chemother. 1997;41:236-41.

Kelly CP, Pothoulakis C, Vavva F, Castagliuolo I, Bostwick EF, O'Keane JC, Keates S, LaMont JT. Anti-Clostridium difficile bovine immunoglobulin concentrate inhibits cytotoxicity and enterotoxicity of C. difficile toxins. Antimicrobial Agents Chemother. 1996;40:373-379.

Mero A, Miikkulainen H, Riski J, Pakkanen R, Aalto J, Takala T. Effects of bovine colostrum supplementation on serum IGF-1, IgG, hormone and saliva IgA during training. J Appl Physiol. 1997;83(4):1144-51.

Playford RJ, Floyd DN, Macdonald CE, Calnan DP, Adenekan RO, Johnson W, Goodlad RA, Marchbank T. Bovine colostrum is a health food supplement which prevents NSAID induced gut damage. Gut. 1999 May; 44(5):653-8.

Tacket CO, Binion SB, Bostwick E, Losonsky G, Roy MJ, Edelman R. Efficacy of bovine milk immunoglobulins concentrate in preventing illness after Shigella flexneri challenge. Amer J Trop Med Hyg. 1992;47:276-83.

Takahashi N, Eisenhuth G, Lee I, Schachtele C, Laible N, Binion S. Nonspecific antibacterial factors in milk from cows immunized with human oral bacterial pathogens. J Dairy Sci. 1992;75:1810-20.

Tollemar J, Gross N, Dolgiras N, Jarstrand C, Ringden O, Hammarstrom L. Fungal prophylaxis by reduction of fungal colonization by oral administration of bovine anti-Candida antibodies in bone marrow transplant recipients. Bone Marrow Transpl. 1999;23:283-90.

Warny M, Fatimi A, Bostwick EF, Laine DC, Lebel F, LaMont JT, Pothoulakis C, Kelly CP. Bovine immunoglobulins concentrate-Clostridium difficile retains C. difficile toxin neutralizing activity after passage through the human stomach and small intestine. Gut. 1999;44:212-17.

BETA-GLUCANS

What Is It?

Glucan is a beta 1,3-linked polyglucose (a long chain of simple sugars) that has been shown to have general immunostimulatory properties in animal and test-tube studies. Among its effects are macrophage activation, tumor inhibition, and decreased infection rates. Commercial products are marketed for maintaining a strong immune system.

Claims

- Immune system stimulation
- Cancer treatment/prevention

Theory

Glucans are hypothesized to stimulate immune system strength by activating white blood cells to attack infections and tumors.

Scientific Support

A review of the relevant literature on beta-glucans and immune function suggests a clear effect of glucan administration on prophylaxis against infections, activation of macrophages, and tumoricidal activity. Numerous studies suggest an effect of the glucans in preventing infection and destroying tumors—provided that you're either a lab rat or a cell living in a test tube. A number of in vitro (test tube) studies have confirmed that beta-glucan stimulates production of monocyte cytokines, which may help promote regression of certain tumors. A significant drawback of the existing literature, however, is a lack of studies that examine *oral* delivery of beta-glucans in animals or humans—as in a *dietary* supplement. Because the vast majority of studies showing positive immune benefits have delivered the glucans by injection rather than orally, we do not know whether their activity persists following digestion or whether they are absorbed (very likely they are not absorbed).

Only four studies were identified in which beta-glucans were administered orally to mice. Enhanced immune function was demonstrated, as measured by natural killer cell activity, lysosomal enzyme activity of macrophages, and inhibition of tumor growth. Two significant drawbacks with these studies are that the administered doses are high (80 mg/kg) and that only a single laboratory (Tokyo College of Pharmacy) has shown positive results with oral delivery of beta-glucans. These results need to be replicated by other laboratories and need to be conducted in humans at safe doses before we can be sure that they are indeed effective.

Safety

Although no long-term (or short-term) safety studies have been done, beta-glucans are probably as safe as other polysaccharide-type herbs for temporary immune system stimulation (such as echinacea, goldenseal, astragalus, and others).

Value

Because of the lack of evidence that beta-glucans are effective immune system stimulators when taken orally, they have to be classified as providing less value than scientifically validated supplements such as echinacea, goldenseal, astragalus, and others.

Dosage

Typical dosage recommendations may range anywhere from 10 mg to upwards of several hundred mg per day—although no credible scientific evidence supports any dosage recommendation for oral use.

WORKS CONSULTED

Estrada A, Yun CH, Van Kessel A, Li B, Hauta S, Laarveld B. Immunomodulatory activities of oat beta-glucan in vitro and in vivo. Microbiol Immunol. 1997; 41(12):991-8.

Figueras A, Santarem MM, Novoa B. Influence of the sequence of administration of beta-glucans and a Vibrio damsela vaccine on the immune response of turbot (Scophthalmus maximus L.). Vet Immunol Immunopathol. 1998 Jun 30;64(1):59-68.

Kim HM, Han SB, Oh GT, Kim YH, Hong DH, Hong ND, Yoo ID. Stimulation of humoral and cell mediated immunity by polysaccharide from mushroom Phellinus linteus. Int J Immunopharmacol. 1996 May;18(5):295-303.

Ooi VE, Liu F. Immunomodulation and anti-cancer activity of polysaccharide-protein complexes. Curr Med Chem. 2000 Jul;7(7):715-29.

Yan J, Vetvicka V, Xia Y, Coxon A, Carroll MC, Mayadas TN, Ross GD. Beta-glucan, a "specific" biologic response modifier that uses antibodies to target tumors for cytotoxic recognition by leukocyte complement receptor type 3 (CD11b/CD18). J Immunol. 1999 Sep 15;163(6):3045-52.

Yan J, Vetvicka V, Xia Y, Hanikyrova M, Mayadas TN, Ross GD. Critical role of Kupffer cell CR3 (CD11b/CD18) in the clearance of IgM-opsonized erythrocytes or soluble beta-glucan. Immunopharmacology. 2000 Jan;46(1):39-54.

Yoshioka S, Ohno N, Miura T, Adachi Y, Yadomae T. Immunotoxicity of soluble beta-glucans induced by indomethacin treatment. FEMS Immunol Med Microbiol. 1998 Jul;21(3):171-9.

PERILLA SEED

What Is It?

Perilla seed *(Perilla frutescens)* is a common annual weed found across the eastern and southern United States. In Asia, perilla is considered a commercial crop. Perilla food products are available in the United States in many Korean ethnic markets.

Claims

- Reduces allergic symptoms and asthma
- Pain reliever and anti-inflammatory
- Stimulates immune function
- Protects heart health (reduces blood clotting)

Theory

Asian herbalists prescribe perilla for relieving coughing and for support of lung health and protection from colds and flu. The oil from perilla seeds is relatively high in omega-3 fatty acids, specifically alpha-linolenic acid, as well as several phenolic compounds (rosemarinic acid, luteolin, chrysoeriol, quercetin, catechin, and apigenin). Perilla seed extracts are known to suppress the production of key chemical mediators in the allergic and inflammatory response (leukotrienes, histamine, thromboxanes, and prostaglandins), possibly via an inhibition of the 5-lipoxygenase enzyme. A cardiovascular benefit of perilla seed oil is thought to be provided through a reduction in the activity of platelet activating factor and production of thromboxane A2 (which could reduce blood clotting and atherosclerotic plaque formation).

Scientific Support

In a variety of rodent studies, perilla seed oil has been shown to decrease blood clotting by about 50 percent when compared to other plant oils such as safflower and soybean oils. Incidence of tumors of the mammary gland, colon, and kidney have also been reduced in rats following feeding of perilla seed oil (for about eight to ten weeks) when compared to soybean oil.

As an anti-inflammatory compound, the essential fatty acids have been associated with benefits in a wide range of inflammatory conditions, including heart disease, colitis and Crohn's disease, and allergy. Fish oil appears to be especially beneficial, but many people avoid fish oils due to smell and flavor concerns.

In a handful of animal studies, perilla seed oil appears to suppress a wide range of allergic mediators (leukotrienes, immunoglobulins) in mice and rats fed either perilla seed oil or safflower oil (which is rich in omega-6 fatty acids) for two to eight weeks. These findings raise the potential for perilla oil to be effective in reducing allergic hypersensitivity in humans. To evaluate this hypothesis, one study looked at fourteen asthmatics, seven of whom received perilla seed oil supplements and seven received corn oil supplements. Results showed that allergic mediators (leukotrienes B4 and C4) were elevated in the corn oil group but decreased in the perilla seed group. The perilla seed group also showed benefits in terms of lung function and breathing parameters (forced vital capacity, expiratory volume, and lung volume) within two to four weeks. These results suggest that perilla seed oil may be useful for the treatment of asthma and for improving lung function.

Safety

Because the majority of the studies on perilla seed oil have been conducted in animals, not a great deal of information is available on long-term safety in humans. It is encouraging to note, however, that perilla seed oil is widely consumed in a variety of Asian food products and has not been associated with any adverse side effects.

Value

In general, the consensus from both animal and human experiments has led to the public health recommendation that, for most people, dietary intake of omega-6 fatty acids should be decreased and consumption of omega-3 oils should be increased. As a dietary source of omega-3 fatty acids and many phenolic compounds, perilla seed oil appears to be beneficial for reducing some of the chemical mediators of allergy, asthma, and inflammation. As such, perilla seed oil may be helpful in alleviating symptoms of asthma and promoting optimal lung function. Because perilla seed oil is quite inexpensive, this may be a particularly economical route for many people to increase their daily intake of omega-3 oils.

Dosage

Typical dosage recommendations for omega-3 fatty acid supplementation from perilla seed oil are in the range of 6 g per day (which would provide about 3 g of the essential omega-3 oil, alpha-linolenic acid).

WORKS CONSULTED

Gu JY, Wakizono Y, Dohi A, Nonaka M, Sugano M, Yamada K. Effect of dietary fats and sesamin on the lipid metabolism and immune function of Sprague-Dawley rats. Biosci Biotechnol Biochem. 1998 Oct;62(10):1917-24.

Hashimoto A, Katagiri M, Torii S, Dainaka J, Ichikawa A, Okuyama H. Effect of the dietary alpha-linolenate/linoleate balance on leukotriene production and histamine release in rats. Prostaglandins. 1988 Jul;36(1):3-16.

Hirose M, Masuda A, Ito N, Kamano K, Okuyama H. Effects of dietary perilla oil, soybean oil and safflower oil on 7,12-dimethylbenz[a]anthracene (DMBA) and 1,2-dimethyl-hydrazine (DMH)-induced mammary gland and colon carcinogenesis in female SD rats. Carcinogenesis. 1990 May;11(5):731-5.

Ide T, Murata M, Sugano M. Stimulation of the activities of hepatic fatty acid oxidation enzymes by dietary fat rich in alpha-linolenic acid in rats. J Lipid Res. 1996 Mar;37(3):448-63.

Ihara M, Umekawa H, Takahashi T, Furuichi Y. Comparative effects of short- and long-term feeding of safflower oil and perilla oil on lipid metabolism in rats. Comp Biochem Physiol B Biochem Mol Biol. 1998 Oct;121(2):223-31.

Nagatsu A, Tenmaru K, Matsuura H, Murakami N, Kobayashi T, Okuyama H, Sakakibara J. Novel antioxidants from roasted perilla seed. Chem Pharm Bull (Tokyo). 1995 May;43(5):887-9.

Narisawa T, Fukaura Y, Yazawa K, Ishikawa C, Isoda Y, Nishizawa Y. Colon cancer prevention with a small amount of dietary perilla oil high in alpha-linolenic acid in an animal model. Cancer. 1994 Apr 15;73(8):2069-75.

Ohhashi K, Takahashi T, Watanabe S, Kobayashi T, Okuyama H, Hata N, Misawa Y. Effect of replacing a high linoleate oil with a low linoleate, high alpha-linolenate oil, as compared with supplementing EPA or DHA, on reducing lipid mediator production in rat polymorphonuclear leukocytes. Biol Pharm Bull. 1998 Jun;21(6):558-64.

Okamoto M, Mitsunobu F, Ashida K, Mifune T, Hosaki Y, Tsugeno H, Harada S, Tanizaki Y. Effects of dietary supplementation with n-3 fatty acids compared with n-6 fatty acids on bronchial asthma. Intern Med. 2000 Feb;39(2):107-11.

Okuno M, Kajiwara K, Imai S, Kobayashi T, Honma N, Maki T, Suruga K, Goda T, Takase S, Muto Y, Moriwaki H. Perilla oil prevents the excessive growth of visceral adipose tissue in rats by down-regulating adipocyte differentiation. J Nutr. 1997 Sep;127(9):1752-7.

Sadi AM, Toda T, Oku H, Hokama S. Dietary effects of corn oil, oleic acid, perilla oil, and evening primrose oil on plasma and hepatic lipid level and atherosclerosis in Japanese quail. Exp Anim. 1996 Jan;45(1):55-62.

Suzuki H, Ishigaki A, Hara Y. Long-term effect of a trace amount of tea catechins with perilla oil on the plasma lipids in mice. Int J Vitam Nutr Res. 1998;68(4):272-4.

Umezawa M, Kogishi K, Tojo H, Yoshimura S, Seriu N, Ohta A, Takeda T, Hosokawa M. High-linoleate and high-alpha-linolenate diets affect learning ability and natural behavior in SAMR1 mice. J Nutr. 1999 Feb;129(2):431-7.

CAT'S CLAW

What Is It?

The terms "cat's claw" and "claw vine" are used to refer to about two dozen related plant species native to Peru and surrounding rain forests (the hooks of the plant look a bit like a cat's claw). The root of the *Uncaria tomentosa* variety is traditionally used as a treatment for a variety of infections and to promote wound healing. Its use as a modern dietary supplement is generally targeted toward immune system support.

Claims

- Stimulates/modulates the immune system
- Prevents/treats infections
- Alleviates intestinal/gastric ulcers
- Relieves arthritis pain (rheumatoid arthritis)

Theory

Chemical analysis shows that the bark of the root contains oxindole alkaloids (probably the major "active" compound) along with a variety of catechin/polyphenols, triterpenes, and sterols. It is theorized that a higher content of *pentacyclic* oxindole alkaloids versus the *tetracyclic* alkaloids will deliver a more powerful stimulation or modulation of the immune system (based on the concept that the tetracyclics may block the effects of the pentacyclics). In addition, the quinovic acid glycoside found in cat's claw may provide an additional benefit in wound healing via its effects in reducing inflammation.

Scientific Support

About half a dozen clinical trials suggest beneficial immune-modulating activities of cat's claw. Test-tube studies support the theory that the pentacyclic alkaloids can stimulate white blood cells to engulf and destroy pathogens and cellular debris (phagocytosis), laying the foundation for clinical studies of cat's claw extracts for immune system and wound-healing bene-

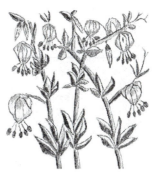

fits. In a small group of subjects, cat's claw has been shown to reduce the occurrence of upper respiratory tract infections. In a six-month study of rheumatoid arthritis, an autoimmune disease, cat's claw was shown to produce significant improvements on measures of joint swelling and tenderness in seventeen out of eighteen of the subjects receiving the supplement (versus only ten of the seventeen subjects taking placebo). These results suggest that cat's claw may actually modulate immune system activity in some way rather than simply stimulating immune system cells.

Safety

Cat's claw has not been fully evaluated for safety during pregnancy, so pregnant or lactating women should avoid its use. During the initial period of consumption, mild to moderate gastrointestinal side effects (gas, bloating, nausea, diarrhea) have been reported.

Value

Cat's claw appears to provide some beneficial immune-modulating effects—especially for those suffering from rheumatoid arthritis. It is important to note that many forms of cat's claw supplements may use parts of the plant other than the root, where the primary active compounds are concentrated. In addition, test-tube studies suggest that extracts containing more of the *pentacyclic* oxindole alkaloids (POAs) may be more potent than extracts that also contain the *tetracyclic* form (TOAs).

Dosage

Dosage is generally based on the total content of oxindole alkaloids (OAs)—but the tetracyclic form is thought to interfere with the more active pentacyclic form. Typical dosage recommendations are in the range of 20 to 60 mg per day (20 mg, three times per day for seven to ten days, followed by 20 mg per day as a maintenance dose).

WORKS CONSULTED

Budzinski JW, Foster BC, Vandenhoek S, Arnason JT. An in vitro evaluation of human cytochrome P450 3A4 inhibition by selected commercial herbal extracts and tinctures. Phytomedicine. 2000 Jul;7(4):273-82.

Hilepo JN, Bellucci AG, Mossey RT. Acute renal failure caused by "cat's claw" herbal remedy in a patient with systemic lupus erythematosus. Nephron. 1997; 77(3):361.

Reinhard KH. Uncaria tomentosa (Willd.) D.C.: Cat's claw, una de gato, or saventaro. J Altern Complement Med. 1999 Apr;5(2):143-51.

Sandoval M, Charbonnet RM, Okuhama NN, Roberts J, Krenova Z, Trentacosti AM, Miller MJ. Cat's claw inhibits TNFalpha production and scavenges free radicals: Role in cytoprotection. Free Radic Biol Med. 2000 Jul 1;29(1):71-8.

Sandoval-Chacon M, Thompson JH, Zhang XJ, Liu X, Mannick EE, Sadowska-Krowicka H, Charbonnet RM, Clark DA, Miller MJ. Anti-inflammatory actions of cat's claw: The role of NF-kappaB. Aliment Pharmacol Ther. 1998 Dec; 12(12):1279-89.

Sheng Y, Bryngelsson C, Pero RW. Enhanced DNA repair, immune function and reduced toxicity of C-MED-100, a novel aqueous extract from Uncaria tomentosa. J Ethnopharmacol. 2000 Feb;69(2):115-26.

Chapter 12

Supplements for Antioxidant Protection and Eye Health

ANTIOXIDANTS—RIGHT WHERE YOU NEED THEM MOST

The vast majority of supplement users are probably aware of the term "antioxidant" and the concept that such compounds can help protect cell membranes and other structures from the damaging effects of free radicals. Those very same supplement users, however, often fail to stop and ask themselves which of their body's systems might benefit the *most* from an increased dietary intake of antioxidants. To answer this question, think about which parts of your body are exposed to the highest levels of free radicals. For example, the *lungs and muscles* of endurance athletes are subjected to high free radical loads as a result of the increased oxygen demands of exercise. For sunbathers, the *skin* can benefit from the increased protection that antioxidants provide against the oxidizing ultraviolet radiation of the sun. Likewise, anybody that spends time outdoors exposed to the sun should be concerned with the potential for ultraviolet radiation to damage *eye health*.

Sunlight exposure has been linked to premature vision loss, development of cataracts, and an increased risk of age-related macular degeneration (ARMD)—the leading cause of blindness in people over sixty-five years of age. In the United States, about 13 to 14 million people have evidence of ARMD, and almost 30 percent of those over the age of seventy-five are affected. With regard to cataract development, with age, virtually everybody will develop some degree of oxidative damage to the lenses of their eyes (the first step in cataract development).

The macula is a specialized region in the back of the eye (retina) that allows you to see fine details. As cells in the macula region begin to break down, you begin to lose sight in the center of your field of vision and may develop problems seeing in bright or dark conditions. In addition to sunlight exposure, age, smoking, and diet have been identified as risk factors for ARMD.

Although there isn't much you can do about your age as a risk factor for ARMD or cataracts, you *can* modify your risk from the sun (by wearing UV-blocking sunglasses or wide-brimmed hats), smoking (don't), and diet (consume enough antioxidants). In terms of diet, it is clear that individuals who consume fruits and vegetables at least once per day have a significantly reduced risk of developing ARMD and cataracts. It is also well known that higher levels of antioxidants in the blood are associated with reduced rates of these conditions. Among the dozens of dietary antioxidants, however, carotenoids appear to provide the greatest benefit—two carotenoids in particular, lutein and zeaxanthin, seem to be most effective.

DIETARY SUPPLEMENTS

Lutein—Specific Eye Nutrition

The best dietary sources of antioxidants in general, and carotenoids specifically, are fruits and vegetables—and the more brightly colored, the better. Lutein and zeaxanthin are yellow pigments found in high concentrations in yellow fruits and vegetables (obviously) as well as in dark green, leafy vegetables. In particular, spinach, kale, and collard greens contain high levels of these two carotenoids—so high that individuals with the highest spinach consumption reduce their risk of developing ARMD by almost 90 percent!

Both lutein and zeaxanthin seem to reduce the risk of ARMD and protect overall eye health by at least two different routes. These routes are (1) concentration in the macula, which helps absorb blue light radiation, and (2) general antioxidant function in the retina (not related to light radiation). First, both of these carotenoids are absorbed from the diet into the circulation and eventually end up concentrated specifically in the eye (in the macular region of the retina). It is interesting to note that lutein and zeaxanthin are the only carotenoids known to concentrate specifically in the eye tissues. High levels of these carotenoids in the eye serve to protect tissues by minimizing free radical damage and by absorbing damaging blue light rays. Because the eyes are subjected to such a high degree of oxidizing radiation each day, adequate dietary intake of lutein is a crucial component of providing optimal protection to the delicate tissues of the eye (lutein is only obtained through the diet, while zeaxanthin is theorized to be also produced by conversion from lutein in the eye).

Other Supplements

Aside from the very specific effect of lutein and zeaxanthin on maintaining the integrity of the macular region of the eye, a wide variety of additional antioxidant nutrients can help support other important structures and functions within the eye. For example, development of cataracts (clouding) can occur when proteins in the lens of the eye become damaged by free radicals. In general, the greater your exposure to oxidative damage induced by free radicals (higher in smokers, diabetics, and "sun worshipers"), the greater are your chances to develop cataracts and impaired vision.

The good news, however, is that a number of dietary supplements may be able to offer some degree of protection—especially for individuals who consume low levels of fruits and vegetables (which are rich in antioxidants) and are at an increased risk for developing cataracts later in life.

In the eye, antioxidant vitamins such as C and E, bioflavonoids, beta-carotene, cysteine, and alpha lipoic acid may be especially beneficial in protecting delicate structures from damage as well as promoting repair processes by supporting collagen synthesis. For example, vitamin C levels in the eye are known to decrease somewhat with age—a situation that can reduce capillary integrity and increase the risk of cataracts.

Synthesis of one of the major antioxidant enzymes in the eye, glutathione, can be stimulated by a combination of cysteine, alpha-lipoic acid, and vitamins C and E. Direct supplementation with glutathione does not appear to have the same effect in raising glutathione levels in the tissues (probably due to poor dietary absorption of glutathione supplements and destruction during digestion).

Because B-complex vitamins are involved in amino acid metabolism, riboflavin (B_2) and niacin (B_3) have been suggested as useful support nutrients to help maintain glutathione synthesis. This may be a good recommendation, as deficiency of riboflavin is associated with increased risk of cataracts.

Remember how your mother always told you to eat your carrots for good eyesight? Well, dear old Mom knew what she was talking about. Carrots are a rich source of beta-carotene, which can be converted into vitamin A—both of which can be beneficial for eye health (vitamin A for maintaining night vision and beta-carotene for its antioxidant properties). At least a few small studies have suggested that eating food rich in beta-carotene and vitamin A (carrots, sweet potatoes, cantaloupes) may lower the risk of cataracts.

Bioflavonoids, typically found in blueberries, bilberries, red or purple grapes, citrus fruits, and cranberries, are known to act as powerful antioxidants to help protect the lens of the eye as well as strengthen the collagen-containing structures of the eye such as the cornea and capillaries. One flavonoid in particular, quercetin, can help by inhibiting accumulation of sugar alcohols such as sorbitol in the eyes of diabetics. Bilberry extract is probably the most popular eye supplement (after lutein)—primarily due to its high bioflavonoid content. In addition to its benefits in protecting the eye, bilberry is often touted as a supplement to improve visual acuity in low light conditions (increased ability to see in the dark), although there is little direct evidence to support these claims.

For a list of supplements, see Table 12.1.

KEY POINTS REGARDING DIETARY SUPPLEMENTS FOR EYE HEALTH

- Age-related macular degeneration is the leading cause of blindness in people over age sixty-five.
- ARMD affects approximately 13 to 14 million people in the United States (25 to 40 percent of all people over age sixty-five).
- Females have a higher risk of ARMD than males.
- People with light-colored eyes (blue, green, hazel) have an increased risk of ARMD.
- ARMD and cataract risk are both related to total sunlight exposure, cigarette smoking, and dietary intake of antioxidants.
- Antioxidant-rich fruits and vegetables are linked with lower rates of ARMD and cataracts.
- Among antioxidant nutrients, the carotenoids lutein and zeaxanthin appear to be the most effective in directly protecting eye health, while other antioxidant nutrients, such as bioflavonoids, cysteine, alpha lipoic acid, beta-carotene, and vitamins C and E can provide additional support.
- Lutein and zeaxanthin are the only carotenoids that concentrate specifically in the eye tissues (the macula region of the retina).
- Lutein is theorized to be converted to zeaxanthin in the retina.
- In the macula region of the eye, lutein and zeaxanthin serve to protect eye tissues from free radical damage and from photooxidizing damage of light rays (by filtering blue light).

TABLE 12.1. Dietary Supplements for Eye Health

Ingredient	Dose (per day)	Primary claims/notes
Alpha-lipoic acid	100-300 mg	Glutathione support, can be boosted with added cysteine or NAC
Beta-carotene	5-6 mg	Best as part of a mixed carotenoid blend
Bilberry	100-500 mg	Promotes better night vision—look for anthocyanoside content of 25 percent or more
Bioflavonoids	100-300 mg	Look for extracts standardized for anthocyanidin and/or polyphenol content
Ginkgo biloba	60-120 mg	Look for an extract standardized to at least "24/6"—24 percent flavone glycosides and 6 percent terpene lactones.
Grape seed/pine bark extracts	50-100 mg	General antioxidant benefits
Lutein/zeaxanthin	3-6 mg	Especially for lightly pigmented eyes (blue, green, hazel)
N-acetylcysteine (NAC)	250-1,500 mg	General antioxidant benefit, increases cellular glutathione levels
Quercetin	50-100 mg	General antioxidant benefits
Selenium	70-200 mcg	Look for organic form (selenomethionine) versus inorganic form (sodium selenite)
Vitamin C	200-1,000 mg	Collagen support
Vitamin E	100-800 IU	Look for natural source d-alpha-tocopherol versus synthetic dl-form

ANTIOXIDANTS

What Is It?

The term "antioxidant" refers to the ability possessed by numerous vitamins, minerals, and other phytochemicals to protect against the damaging effects of highly reactive molecules known as free radicals. Free radicals have the ability to chemically react with, and damage, many structures in the body. Particularly susceptible to oxidative damage are the cell membranes of virtually all cells and the very source of our genetic material—DNA. Free radical reactions and oxidative damage have been linked to many of the "diseases of aging" such as heart disease and cancer.

Claims

- Cellular protection
- Antiaging
- Cancer prevention
- Heart disease prevention
- Antiwrinkle (applied topically or taken orally)
- Promotes vision and eyesight
- Enhances immune function

Theory

The free radical theory of aging (and disease promotion) holds that through a gradual accumulation of microscopic damage to our cell membranes, DNA, tissue structures, and enzyme systems, we begin to lose function and are predisposed to disease. In response to free radical exposure, the body increases its production of endogenous antioxidant enzymes (glutathione peroxidase, catalase, superoxide dismutase), but it has been theorized that supplemental levels of dietary antioxidants may be warranted in some situations to help prevent excessive oxidative damage to muscles, mitochondria, and other tissues (such as during or following intense exercise and exposure to pollutants such as secondhand smoke).

Scientific Support

Thousands of studies have clearly documented the beneficial effects of dozens of antioxidant nutrients—and thousands of nutrients and phytochemicals possess significant antioxidant activity in the test tube. Increased dietary intake of antioxidant nutrients such as vitamins C and E, minerals such as selenium, and various phytonutrients such as extracts from grape seed, pine bark, and green tea have all been linked to reduced rates of oxidative damage and may help reduce the incidence of chronic diseases such as heart disease and cancer.

Safety

At the typically recommended levels, the majority of antioxidants appear to be quite safe. For example, vitamin E, one of the most powerful membrane-bound antioxidants, also has one of the best safety profiles. Doses of 100 to 400 IU of vitamin E have been linked to significant cardiovascular benefits with no side effects. Vitamin C, another powerful antioxidant, can help to protect and restore the antioxidant activity of vitamin E and is considered safe up to doses of 500 to 1,000 mg. Higher doses of vitamin C are not recommended because of concerns that such levels may cause an "unbalancing" of the oxidative systems and actually *promote* oxidative damage instead of preventing it. Another popular antioxidant, beta-carotene, is somewhat controversial as a dietary supplement. Although diets high in fruits and vegetables might deliver approximately 5 to 6 mg of carotenes daily, these would be a mixture of beta-carotene and other naturally occurring carotenoids. Concern was raised several years ago by studies in which high-dose beta-carotene supplements appeared to promote lung cancer in heavy smokers. Those studies provided beta-carotene supplements of 20 to 60 mg per day—about five to ten times the levels that could reasonably be expected in the diet.

Value

The four key nutritional antioxidants, vitamins C and E, beta-carotene, and selenium, are well studied, relatively inexpensive, and widely available as dietary supplements. As mentioned, a multitude of fruit and vegetable phytonutrient extracts also possess significant antioxidant activity. In most cases, phytonutrient extracts tend to be quite expensive, although their potent antioxidant activity may allow dosages to be fairly small. Some of the more popular antioxidant nutrients found in commercial dietary supplements also include zinc, copper, *Ginkgo biloba,* grape seed extract, pine bark extract, lycopene, lutein, quercetin, and alpha-lipoic acid as well as dozens of others.

Dosage

- Vitamin E—100 to 400 IU per day
- Vitamin C—250 to 1,000 mg per day
- Beta-carotene—5 to 6 mg per day
- Selenium—70 to 200 mcg per day

WORKS CONSULTED

Applegate E. Effective nutritional ergogenic aids. Int J Sport Nutr. 1999 Jun; 9(2):229-39.

Balakrishnan SD, Anuradha CV. Exercise, depletion of antioxidants and antioxidant manipulation. Cell Biochem Funct. 1998 Dec;16(4):269-75.

Bazzarre TL, Kleiner SM, Ainsworth BE. Vitamin C intake and lipid profiles of competitive male and female bodybuilders. Int J Sport Nutr. 1992 Sep;2(3):260-71.

Brites FD, Evelson PA, Christiansen MG, Nicol MF, Basilico MJ, Wikinski RW, Llesuy SF. Soccer players under regular training show oxidative stress but an improved plasma antioxidant status. Clin Sci (Colch). 1999 Apr;96(4):381-5.

Bruckner G. Microcirculation, vitamin E and omega 3 fatty acids: An overview. Adv Exp Med Biol. 1997;415:195-208.

Bunker VW. Free radicals, antioxidants and ageing. Med Lab Sci. 1992 Dec;49(4):299-312.

Chatard JC, Boutet C, Tourny C, Garcia S, Berthouze S, Guezennec CY. Nutritional status and physical fitness of elderly sportsmen. Eur J Appl Physiol Occup Physiol. 1998;77(1-2):157-63.

Child RB, Wilkinson DM, Fallowfield JL. Resting serum antioxidant status is positively correlated with peak oxygen uptake in endurance trained runners. J Sports Med Phys Fitness. 1999 Dec;39(4):282-4.

Child RB, Wilkinson DM, Fallowfield JL, Donnelly AE. Elevated serum antioxidant capacity and plasma malondialdehyde concentration in response to a simulated half-marathon run. Med Sci Sports Exerc. 1998 Nov;30(11):1603-7.

Clarkson PM. Micronutrients and exercise: Anti-oxidants and minerals. J Sports Sci. 1995 Summer;13 (Spec No):S11-24.

Clarkson PM, Thompson HS. Antioxidants: What role do they play in physical activity and health? Am J Clin Nutr. 2000 Aug;72(2 Suppl):637S-46S.

Davison A, Rousseau E, Dunn B. Putative anticarcinogenic actions of carotenoids: Nutritional implications. Can J Physiol Pharmacol. 1993 Sep;71(9):732-45.

Dragan I, Dinu V, Mohora M, Cristea E, Ploesteanu E, Stroescu V. Studies regarding the antioxidant effects of selenium on top swimmers. Rev Roum Physiol. 1990 Jan-Mar;27(1):15-20.

Dufaux B, Heine O, Kothe A, Prinz U, Rost R. Blood glutathione status following distance running. Int J Sports Med. 1997 Feb;18(2):89-93.

Duthie GG, Robertson JD, Maughan RJ, Morrice PC. Blood antioxidant status and erythrocyte lipid peroxidation following distance running. Arch Biochem Biophys. 1990 Oct;282(1):78-83.

Evans JR, Henshaw K. Antioxidant vitamin and mineral supplementation for preventing age-related macular degeneration. Cochrane Database Syst Rev. 2000;(2):CD000253.

Gerster H. The role of vitamin C in athletic performance. J Am Coll Nutr. 1989 Dec;8(6):636-43.

Ginsburg GS, Agil A, O'Toole M, Rimm E, Douglas PS, Rifai N. Effects of a single bout of ultraendurance exercise on lipid levels and susceptibility of lipids to peroxidation in triathletes. JAMA. 1996 Jul 17;276(3):221-5.

Grievink L, Jansen SM, van't Veer P, Brunekreef B. Acute effects of ozone on pulmonary function of cyclists receiving antioxidant supplements. Occup Environ Med. 1998 Jan;55(1):13-7.

Grievink L, Smit HA, Veer P, Brunekreef B, Kromhout D. Plasma concentrations of the antioxidants beta-carotene and alpha-tocopherol in relation to lung function. Eur J Clin Nutr. 1999 Oct;53(10):813-7.

Grievink L, Zijlstra AG, Ke X, Brunekreef B. Double-blind intervention trial on modulation of ozone effects on pulmonary function by antioxidant supplements. Am J Epidemiol. 1999 Feb 15;149(4):306-14.

Hellsten Y, Apple FS, Sjodin B. Effect of sprint cycle training on activities of antioxidant enzymes in human skeletal muscle. J Appl Physiol. 1996 Oct;81(4):1484-7.

Jenkins DJ. Optimal diet for reducing the risk of arteriosclerosis. Can J Cardiol. 1995 Oct;11(Suppl G):118G-22G.

Ji LL. Oxidative stress during exercise: Implication of antioxidant nutrients. Free Radic Biol Med. 1995 Jun;18(6):1079-86.

Jonat W. Nonhormonal prevention of breast cancer. Med Klin. 2000 Jun;95 (Suppl 1):9-13.

Kaikkonen J, Kosonen L, Nyyssonen K, Porkkala-Sarataho E, Salonen R, Korpela H, Salonen JT. Effect of combined coenzyme Q10 and d-alpha-tocopheryl acetate supplementation on exercise-induced lipid peroxidation and muscular damage: A placebo-controlled double-blind study in marathon runners. Free Radic Res. 1998 Jul;29(1):85-92.

Kanter M. Free radicals, exercise and antioxidant supplementation. Proc Nutr Soc. 1998 Feb;57(1):9-13.

Kostka T, Drai J, Berthouze SE, Lacour JR, Bonnefoy M. Physical activity, fitness and integrated antioxidant system in healthy active elderly women. Int J Sports Med. 1998 Oct;19(7):462-7.

Liu ML, Bergholm R, Makimattila S, Lahdenpera S, Valkonen M, Hilden H, Yki-Jarvinen H, Taskinen MR. A marathon run increases the susceptibility of LDL to oxidation in vitro and modifies plasma antioxidants. Am J Physiol. 1999 Jun; 276(6 Pt 1):E1083-91.

Marzatico F, Pansarasa O, Bertorelli L, Somenzini L, Della Valle G. Blood free radical antioxidant enzymes and lipid peroxides following long-distance and lactacidemic performances in highly trained aerobic and sprint athletes. J Sports Med Phys Fitness. 1997 Dec;37(4):235-9.

McKeown-Eyssen G, Holloway C, Jazmaji V, Bright-See E, Dion P, Bruce WR. A randomized trial of vitamins C and E in the prevention of recurrence of colorectal polyps. Cancer Res. 1988 Aug 15;48(16):4701-5.

Nielsen AN, Mizuno M, Ratkevicius A, Mohr T, Rohde M, Mortensen SA, Quistorff B. No effect of antioxidant supplementation in triathletes on maximal oxygen uptake, 31P-NMRS detected muscle energy metabolism and muscle fatigue. Int J Sports Med. 1999 Apr;20(3):154-8.

Okamura K, Doi T, Hamada K, Sakurai M, Yoshioka Y, Mitsuzono R, Migita T, Sumida S, Sugawa-Katayama Y. Effect of repeated exercise on urinary 8-hydroxy-deoxyguanosine excretion in humans. Free Radic Res. 1997 Jun;26(6):507-14.

Oostenbrug GS, Mensink RP, Hardeman MR, De Vries T, Brouns F, Hornstra G. Exercise performance, red blood cell deformability, and lipid peroxidation: Effects of fish oil and vitamin E. J Appl Physiol. 1997 Sep;83(3):746-52.

Ortenblad N, Madsen K, Djurhuus MS. Antioxidant status and lipid peroxidation after short-term maximal exercise in trained and untrained humans. Am J Physiol. 1997 Apr;272(4 Pt 2):R1258-63.

Peters EM, Goetzsche JM, Grobbelaar B, Noakes TD. Vitamin C supplementation reduces the incidence of postrace symptoms of upper-respiratory-tract infection in ultramarathon runners. Am J Clin Nutr. 1993 Feb;57(2):170-4.

Pierson WE, Covert DS, Koenig JQ, Namekata T, Kim YS. Implications of air pollution effects on athletic performance. Med Sci Sports Exerc. 1986 Jun; 18(3):322-7.

Pincemail J, Lecomte J, Castiau J, Collard E, Vasankari T, Cheramy-Bien J, Limet R, Defraigne J. Evaluation of autoantibodies against oxidized LDL and antioxidant status in top soccer and basketball players after 4 months of competition. Free Radic Biol Med. 2000 Feb 15;28(4):559-65.

Powers SK, Hamilton K. Antioxidants and exercise. Clin Sports Med. 1999 Jul;18(3):525-36.

Rautalahti M, Huttunen J. Antioxidants and carcinogenesis. Ann Med. 1994 Dec;26(6):435-41.

Rokitzki L, Hinkel S, Klemp C, Cufi D, Keul J. Dietary, serum and urine ascorbic acid status in male athletes. Int J Sports Med. 1994 Oct;15(7):435-40.

Rokitzki L, Logemann E, Huber G, Keck E, Keul J. alpha-Tocopherol supplementation in racing cyclists during extreme endurance training. Int J Sport Nutr. 1994 Sep;4(3):253-64.

Sanchez-Quesada JL, Jorba O, Payes A, Otal C, Serra-Grima R, Gonzalez-Sastre F, Ordonez-Llanos J. Ascorbic acid inhibits the increase in low-density lipoprotein (LDL) susceptibility to oxidation and the proportion of electronegative LDL induced by intense aerobic exercise. Coron Artery Dis. 1998;9(5):249-55.

Schroder H, Navarro E, Tramullas A, Mora J, Galiano D. Nutrition antioxidant status and oxidative stress in professional basketball players: Effects of a three compound antioxidative supplement. Int J Sports Med. 2000 Feb;21(2):146-50.

Taylor PR, Li B, Dawsey SM, Li JY, Yang CS, Guo W, Blot WJ. Prevention of esophageal cancer: The nutrition intervention trials in Linxian, China. Linxian Nutrition Intervention Trials Study Group. Cancer Res. 1994 Apr 1;54(7 Suppl):2029S-31S.

Tiidus PM. Radical species in inflammation and overtraining. Can J Physiol Pharmacol. 1998 May;76(5):533-8.

Tiidus PM, Houston ME. Vitamin E status and response to exercise training. Sports Med. 1995 Jul;20(1):12-23.

Tiidus PM, Pushkarenko J, Houston ME. Lack of antioxidant adaptation to short-term aerobic training in human muscle. Am J Physiol. 1996 Oct;271(4 Pt 2): R832-6.

Vasankari TJ, Kujala UM, Rusko H, Sarna S, Ahotupa M. The effect of endurance exercise at moderate altitude on serum lipid peroxidation and antioxidative functions in humans. Eur J Appl Physiol Occup Physiol. 1997;75(5):396-9.

Vasankari T, Kujala U, Sarna S, Ahotupa M. Effects of ascorbic acid and carbohydrate ingestion on exercise induced oxidative stress. J Sports Med Phys Fitness. 1998 Dec;38(4):281-5.

Vasankari TJ, Kujala UM, Vasankari TM, Vuorimaa T, Ahotupa M. Increased serum and low-density-lipoprotein antioxidant potential after antioxidant supplementation in endurance athletes. Am J Clin Nutr. 1997 Apr;65(4):1052-6.

Ward JA. Should antioxidant vitamins be routinely recommended for older people? Drugs Aging. 1998 Mar;12(3):169-75.

Williams MH. Vitamin supplementation and athletic performance. Int J Vitam Nutr Res Suppl. 1989;30:163-91.

Woteki CE. Applications of antioxidants in physiologically functional foods. Consumption, intake patterns, and exposure. Crit Rev Food Sci Nutr. 1995 Jan;35(1-2):143-7.

Yu BP, Kang CM, Han JS, Kim DS. Can antioxidant supplementation slow the aging process? Biofactors. 1998;7(1-2):93-101.

LUTEIN/ZEAXANTHIN

What Is It?

Lutein and zeaxanthin are carotenoids found in highest concentrations in the macular region of the eyes (the back of the eye where the retina is located), where they are believed to help filter out damaging blue light and prevent free radical damage to the delicate structures in the back of the eye.

Claims

- Prevents age-related macular degeneration (ARMD)
- May help prevent glaucoma and cataracts
- Supports normal eye health
- Antioxidant

Theory

Anybody who spends time outdoors exposed to the sun should be concerned with the potential for ultraviolet radiation to damage eye health and impact vision. Antioxidants can provide increased protection against the oxidizing ultraviolet radiation of the sun. Lutein and zeaxanthin are the only carotenoids that become concentrated in the retinal region of the eye, known as the macula. High dietary intake of lutein-rich fruits and vegetables has been associated with a significant reduction in macular degeneration, the leading cause of blindness in Americans over the age of sixty-five.

Scientific Support

It is thought that a low macular pigment density may increase the risk of ARMD and cataracts (by allowing more damage from blue light). Several observational studies have shown that high dietary intakes of lutein and zeaxanthin (from spinach, broccoli, and eggs) are associated with a significant reduction in the risk for cataracts (up to 20 percent) and for age-related macular degeneration (up to 40 percent). One study has shown that dietary supplementation with lutein (30 mg per day for 140 days) ele-

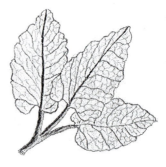

Spinach

vates serum lutein levels by ten times, increases macular pigment density by 20 to 40 percent, and reduces transmission of blue light to the eye's photoreceptors by 30 to 40 percent. Another study showed that daily egg yolk consumption can increase plasma levels of lutein by 28 to 50 percent and zeaxanthin by 114 to 142 percent. A multicenter clinical study (Eye Disease Case-Control Study) compared 356 patients with advanced ARMD (ages fifty-five to eighty years) to 520 control subjects—finding that the risk for ARMD was reduced by over 40 percent by a high dietary intake of carotenoids. In particular, both lutein and zeaxanthin were strongly associated with a reduced risk for macular degeneration.

Safety

No known adverse side effects are associated with dietary supplements containing lutein or zeaxanthin when used at recommended levels. Most supplements should be taken with a meal to lessen the chance of causing stomach upset and to increase their digestion and absorption (bioavailability).

Value

Dietary supplements containing lutein and zeaxanthin are available from a number of manufacturers as an alternative for people not able or willing to increase their vegetable consumption. When choosing a supplement, be sure to select one that delivers an effective level of lutein (about 4 to 6 mg per day). Lutein is now being added to national brands of multivitamins— but most provide only 250 mcg or less of lutein, or more than twenty times less than the levels shown to be effective in preventing ARMD and even several times below levels that could reasonably be achieved in the diet from a high intake of fruits and vegetables.

Dosage

From studies of ARMD rates and dietary intake, it appears that diets providing about 6 mg of lutein per day can reduce ARMD prevalence by nearly half. Eating more carotenoid-rich foods should be your first step to increase lutein intake. Unfortunately, recent diet surveys have indicated that consumption of these foods has dropped more than 20 percent in the two groups at highest risk for ARMD (women and elderly). As many carotenoids are rapidly cleared from the body, you may also want to consider splitting your daily intake into two doses (3 mg with breakfast and 3 mg with dinner).

WORKS CONSULTED

Bone RA, Landrum JT, Dixon Z, Chen Y, Llerena CM. Lutein and zeaxanthin in the eyes, serum and diet of human subjects. Exp Eye Res. 2000 Sep;71(3):239-45.

Bone RA, Landrum JT, Friedes LM, Gomez CM, Kilburn MD, Menendez E, Vidal I, Wang W. Distribution of lutein and zeaxanthin stereoisomers in the human retina. Exp Eye Res. 1997 Feb;64(2):211-8.

Castenmiller JJ, West CE, Linssen JP, van het Hof KH, Voragen AG. The food matrix of spinach is a limiting factor in determining the bioavailability of beta-carotene and to a lesser extent of lutein in humans. J Nutr. 1999 Feb;129(2):349-55.

Dugas TR, Morel DW, Harrison EH. Dietary supplementation with beta-carotene, but not with lycopene, inhibits endothelial cell-mediated oxidation of low-density lipoprotein. Free Radic Biol Med. 1999 May;26(9-10):1238-44.

Hammond BR Jr, Curran-Celentano J, Judd S, Fuld K, Krinsky NI, Wooten BR, Snodderly DM. Sex differences in macular pigment optical density: Relation to plasma carotenoid concentrations and dietary patterns. Vision Res. 1996 Jul;36(13):2001-12.

Hammond BR Jr, Johnson EJ, Russell RM, Krinsky NI, Yeum KJ, Edwards RB, Snodderly DM. Dietary modification of human macular pigment density. Invest Ophthalmol Vis Sci. 1997 Aug;38(9):1795-801.

Handelman GJ, Nightingale ZD, Lichtenstein AH, Schaefer EJ, Blumberg JB. Lutein and zeaxanthin concentrations in plasma after dietary supplementation with egg yolk. Am J Clin Nutr. 1999 Aug;70(2):247-51.

Jewell C, O'Brien NM. Effect of dietary supplementation with carotenoids on xenobiotic metabolizing enzymes in the liver, lung, kidney and small intestine of the rat. Br J Nutr. 1999 Mar;81(3):235-42.

Johnson EJ, Hammond BR, Yeum KJ, Qin J, Wang XD, Castaneda C, Snodderly DM, Russell RM. Relation among serum and tissue concentrations of lutein and zeaxanthin and macular pigment density. Am J Clin Nutr. 2000 Jun;71(6):1555-62.

Kim HW, Chew BP, Wong TS, Park JS, Weng BB, Byrne KM, Hayek MG, Reinhart GA. Dietary lutein stimulates immune response in the canine. Vet Immunol Immunopathol. 2000 May 23;74(3-4):315-27.

Kim HW, Chew BP, Wong TS, Park JS, Weng BB, Byrne KM, Hayek MG, Reinhart GA. Modulation of humoral and cell-mediated immune responses by dietary lutein in cats. Vet Immunol Immunopathol. 2000 Mar 15;73(3-4):331-41.

Landrum JT, Bone RA, Joa H, Kilburn MD, Moore LL, Sprague KE. A one year study of the macular pigment: The effect of 140 days of a lutein supplement. Exp Eye Res. 1997 Jul;65(1):57-62.

Michaud DS, Feskanich D, Rimm EB, Colditz GA, Speizer FE, Willett WC, Giovannucci E. Intake of specific carotenoids and risk of lung cancer in 2 prospective US cohorts. Am J Clin Nutr. 2000 Oct;72(4):990-7.

Moeller SM, Jacques PF, Blumberg JB. The potential role of dietary xanthophylls in cataract and age-related macular degeneration. J Am Coll Nutr. 2000 Oct; 19(5 Suppl):522S-7S.

Muller H, Bub A, Watzl B, Rechkemmer G. Plasma concentrations of carotenoids in healthy volunteers after intervention with carotenoid-rich foods. Eur J Nutr. 1999 Feb;38(1):35-44.

Paiva SA, Yeum KJ, Cao G, Prior RL, Russell RM. Postprandial plasma carotenoid responses following consumption of strawberries, red wine, vitamin C or spinach by elderly women. J Nutr. 1998 Dec;128(12):2391-4.

Park JS, Chew BP, Wong TS, Zhang JX, Magnuson NS. Dietary lutein but not astaxanthin or beta-carotene increases pim-1 gene expression in murine lymphocytes. Nutr Cancer. 1999;33(2):206-12.

Pratt S. Dietary prevention of age-related macular degeneration. J Am Optom Assoc. 1999 Jan;70(1):39-47.

Richer S. ARMD—pilot (case series) environmental intervention data. J Am Optom Assoc. 1999 Jan;70(1):24-36.

Roodenburg AJ, Leenen R, van het Hof KH, Weststrate JA, Tijburg LB. Amount of fat in the diet affects bioavailability of lutein esters but not of alpha-carotene, beta-carotene, and vitamin E in humans. Am J Clin Nutr. 2000 May;71(5):1187-93.

Rumi G Jr, Szabo I, Vincze A, Matus Z, Toth G, Rumi G, Mozsik G. Decrease in serum levels of vitamin A and zeaxanthin in patients with colorectal polyp. Eur J Gastroenterol Hepatol. 1999 Mar;11(3):305-8.

Seddon JM, Ajani UA, Sperduto RD, Hiller R, Blair N, Burton TC, Farber MD, Gragoudas ES, Haller J, Miller DT, et al. Dietary carotenoids, vitamins A, C, and E, and advanced age-related macular degeneration. Eye Disease Case-Control Study Group. JAMA. 1994 Nov 9;272(18):1413-20.

Sommerburg O, Keunen JE, Bird AC, van Kuijk FJ. Fruits and vegetables that are sources for lutein and zeaxanthin: The macular pigment in human eyes. Br J Ophthalmol. 1998 Aug;82(8):907-10.

Sommerburg OG, Siems WG, Hurst JS, Lewis JW, Kliger DS, van Kuijk FJ. Lutein and zeaxanthin are associated with photoreceptors in the human retina. Curr Eye Res. 1999 Dec;19(6):491-5.

van het Hof KH, Brouwer IA, West CE, Haddeman E, Steegers-Theunissen RP, van Dusseldorp M, Weststrate JA, Eskes TK, Hautvast JG. Bioavailability of lutein from vegetables is 5 times higher than that of beta-carotene. Am J Clin Nutr. 1999 Aug;70(2):261-8.

Voorrips LE, Goldbohm RA, Brants HA, van Poppel GA, Sturmans F, Hermus RJ, van den Brandt PA. A prospective cohort study on antioxidant and folate intake and male lung cancer risk. Cancer Epidemiol Biomarkers Prev. 2000 Apr;9(4):357-65.

ALPHA-LIPOIC ACID

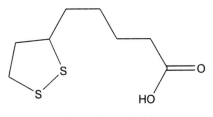

Alpha-Lipoic Acid

What Is It?

Alpha-lipoic acid is a compound found in the mitochondria—the energy-producing structures found in our cells. As a dietary supplement, alpha-lipoic acid may act as a powerful antioxidant, where it may work in synergy with other nutritional antioxidants such as vitamins C and E.

Claims

- Prevents cellular damage (from free radicals)
- Reduces oxidative stress
- Lowers blood sugar
- Increases energy levels

Theory

Although alpha-lipoic acid is involved in cellular energy production, its chief role as a dietary supplement may be as a powerful antioxidant. The body appears to be able to manufacture enough alpha-lipoic acid for its metabolic functions (as a cofactor for a number of enzymes involved in converting fat and sugar to energy), but the excess levels provided by supplements allow alpha-lipoic acid to circulate in a free state. In this state, alpha-lipoic acid has functions as both a water- and fat-soluble antioxidant. This unique ability of alpha-lipoic acid to be active in both water and lipid compartments of the body is important because most antioxidants, such as vitamins C and E, are effective in only one area or the other. For instance, vitamin C is usually restricted to the interior compartment of cells and the aqueous ("watery") portion of blood, while vitamin E embeds itself in the lipid ("fatty") portion of cell membranes. Adding to the potential importance of alpha-lipoic acid is its role in the production of glutathione, one of the chief anti-oxidants produced directly by the body.

Scientific Support

In animal studies, alpha-lipoic acid supplementation has been shown to improve several indices of metabolic activity and lower the degree of oxidative stress. Alpha-lipoic acid supplementation may also help to reverse the decline in mitochondrial energy production that is commonly observed during the normal aging process. Activity levels can be increased approximately threefold in animals supplemented with alpha-lipoic acid, suggesting a beneficial effect on energy metabolism. Levels of other antioxidants, such as glutathione and ascorbic acid, are also elevated in animals consuming alpha-lipoic acid, suggesting that the supplement may help protect and/or recycle these antioxidants and contribute to the overall capacity of the body to neutralize free radical damage.

In conjunction with other antioxidants, such as vitamin E, alpha-lipoic acid may be doubly helpful in patients with diabetes. By promoting the production of energy from fat and sugar in the mitochondria, glucose removal from the bloodstream may be enhanced and insulin function improved. Indeed, alpha-lipoic acid has been shown to decrease insulin resistance and is prescribed frequently in Europe as a treatment for peripheral neuropathy (nerve damage) associated with diabetes. In the United States, the American Diabetes Association has suggested that alpha-lipoic acid plus vitamin E may be helpful in combating some of the health complications associated with diabetes, including heart disease, vision problems, nerve damage, and kidney disease. Alpha-lipoic acid also may be involved in helping to protect the brain from damage following a stroke.

Safety

Although relatively few studies have been conducted with alpha-lipoic acid in humans, it appears to be safe as a dietary supplement. Intakes of as much as 600 mg per day have been used for treatment of diabetic neuropathy with no serious side effects.

Value

If alpha-lipoic acid were just another antioxidant, then its value would be far less. After all, there are dozens of ingredients on the market that have powerful antioxidant functions. The unique qualities possessed by alpha-lipoic acid, functioning as both a water- and fat-soluble antioxidant, as well as its role in increasing the overall function of other dietary antioxidants make it an intriguing supplement worthy of serious consideration.

Dosage

General recommendations for antioxidant benefits typically call for 50 to 100 mg per day.

WORKS CONSULTED

Arivazhagan P, Panneerselvam C. Effect of DL-alpha-lipoic acid on neural antioxidants in aged rats. Pharmacol Res. 2000 Sep;42(3):219-22.

Biewenga GP, Haenen GR, Bast A. The pharmacology of the antioxidant lipoic acid. Gen Pharmacol. 1997 Sep;29(3):315-31.

Dovinova I. Alpha-lipoic acid—a natural disulfide cofactor and antioxidant with anticarcinogenic effects. Ceska Slov Farm. 1996 Sep;45(5):237-41.

Hagen TM, Ingersoll RT, Lykkesfeldt J, Liu J, Wehr CM, Vinarsky V, Bartholomew JC, Ames AB. (R)-alpha-lipoic acid-supplemented old rats have improved mitochondrial function, decreased oxidative damage, and increased metabolic rate. FASEB J. 1999 Feb;13(2):411-8.

Khanna S, Atalay M, Lodge JK, Laaksonen DE, Roy S, Hanninen O, Packer L, Sen CK. Skeletal muscle and liver lipoyllysine content in response to exercise, training and dietary alpha-lipoic acid supplementation. Biochem Mol Biol Int. 1998 Oct;46(2):297-306.

Konrad T, Vicini P, Kusterer K, Hoflich A, Assadkhani A, Bohles HJ, Sewell A, Tritschler HJ, Cobelli C, Usadel KH. Alpha-lipoic acid treatment decreases serum lactate and pyruvate concentrations and improves glucose effectiveness in lean and obese patients with type 2 diabetes. Diabetes Care. 1999 Feb;22(2):280-7.

Nickander KK, McPhee BR, Low PA, Tritschler H. Alpha-lipoic acid: Antioxidant potency against lipid peroxidation of neural tissues in vitro and implications for diabetic neuropathy. Free Radic Biol Med. 1996;21(5):631-9.

Packer L. Alpha-lipoic acid: A metabolic antioxidant which regulates NF-kappa B signal transduction and protects against oxidative injury. Drug Metab Rev. 1998 May;30(2):245-75.

Packer L, Tritschler HJ, Wessel K. Neuroprotection by the metabolic antioxidant alpha-lipoic acid. Free Radic Biol Med. 1997;22(1-2):359-78.

Packer L, Witt EH, Tritschler HJ. Alpha-lipoic acid as a biological antioxidant. Free Radic Biol Med. 1995 Aug;19(2):227-50.

Panigrahi M, Sadguna Y, Shivakumar BR, Kolluri SV, Roy S, Packer L, Ravindranath V. Alpha-lipoic acid protects against reperfusion injury following cerebral ischemia in rats. Brain Res. 1996 Apr 22;717(1-2):184-8.

Podda M, Tritschler HJ, Ulrich H, Packer L. Alpha-lipoic acid supplementation prevents symptoms of vitamin E deficiency. Biochem Biophys Res Commun. 1994 Oct 14;204(1):98-104.

Roy S, Sen CK, Tritschler HJ, Packer L. Modulation of cellular reducing equivalent homeostasis by alpha-lipoic acid. Mechanisms and implications for diabetes and ischemic injury. Biochem Pharmacol. 1997 Feb 7;53(3):393-9.

Scholz RW, Reddy PV, Wynn MK, Graham KS, Liken AD, Gumpricht E, Reddy CC. Glutathione-dependent factors and inhibition of rat liver microsomal lipid peroxidation. Free Radic Biol Med. 1997;23(5):815-28.

Serbinova E, Khwaja S, Reznick AZ, Packer L. Thioctic acid protects against ischemia-reperfusion injury in the isolated perfused Langendorff heart. Free Radic Res Commun. 1992;17(1):49-58.

Vasdev S, Ford CA, Parai S, Longerich L, Gadag V. Dietary alpha-lipoic acid supplementation lowers blood pressure in spontaneously hypertensive rats. J Hypertens. 2000 May;18(5):567-73.

Ziegler D, Gries FA. Alpha-lipoic acid in the treatment of diabetic peripheral and cardiac autonomic neuropathy. Diabetes. 1997 Sep;46 (Suppl 2):S62-6.

BILBERRY/BLUEBERRY

What Is It?

Bilberries are basically the European version of the American blueberry. Bilberries are grown in Europe, Canada, and the United States, and extracts of the ripe berry contain flavonoid pigments known as anthocyanins, which act as powerful antioxidants. For you history buffs, some of the mythology behind eating bilberries to promote good vision originated during World War II when English bomber pilots reported an increase in their night vision after eating bilberry jam. Bilberry extracts are now promoted for a number of vision and vein health benefits such as diabetic retinopathy, cataracts, glaucoma, macular degeneration, varicose veins, and hemorrhoids. Commercial supplements are typically standardized to at least 25 percent anthocyanosides.

Claims

- Strengthens capillaries
- Reduces bruising and promotes wound healing
- Promotes good vision
- Prevents diabetic retinopathy and cataracts
- Prevents varicose veins and hemorrhoids

Theory

Bilberries are a rich source of anthocyanosides, compounds that possess potent antioxidant properties which can protect capillaries from free radical damage. Because capillary damage is a primary factor in a number of diseases such as diabetic retinopathy, glaucoma, and cataracts, bilberry extracts are often promoted as a way to protect against these problems. Anthocyanosides may also promote the formation of connective tissue through their protective effects on collagen synthesis and repair and thus may also improve vascular circulation.

Scientific Support

A number of venous disorders have been treated with bilberry extracts, showing anti-inflammatory benefits and reduction in hemorrhoidal symptoms. Improved visual acuity has been noted in anecdotal reports of night vision (as in the bomber pilot story) and diabetic retinopathy. A 20 percent reduction in capillary lesions was noted in one study following daily intake of 600 mg of bilberry extract for six months.

As for the most frequent product claims of improved visual acuity attributed to either blueberry or bilberry extract, one study investigated the effect of bilberry on night visual acuity and night contrast sensitivity. Each phase of the double-blind, placebo-controlled, crossover design lasted three weeks (with a four-week washout period) and looked at fifteen young males with good vision (eight received placebo and seven received bilberry). Subjects consumed three bilberry capsules (or placebo) daily, with each bilberry capsule providing 160 mg of extract and 25 percent anthocyanosides (comparable to commercially available supplements). Results showed no differences in visual acuity or contrast sensitivity—and call into doubt many of the anecdotal reports of bilberry supplementation (at these doses, 480 mg per day) as an aid for improving various aspects of vision.

Safety

Under recommended intakes, bilberry extract is safe. In some cases, it may even be recommended for use during pregnancy for prevention and treatment of varicose veins and hemorrhoids. *All* women, however, who are pregnant or breast-feeding should check with their personal physician before taking this, or any, dietary supplement.

Value

Bilberry extract, as a stand-alone supplement, probably does not offer a great deal of value as a powerful eye health supplement, but it may be viewed as a nice addition to a blend of other ingredients with stronger evidence of benefits for eye health (such as lutein).

Dosage

You can get all the anthocyanins you need by eating ½ to 1 cup of fresh bilberries or blueberries with your breakfast. Standardized extracts are often more convenient, and doses should approximate 100 to 500 mg per day (25 percent anthocyanosides), taken in two to three divided doses.

WORKS CONSULTED

Bomser J, Madhavi DL, Singletary K, Smith MA. In vitro anticancer activity of fruit extracts from Vaccinium species. Planta Med. 1996 Jun;62(3):212-6.

Cantarelli G, Panelli M. Isolation of bilberry anthocyanines and their pharmacologic activity. Boll Chim Farm. 1968 Dec;107(12):792-6.

Fraisse D, Carnat A, Lamaison JL. Polyphenolic composition of the leaf of bilberry. Ann Pharm Fr. 1996;54(6):280-3.

Friedrich H, Schonert J. Tannin-producing substances in the leaves and fruits of the bilberry. Arch Pharm (Weinheim). 1973 Aug;306(8):611-8.

Hakkinen SH, Karenlampi SO, Heinonen IM, Mykkanen HM, Torronen AR. Content of the flavonols quercetin, myricetin, and kaempferol in 25 edible berries. J Agric Food Chem. 1999 Jun;47(6):2274-9.

Hakkinen SH, Karenlampi SO, Mykkanen HM, Torronen AR. Influence of domestic processing and storage on flavonol contents in berries. J Agric Food Chem. 2000 Jul;48(7):2960-5.

Ichiyanagi T, Tateyama C, Oikawa K, Konishi T. Comparison of anthocyanin distribution in different blueberry sources by capillary zone electrophoresis. Biol Pharm Bull. 2000 Apr;23(4):492-7.

Muth ER, Laurent JM, Jasper P. The effect of bilberry nutritional supplementation on night visual acuity and contrast sensitivity. Altern Med Rev. 2000 Apr;5(2):164-73.

Petri G, Krawczyk U, Kery A. Spectrophotometric and chromatographic investigation of bilberry anthocyanins for qualification purposes. Acta Pharm Hung. 1994 Jul;64(4):117-22.

Schonert J, Friedrich H. Determination of tannin in leaves of bilberry. Pharmazie. 1970 Dec;25(12):775-6.

Tolan L, Barna V, Szigeti I, Tecsa D, Gavris C, Csernatony O, Buchwald I. The use of bilberry powder in dyspepsia in infants. Pediatria (Bucur). 1969 Jul-Aug;18(4):375-9.

Zaitsev AN, Sorokina EI, Aksiuk IN, Levin LG. Cranberries: Chemical composition, nutritional and medicinal properties. Vopr Pitan. 1997;(2):38-40.

BETA-CAROTENE

What Is It?

Beta-carotene is part of a large family of compounds known as carotenoids (which includes over 600 members such as lycopene and lutein). Carotenoids are widely distributed in fruits and vegetables and are responsible, along with flavonoids, for contributing the color to many plants (a rule of thumb is the brighter the fruit or vegetable, the higher the content of flavonoids and carotenoids). In terms of nutrition, beta-carotene's primary role is as a precursor to vitamin A (the body can convert beta-carotene into vitamin A as it is needed). It is important to note that beta-carotene and vitamin A are often described in the same breath, almost as if they were the same compound (they are not). Although beta-carotene can be converted to vitamin A in the body, there are important differences in terms of action and safety between the two compounds. Beta-carotene, like most carotenoids, is also a powerful antioxidant—so it has been recommended to protect against a variety of diseases such as cancer, cataracts, and heart disease. The best food sources are brightly colored fruits and veggies such as cantaloupe, apricots, carrots, red peppers, sweet potatoes, and dark leafy greens.

Claims

- Antioxidant
- Cancer prevention
- Skin protection (from sunburns)
- Heart disease prevention
- Prevention of cataracts and macular degeneration

Theory

Evidence from population studies suggests that mixed sources of carotenoids from foods (eating lots of fruits and veggies) can help protect against many forms of cancer and heart disease as well as slow the progression of eye diseases such as cataracts and macular degeneration. As an antioxidant, it is logical (perhaps) to assume that beta-carotene (which is the primary carotenoid in the

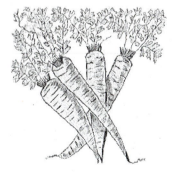

diet) may be responsible for a significant portion of the observed beneficial health effects of carotenoid-rich diets.

Scientific Support

It is important to note that the vast majority of the scientific evidence for the health benefits of beta-carotene comes from studies that looked at *food* sources of beta-carotene (and other carotenoids, often referred to as "mixed" carotenoids)—not supplements. From population (epidemiological) studies, we know that a high consumption of fruits and vegetables is associated with a significant reduction in many diseases, especially several forms of cancer (lung, stomach, colon, breast, prostate, and bladder). Because the data suggested that the active components in a plant-based diet may be carotenoids, and because beta-carotene is the chief carotenoid in our diets, it was widely believed (until about the mid-1990s) that the majority of the health benefits attributable to fruits and vegetables may be due to beta-carotene.

One of the largest epidemiological studies, the Physicians' Health Study (PHS—over 22,000 male physicians) found that while high levels of carotenoids obtained from the diet were associated with reduced cancer risk, beta-carotene from supplements (about 25 mg per day) had no effect on cancer risk. A possible explanation for this finding may be that while purified beta-carotene may contribute some antioxidant benefits, a blend of carotenoids (and/or other compounds in fruits and veggies) is probably even more important for preventing cancer. It may even be possible that isolated beta-carotene supplements could interfere with absorption or metabolism of other beneficial carotenoids from the diet.

Unfortunately, intervention studies that have looked at purified beta-carotene supplements (not mixed carotenoids) have not cleared up any of the confusion. In 1994, the results from a large (almost 30,000 subjects) supplementation study (ATBC, the Alpha-Tocopherol and Beta-Carotene study) showed not only that beta-carotene supplements (20 mg per day for five to eight years) did *not* prevent lung cancer in high-risk subjects (long-time male smokers), they actually caused an increase in lung cancer risk by almost 20 percent. The same study also found a 10 percent increase in heart disease and a 20 percent increase in strokes among the beta-carotene users. In 1996, another large study (CARET, the Beta-Carotene and Retinol Efficacy Trial) found virtually the same thing—subjects receiving beta-carotene showed almost 50 percent more cases of lung cancer. These results were so alarming that the National Cancer Institute decided to halt the $40 million study nearly two years early. The ATBC study examined long-time heavy smokers, while the CARET study looked at present and former smokers as well as workers exposed to asbestos, all of which can be considered high-risk populations for developing lung cancer (which may or may not have contributed to the surprising study results).

On the positive side, beta-carotene has been successfully used for nearly twenty years to treat photosensitivity diseases, such as erythropoietic protoporphyria (EPP) and other skin conditions. As such, beta-carotene has found its way into a variety of topical and internally consumed products meant for skin protection. In Europe, one of the most popular uses for carotenoid supplements (primarily beta-carotene and lycopene) is for skin protection during the summer sunbathing months (for "inside-out" sun protection).

Overall, it is interesting to note that of the three large-scale clinical trials on beta-carotene supplementation and cancer risk (ATBC, CARET, and PHS), all three concluded that beta-carotene provided no protection against lung cancer, while two of them found a *higher* risk for lung cancer. However, the association between eating a diet high in fruits and vegetables and a reduced risk for cancer and heart disease remains strong—and there is no current evidence that small amounts of supplemental beta-carotene (such as a multivitamin) is unsafe. A prudent approach to carotenoid supplementation for disease prevention may be to strive to obtain a balanced blend of mixed carotenoids from foods, while reserving purified beta-carotene supplements for skin protection and as a source of vitamin A (see Dosage).

Safety

At recommended dosages, beta-carotene is thought to be quite safe—although at least two large studies have shown that high-dose beta-carotene (20 to 50 mg per day) can increase the risk of heart disease and cancer in smokers. Other reported side effects from high dose beta-carotene supplements (100,000 IU or 60 mg per day) include nausea, diarrhea, and a yellow-orange tinge to the skin (especially hands and feet), which fades at lower doses of beta-carotene. The safest way to get your beta-carotene and other carotenoids is from eating a wide variety of fruits and vegetables.

Value

Beta-carotene supplements are relatively inexpensive and widely available, from synthetic and natural sources. The natural forms typically come from algae *(Dunaliella salina),* fungi *(Blakeslea trispora),* or palm oil. In terms of conversion to vitamin A, the *trans-* form of beta-carotene has the maximum conversion rate. Synthetic beta-carotene is nearly all in the *trans-*form (98 percent), while natural forms vary in the form of beta-carotene that they provide (the different forms are known as isomers). Among natural forms of beta-carotene, the fungal form provides the highest concentration of *trans*-beta-carotene (94 percent), followed by algae sources (64 percent) and palm oil sources (34 percent)—so from the perspective of vitamin A conversion, either the synthetic form or the fungal form of beta-carotene will provide the highest conversion into active vitamin A. For mixed carotenoids, however, beta-carotene derived from algae also provides the *cis*-isomer of beta-carotene (about 31 percent) as well as alpha-carotene (3 to 4 percent) and other carotenoids (1 to 2 percent). Beta-carotene derived from palm oil provides the most balanced mixture of carotenoid isomers (34 percent *trans*-beta, 27 percent *cis*-beta, 30 percent alpha, and 9 percent other carotenoids), but it also has the lowest vitamin A conversion (because it only provides 34 percent as the *trans-* form).

Based on current scientific evidence, beta-carotene supplements should be utilized and recommended primarily as a way to supply adequate levels of vitamin A for proper nutrition—*not* for prevention of cancer, heart disease, or eye problems (although a dietary level of mixed carotenoids of up to 10 mg per day probably poses no significant health risk). There may also be some benefit in consuming beta-carotene supplements for skin protection, but this effect may be more pronounced when taken in conjunction with other antioxidants such as lycopene, selenium, and vitamins C and E.

Dosage

Beta-carotene (the *trans-* form) can be converted to vitamin A (3 mg of beta-carotene supplies 5,000 IU of vitamin A). Although beta-carotene supplements are commonly available in doses of 25,000 IU (15 mg) per day, and many people consume as much as 100,000 IU (60 mg) per day, the current state of the scientific literature does not support doses of beta-carotene much higher than the levels recommended for supplying vitamin A precursors (about 5,000 to 10,000 IU per day of beta-carotene equals 3 to 6 mg).

WORKS CONSULTED

Botterweck AA, van den Brandt PA, Goldbohm RA. Vitamins, carotenoids, dietary fiber, and the risk of gastric carcinoma: Results from a prospective study after 6.3 years of follow-up. Cancer. 2000 Feb 15;88(4):737-48.

Collins AR, Olmedilla B, Southon S, Granado F, Duthie SJ. Serum carotenoids and oxidative DNA damage in human lymphocytes. Carcinogenesis. 1998 Dec;19(12):2159-62.

Comstock GW, Alberg AJ, Huang HY, Wu K, Burke AE, Hoffman SC, Norkus EP, Gross M, Cutler RG, Morris JS, Spate VL, Helzlsouer KJ. The risk of developing lung cancer associated with antioxidants in the blood: Ascorbic acid, carotenoids, alpha-tocopherol, selenium, and total peroxyl radical absorbing capacity. Cancer Epidemiol Biomarkers Prev. 1997 Nov;6(11):907-16.

Daviglus ML, Dyer AR, Persky V, Chavez N, Drum M, Goldberg J, Liu K, Morris DK, Shekelle RB, Stamler J. Dietary beta-carotene, vitamin C, and risk of prostate cancer: Results from the Western Electric Study. Epidemiology. 1996 Sep;7(5):472-7.

Freeman VL, Meydani M, Yong S, Pyle J, Wan Y, Arvizu-Durazo R, Liao Y. Prostatic levels of tocopherols, carotenoids, and retinol in relation to plasma levels and self-reported usual dietary intake. Am J Epidemiol. 2000 Jan 15;151(2):109-18.

Gandini S, Merzenich H, Robertson C, Boyle P. Meta-analysis of studies on breast cancer risk and diet: The role of fruit and vegetable consumption and the intake of associated micronutrients. Eur J Cancer. 2000 Mar;36(5):636-46.

Goodman GE, Thornquist M, Kestin M, Metch B, Anderson G, Omenn GS. The association between participant characteristics and serum concentrations of beta-carotene, retinol, retinyl palmitate, and alpha-tocopherol among participants in the Carotene and Retinol Efficacy Trial (CARET) for prevention of lung cancer. Cancer Epidemiol Biomarkers Prev. 1996 Oct;5(10):815-21.

Jumaan AO, Holmberg L, Zack M, Mokdad AH, Ohlander EM, Wolk A, Byers T. Beta-carotene intake and risk of postmenopausal breast cancer. Epidemiology. 1999 Jan;10(1):49-53.

Pietinen P, Ascherio A, Korhonen P, Hartman AM, Willett WC, Albanes D, Virtamo J. Intake of fatty acids and risk of coronary heart disease in a cohort of Finnish men. The Alpha-Tocopherol, Beta-Carotene Cancer Prevention Study. Am J Epidemiol. 1997 May 15;145(10):876-87.

Pryor WA, Stahl W, Rock CL. Beta carotene: From biochemistry to clinical trials. Nutr Rev. 2000 Feb;58(2 Pt 1):39-53.

Slattery ML, Benson J, Curtin K, Ma KN, Schaeffer D, Potter JD. Carotenoids and colon cancer. Am J Clin Nutr. 2000 Feb;71(2):575-82.

Tornwall ME, Virtamo J, Haukka JK, Aro A, Albanes D, Huttunen JK. Prospective study of diet, lifestyle, and intermittent claudication in male smokers. Am J Epidemiol. 2000 May 1;151(9):892-901.

Vainio H. Chemoprevention of cancer: Lessons to be learned from beta-carotene trials. Toxicol Lett. 2000 Mar 15;112-113:513-7.

van Poppel G. Epidemiological evidence for beta-carotene in prevention of cancer and cardiovascular disease. Eur J Clin Nutr. 1996 Jul;50(Suppl 3):S57-61.

Woutersen RA, Wolterbeek AP, Appel MJ, van den Berg H, Goldbohm RA, Feron VJ. Safety evaluation of synthetic beta-carotene. Crit Rev Toxicol. 1999 Nov; 29(6):515-42.

SELENIUM

What Is It?

Selenium is a trace mineral that is found in supplements in several forms such as sodium selenite, selenomethionine, and high-selenium yeast (which contains selenomethionine). In general, the organic form of selenium (selenomethionine) is absorbed somewhat better than the inorganic (selenite) form. In the body, selenium functions as part of an antioxidant enzyme called glutathione peroxidase as well as being necessary for normal growth and proper utilization of iodine in thyroid function. Selenium also supports the antioxidant effect of vitamin E. The best dietary sources of selenium include nuts, unrefined grains, brown rice, wheat germ, and seafood.

Claims

- Antioxidant
- Cancer prevention
- Prevents heart disease
- Skin protection
- Male fertility and prostate support
- Immune system support

Theory

Population studies in China have shown that people living in areas in which soil is depleted of selenium have higher rates of certain cancers— leading to the obvious suggestion that optimal selenium consumption may help protect against cancer. As part of the antioxidant glutathione peroxidase system, selenium plays a direct role in the body's ability to protect cells from damage by free radicals.

Scientific Support

The strongest scientific evidence for a beneficial effect of selenium supplementation comes from studies of cancer risk. In one of the largest well-controlled studies, 200 mcg of selenium (from high-selenium yeast) was found to reduce the risk of several cancers, including cancer of the prostate (66 percent), colon (50 percent), and lung (40 percent) when compared to a group receiving a placebo. There was no significant difference in the risk of skin cancer between groups (which is what the study was originally designed to look at). A number of animal studies have shown that selenium supplementation can reduce tumor growth in mice and rats.

Safety

Although selenium can be considered quite toxic at high doses, its important role in supporting the body's own internal antioxidant defense systems cannot be disputed. At the recommended dosage, 50 to 200 mcg per day, selenium is considered safe, whereas doses of 900 to 1,000 mcg per day may cause selenium toxicity (nausea, vomiting, depression, irritability, nervousness, skin rashes, and loss of hair and fingernails).

Value

Although most people don't take in enough selenium, gross deficiencies are rare (unless you consume primarily fruits and vegetables grown in selenium-depleted soil). As part of an overall antioxidant support regimen, selenium should be included at 50 to 200 mcg per day. Virtually all multivitamin/mineral products include selenium (even a basic multi should provide 20 mcg or so).

Dosage

The recommended intake (DRI or Dietary Reference Intake) for selenium is 55 to 70 mcg for adults and 65 to 75 mcg for pregnant and nursing women. In most clinical trials of selenium, doses are typically in the range of 100 to 200 mcg per day. Daily selenium intake should be limited to 200 mcg.

WORKS CONSULTED

Comstock GW, Alberg AJ, Huang HY, Wu K, Burke AE, Hoffman SC, Norkus EP, Gross M, Cutler RG, Morris JS, Spate VL, Helzlsouer KJ. The risk of developing lung cancer associated with antioxidants in the blood: Ascorbic acid, carotenoids, alpha-tocopherol, selenium, and total peroxyl radical absorbing capacity. Cancer Epidemiol Biomarkers Prev. 1997 Nov;6(11):907-16.

Dorgan JF, Schatzkin A. Antioxidant micronutrients in cancer prevention. Hematol Oncol Clin North Am. 1991 Feb;5(1):43-68.

Guo WD, Chow WH, Zheng W, Li JY, Blot WJ. Diet, serum markers and breast cancer mortality in China. Jpn J Cancer Res. 1994 Jun;85(6):572-7.

Hughes K, Chua LH, Ong CN. Serum selenium in the general population of Singapore, 1993 to 1995. Ann Acad Med Singapore. 1998 Jul;27(4):520-3.

Knekt P, Jarvinen R, Seppanen R, Rissanen A, Aromaa A, Heinonen OP, Albanes D, Heinonen M, Pukkala E, Teppo L. Dietary antioxidants and the risk of lung cancer. Am J Epidemiol. 1991 Sep 1;134(5):471-9.

Lamberg L. Diet may affect skin cancer prevention. JAMA. 1998 May 13;279(18): 1427-8.

Luoma P. Antioxidants, infections and environmental factors in health and disease in northern Finland. Int J Circumpolar Health. 1998 Jul;57(2-3):109-13.

Stahelin HB. Critical reappraisal of vitamins and trace minerals in nutritional support of cancer patients. Support Care Cancer. 1993 Nov;1(6):295-7.

Taylor PR, Li B, Dawsey SM, Li JY, Yang CS, Guo W, Blot WJ. Prevention of esophageal cancer: The nutrition intervention trials in Linxian, China. Linxian Nutrition Intervention Trials Study Group. Cancer Res. 1994 Apr 1;54(7 Suppl):2029S-31S.

van den Brandt PA, Goldbohm RA, van't Veer P, Bode P, Dorant E, Hermus RJ, Sturmans F. A prospective cohort study on selenium status and the risk of lung cancer. Cancer Res. 1993 Oct 15;53(20):4860-5.

Zhou B, Wang T, Sun G, Guan P, Wu JM. A case-control study of the relationship between dietary factors and risk of lung cancer in women of Shenyang, China. Oncol Rep. 1999 Jan-Feb;6(1):139-43.

POLYPHENOLS/BIOFLAVONOIDS

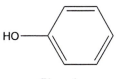

Phenol

What Is It?

Polyphenols are a class of phytochemicals found in high concentrations in wine, tea, grapes, and a wide variety of other plants that have been associated with heart disease and cancer prevention. In general terms, phenolic compounds or polyphenols have a similar basic structural chemistry, including an "aromatic" or "phenolic" ring structure. That said, it is also important to note that at least 8,000 phenolic compounds have already been identified in a dozen chemical subcategories. Phenolic compounds are responsible for the brightly colored pigments of many fruits and vegetables, and they protect plants from diseases and ultraviolet light by helping prevent damage to seeds until they germinate. One of the more nutritionally important classes of polyphenols, the flavonoids, are widely distributed in plant foods and include the following:

- Lignins (nuts, whole-grain cereals)
- Proanthocyanins (grapes, pine bark)
- Anthocyanins/anthocyanidins (brightly colored fruits and vegetables, berries)
- Isoflavones—genistein, daidzein (soybeans)
- Catechins (tea, grapes, wine)
- Tannins (tea, nuts)
- Quercetin (grapes, wine, onions)
- Naringenin/hesperidin (citrus fruits)

Natural polyphenols can range from simple molecules such as phenolic acid to large and highly polymerized compounds such as tannins. Conjugated forms of polyphenols are the most common, in which various sugar molecules, organic acids, and lipids (fats) are linked with the phenolic ring structure. Differences in this conjugated chemical structure account for variations in chemical classification and in mode of action and health properties between the various compounds.

Claims

- Antioxidant
- Cancer prevention
- Protection from heart disease and hypertension
- Antibiotic/antiviral activity
- Anti-inflammatory activity
- Protects and strengthens blood vessels

Theory

Polyphenols, particularly the flavonoids, are among the most potent plant antioxidants. Polyphenols can form complexes with reactive metals such as iron, zinc, and copper—reducing their absorption. At first glance, this may seem to be a negative side effect (reducing nutrient absorption), but excess levels of such elements (metal cations) in the body can promote the generation of free radicals and contribute to the oxidative damage of cell membranes and cellular DNA. In addition to their chelating effect on metal cations, polyphenols also function as potent free radical scavengers within the body, where they can neutralize free radicals before they can cause cellular damage.

Epidemiological studies have shown a relationship between high dietary intakes of phenols (in foods) and reduced risk of cardiovascular disease and cancer. You've undoubtedly heard of the "French paradox," in which regular moderate consumption of red wine (which is rich in polyphenols) is associated with low rates of coronary artery disease. In general, polyphenols (flavonoids) are thought to deliver health benefits by several mechanisms, including the following:

- Direct free radical quenching
- Protection and regeneration of other dietary antioxidants (such as vitamin E)
- Chelation of metal ions

Scientific Support

Numerous in vitro (test-tube) studies have shown that polyphenolic compounds are powerful antioxidants that can protect cell membranes and cellular DNA from the damaging effects of free radical-induced oxidative damage. Several epidemiological studies have indicated that regular consumption of foods rich in polyphenolic compounds (fruits, vegetables, nuts, whole grain cereals, red wine, green tea) is associated with reduced risk of developing cardiovascular disease and certain cancers. Recent experimental studies in both animals and humans have shown that increasing polyphenol intake can protect LDL cholesterol from becoming oxidized (a key step in developing atherosclerosis), lower blood pressure in hypertensive subjects, reduce the tendency of the blood to clot, and elevate total antioxidant capacity of the blood.

Unfortunately, although the epidemiological data for regular fruit and vegetable intake and disease prevention are strong, dietary supplements containing isolated phenolic antioxidants have not been extensively studied in terms of disease prevention. The studies that do exist, however, provide strong indications that such supplements are likely to be beneficial for long-term health by acting as potent antioxidants.

Safety

No significant side effects are evident from regular consumption of polyphenol- or flavonoid-containing dietary supplements.

Value

As general antioxidants, polyphenolic compounds are a useful addition to an overall healthy diet. Whenever possible, it is advisable to obtain the widest possible range of antioxidant compounds from mixed sources such as fruits, vegetables, nuts, and whole grain cereals. Dietary supplements should be added as a second step to broader antioxidant support.

Dosage

Fruits and vegetables can vary significantly in total polyphenol content, depending on the part of the plant used (leaves are highest), cultivation and harvesting methods, degree of ripeness, storage conditions, and processing methods. Dietary recommendations for five or more servings of fruits and vegetables daily would result in a total flavonoid intake of about 150 to 300 mg per day. Supplemental intake should be in this range, and specific recommendations vary depending on the compound in question (e.g., grape seed, pine bark, green tea, etc.).

WORKS CONSULTED

Bravo L. Polyphenols: Chemistry, dietary sources, metabolism, and nutritional significance. Nutr Rev.1998 Nov;56(11):317-33.

Damianaki A, Bakogeorgou E, Kampa M, Notas G, Hatzoglou A, Panagiotou S, Gemetzi C, Kouroumalis E, Martin PM, Castanas E. Potent inhibitory action of red wine polyphenols on human breast cancer cells. J Cell Biochem. 2000 Jun 6;78(3):429-41.

Fuhrman B, Lavy A, Aviram M. Consumption of red wine with meals reduces the susceptibility of human plasma and low-density lipoprotein to lipid peroxidation. Am J Clin Nutr. 1995 Mar;61(3):549-54.

Goldbohm RA, Hertog MG, Brants HA, van Poppel G, van den Brandt PA. Consumption of black tea and cancer risk: A prospective cohort study. J Natl Cancer Inst. 1996 Jan 17;88(2):93-100.

Kuo SM. Dietary flavonoid and cancer prevention: Evidence and potential mechanism. Crit Rev Oncog. 1997;8(1):47-69.

Siegenberg D, Baynes RD, Bothwell TH, Macfarlane BJ, Lamparelli RD, Car NG, MacPhail P, Schmidt U, Tal A, Mayet F. Ascorbic acid prevents the dose-dependent inhibitory effects of polyphenols and phytates on nonheme-iron absorption. Am J Clin Nutr. 1991 Feb;53(2):537-41.

Soleas GJ, Diamandis EP, Goldberg DM. Resveratrol: A molecule whose time has come? And gone? Clin Biochem. 1997 Mar;30(2):91-113.

Virgili F, Pagana G, Bourne L, Rimbach G, Natella F, Rice-Evans C, Packer L. Ferulic acid excretion as a marker of consumption of a French maritime pine (Pinus maritima) bark extract. Free Radic Biol Med. 2000 Apr 15;28(8):1249-56.

Wang JF, Schramm DD, Holt RR, Ensunsa JL, Fraga CG, Schmitz HH, Keen CL. A dose-response effect from chocolate consumption on plasma epicatechin and oxidative damage. J Nutr. 2000 Aug;130(8S Suppl):2115S-9S.

N-ACETYLCYSTEINE (NAC)

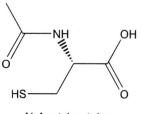

N-Acetylcysteine

What Is It?

N-Acetylcysteine (NAC) is a derivative of the sulfur-containing amino acid cysteine. It is produced naturally in the body and is found in many protein-containing foods. NAC is an intermediary, along with glutamic acid and glycine, in the conversion of cysteine into glutathione, the body's primary cellular antioxidant.

Claims

- General antioxidant/increases cellular glutathione levels
- Immune enhancer/slows progression of HIV
- Prevents/treats cancer
- Detoxifies heavy metals
- Treats smoker's cough and bronchitis
- Prevents heart disease
- Reduces exercise fatigue

Theory

NAC's proposed benefits in human health are thought to originate from either of its two primary actions in the body. First, NAC is rapidly metabolized to intracellular glutathione. Glutathione (GTH) and the enzyme complexes that it forms act as reducing agents and antioxidants in the body. GTH also helps "detoxify" many chemicals into less harmful compounds and accelerates the body's removal of heavy metals such as mercury and lead. GTH is also known to protect cell membranes, especially those of lymphocytes and phagocytes, two of the major classes of immune cells. Although purified glutathione is sold as a dietary supplement, absorption is notoriously low, and NAC is thought to be a better source method of boosting cellular GTH levels. NAC's second beneficial action in the body is to cleave protein disulfide bonds by converting them to two sulfhydryl groups. In the case of smoker's cough and bronchitis, this action results in the breakup of mucoproteins in lung mucus, reducing their chain lengths, thinning the mucus, and easing breathing.

Scientific Support

Several studies have been performed to confirm that NAC is converted to glutathione in the body. A review of these studies showed that oral NAC supplementation was successful in enhancing the levels of glutathione in the liver, in plasma, and in the bronchioles of the lungs. Lack of glutathione has been shown to contribute to a variety of health conditions such as adult respiratory distress syndrome and idiopathic pulmonary fibrosis.

In a double-blind placebo-controlled study of 116 subjects with chronic bronchitis, the therapeutic effects of NAC were investigated over a six-month period. The group receiving NAC experienced a significant reduction in the number of sick days from December to March (173 NAC versus 456 placebo) as well as a greater reduction in days of coughing (204 NAC versus 399 placebo). NAC has also been shown to help reduce levels of fatigue and improve ability for muscle contraction during exhaustive exercise (possibly due to reduced levels of oxidative stress).

A clinical trial of NAC and immune function evaluated the response of the CD4-CD8 lymphocyte system in HIV-positive patients (in whom falling CD4 counts are an indicator of disease progression). The fifteen patients were divided into two groups, one receiving two 400 mg doses of NAC parenterally twice daily and the other receiving 600 mg orally twice daily. During the experiment, eight patients receiving NAC were considered successful, including two patients who became serum negative for the illness and six patients who experienced no opportunistic infections. The researchers involved concluded that NAC was a useful adjunct to antiviral and immunotherapy.

Safety

Toxicological data shows that NAC is safe for consumption in its therapeutic dosage ranges, and high intakes of approximately 60 to 80 g per day are not associated with significant adverse effects—although extended supplementation with high levels of NAC could lead to minor zinc depletion.

Value

Research on NAC has clearly shown value in the treatment of chronic bronchitis and lung ailments as well as for individuals desiring an increase in generalized antioxidant protection and immune system support.

Dosage

Typical dosage recommendations are in the range of 250 to 1,500 mg of NAC daily for the majority of therapeutic benefits.

WORKS CONSULTED

De la Fuente M, Victor VM. Anti-oxidants as modulators of immune function. Immunol Cell Biol. 2000 Feb;78(1):49-54.

Droge W. Cysteine and glutathione in catabolic conditions and immunological dysfunction. Curr Opin Clin Nutr Metab Care. 1999 May;2(3):227-33.

Faintuch J, Aguilar PB, Nadalin W. Relevance of N-acetylcysteine in clinical practice: Fact, myth or consequence? Nutrition. 1999 Feb;15(2):177-9.

Floyd RA. Antioxidants, oxidative stress, and degenerative neurological disorders. Proc Soc Exp Biol Med. 1999 Dec;222(3):236-45.

Grootveld M, Silwood CJ, Lynch EJ, Patel IY, Blake DR. The role of N-acetylcysteine in protecting synovial fluid biomolecules against radiolytically-mediated oxidative damage: A high field proton NMR study. Free Radic Res. 1999 May;30(5):351-69.

Malorni W, Rivabene R, Lucia BM, Ferrara R, Mazzone AM, Cauda R, Paganelli R. The role of oxidative imbalance in progression to AIDS: Effect of the thiol supplier N-acetylcysteine. AIDS Res Hum Retroviruses. 1998 Nov 20;14(17):1589-96.

Marchetti G, Lodola E, Licciardello L, Colombo A. Use of N-acetylcysteine in the management of coronary artery diseases. Cardiologia. 1999 Jul;44(7):633-7.

Martinez M, Martinez N, Hernandez AI, Ferrandiz ML. Hypothesis: Can N-acetylcysteine be beneficial in Parkinson's disease? Life Sci. 1999;64(15):1253-7.

Molnar Z, MacKinnon KL, Shearer E, Lowe D, Watson ID. The effect of N-acetylcysteine on total serum anti-oxidant potential and urinary albumin excretion in critically ill patients. Intensive Care Med. 1998 Mar;24(3):230-5.

Pela R, Calcagni AM, Subiaco S, Isidori P, Tubaldi A, Sanguinetti CM. N-acetylcysteine reduces the exacerbation rate in patients with moderate to severe COPD. Respiration. 1999 Nov-Dec;66(6):495-500.

Rahman Q, Abidi P, Afaq F, Schiffmann D, Mossman BT, Kamp DW, Athar M. Glutathione redox system in oxidative lung injury. Crit Rev Toxicol. 1999 Nov;29(6):543-68.

Ruffmann R. Reactive oxygen species in acute lung injury. Eur Respir J. 1998 Dec;12(6):1486.

Sen CK, Packer L. Thiol homeostasis and supplements in physical exercise. Am J Clin Nutr. 2000 Aug;72(2 Suppl):653S-69S.

Supinski G. Free radical induced respiratory muscle dysfunction. Mol Cell Biochem. 1998 Feb;179(1-2):99-110.

Walsh TS, Lee A. N-acetylcysteine administration in the critically ill. Intensive Care Med. 1999 May;25(5):432-4.

VITAMIN E

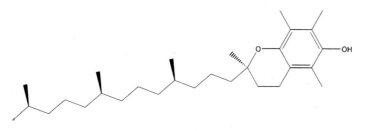

Alpha-Tocopherol

What Is It?

Vitamin E is actually a family of related compounds known as tocopherols and tocotrienols. Although alpha-tocopherol is the most common form found in dietary supplements, vitamin E also exists in foods with slightly different chemical structures, such as beta-, gamma-, and delta-tocopherol as well as alpha-, beta-, gamma-, and delta-tocotrienols. Vitamin E was discovered in the early 1930s when rats fed a diet free of vegetable oils (the primary dietary source of vitamin E) developed reproductive problems. Although vitamin E doesn't have exactly the same reproductive effects in humans, vitamin E is commonly thought of as a "virility vitamin" for men.

Vitamin E can be obtained as a supplement in natural or synthetic form. In most cases, the natural and synthetic form of vitamins and minerals are identical, but in the case of vitamin E, the natural form is clearly superior in terms of absorption and retention in the body. The natural form of alpha-tocopherol is known as "d-alpha tocopherol," whereas the synthetic form is called "dl-alpha tocopherol." The synthetic dl- form is the most common form found in dietary supplements, although many manufacturers are switching over to the more potent (and expensive) natural d- form because consumers are learning to look for it.

Dietary sources of vitamin E include vegetable oils, margarine, nuts, seeds, avocados, and wheat germ. Safflower oil contains a good amount of vitamin E (about two-thirds of the RDA in ¼ cup), but there is very little vitamin E in either corn oil or soybean oil. For individuals watching their dietary fat consumption, vitamin E intake is likely to be low, due to a reduced intake of foods with high fat content (you'd need to eat about sixty almonds to get the RDA for vitamin E and about 400 to 800 to get the amount of vitamin E, 200 to 400 IU, associated with heart health benefits).

Claims

- Reduces risk of cardiovascular disease
- Boosts immune system function
- Antioxidant
- Wound healing (topical)
- Reduces cancer risk

Theory

Vitamin E is one of the most potent fat-soluble antioxidants in the body. As such, vitamin E protects cell membranes from the damage caused by free radicals. High doses of vitamin E have also been linked to a decreased ability of the blood to clot, which may be beneficial in individuals at risk for heart disease by reducing the risk of heart attack.

Scientific Support

Of the different isomers of vitamin E, the alpha-tocopherol form is typically considered the gold standard in terms of antioxidant activity—although the most recent research suggests that the other chemical forms may possess equivalent or superior antioxidant protection (in the test tube). Vitamin E deficiencies are related to a wide variety of health problems, including cataracts, heart disease, lung problems, and liver damage. As mentioned, the role of vitamin E as a fertility enhancer in humans is nonexistent, but is still a part of the folklore surrounding vitamin E as a dietary supplement.

Several studies published over the last two to three years have clearly shown that natural vitamin E, the d- form, is about two to three times more bioavailable than synthetic dl- vitamin E. The natural form of the vitamin is extracted from vegetable oils, mostly from soybeans, which are cheap and plentiful in the United States. Processing soybeans removes most of the vitamin E. Synthetic vitamin E, in contrast, is manufactured from petroleum by-products, resulting in a chemical mixture in which only one-eighth of the mixture is the powerful d- isomer (the other seven-eighths are weaker vitamin E isomers).

A wide variety of epidemiological and prospective studies have associated health benefits with higher than average vitamin E consumption. In most cases, the level of vitamin E intake required for heart, lung, eye, and cancer protection is ten to thirty times higher than the current RDA levels. Although high-dose alpha-tocopherol supplements are clearly a powerful antioxidant measure, concern has recently been raised because such supplements may displace body stores of the other naturally occurring vitamin E forms.

There is a strong inverse relationship between plasma vitamin E levels (which almost exclusively measure only alpha-tocopherol) and the incidence of coronary heart disease. However, several supplementation studies have failed to demonstrate a protective effect when alpha-tocopherol *alone* has been supplemented. In one large study published in the *New England Journal of Medicine,* vitamin E appeared to offer protection only when obtained from the diet (which is primarily *gamma*-tocopherol) and not when taken in supplements (which are primarily *alpha*-tocopherol). The strongest correlation was shown with the consumption of margarine, nuts, and seeds—all of which are excellent sources of gamma-tocopherol. In addition, serum levels of gamma-tocopherol (but not alpha-) are reduced in heart disease patients and rise rapidly when chronic smokers quit. Because alpha-tocopherol supplementation reduces tissue levels of the gamma- form, a mixed tocopherol that better reflects the ratios found in our diet may be more useful as a supplement than the formulations of vitamin E currently available.

In other studies, heart disease patients have been shown to have normal serum alpha-tocopherol levels but much lower gamma-tocopherol levels compared to a group of healthy control subjects. In one of the largest epidemiological studies (21,809 women), vitamin E consumption was inversely associated with the risk of death from coronary heart disease, but this link was strongest in the women who *did not* consume vitamin E supplements—they got their vitamin E from foods.

Overall, at least some studies indicate that a balanced intake of each of the naturally occurring forms of vitamin E may be the most prudent approach in terms of overall health benefits. For example, high-dose alpha-tocopherol supplements can reduce body stores of gamma-tocopherol, whereas a fifty-fifty intake of each maintains elevated tissues stores of both. Such findings are potentially important, given that gamma-tocopherol is the major form of vitamin E in the U.S. diet and has been found to inhibit lipid peroxidation (cell membrane damage) more effectively than alpha-tocopherol (in a test-tube study). This may mean that the different vitamin E forms may complement each other in the body.

Safety

Side effects associated with vitamin E supplements are exceedingly rare. Unlike other fat-soluble vitamins, such as A, D, and K, vitamin E is relatively nontoxic, even at doses many times the current daily value of 30 IU. Caution is advised, however, in individuals at risk for prolonged bleeding, such as those taking anticoagulant medications, because vitamin E supplements can decrease blood-clotting ability (reduce platelet aggregation) and prolong bleeding time.

Value

Natural (d-) alpha-tocopherol is clearly more bioavailable and is preferentially retained by the body compared to the more common synthetic (dl-) form of vitamin E. Unfortunately, although the natural form is two to three times more potent than the synthetic form, it is also about twice the price (although prices are rapidly coming down). For reasons outlined previously, it may be preferable to choose products that offer a balanced source of mixed tocopherols, including the natural forms of all eight of the vitamin E isomers (d-alpha, d-beta, d-gamma, and d-delta forms of both the tocopherols and tocotrienols).

Dosage

The daily value for vitamin E is 30 IU, but most research studies show that optimal intakes associated with health benefits are in the range of 100 to 800 IU—an amount that cannot realistically be obtained from foods.

WORKS CONSULTED

Arlt S, Finckh B, Beisiegel U, Kontush A. Time-course of oxidation of lipids in human cerebrospinal fluid in vitro. Free Radic Res. 2000 Feb;32(2):103-14.

Bates CJ, Chen SJ, Macdonald A, Holden R. Quantitation of vitamin E and a carotenoid pigment in cataractous human lenses, and the effect of a dietary supplement. Int J Vitam Nutr Res. 1996;66(4):316-21.

Behl C. Vitamin E and other antioxidants in neuroprotection. Int J Vitam Nutr Res. 1999 May;69(3):213-9.

Botterweck AA, van den Brandt PA, Goldbohm RA. Vitamins, carotenoids, dietary fiber, and the risk of gastric carcinoma: Results from a prospective study after 6.3 years of follow-up. Cancer. 2000 Feb 15;88(4):737-48.

Boylan LM, Sugerman HJ, Driskell JA. Vitamin E, vitamin B-6, vitamin B-12, and folate status of gastric bypass surgery patients. J Am Diet Assoc. 1988 May;88(5):579-85.

Brown JE, Wahle KW. Effect of fish-oil and vitamin E supplementation on lipid peroxidation and whole-blood aggregation in man. Clin Chim Acta. 1990 Dec 14;193(3):147-56.

Bruckner G. Microcirculation, vitamin E and omega 3 fatty acids: An overview. Adv Exp Med Biol. 1997;415:195-208.

Bunnell RH, De Ritter E, Rubin SH. Effect of feeding polyunsaturated fatty acids with a low vitamin E diet on blood levels of tocopherol in men performing hard physical labor. Am J Clin Nutr. 1975 Jul;28(7):706-11.

Butterfield DA, Koppal T, Subramaniam R, Yatin S. Vitamin E as an antioxidant/free radical scavenger against amyloid beta-peptide-induced oxidative stress in neocortical synaptosomal membranes and hippocampal neurons in culture: Insights into Alzheimer's disease. Rev Neurosci. 1999;10(2):141-9.

Cooney RV, Franke AA, Hankin JH, Custer LJ, Wilkens LR, Harwood PJ, Le Marchand L. Seasonal variations in plasma micronutrients and antioxidants. Cancer Epidemiol Biomarkers Prev. 1995 Apr-May;4(3):207-15.

Copp RP, Wisniewski T, Hentati F, Larnaout A, Ben Hamida M, Kayden HJ. Localization of alpha-tocopherol transfer protein in the brains of patients with ataxia with vitamin E deficiency and other oxidative stress related neurodegenerative disorders. Brain Res. 1999 Mar 20;822(1-2):80-7.

Davis KL. Alzheimer's disease: Seeking new ways to preserve brain function. Geriatrics. 1999 Feb;54(2):42-7.

DeCosse JJ, Miller HH, Lesser ML. Effect of wheat fiber and vitamins C and E on rectal polyps in patients with familial adenomatous polyposis. J Natl Cancer Inst. 1989 Sep 6;81(17):1290-7.

Draczynska-Lusiak B, Doung A, Sun AY. Oxidized lipoproteins may play a role in neuronal cell death in Alzheimer disease. Mol Chem Neuropathol. 1998 Feb;33(2):139-48.

Evans JR, Henshaw K. Antioxidant vitamin and mineral supplementation for preventing age-related macular degeneration. Cochrane Database Syst Rev. 2000;(2):CD000253.

Fairris GM, Perkins PJ, Lloyd B, Hinks L, Clayton BE. The effect on atopic dermatitis of supplementation with selenium and vitamin E. Acta Derm Venereol. 1989;69(4):359-62.

Faulks RM, Hart DJ, Scott KJ, Southon S. Changes in plasma carotenoid and vitamin E profile during supplementation with oil palm fruit carotenoids. J Lab Clin Med. 1998 Dec;132(6):507-11.

Fenech M, Dreosti I, Aitken C. Vitamin-E supplements and their effect on vitamin-E status in blood and genetic damage rate in peripheral blood lymphocytes. Carcinogenesis. 1997 Feb;18(2):359-64.

Fernandes MA, Proenca MT, Nogueira AJ, Grazina MM, Oliveira LM, Fernandes AI, Santiago B, Santana I, Oliveira CR. Influence of apolipoprotein E genotype on blood redox status of Alzheimer's disease patients. Int J Mol Med. 1999 Aug;4(2):179-86.

Floyd RA. Antioxidants, oxidative stress, and degenerative neurological disorders. Proc Soc Exp Biol Med. 1999 Dec;222(3):236-45.

Grundman M. Vitamin E and Alzheimer disease: The basis for additional clinical trials. Am J Clin Nutr. 2000 Feb;71(2):630S-6S.

Jacob RA, Kutnink MA, Csallany AS, Daroszewska M, Burton GW. Vitamin C nutriture has little short-term effect on vitamin E concentrations in healthy women. J Nutr. 1996 Sep;126(9):2268-77.

Jimenez-Jimenez FJ, de Bustos F, Molina JA, Benito-Leon J, Tallon-Barranco A, Gasalla T, Orti-Pareja M, Guillamon F, Rubio JC, Arenas J, Enriquez-de-Salamanca R. Cerebrospinal fluid levels of alpha-tocopherol (vitamin E) in Alzheimer's disease. J Neural Transm. 1997;104(6-7):703-10.

Kanter M. Free radicals, exercise and antioxidant supplementation. Proc Nutr Soc. 1998 Feb;57(1):9-13.

Kanter MM, Nolte LA, Holloszy JO. Effects of an antioxidant vitamin mixture on lipid peroxidation at rest and postexercise. J Appl Physiol. 1993 Feb;74(2):965-9.

Kilander L, Ohrvall M. Alpha-tocopherol and Alzheimer's disease. N Engl J Med. 1997 Aug 21;337(8):572-3.

Knopman DS, Berg JD, Thomas R, Grundman M, Thal LJ, Sano M. Nursing home placement is related to dementia progression: Experience from a clinical trial. Alzheimer's Disease Cooperative Study. Neurology. 1999 Mar 10;52(4):714-8.

Kushi LH, Folsom AR, Prineas RJ, Mink PJ, Wu Y, Bostick RM. Dietary antioxidant vitamins and death from coronary heart disease in postmenopausal women. N Engl J Med. 1996 May 2;334(18):1156-62.

Lyle BJ, Mares-Perlman JA, Klein BE, Klein R, Greger JL. Supplement users differ from nonusers in demographic, lifestyle, dietary and health characteristics. J Nutr. 1998 Dec;128(12):2355-62.

Maehle L, Lystad E, Eilertsen E, Einarsdottir E, Hostmark AT, Haugen A. Growth of human lung adenocarcinoma in nude mice is influenced by various types of dietary fat and vitamin E. Anticancer Res. 1999 May-Jun;19(3A):1649-55.

Masaki KH, Losonczy KG, Izmirlian G, Foley DJ, Ross GW, Petrovitch H, Havlik R, White LR. Association of vitamin E and C supplement use with cognitive function and dementia in elderly men. Neurology. 2000 Mar 28;54(6):1265-72.

McKeown-Eyssen G, Holloway C, Jazmaji V, Bright-See E, Dion P, Bruce WR. A randomized trial of vitamins C and E in the prevention of recurrence of colorectal polyps. Cancer Res. 1988 Aug 15;48(16):4701-5.

Meydani M. Modulation of the platelet thromboxane A2 and aortic prostacyclin synthesis by dietary selenium and vitamin E. Biol Trace Elem Res. 1992 Apr-Jun;33:79-86.

Miller ER 3rd, Appel LJ, Levander OA, Levine DM. The effect of antioxidant vitamin supplementation on traditional cardiovascular risk factors. J Cardiovasc Risk. 1997 Feb;4(1):19-24.

Miller JW. Vitamin E and memory: Is it vascular protection? Nutr Rev. 2000 Apr;58(4):109-11.

Morris MC, Beckett LA, Scherr PA, Hebert LE, Bennett DA, Field TS, Evans DA. Vitamin E and vitamin C supplement use and risk of incident Alzheimer disease. Alzheimer Dis Assoc Disord. 1998 Sep;12(3):121-6.

Moyad MA, Brumfield SK, Pienta KJ. Vitamin E, alpha- and gamma-tocopherol, and prostate cancer. Semin Urol Oncol. 1999 May;17(2):85-90.

Peters SA, Kelly FJ. Vitamin E supplementation in cystic fibrosis. J Pediatr Gastroenterol Nutr. 1996 May;22(4):341-5.

Pietinen P, Ascherio A, Korhonen P, Hartman AM, Willett WC, Albanes D, Virtamo J. Intake of fatty acids and risk of coronary heart disease in a cohort of Finnish men. The Alpha-Tocopherol, Beta-Carotene Cancer Prevention Study. Am J Epidemiol. 1997 May 15;145(10):876-87.

Post SG. Future scenarios for the prevention and delay of Alzheimer disease onset in high-risk groups. An ethical perspective. Am J Prev Med. 1999 Feb;16(2):105-10.

Postaire E, Jungmann H, Bejot M, Heinrich U, Tronnier H. Evidence for antioxidant nutrients-induced pigmentation in skin: Results of a clinical trial. Biochem Mol Biol Int. 1997 Aug;42(5):1023-33.

Riviere S, Birlouez-Aragon I, Nourhashemi F, Vellas B. Low plasma vitamin C in Alzheimer patients despite an adequate diet. Int J Geriatr Psychiatry. 1998 Nov;13(11):749-54.

Sanchez-Lugo L, Mayer-Davis EJ, Howard G, Selby JV, Ayad MF, Rewers M, Haffner S. Insulin sensitivity and intake of vitamins E and C in African American, Hispanic, and non-Hispanic white men and women: The Insulin Resistance and Atherosclerosis Study (IRAS). Am J Clin Nutr. 1997 Nov;66(5):1224-31.

Sano M, Ernesto C, Thomas RG, Klauber MR, Schafer K, Grundman M, Woodbury P, Growdon J, Cotman CW, Pfeiffer E, Schneider LS, Thal LJ. A controlled trial of selegiline, alpha-tocopherol, or both as treatment for Alzheimer's disease. The Alzheimer's Disease Cooperative Study. N Engl J Med. 1997 Apr 24;336(17):1216-22.

Schippling S, Kontush A, Arlt S, Buhmann C, Sturenburg HJ, Mann U, Muller-Thomsen T, Beisiegel U. Increased lipoprotein oxidation in Alzheimer's disease. Free Radic Biol Med. 2000 Feb 1;28(3):351-60.

Sinha R, Patterson BH, Mangels AR, Levander OA, Gibson T, Taylor PR, Block G. Determinants of plasma vitamin E in healthy males. Cancer Epidemiol Biomarkers Prev. 1993 Sep-Oct;2(5):473-9.

Tengerdy RP. Vitamin E, immune response, and disease resistance. Ann N Y Acad Sci. 1989;570:335-44.

Vatassery GT. Vitamin E and other endogenous antioxidants in the central nervous system. Geriatrics. 1998 Sep;53(Suppl 1):S25-7.

Vatassery GT, Bauer T, Dysken M. High doses of vitamin E in the treatment of disorders of the central nervous system in the aged. Am J Clin Nutr. 1999 Nov;70(5):793-801.

Wander RC, Du SH, Ketchum SO, Rowe KE. alpha-Tocopherol influences in vivo indices of lipid peroxidation in postmenopausal women given fish oil. J Nutr. 1996 Mar;126(3):643-52.

Wander RC, Du SH, Ketchum SO, Rowe KE. Effects of interaction of RRR-alpha-tocopheryl acetate and fish oil on low-density-lipoprotein oxidation in postmenopausal women with and without hormone-replacement therapy. Am J Clin Nutr. 1996 Feb;63(2):184-93.

Weight LM, Noakes TD, Labadarios D, Graves J, Jacobs P, Berman PA. Vitamin and mineral status of trained athletes including the effects of supplementation. Am J Clin Nutr. 1988 Feb;47(2):186-91.

Willett W, Sampson L, Bain C, Rosner B, Hennekens CH, Witschie J, Speizer FE. Vitamin supplement use among registered nurses. Am J Clin Nutr. 1981 Jun;34(6):1121-5.

Willett WC, Stampfer MJ, Underwood BA, Taylor JO, Hennekens CH. Vitamins A, E, and carotene: Effects of supplementation on their plasma levels. Am J Clin Nutr. 1983 Oct;38(4):559-66.

Woodall AA, Britton G, Jackson MJ. Dietary supplementation with carotenoids: Effects on alpha-tocopherol levels and susceptibility of tissues to oxidative stress. Br J Nutr. 1996 Aug;76(2):307-17.

VITAMIN C

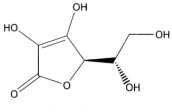

Ascorbic Acid

What Is It?

Vitamin C, also known as ascorbic acid, is a water-soluble vitamin needed by the body for hundreds of vital metabolic reactions. The vitamin C deficiency disease, scurvy, is prevented by adequate intake of ascorbic acid ("ascorbic" actually means "without scurvy"). As a dietary supplement, vitamin C is consumed by more people than any other vitamin, mineral, or herbal product. Good food sources of vitamin C include all citrus fruits (oranges, grapefruit, lemons) as well as many other fruits and vegetables such as strawberries, tomatoes, broccoli, Brussels sprouts, peppers, and cantaloupe. Vitamin C is fairly fragile and can be easily destroyed by cooking or exposure of food to oxygen.

Claims

- Antioxidant
- Prevents colds/boosts immunity
- Promotes wound healing
- Protects against effects of stress
- Cancer prevention

Theory

Because of the wide variety of reactions in which vitamin C plays a role, many structure/function claims can be made for supplements. Perhaps the most well-known function of vitamin C is as one of the key nutritional antioxidants—it protects the body from free radical damage. As a water-soluble vitamin, ascorbic acid performs its antioxidant functions within the aqueous compartments of the blood and inside cells and can help restore the antioxidant potential of vitamin E (a fat-soluble antioxidant).

Vitamin C also functions as an essential cofactor for the enzymes involved in the synthesis of collagen—the chief structural protein in connective tissues such as bones, cartilage, and skin. As such, vitamin C is often recommended for wound healing and as an ingredient in supplements for healthy skin.

As a preventive against infections such as influenza and other viruses, vitamin C is thought to strengthen cell membranes, thereby preventing entrance of the virus into the cell. Support of immune cell function is also a key role performed by vitamin C, an effect that may help fight infections in their early stages. The combined effects of cellular strengthening, collagen synthesis, and antioxidant protection are thought to account for the multifaceted way in which vitamin C helps to maintain health.

Scientific Support

As a way to prevent or reduce the symptoms associated with the common cold, over 100 vitamin C studies have been conducted. In several of the largest studies, no effect on common cold incidence is observed, indicating to many scientists that vitamin C has no preventive effects in normally nourished subjects. However, a number of smaller, targeted studies, conducted in subjects under acute physical stress, show that vitamin C decreases the incidence of the common cold by half. In other studies, healthy subjects consuming low levels of vitamin C (below 60 mg per day) have a cold incidence that is about one-third lower following vitamin C supplementation.

In general, regular vitamin C supplementation at levels at or slightly above 1,000 mg per day has consistently reduced the incidence and duration of colds (although the degree of benefit has varied significantly). For example, in some of the larger studies, duration of infection was reduced by only about 5 percent, but absentee reports were reduced by nearly 20 percent. At least three controlled studies have shown an 80 percent reduction in the incidence of pneumonia among vitamin C users. In one large study (over 700 students), vitamin C (1,000 mg per hour for the first six hours followed by 3,000 mg per day) reduced cold and flu symptoms by 85 percent.

In most cases, it appears that while the most important and dramatic preventive effects of vitamin C supplementation will be experienced by individuals with low vitamin C intakes, those with average daily consumption from foods may also benefit from supplemental levels. In support of an elevated vitamin C intake, an expert scientific panel recently recommended increasing the current RDA for vitamin C from 60 mg to at least 100 to 200 mg per day. This same panel also cautioned that taking more than 1,000 mg of vitamin C daily could have adverse effects (read more under Safety). The report of this expert panel was published in the April 21, 1999, issue of *The Journal of the American Medical Association (JAMA)*. In the report, the expert panel recommended that "whenever possible, vitamin C intake should come from fruits and vegetables" (at least five servings of fruits and vegetables daily). The current RDA of 60 mg per day was established in 1980, but since the last RDA review (in 1989), scientists have learned a great deal more about the functions of vitamin C in the body and the need for elevated vitamin C consumption.

Safety

As a water-soluble vitamin, ascorbic acid is extremely safe even at relatively high doses (because most of the excess is excreted in the urine). At high doses (over 1,000 mg per day), some people can experience gastrointestinal side effects such as stomach cramps, nausea, and diarrhea. In addition, vitamin C intakes above 1,000 mg per day may increase the risk of developing kidney stones for some people.

Value

Vitamin C is the most popular single nutrient supplement. It is typically included in all multivitamin blends, but at widely varying levels from less than 30 mg to over 1,000 mg—so check your labels. As a single-nutrient supplement, typical doses range from 100 to 500 mg per tablet. The body, however, can only absorb and retain about 200 mg of vitamin C at one time—the rest is quickly washed out in the urine. This means that the most effective approach to supplementing with vitamin C is to take it in divided doses throughout the day.

Vitamin C is one of the least expensive dietary supplements available—don't worry about paying more than a few dollars for a one-month supply. Also, beware of expensive "natural" forms of ascorbic acid, as there is no reliable evidence to show that these forms (derived from rose hips or acerola) are any better absorbed or utilized by the body than synthetic vitamin C (but this is not the case with vitamin E, where the natural form is clearly superior to the synthetic form).

Dosage

Although the RDA for vitamin C has recently been raised from 60 mg to 75 to 90 mg (higher for men), it is well established that almost everybody can benefit from higher levels. For example, the vitamin C recommendation for cigarette smokers is 100 to 200 mg per day because smoking destroys vitamin C in the body. You need not worry about developing scurvy (as long as you consume at least 10 mg of vitamin C daily), but be sure to increase your intake if you're exposed to stress (physical or psychological) or infection (such as a sick friend or family member).

Although vitamin C is well absorbed, the percentage absorbed from supplements decreases with increasing dosages, and optimal absorption is achieved by taking several small doses throughout the day (100 mg per dose for a total daily intake of 200 to 1,000 mg). Full blood and tissue saturation is typically achieved with daily intakes of 200 to 500 mg per day (in two to three divided doses).

WORKS CONSULTED

Ames BN, Shigenaga MK, Hagen TM. Oxidants, antioxidants, and the degenerative diseases of aging. Proc Natl Acad Sci USA. 1993 Sep 1;90(17):7915-22.

Armstrong AM, Chestnutt JE, Gormley MJ, Young IS. The effect of dietary treatment on lipid peroxidation and antioxidant status in newly diagnosed noninsulin dependent diabetes. Free Radic Biol Med. 1996;21(5):719-26.

Bates CJ, Walmsley CM, Prentice A, Finch S. Does vitamin C reduce blood pressure? Results of a large study of people aged 65 or older. J Hypertens. 1998 Jul;16(7):925-32.

Benzie IF, Janus ED, Strain JJ. Plasma ascorbate and vitamin E levels in Hong Kong Chinese. Eur J Clin Nutr. 1998 Jun;52(6):447-51.

Bodner C, Godden D, Brown K, Little J, Ross S, Seaton A. Antioxidant intake and adult-onset wheeze: A case-control study. Aberdeen WHEASE Study Group. Eur Respir J. 1999 Jan;13(1):22-30.

Cadenas S, Barja G, Poulsen HE, Loft S. Oxidative DNA damage estimated by oxo8dG in the liver of guinea-pigs supplemented with graded dietary doses of ascorbic acid and alpha-tocopherol. Carcinogenesis. 1997 Dec;18(12):2373-7.

Eastwood MA. Interaction of dietary antioxidants in vivo: How fruit and vegetables prevent disease? QJM. 1999 Sep;92(9):527-30.

Eiserich JP, van der Vliet A, Handelman GJ, Halliwell B, Cross CE. Dietary antioxidants and cigarette smoke-induced biomolecular damage: A complex interaction. Am J Clin Nutr. 1995 Dec;62(6 Suppl):1490S-1500S.

Fuller CJ, Grundy SM, Norkus EP, Jialal I. Effect of ascorbate supplementation on low density lipoprotein oxidation in smokers. Atherosclerosis. 1996 Jan 26;119(2):139-50.

Giugliano D. Dietary antioxidants for cardiovascular prevention. Nutr Metab Cardiovasc Dis. 2000 Feb;10(1):38-44.

Halliwell B. Oxidative stress, nutrition and health. Experimental strategies for optimization of nutritional antioxidant intake in humans. Free Radic Res. 1996 Jul;25(1):57-74.

Halliwell B. Antioxidant defence mechanisms: From the beginning to the end (of the beginning). Free Radic Res. 1999 Oct;31(4):261-72.

Jacob RA, Kutnink MA, Csallany AS, Daroszewska M, Burton GW. Vitamin C nutriture has little short-term effect on vitamin E concentrations in healthy women. J Nutr. 1996 Sep;126(9):2268-77.

Jacob RA, Pianalto FS, Agee RE. Cellular ascorbate depletion in healthy men. J Nutr. 1992 May;122(5):1111-8.

Jialal I, Grundy SM. Effect of combined supplementation with alpha-tocopherol, ascorbate, and beta carotene on low-density lipoprotein oxidation. Circulation. 1993 Dec;88(6):2780-6.

Johnston CS, Meyer CG, Srilakshmi JC. Vitamin C elevates red blood cell glutathione in healthy adults. Am J Clin Nutr. 1993 Jul;58(1):103-5.

Lykkesfeldt J, Christen S, Wallock LM, Chang HH, Jacob RA, Ames BN. Ascorbate is depleted by smoking and repleted by moderate supplementation: A study in male smokers and nonsmokers with matched dietary antioxidant intakes. Am J Clin Nutr. 2000 Feb;71(2):530-6.

Nyyssonen K, Parviainen MT, Salonen R, Tuomilehto J, Salonen JT. Vitamin C deficiency and risk of myocardial infarction: Prospective population study of men from eastern Finland. BMJ. 1997 Mar 1;314(7081):634-8.

Prasad KN, Kumar A, Kochupillai V, Cole WC. High doses of multiple antioxidant vitamins: Essential ingredients in improving the efficacy of standard cancer therapy. J Am Coll Nutr. 1999 Feb;18(1):13-25.

Rokitzki L, Hinkel S, Klemp C, Cufi D, Keul J. Dietary, serum and urine ascorbic acid status in male athletes. Int J Sports Med. 1994 Oct;15(7):435-40.

Schectman G, Byrd JC, Hoffmann R. Ascorbic acid requirements for smokers: Analysis of a population survey. Am J Clin Nutr. 1991 Jun;53(6):1466-70.

Sharma DC, Mathur R. Correction of anemia and iron deficiency in vegetarians by administration of ascorbic acid. Indian J Physiol Pharmacol. 1995 Oct;39(4):403-6.

Sinclair AJ, Taylor PB, Lunec J, Girling AJ, Barnett AH. Low plasma ascorbate levels in patients with type 2 diabetes mellitus consuming adequate dietary vitamin C. Diabet Med. 1994 Nov;11(9):893-8.

Taylor A, Jacques PF, Nadler D, Morrow F, Sulsky SI, Shepard D. Relationship in humans between ascorbic acid consumption and levels of total and reduced ascorbic acid in lens, aqueous humor, and plasma. Curr Eye Res. 1991 Aug; 10(8):751-9.

VanderJagt DJ, Garry PJ, Bhagavan HN. Ascorbic acid intake and plasma levels in healthy elderly people. Am J Clin Nutr. 1987 Aug;46(2):290-4.

Varma SD, Devamanoharan PS, Morris SM. Prevention of cataracts by nutritional and metabolic antioxidants. Crit Rev Food Sci Nutr. 1995 Jan;35(1-2):111-29.

Vatassery GT, Smith WE, Quach HT. Ascorbic acid, glutathione and synthetic antioxidants prevent the oxidation of vitamin E in platelets. Lipids. 1989 Dec;24(12):1043-7.

GRAPE SEED EXTRACT (GSE)/PINE BARK EXTRACT

What Is It?

Grape seed extract (GSE) is just what it sounds like—an extract from grape seeds. The seeds are typically from red grapes (not white), which have a high content of compounds known as oligomeric proanthocyanidins (OPCs). The OPCs are also present in a wide variety of fruits and vegetables, plus pine bark (pycnogenol) and green tea, and possess potent antioxidant properties.

The OPCs are chemically known as flavonoids or polyphenols, which can differ substantially based on their polymer arrangement. For example, polyphenols can exist in single (monomer), double (dimer), triple (trimer), quadruple (tetramer), and even longer cyanidin chains (tannins). Any chain length from two to seven or so is termed an "oligomer" and longer chains are called "polymers." It is generally assumed that the longer the cyanidin chain length, the less bioavailable and less active the molecule becomes. It may even be possible for the longer-chain compounds (tannins) to interfere with the absorption of other nutrients consumed at the same time. Many commercial grape seed extracts are standardized to a *total* OPC content, which may or may not take into account the assortment of various chain lengths present in the final product.

Claims

- Antioxidant
- Cardioprotection (reduces risk of atherosclerosis)
- Reduces cancer risk
- Improves vascular strength (stronger blood vessels)
- Reduces edema (inflammation/swelling)
- Promotes eye health (reduces risk of macular degeneration and cataracts)

Theory

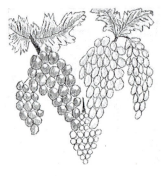

The "French paradox" attributes the low incidence of heart disease in France, despite their high fat intake, to a hearty consumption of red wine. It has been further speculated that the cardioprotective effects of red wine (and possibly of red/purple grape juice) derive from a group of compounds variously called flavonoids, catechins, tannins, and proanthocyanidins, which are found at high concentrations in red wine. These compounds are found at especially high levels in grape seeds, where they can be extracted and concentrated for use as a dietary supplement. Research on the chemical properties of grape seed extract has shown them to be powerful antioxidants, or free radical scavengers—even more potent than the more commonly used antioxidant vitamins such as C and E.

Scientific Support

Grape seed extract and oligomeric proanthocyanidins clearly possess remarkable antioxidant properties. Their effects in reducing free radical damage and oxidative stress suggest that they may be particularly effective in reducing the risk of cancer, cardiovascular disease, and a number of the chronic diseases associated with aging and due in part to free radical damage. Although the majority of the studies conducted on GSE have been done in cell culture (test tube) and animals, the results are extremely promising.

In one laboratory study, the chemoprotective (cancer fighting) properties of GSE were tested in human breast cancer and lung cancer cells. Results indicated that GSE was effective in promoting cytotoxicity (cell death) in the cancer cells, but that the growth and viability of the normal cells was maintained. Another cell study examined the effects of GSE on preventing the DNA damage and cell death that occurs when cells are exposed to tobacco. The results showed that tobacco exposure causes oxidative tissue damage and apoptosis (cell death), which can be reduced 10 to 85 percent by antioxidants such as vitamins C and E and grape seed extract. GSE was about two to five times more effective than vitamins C or E alone, and the combination of the vitamins with GSE is even more effective in preventing cell damage and death.

A number of animal studies have confirmed the antioxidant potential of grape seed extract. In one study, rabbits were fed a high-cholesterol diet with and without GSE. Although there was no change in cholesterol levels in the rabbits, those receiving the GSE showed a reduced level of damaging cholesteryl ester hydroperoxides and aortic malondialdehyde (MDA), both of which can induce significant damage to blood vessel linings and lead to atherosclerosis. Immunohistochemical analysis revealed a decrease in oxidized LDL—the type of cholesterol that forms atherosclerotic lesions. In another experiment using human plasma, GSE added to the plasma also inhibited the oxidation of LDL, suggesting a possible benefit in preventing atherosclerosis.

In one of the few human studies to be conducted directly on GSE, 300 mg given daily for five days caused a significant increase in the total antioxidant capacity of the blood. A number of epidemiological and case-control studies have shown that individuals who consume one to two glasses of red wine per day are at reduced risk for heart disease and possibly for certain cancers. Such studies only suggest possible health effects, but other studies have shown that many of the phenolic compounds in red wine are absorbed into the blood, become associated with LDL cholesterol, and reduce the susceptibility of LDL to oxidation—a logical chain of events for the cardioprotective effect of red wine. Finally, some small studies, primarily conducted in rabbits and rats, suggest that GSE may also possess activity in reducing inflammation, increasing circulation (vasodilation), and enhancing blood vessel integrity.

Safety

Grape seed extract is safe when used as directed. No adverse effects have been associated with its use.

Value

At $15 to $20 per month, grape seed extract may be a logical and economical choice for a potent antioxidant supplement. Consumers interested in dietary protection from heart disease, cancer, edema, and general oxidative damage (athletes) should consider adding grape seed extract to their dietary regime.

Dosage

As a general antioxidant, approximately 50 to 100 mg per day of an extract standardized to contain 80 to 90 percent oligomeric proanthocyanidins is recommended.

WORKS CONSULTED

Ariga T. Radical scavenging action and its mode in procyanidins B-1 and B-3 from Azuki beans to peroxyl radicals. Agric Biol Chem. 1990; 54(10):2499-504.
Bagchi D, Bagchi M, Stohs SJ, Das DK, Ray SD, Kuszynski CA, Joshi SS, Pruess HG. Free radicals and grape seed proanthocyanidin extract: Importance in human health and disease prevention. Toxicology. 2000 Aug 7;148(2-3):187-97.

Bagchi D, Garg A, Krohn RL, Bagchi M, Bagchi DJ, Balmoori J, Stohs SJ. Protective effects of grape seed proanthocyanidins and selected antioxidants against TPA-induced hepatic and brain lipid peroxidation and DNA fragmentation, and peritoneal macrophage activation in mice. Gen Pharmacol. 1998 May;30(5):771-6.

Bagchi D, Garg A, Krohn RL, Bagchi M, Tran MX, Stohs SJ. Oxygen free radical scavenging abilities of vitamins C and E, and a grape seed proanthocyanidin extract in vitro. Res Commun Mol Pathol Pharmacol. 1997 Feb;95(2):179-89.

Blazsó G, Gábor M. Oedema-inhibiting effect of procyanidin. Acta Physiol Acad Sci Hung. 1980;56(2): 235-240.

Bouhamidi R, Prevost V, Nouvelot A. High protection by grape seed proanthocyanidins (GSPC) of polyunsaturated fatty acids against UV-C induced peroxidation. C R Acad Sci III. 1998 Jan;321(1):31-8.

Cheshier JE, Ardestani-Kaboudanian S, Liang B, Araghiniknam M, Chung S, Lane L, Castro A, Watson RR. Immunomodulation by pycnogenol in retrovirus-infected or ethanol-fed mice. Life Sci. 1996;58(5):PL 87-96.

Cho KJ, Yun CH, Yoon DY, Cho YS, Rimbach G, Packer L, Chung AS. Effect of bioflavonoids extracted from the bark of Pinus maritima on proinflammatory cytokine interleukin-1 production in lipopolysaccharide-stimulated RAW 264.7. Toxicol Appl Pharmacol. 2000 Oct 1;168(1):64-71.

Cossins E, Lee R, Packer L. ESR studies of vitamin C regeneration, order of reactivity of natural source phytochemical preparations. Biochem Mol Biol Int. 1998 July;45(3):583-97.

Da Silva JMR, Darmon N, Fernandez Y, Mitjavila S. Radical scavenger capacity of different procyanidins from grape seeds. Presented at a symposium Free Radicals in Biotechnology and Medicine. Royal Society of Chemistry, London, January 1990, pp. 79-80.

Devi M, Ambika Das NP. In vitro effects of natural plant polyphenols on the proliferation of normal and abnormal human lymphocytes and their secretions of interleukin-2. Cancer Letters. 1993;69(3):191-6.

Fitzpatrick DF, Bing B, Rohdewald P. Endothelium-dependent vascular effects of pycnogenol. J Cardiovasc Pharmacol. 1998 Oct;32(4):509-15.

Greenblatt J. Nutritional supplements in ADHD. J Am Acad Child Adolesc Psychiatry. 1999 Oct;38(10):1209-11.

Habtemariam S. Flavonoids as inhibitors or enhancers of the cytotoxicity of tumor necrosis factor-alpha in L-929 tumor cells. J Nat Prod. 1997;60(8):775-8.

Hasegawa N. Inhibition of lipogenesis by pycnogenol. Phytother Res. 2000 Sep;14(6):472-3.

Hasegawa N. Stimulation of lipolysis by pycnogenol. Phytother Res. 1999 Nov;13(7):619-20.

Heimann SW. Pycnogenol for ADHD? J Am Acad Child Adolesc Psychiatry. 1999 Apr;38(4):357-8.

Huynh HT, Teel RW. Selective induction of apoptosis in human mammary cancer cells (MCF-7) by pycnogenol. Anticancer Res. 2000 Jul-Aug;20(4):2417-20.

Kakegawa H, Matsumoto H, Endo K, Satoh T, Nonaka G, Mishioka I. Inhibitory effects of tannins on hyaluronidase activation and on the degranulation from rat mesentery mast cells. Chem Pharm Bull. 1985;33(11):5079-82.

Kandaswami C, Perkin E, Soloniuk DS, Drzeweicki G, Middleton E Jr. Antiproliferative effects of citrus flavonoids on a human squamous cell carcinoma in vitro. Cancer Letters. 1991;56(2):147-52.

Liu F, Lau BH, Peng Q, Shah V. Pycnogenol protects vascular endothelial cells from beta-amyloid-induced injury. Biol Pharm Bull. 2000 Jun;23(6):735-7.

Liu FJ, Zhang YX, Lau BH. Pycnogenol enhances immune and haemopoietic functions in senescence-accelerated mice. Cell Mol Life Sci. 1998 Oct;54(10):1168-72.

Manach C, Texier O, Morand C, Crespy V, Regerat F, Demigne C, Remesy C. Bioavailability, metabolism, and physicological impact of 4-oxo-flavonoids. Nutrition Res. 1996;16(3):517-44.

Masquelier J, Dumon MC, Dumas J. Stabilization du collagene par les oligomeres procyanidoliques. Acta Therapeutica. 1981;7:101-5.

Morel I, Lescoat G, Cogrel P, Sergent O, Pasdeloup N, Brissot P, Cillard P, Cillard J. Antioxidant and iron-chelating activities of the flavonoids catechin, quercetin, and diosmetin on iron-loaded rat hepatocyte cultures. Biochem Pharmacology. 1993;45(1):13-19.

Nuttall SL, Kendall MJ, Bombardelli E, Morazzoni P. An evaluation of the antioxidant activity of a standardized grape seed extract, Leucoselect. J Clin Pharm Ther. 1998 Oct;23(5):385-9.

Packer L, Rimbach G, Virgili F. Antioxidant activity and biologic properties of a procyanidin-rich extract from pine (Pinus maritima) bark, pycnogenol. Free Radic Biol Med. 1999 Sep;27(5-6):704-24.

Palma M, Taylor LT. Extraction of polyphenolic compounds from grape seeds with near critical carbon dioxide. J Chromatogr A. 1999 Jul 16;849(1):117-24.

Peng Q, Wei Z, Lau BH. Pycnogenol inhibits tumor necrosis factor-alpha-induced nuclear factor kappa B activation and adhesion molecule expression in human vascular endothelial cells. Cell Mol Life Sci. 2000 May;57(5):834-41.

Putter M, Grotemeyer KH, Wurthwein G, Araghi-Niknam M, Watson RR, Hosseini S, Rohdewald P. Inhibition of smoking-induced platelet aggregation by aspirin and pycnogenol. Thromb Res. 1999 Aug 15;95(4):155-61.

Robert AM, Groult N, Six C, Robert L. Study of the effect of procyanidolic oligomers on mesenchymal cells in culture. Pat Biol. 1990;38(6):601-7.

Rong Y, Li L, Shah V, Lau BH. Pycnogenol protects vascular endothelial cells from t-butyl hydroperoxide induced oxidant injury. Biotechnol Ther. 1994-95;5(3-4):117-26.

Salah N, Miller NJ, Paganga G, Tijburg L, Bolwell GP, Rice-Evans C. Polyphenolic flavanols as scavengers of aqueous phase radicals and as chain-breaking antioxidants. Arch Biochem Biophys. 1995;322(2):339-46.

Tixier JM, Godeau G, Robert AM, Hornebeck W. Evidence by in vivo and in vitro studies that binding of pycnogenols to elastin affects its rate of degradation by elastases. Biochem Pharmacol. 1984 Dec 15;33(24):3933-9.

van Jaarsveld H, Kuyl JM, Schulenburg DH, Wiid NM. Effect of flavonoids on the outcome of myocardial mitochondrial ischemia/reperfusion injury. Res Commun Mol Pathol Pharmacol. 1996 Jan;91(1):65-75.

Virgili F, Kobuchi H, Packer L. Procyanidins extracted from Pinus maritima (pycnogenol): Scavengers of free radical species and modulators of nitrogen monoxide metabolism in activated murine RAW 264.7 macrophages. Free Radic Biol Med. 1998 May;24(7-8):1120-9.

Virgili F, Pagana G, Bourne L, Rimbach G, Natella F, Rice-Evans C, Packer L. Ferulic acid excretion as a marker of consumption of a french maritime pine (Pinus maritima) bark extract. Free Radic Biol Med. 2000 Apr 15;28(8):1249-56.

Yamakoshi J, Kataoka S, Koga T, Ariga T. Proanthocyanidin-rich extract from grape seeds attenuates the development of aortic atherosclerosis in cholesterol-fed rabbits. Atherosclerosis. 1999 Jan;142(1):139-49.

QUERCETIN

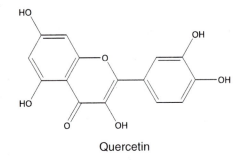

Quercetin

What Is It?

Quercetin is a water-soluble flavonoid typically found in red wine, green tea, onions, apples, and leafy vegetables. In the body, quercetin has potent antioxidant and anti-inflammatory activity, where it can protect cellular structures and blood vessels from the damaging effects of free radicals. There is some evidence that quercetin also acts as an antihistamine and may play a role in elevating norepinephrine levels—effects that have been linked to relief of allergies and asthma as well as increased energy expenditure and thermogenesis.

Claims

- Antioxidant
- Protects from heart disease (reduced LDL oxidation)
- Relieves allergic symptoms (antihistamine activity)
- Improves blood vessel strength (capillary fragility)
- Helps prevent cataracts (antioxidant function)
- Enhances thermogenesis and energy expenditure (via increased norepinephrine levels)

Theory

Flavonoids such as catechins from green tea, polyphenols from pine bark, and resveratrol from red wine are generally acknowledged as potent antioxidants and vasodilators. As such, they are typically included in dietary supplements targeted to cellular protection from free radical damage and re-duction of heart disease risk. In addition to these beneficial health effects, quercetin, a flavonoid found in both green tea and red wine, also inhibits the activity of an enzyme (catechol-O-methyltransferase) that breaks down the neurotransmitter norepinephrine. This effect may lead to elevated levels of norepinephrine and an increase in energy expenditure (thermogenesis) and fat oxidation.

Scientific Support

The majority of the scientific evidence for quercetin's health benefits is drawn from cellular and animal studies. It is well accepted that flavonoids in general, and quercetin in particular, are extremely effective antioxidants and vasodilators. These effects are thought to provide a distinct cardioprotective effect by preventing LDL cholesterol oxidation, protecting the inner lining of blood vessels from damage, and promoting vascular relaxation and lower blood pressure. In test-tube studies, both quercetin and green tea catechins have been shown to inhibit the activity of catechol-O-methyltransferase (COMT) and elevate the level and activity of norepinephrine. Given the im-portant role that norepinephrine plays in regulating thermogenesis and fat oxidation, it is conceivable that inhibition of COMT may result in a more prolonged effect of norepinephrine and an increase in energy expenditure and fat metabolism. In cellular studies, it is clear that quercetin can also in-teract with norepinephrine to stimulate cellular energy expenditure.

Safety

No adverse side effects have been identified relating to typical doses of quercetin in dietary supplements. Because of a general effect of many flavonoids on blood vessel dilation and blood thinning, however, high doses of any flavonoid, including quercetin, should be avoided—especially by in-dividuals at risk for hypotension (low blood pressure) or problems with blood clotting.

Value

Quercetin has been shown to be effective as a general-purpose antioxi-dant, vasodilator, and blood thinner. Although the thermogenic properties of quercetin have yet to be fully evaluated in human trials, evidence from test-tube studies suggests that flavonoids such as quercetin and green tea catechins are effective in elevating norepinephrine levels and stimulating fat oxidation.

Dosage

Although there are no widely recognized standard dosage recommendations for quercetin, intakes of as high as 100 to 1,000 mg per day, consumed in two to three divided doses, have been used with no apparent adverse side effects. For general antioxidant benefits and support of norepinephrine levels and thermogenesis, much lower doses are likely to be effective.

WORKS CONSULTED

Akagi K, Hirose M, Hoshiya T, Mizoguchi Y, Ito N, Shirai T. Modulating effects of ellagic acid, vanillin and quercetin in a rat medium term multi-organ carcinogenesis model. Cancer Lett. 1995 Jul 20;94(1):113-21.

Arai Y, Watanabe S, Kimira M, Shimoi K, Mochizuki R, Kinae N. Dietary intakes of flavonols, flavones and isoflavones by Japanese women and the inverse correlation between quercetin intake and plasma LDL cholesterol concentration. J Nutr. 2000 Sep;130(9):2243-50.

Ballmer PE. The Mediterranean diet—healthy but still delicious. Ther Umsch. 2000 Mar;57(3):167-72.

Blardi P, De Lalla A, Volpi L, Di Perri T. Stimulation of endogenous adenosine release by oral administration of quercetin and resveratrol in man. Drugs Exp Clin Res. 1999;25(2-3):105-10.

Conquer JA, Maiani G, Azzini E, Raguzzini A, Holub BJ. Supplementation with quercetin markedly increases plasma quercetin concentration without effect on selected risk factors for heart disease in healthy subjects. J Nutr. 1998 Mar;128(3):593-7.

Damianaki A, Bakogeorgou E, Kampa M, Notas G, Hatzoglou A, Panagiotou S, Gemetzi C, Kouroumalis E, Martin PM, Castanas E. Potent inhibitory action of red wine polyphenols on human breast cancer cells. J Cell Biochem. 2000 Jun 6;78(3):429-41.

Day AJ, Williamson G. Human metabolism of dietary quercetin glycosides. Basic Life Sci. 1999;66:415-34.

De Santi C, Pietrabissa A, Spisni R, Mosca F, Pacifici GM. Sulphation of resveratrol, a natural product present in grapes and wine, in the human liver and duodenum. Xenobiotica. 2000 Jun;30(6):609-17.

de Vries JH, Hollman PC, Meyboom S, Buysman MN, Zock PL, van Staveren WA, Katan MB. Plasma concentrations and urinary excretion of the antioxidant flavonols quercetin and kaempferol as biomarkers for dietary intake. Am J Clin Nutr. 1998 Jul;68(1):60-5.

de Vries JH, Janssen PL, Hollman PC, van Staveren WA, Katan MB. Consumption of quercetin and kaempferol in free-living subjects eating a variety of diets. Cancer Lett. 1997 Mar 19;114(1-2):141-4.

Formica JV, Regelson W. Review of the biology of Quercetin and related bioflavonoids. Food Chem Toxicol. 1995 Dec;33(12):1061-80.

Galijatovic A, Walle UK, Walle T. Induction of UDP-glucuronosyltransferase by the flavonoids chrysin and quercetin in Caco-2 cells. Pharm Res. 2000 Jan;17(1):21-6.

Garcia R, Gonzalez CA, Agudo A, Riboli E. High intake of specific carotenoids and flavonoids does not reduce the risk of bladder cancer. Nutr Cancer. 1999; 35(2):212-4.

Graefe EU, Derendorf H, Veit M. Pharmacokinetics and bioavailability of the flavonol quercetin in humans. Int J Clin Pharmacol Ther. 1999 May;37(5):219-33.

Gross M, Pfeiffer M, Martini M, Campbell D, Slavin J, Potter J. The quantitation of metabolites of quercetin flavonols in human urine. Cancer Epidemiol Biomarkers Prev. 1996 Sep;5(9):711-20.

Hertog MG, Hollman PC. Potential health effects of the dietary flavonol quercetin. Eur J Clin Nutr. 1996 Feb;50(2):63-71.

Hollman PC, de Vries JH, van Leeuwen SD, Mengelers MJ, Katan MB. Absorption of dietary quercetin glycosides and quercetin in healthy ileostomy volunteers. Am J Clin Nutr. 1995 Dec;62(6):1276-82.

Hollman PC, Katan MB. Dietary flavonoids: Intake, health effects and bioavailability. Food Chem Toxicol. 1999 Sep-Oct;37(9-10):937-42.

Hollman PC, Katan MB. Health effects and bioavailability of dietary flavonols. Free Radic Res. 1999 Dec;31(Suppl):S75-80.

Hollman PC, van Trijp JM, Buysman MN, van der Gaag MS, Mengelers MJ, de Vries JH, Katan MB. Relative bioavailability of the antioxidant flavonoid quercetin from various foods in man. FEBS Lett. 1997 Nov 24;418(1-2):152-6.

Janssen K, Mensink RP, Cox FJ, Harryvan JL, Hovenier R, Hollman PC, Katan MB. Effects of the flavonoids quercetin and apigenin on hemostasis in healthy volunteers: Results from an in vitro and a dietary supplement study. Am J Clin Nutr. 1998 Feb;67(2):255-62.

Kang ZC, Tsai SJ, Lee H. Quercetin inhibits benzo[a]pyrene-induced DNA adducts in human Hep G2 cells by altering cytochrome P-450 1A1 gene expression. Nutr Cancer. 1999;35(2):175-9.

Knekt P, Isotupa S, Rissanen H, Heliovaara M, Jarvinen R, Hakkinen S, Aromaa A, Reunanen A. Quercetin intake and the incidence of cerebrovascular disease. Eur J Clin Nutr. 2000 May;54(5):415-7.

Manach C, Morand C, Crespy V, Demigne C, Texier O, Regerat F, Remesy C. Quercetin is recovered in human plasma as conjugated derivatives which retain antioxidant properties. FEBS Lett. 1998 Apr 24;426(3):331-6.

Manach C, Morand C, Texier O, Favier ML, Agullo G, Demigne C, Regerat F, Remesy C. Quercetin metabolites in plasma of rats fed diets containing rutin or quercetin. J Nutr. 1995 Jul;125(7):1911-22.

Manach C, Texier O, Morand C, Crespy V, Regerat F, Demigne C, Remesy C. Comparison of the bioavailability of quercetin and catechin in rats. Free Radic Biol Med. 1999 Dec;27(11-12):1259-66.

Moon JH, Nakata R, Oshima S, Inakuma T, Terao J. Accumulation of quercetin conjugates in blood plasma after the short-term ingestion of onion by women. Am J Physiol Regul Integr Comp Physiol. 2000 Aug;279(2):R461-7.

Oliveira EJ, Watson DG. In vitro glucuronidation of kaempferol and quercetin by human UGT-1A9 microsomes. FEBS Lett. 2000 Apr 7;471(1):1-6.

O'Reilly JD, Sanders TA, Wiseman H. Flavonoids protect against oxidative damage to LDL in vitro: Use in selection of a flavonoid rich diet and relevance to LDL oxidation resistance ex vivo? Free Radic Res. 2000 Oct;33(4):419-26.

Rodgers EH, Grant MH. The effect of the flavonoids, quercetin, myricetin and epicatechin on the growth and enzyme activities of MCF7 human breast cancer cells. Chem Biol Interact. 1998 Nov 27;116(3):213-28.

Saito D, Shirai A, Matsushima T, Sugimura T, Hirono I. Test of carcinogenicity of quercetin, a widely distributed mutagen in food. Teratog Carcinog Mutagen. 1980;1(2):213-21.

Stavric B. Quercetin in our diet: From potent mutagen to probable anticarcinogen. Clin Biochem. 1994 Aug;27(4):245-8.

Terao J. Dietary flavonoids as antioxidants in vivo: Conjugated metabolites of (-)-epicatechin and quercetin participate in antioxidative defense in blood plasma. J Med Invest. 1999 Aug;46(3-4):159-68.

Wiseman H. The bioavailability of non-nutrient plant factors: Dietary flavonoids and phyto-oestrogens. Proc Nutr Soc. 1999 Feb;58(1):139-46.

Wiseman H, O'Reilly J. Influence of the dietary flavonoid quercetin on the cardioprotective antioxidant action of oestrogen and phytoestrogens. Biochem Soc Trans. 1997 Feb;25(1):108S.

Young JF, Nielsen SE, Haraldsdottir J, Daneshvar B, Lauridsen ST, Knuthsen P, Crozier A, Sandstrom B, Dragsted LO. Effect of fruit juice intake on urinary quercetin excretion and biomarkers of antioxidative status. Am J Clin Nutr. 1999 Jan;69(1):87-94.

Chapter 13

Supplements for Gastrointestinal Health

INTRODUCTION

Well over 100 million Americans use an antacid or laxative on a regular basis, and over-the-counter digestive aids account for more than a billion dollars in annual sales (with another billion or so spent on similar products in the Japanese market). Remember those old Alka-Seltzer commercials—the "I can't believe I ate the whole thing" ads? Well, the whole idea behind them was to promote the concept that there were simple remedies for treating heartburn, indigestion, and general stomach upset (by using Alka-Seltzer, of course). Now, with the rise in mainstream use of dietary supplements, there are a number of effective herbal remedies and other natural alternatives to help combat some of the minor annoyances associated with the gastrointestinal tract.

Although a great many factors can affect proper functioning of the digestive tract (diet, medications, exercise level, and stress), many cases of upset stomach and general gastrointestinal distress can be alleviated with simple changes in diet and lifestyle. It is important to note that a simple stomachache or indigestion can be caused by a wide variety of related conditions—everything from a mild touch of gas or bout of heartburn to a potentially serious case of acid reflux or ulcer.

COMMON GASTROINTESTINAL CONDITIONS

Constipation refers to the common situation in which stools become hard and difficult to pass. Two dietary changes that are highly effective in relieving constipation are drinking more water and eating more soluble fiber (fruits and vegetables). A popular method of accomplishing both of these recommendations is to consume a psyllium-based laxative (which will provide both soluble and insoluble fiber) mixed with water. Exercise can also be quite effective in stimulating the intestinal muscles to contract and "get things moving."

Irritable bowel syndrome (IBS) is one of the most common gastrointestinal disorders. Symptoms can change over time, but generally include a mix of diarrhea, gas, constipation, bloating, and pain as well as general feelings of fatigue and lethargy. Although the cause of IBS remains unknown in most people, stress is known to be highly related to the development and flare-up of IBS. Relaxation techniques and stress management may be helpful, and dietary changes such as the elimination of caffeine and other stimulants as well as dairy products (yogurt may still be tolerated in some people) may offer some relief. Adding fiber, such as psyllium, to the diet can facilitate regular bowel movements (although wheat bran can be problematic in some IBS patients), and the addition of peppermint oil (enteric coated) and probiotic bacteria may be helpful.

Ulcerative colitis (UC) is a serious inflammatory condition in which inflammation damages the lining of the colon (large intestine) and leads to bloody diarrhea and intense pain. Treatment by a gastroenterologist often involves anti-inflammatory steroid medications to control the inflammation and tissue damage. In more severe cases of UC, removal of all or part of the colon may be necessary. *Crohn's disease* is related to UC, but the inflammation in Crohn's can involve the entire wall of the colon (not just the lining) and can even involve the small intestine as well. As with IBS, several dietary changes may be beneficial in relieving some of the symptoms of UC and Crohn's disease. Avoidance of caffeine and other stimulants as well as dairy products may be helpful in many people. Although fiber may be beneficial in IBS, raw fruits and vegetables and some seeds may cause additional irritation during an active phase or flare-up of colitis. Slippery elm and aloe vera juice may be soothing to irritated mucous membranes. Because UC may increase the risk of colon cancer, it may be prudent to supplement the diet with 400 to 800 mcg of folic acid to reduce the risk of colon cancer and its precursor, adenomatous polyps.

Low stomach acid, a condition that becomes more common with age, can result in varying degrees of indigestion and a general feeling of fatigue. Because adequate levels of stomach acid are needed for the proper digestion of proteins and for optimal absorption of several vitamins and minerals, it is logical for low stomach acid (hypochlorhydria) to lead to suboptimal energy levels and general feelings of lethargy. One of the most popular supplements for increasing stomach acid is betaine HCl (200 to 600 mg per day), but caution should be used to prevent an overproduction of acid—especially in individuals at high risk for ulcers. Other popular digestive stimulants include capsaicin (cayenne), devil's claw, bromelain, papain, and horseradish.

Heartburn, the condition that is the opposite of low stomach acid is, of course, high stomach acid. Perhaps everybody reading this has experienced

the unpleasant sensation of burning in the center of the chest that is characteristic of the acid reflux of heartburn. Most causes of heartburn can be
traced back to too much food, too much of the *wrong* foods, or too much
stress. If you suffer from chronic heartburn, regular consumption of antac-
ids is not the solution—but lifestyle and dietary modifications can be helpful (although the occasional use of a calcium carbonate-based antacid such
as Tums is OK). Chronic heartburn should be evaluated by a physician to
rule out a more serious condition such as acid reflux disease. The first dietary approach to controlling heartburn is to avoid or cut down on coffee, alcohol, and tobacco—each of which can be a potent stomach irritant. Herbs
such as chamomile, ginger, and meadowsweet may also be helpful in reducing stomach acid and soothing irritated membranes.

SUPPLEMENTS THAT MAY BE HELPFUL

Juice from the aloe vera plant is frequently used as a general digestive aid
due to its mild anti-inflammatory activity and soothing qualities for mucous
membranes.

Ginger is one of the most commonly used stomach soothers—most typically used to treat or prevent motion sickness or sea sickness.

Bioflavonoids, such as those found in grape seed extract and green tea,
have both antioxidant and anti-inflammatory activity.

The sap of the *Boswellia serrata* plant has powerful anti-inflammatory
activity that may be helpful in relieving inflammation of the digestive tract.

Chamomile, the same herb that you may know from your Sleepytime tea,
is also quite effective in calming the stomach and relieving inflammation
along the digestive tract, as are barberry, dandelion, fennel, and melissa
(lemon balm).

Fiber, whether insoluble such as wheat bran or soluble such as oat bran or
pectin, is known to increase digestion time by slowing the movement of
food and acid from the stomach into the intestines—an effect that can help
accelerate healing of duodenal ulcers.

Glutamine is an amino acid that intestinal cells use as a primary source of
energy. Maintaining an optimal energy state within intestinal cells helps to
promote healing of damaged cells and may help treat ulcers. Glutamine has
been shown effective, at several grams per day, in stimulating immune system integrity and reducing inflammation (a potential benefit in inflammatory conditions of the digestive tract).

Goldenseal, which most people think of simply as an immune-stimulating herb, may also be helpful in relieving heartburn, indigestion, and nau-

sea. It is thought that other berberine-containing herbs such as Oregon grape and barberry also possess similar gastrointestinal benefits.

Licorice (no, not the Twizzler kind) can increase the production of mucin and help protect the lining of the digestive tract (be sure to look for the "deglycyrrhizinated" or DGL form of licorice, which has the hypertensive glycyrrhizic acid removed). There is some evidence that licorice root can promote the healing of ulcers. Taken before meals and bedtime, 500 mg or so of licorice root extract can help relieve some of the discomfort associated with heartburn (and may be as effective as the prescription medication Tagamet in many people).

Marshmallow, fenugreek, Irish moss, and slippery elm are all rich sources of mucilages, with potential benefits in relieving inflammation and soothing mucous membranes along the digestive tract.

Probiotic bacteria and prebiotic oligosaccharides are well known to help promote a healthy digestive system and may help reduce some of the symptoms associated with conditions such as IBS, constipation, and diarrhea.

Peppermint oil (taken as enteric-coated capsules) may help treat inflammation of the digestive tract lining as well as help calm the stomach and reduce gas and bloating (do not use it if you are experiencing heartburn). The main effect of peppermint is likely due to the presence of menthol and polyphenol/flavonoids that may help relax the esophageal sphincter in the stomach and promote release of gas. Peppermint also possesses various antispasmodic effects and has been shown in at least one clinical study to reduce abdominal pain, bloating, and flatulence. Many commercial forms of peppermint oil for intestinal health are enteric coated (to prevent release in the stomach and deliver the active compounds to the intestine).

Omega-3 fatty acids, such as those found in fish oil, have strong anti-inflammatory activity, which may be helpful in reducing inflammation of the colon and digestive tract. Doses of fish oil from 5 to 10 g per day may reduce the need (somewhat) for anti-inflammatory steroid medications in people experiencing such conditions.

Artichoke extract *(Cynara scolymus)* is a popular natural remedy used in Europe to calm upset stomachs. A number of European brands are marketed to increase bile flow, which is thought to help stimulate digestion and reduce constipation. Several studies have documented the increase in bile secretion following consumption of artichoke extract (versus a placebo) as well as reduced reports of nausea, constipation, and flatulence. Artichoke extracts may be standardized to 5 to 18 percent caffeylquinic acids, with doses ranging from 150 to 300 mg taken with each meal.

For a list of supplements, see Table 13.1.

TABLE 13.1. Common Dietary Supplements for Promoting Gastrointestinal Health

Supplement	Dose (per day)	Primary claims
Aloe vera	50-200 mg	Mild anti-inflammatory for irritated membranes
Artichoke extract	450-900 mg	Reduces constipation and bloating
Betaine HCl	Follow label directions	Source of hydrochloric acid (stomach acid)
Bioflavonoids	100-300 mg	Antioxidant and anti-inflammatory activity
Boswellia serrata	600-1,200 mg	Anti-inflammatory activity
Bromelain and papain	500-1,500 mg	Proteolytic enzymes that promote digestion
Capsicum	50-200 mg	Digestive aid, stimulates stomach acid
Chamomile	Follow label directions	Relieves inflammation and promotes digestion
Fenugreek seed	15-20 g	Source of mucilage to soothe pain and irritation
Fiber	20-40 g	Provides stool bulk and relieves constipation
Ginger	500-1,000 mg	Relieves nausea
Glutamine	1-10 g	Important fuel source for intestinal cells
Goldenseal	250-500 mg	Mild anti-inflammatory and calms stomach
Irish moss	Follow label directions	Mucilage soothes irritated membranes
Lactase	Follow label directions	Enzyme that degrades lactose (milk sugar)
Licorice	500 mg	Protects mucosal lining of digestive tract
Marshmallow	Follow label directions	Relieves inflammation/soothes mucous membranes
Mastic	1-3 g	Antiulcer
Meadowsweet	Follow label directions	Reduces stomach acid

TABLE 13.1 *(continued)*

Supplement	Dose (per day)	Primary claims
Omega-3 fatty acids	2-10 g	Anti-inflammatory activity
Peppermint oil	10-100 mg	Anti-inflammatory, calms stomach, reduces gas
Prebiotics (FOS)	2-10 g	Provides energy source for probiotics
Probiotic organisms	1-8 billion CFUs	Displaces pathogenic organisms in the lower intestine
Slippery elm	400-1,600 mg	Soothes mucous membranes
Yellow dock	500-1,000 mg	Laxative

FIBER

What Is It?

Fiber is found in the stems, seeds, and leaves of plants. Fiber is made up of long chains of sugar, but humans do not have the enzymes in their digestive tract to be able to break these chains down (although a small amount of ingested fiber can be partially broken down by enzymes produced by bacteria in the intestines). Most of the fiber, however, is not broken down and goes out of the body in the feces. "Fiber" is a very broad term. More precise terms are soluble and insoluble fiber. Soluble fiber dissolves in water and can be broken down by bacterial enzymes, while insoluble fiber cannot. The distinction is important because the solubility of the fiber determines its health benefit. Fiber found in food is usually a mixture of both types of fiber, while purified fiber supplements may contain just one type of fiber.

Dietary sources of fiber are plentiful. Fruits, vegetables, seeds, and legumes (dried peas and beans such as lentils, split peas, red beans, and pinto beans) contain both types of fiber. Barley, oats, oat bran, and rye contain predominantly soluble fiber. Wheat bran, brown rice, and whole grains (grains that have not been refined) are excellent sources of insoluble fiber.

Supplemental sources of fiber include psyllium, methylcellulose, or polycarbophil as well as fiber extracted from fruits, vegetables, and grains. Psyllium is a concentrated source of fiber from the husks of the psyllium plant. Methylcellulose and polycarbophil are chemically altered forms of cellulose (the cell wall of many plants). The chemical alterations make them resistant to bacterial breakdown.

General health recommendations call for a daily consumption of 20 to 40 g of fiber, but the average American consumes less than 15 g. Although the amounts of soluble and insoluble fiber are not specified, it is assumed that people will receive both types of fiber.

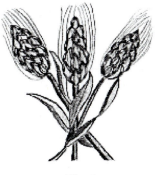

Wheat

Claims

Soluble Fiber

- Reduces the risk of heart disease by lowering total and LDL cholesterol levels
- Prevents constipation

Insoluble Fiber

- Reduces the risk of colon cancer
- Prevents constipation

Theory

Soluble Fiber Reduces the Risk of Heart Disease by Lowering Cholesterol and LDL

Although the mechanism is not entirely known, soluble fiber is thought to decrease the absorption of bile. Bile, which contains cholesterol, is necessary for the digestion of fat. It is secreted into the intestine in response to food intake and most is reabsorbed after digestion is complete. When soluble fiber is present in the digestive tract, not as much bile is reabsorbed, and more must be made by the liver. Some of the cholesterol that would have circulated in the blood is used to make the bile. In addition, soluble fiber can be partially broken down by intestinal bacteria, which produce fatty acids that keep the liver from making cholesterol. It is generally accepted by nutrition scientists that soluble fiber intake can help reduce cholesterol levels.

Insoluble Fiber Reduces the Risk of Colon Cancer

If, and how, fiber reduces the risk of cancer is not completely known and is undoubtedly complicated. The theory that supports the role of a high-fiber diet in the prevention of colon cancer is controversial. It is suggested that insoluble fiber may work by helping to excrete bile from the body. Bile, which is necessary for the digestion of fat, is also thought to promote tumor growth. Insoluble fiber may bind with the bile, thus preventing it from being a promoter. Insoluble fiber also reduces the amount of time that fecal material is in the colon. Exposure to potential cancer-causing compounds is reduced because the fiber binds and removes these compounds quickly. Researchers who question whether insoluble fiber actually reduces colon cancer risk do so because they are not convinced that the fiber itself is responsible. They suggest that foods that contain insoluble dietary fiber also contain substances such as antioxidants, folate, or dozens of other phytonutrients. They argue that it is these compounds, not the dietary fiber, that help to protect against colon cancer.

Fiber Prevents Constipation

Constipation is a condition in which bowel movements (feces) are hard and dry. The strain of trying to pass the hard, dry feces may result in hemorrhoids (swollen veins in the rectum). Adequate fiber, fluid, and exercise help prevent constipation. Both soluble and insoluble fibers help the feces stay moist because fiber attracts water. Insoluble fiber also has a laxative effect and helps speed up the time it takes for feces to move out of the body. This theory is well accepted.

Scientific Support

Soluble Fiber and Heart Disease Risk

Hundreds of studies have been conducted to examine the role of soluble fiber in reducing the risk of heart disease by lowering cholesterol levels. Although it is difficult to compare the studies because of differences in the type and amount of soluble fiber, the number of people studied, and the initial cholesterol levels of the subjects, some general conclusions can be drawn. It is generally accepted by nutrition scientists that approximately 2 to 10 g of soluble fiber daily appears to reduce blood cholesterol and LDL cholesterol. The reduction is small, but makes a substantial contribution to reducing heart disease risk. The source of the fiber (oats, pectin found in fruits, or psyllium) seems to make little difference, as all types have been shown to be effective. The inclusion of soluble fibers in the diet is both practical and safe as long as the individual is not allergic to the source of the fiber.

Insoluble Fiber and Colon Cancer Risk

For nearly thirty years, researchers have been studying the effect of fiber on colon cancer. People who consume diets high in fiber tend to also consume diets that are low in total fat, low in animal fat, and high in fruits and vegetables—all of which are factors that might reduce colon cancer risk. Fiber is also a vehicle for other compounds such as phytic acid, an antioxidant thought to prevent colon cancer. Researchers are trying to determine whether fiber should be considered an independent factor in reducing colon cancer risk or whether the effect of fiber is due to a combination of other factors. Results of human studies have been mixed, but three large studies suggest that fiber is not protective against colon cancer. A 1999 study by highly regarded researchers found that the intake of dietary fiber did *not* protect against colon cancer. This study is considered a strong study because of its large size (more than 88,000 women) and ability to observe changes over time (data were first collected in 1976). Two studies published in April 2000 also found no correlation between fiber intake and reduced risk for colon cancer. Although there is support for a high-fiber diet as a general dietary recommendation, it does not appear to *directly* protect against colon cancer.

Constipation

Scientific studies support the role of dietary fiber in relieving constipation. Fluid and exercise are also mentioned as important factors. Both dietary fiber and fiber supplements are beneficial.

Safety

The intake of dietary fiber or fiber supplements within the recommended doses (see Dosage) is considered safe. To prevent dehydration, adequate fluid must be consumed. Side effects such as excessive gas or bloating may occur. Some individuals may be allergic to the source of the fiber, for example, wheat or psyllium.

Value

There is no question that adequate fiber is necessary for good health. Consumption of 20 to 40 g of fiber per day is possible from food sources alone. However, it is recognized that in the United States, the average fiber intake is less than 15 g per day. In light of average intake, fiber supplements are often recommended.

Dosage

- Total dietary fiber, 20 to 40 g per day
- Psyllium supplements, 7 g in 8 oz of liquid (up to three times per day)
- Methylcellulose, 10 g in 8 oz of liquid (up to three times per day)
- Polycarbophil, 1 g (two caplets) per day with a glass of water (maximum of 4 g daily)

WORKS CONSULTED

Anderson JW, Smith BM, Gustafson NJ. Health benefits and practical aspects of high-fiber diets. Am J Clin Nutr. 1994 May;59(5 Suppl):1242S-7S.

Auld GW, Bruhn CM, McNulty J, Bock MA, Gabel K, Lauritzen G, Medeiros D, Newman R, Nitzke S, Ortiz M, Read M, Schutz H, Sheehan ET. Reported adoption of dietary fat and fiber recommendations among consumers. J Am Diet Assoc. 2000 Jan;100(1):52-8.

Correa P. Epidemiological correlations between diet and cancer frequency. Cancer Res. 1981 Sep;41(9 Pt 2):3685-90.

DeVries JW. Overview on complex carbohydrates. Adv Exp Med Biol. 1997;427:43-50.

Dietary fiber and health. AMA Council on Scientific Affairs. Conn Med. 1989 Sep;53(9):529-34.

Floch MH, Maryniuk MD, Bryant C, Franz MJ, Tietyen-Clark J, Marotta RB, Wolever T, Maillet JO, Jenkins AL. Practical aspects of implementing increased dietary fiber intake. Am J Gastroenterol. 1986 Oct;81(10):936-9.

Geil PB, Anderson JW. Nutrition and health implications of dry beans: A review. J Am Coll Nutr. 1994 Dec;13(6):549-58.

Jacobs DR Jr, Meyer KA, Kushi LH, Folsom AR. Whole-grain intake may reduce the risk of ischemic heart disease death in postmenopausal women: The Iowa Women's Health Study. Am J Clin Nutr. 1998 Aug;68(2):248-57.

Kritchevsky D. The role of dietary fiber in health and disease. J Environ Pathol Toxicol Oncol. 1986 Mar-Apr;6(3-4):273-84.

Saldanha LG. Fiber in the diet of US children: Results of national surveys. Pediatrics. 1995 Nov;96(5 Pt 2):994-7.

Sali A. Dietary fibre and fats in health and disease. Aust Fam Physician. 1990 Mar;19(3):315-7, 320-2, 325-32.

Stampfer MJ, Hu FB, Manson JE, Rimm EB, Willett WC. Primary prevention of coronary heart disease in women through diet and lifestyle. N Engl J Med. 2000 Jul 6;343(1):16-22.

Thompson LU. Antioxidants and hormone-mediated health benefits of whole grains. Crit Rev Food Sci Nutr. 1994;34(5-6):473-97.

Vuksan V, Korsic M, Posavi-Antonovic A. Metabolic diseases and the high-fiber diet. Lijec Vjesn. 1997 Mar-Apr;119(3-4):125-7.

Weisburger JH. Worldwide prevention of cancer and other chronic diseases based on knowledge of mechanisms. Mutat Res. 1998 Jun 18;402(1-2):331-7.

Wolk A, Manson JE, Stampfer MJ, Colditz GA, Hu FB, Speizer FE, Hennekens CH, Willett WC. Long-term intake of dietary fiber and decreased risk of coronary heart disease among women. JAMA. 1999 Jun 2;281(21):1998-2004.

ALOE VERA

What Is It?

The gel of the aloe vera leaf has been used for centuries as a topical remedy for minor burns, cuts, and other skin irritations. Taken internally, aloe juice or encapsulated powder is used as a laxative. Some of the sugar compounds found in aloe have been promoted as immune system stimulants, although the data in this regard are limited.

Claims

- Treats minor burns and skin irritation (topically)
- Relieves constipation
- Lowers blood sugar (diabetes)
- Immune system support

Theory

The active constituents for aloe's laxative effect are known as anthraquinone glycosides, which are converted by intestinal bacteria into aglycones. The active compounds responsible for aloe's wound-healing properties are less well-described but are likely a combination of several saccharide molecules. When the leaf is consumed, the high fiber content of the plant has been shown to exert beneficial effects on cardiac disease risk factors by reducing blood levels of cholesterol, triglycerides, and glucose.

Scientific Support

In animal experiments, aloe vera gel clearly promotes the healing of minor burns and small wounds. Aloe vera juice or encapsulated powder results in reduced intestinal transit time. In one study of heart disease patients, aloe vera leaf added to the diet reduced serum levels of cholesterol, triglycerides, and blood sugar.

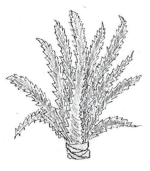

Safety

No significant side effects are noted with aloe vera as an internal or topical agent, except in rare cases of aloe latex allergy. Pregnant women, however, should avoid aloe-derived laxatives during pregnancy. Excess consumption of oral aloe juice products (12 to 16 oz per day) may lead to nausea, vomiting, and diarrhea.

Value

As a topical agent for minor skin irritations (cuts, burns, and sunburn), aloe vera gel is an effective treatment to reduce pain and inflammation and speed wound healing. Be sure to select the freshest gel available, as prolonged storage of gel products can result in appreciable loss of the wound-healing properties. As an internal (oral) agent, aloe vera juice or powder is an effective laxative.

Dosage

As a laxative, encapsulated dietary supplements of 50 to 200 mg per day or about 1 to 3 oz of aloe gel can be taken by mouth for constipation relief. Do not use for more than two weeks. As topical relief for minor skin irritations, aloe gel can be applied as needed throughout the day.

WORKS CONSULTED

Atherton P. Aloe vera: Magic or medicine? Nurs Stand. 1998 Jul 1-7;12(41):49-52, 54.

Davis RH, Agnew PS, Shapiro E. Antiarthritic activity of anthraquinones found in aloe for podiatric medicine. J Am Podiatr Med Assoc. 1986 Feb;76(2):61-6.

Dykman KD, Tone C, Ford C, Dykman RA. The effects of nutritional supplements on the symptoms of fibromyalgia and chronic fatigue syndrome. Integr Physiol Behav Sci. 1998 Jan-Mar;33(1):61-71.

Fairbairn JW. The anthraquinone laxatives. Biological assay and its relation to chemical structure. Pharmacology. 1976;14(Suppl 1):48-61.

Ghannam N, Kingston M, Al-Meshaal IA, Tariq M, Parman NS, Woodhouse N. The antidiabetic activity of aloes: Preliminary clinical and experimental observations. Horm Res. 1986;24(4):288-94.

Graf J. Herbal anti-inflammatory agents for skin disease. Skin Therapy Lett. 2000;5(4):3-5.

Grindlay D, Reynolds T. The Aloe vera phenomenon: A review of the properties and modern uses of the leaf parenchyma gel. J Ethnopharmacol. 1986 Jun; 16(2-3):117-51.

Hadley SK, Petry JJ. Medicinal herbs: A primer for primary care. Hosp Pract (Off Ed). 1999 Jun 15;34(6):105-6.

Hart LA, van Enckevort PH, van Dijk H, Zaat R, de Silva KT, Labadie RP. Two functionally and chemically distinct immunomodulatory compounds in the gel of Aloe vera. J Ethnopharmacol. 1988 May-Jun;23(1):61-71.

Iena IM. The therapeutic properties of aloe. Lik Sprava. 1993 Feb-Mar;(2-3):142-5.

Kivett WF. Aloe vera for burns. Plast Reconstr Surg. 1989 Jan;83(1):195.

Laurie JA, Shanahan TG, Moore RL, Urias RE, Kuske RR, Engel RE, Eggleston WD, Williams MS, Burk M, Loprinzi CL, et al. Phase III double-blind evaluation of an aloe vera gel as a prophylactic agent for radiation-induced skin toxicity. Int J Radiat Oncol Biol Phys. 1996 Sep 1;36(2):345-9.

Lutomski J. Aloe, a succulent plant with therapeutic action. Pharm Unserer Zeit. 1984 Nov;13(6):172-6.

Mapp RK, McCarthy TJ. The assessment of purgative principles in aloes. Planta Med. 1970 Aug;18(4):361-5.

Morton J. The detection of laxative abuse. Ann Clin Biochem. 1987 Jan;24(Pt 1): 107-8.

Natow AJ. Aloe vera, fiction or fact. Cutis. 1986 Feb;37(2):106, 108.

Reynolds T, Dweck AC. Aloe vera leaf gel: A review update. J Ethnopharmacol. 1999 Dec 15;68(1-3):3-37.

Robinson M. Medical therapy of inflammatory bowel disease for the 21st century. Eur J Surg Suppl. 1998;(582):90-8.

Salcido R. Complementary and alternative medicine in wound healing. Adv Wound Care. 1999 Nov-Dec;12(9):438.

Shelton RM. Aloe vera. Its chemical and therapeutic properties. Int J Dermatol. 1991 Oct;30(10):679-83.

Shida T, Yagi A, Nishimura H, Nishioka I. Effect of Aloe extract on peripheral phagocytosis in adult bronchial asthma. Planta Med. 1985 Jun;(3):273-5.

Spoerke DG, Ekins BR. Aloe vera—fact or quackery. Vet Hum Toxicol. 1980 Dec;22(6):418-24.

Sturm PG, Hayes SM. Aloe Vera in dentistry. J Bergen Cty Dent Soc. 1984 May;50(8):11-4.

t'Hart LA, Nibbering PH, van den Barselaar MT, van Dijk H, van den Berg AJ, Labadie RP. Effects of low molecular constituents from Aloe vera gel on oxidative metabolism and cytotoxic and bactericidal activities of human neutrophils. Int J Immunopharmacol. 1990;12(4):427-34.

t'Hart LA, van den Berg AJ, Kuis L, van Dijk H, Labadie RP. An anti-complementary polysaccharide with immunological adjuvant activity from the leaf parenchyma gel of Aloe vera. Planta Med. 1989 Dec;55(6):509-12.

van Os FH. Anthraquinone derivatives in vegetable laxatives. Pharmacology. 1976;14(Suppl 1):7-17.

Visuthikosol V, Chowchuen B, Sukwanarat Y, Sriurairatana S, Boonpucknavig V. Effect of aloe vera gel to healing of burn wound a clinical and histologic study. J Med Assoc Thai. 1995 Aug;78(8):403-9.

Vogler BK, Ernst E. Aloe vera: A systematic review of its clinical effectiveness. Br J Gen Pract. 1999 Oct;49(447):823-8.

GINGER

What Is It?

Ginger *(Zingiber officinale)* is native to coastal India, but it now grows and is harvested commonly in Jamaica, China, Africa, and the West Indies. The root is the source of ginger's familiar aroma, and the spice is made by drying the root and grinding it into a powder. Ginger has been used throughout history as an aid for many gastrointestinal disturbances as well as to relieve inflamed joints. In addition, the Chinese still use ginger as a tasty marinade to detoxify meats.

Claims

- Alleviates motion sickness and nausea
- Combats indigestion, flatulence, and diarrhea
- Treats pain from rheumatoid and osteoarthritis
- Acts as a heart tonic

Theory

The most active chemical compounds in ginger are known as the gingerols, which are also the most aromatic compounds in this root. Ginger also contains shogaols, which are formed during the drying process. These substances are thought to help break down gastric substances that could cause nausea. Ginger is also thought to increase the tone and movement of the intestines and to promote heart health. Furthermore, ginger may inhibit substances that could cause the pain and inflammation associated with osteoarthritis.

Scientific Support

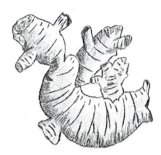

Ginger's most renowned use is its tendency to counteract nausea and other symptoms caused by excessive motion during travel, including seasickness. It is believed that whereas medications such as Dramamine act on the brain, ginger acts within the gastrointestinal tract to slow feedback from the stomach to the brain where the feelings of nausea are realized. In one particularly *extreme* study, thirty-six volunteers with a history of severe motion sickness received either Dramamine, powdered ginger, or a placebo. A short while later, they were blindfolded and spun in a mechanical chair until they either asked to stop or vomited (seriously). Those who received ginger remained in the chair for 5.5 minutes, while those who received Dramamine begged for mercy after 3.5 minutes. The unfortunate subjects who did not receive either therapeutic agent lasted a mere minute and a half. In other less extreme studies, subjects receiving ginger tend to fare significantly better in terms of symptoms of nausea and vertigo, and in most cases ginger is rated similarly to or better than prescription medications.

Safety

Although no adverse effects of ginger have been reported, and it does not have any reported interactions with medications, excessive doses could theoretically interfere with cardiac, antidiabetic, or anticoagulant (clotting) therapies. Those who have gallstone conditions should not take ginger. At 3,500 to 9,000 times the human dose, an alcohol extract of ginger caused death via involuntary contractions of skeletal muscle in mice after 72 hours of administration, although this hardly seems to be an attainable human dose. Pregnant women have often used ginger to abate nausea and other symptoms of morning sickness. Although negative consequences of this treatment are not documented, it is important to consult with a physician before self-medicating.

Value

Ginger is a relatively inexpensive supplement and can be enjoyed as a spice in many forms, including ginger beer (a Jamaican treat), candied ginger, sautéed ginger, etc. Most forms of ginger ale contain synthetic ginger flavors rather than real ginger and should not be expected to aid an upset stomach. Ginger supplements for therapeutic purposes can be found in powder, capsule, oil, and tea form for as little as $5 for sixty capsules. Because it is comparable to or even better than synthetic prescription or over-the-counter medications, ginger represents a good value for relief of nausea and indigestion.

Dosage

Most studies have used 1 g of powdered dried root per day, which is generally considered to be the preferred form. Ginger should be taken on an "as needed" basis.

WORKS CONSULTED

Aikins Murphy P. Alternative therapies for nausea and vomiting of pregnancy. Obstet Gynecol. 1998 Jan;91(1):149-55.

Arfeen Z, Owen H, Plummer JL, Ilsley AH, Sorby-Adams RA, Doecke CJ. A double-blind randomized controlled trial of ginger for the prevention of postoperative nausea and vomiting. Anaesth Intensive Care. 1995 Aug;23(4):449-52.

Backon J. Ginger as an antiemetic: Possible side effects due to its thromboxane synthetase activity. Anaesthesia. 1991 Aug;46(8):705-6.

Backon J. Ginger in preventing nausea and vomiting of pregnancy; a caveat due to its thromboxane synthetase activity and effect on testosterone binding. Eur J Obstet Gynecol Reprod Biol. 1991 Nov 26;42(2):163-4.

Bliddal H, Rosetzsky A, Schlichting P, Weidner MS, Andersen LA, Ibfelt HH, Christensen K, Jensen ON, Barslev J. A randomized, placebo-controlled, cross-over study of ginger extracts and ibuprofen in osteoarthritis. Osteoarthritis Cartilage. 2000 Jan;8(1):9-12.

Bone ME, Wilkinson DJ, Young JR, McNeil J, Charlton S. Ginger root—a new antiemetic. The effect of ginger root on postoperative nausea and vomiting after major gynaecological surgery. Anaesthesia. 1990 Aug;45(8):669-71.

Chun KS, Sohn Y, Kim HS, Kim OH, Park KK, Lee JM, Moon A, Lee SS, Surh YJ. Anti-tumor promoting potential of naturally occurring diarylheptanoids structurally related to curcumin. Mutat Res. 1999 Jul 16;428(1-2):49-57.

Denyer CV, Jackson P, Loakes DM, Ellis MR, Young DA. Isolation of anti-rhinoviral sesquiterpenes from ginger (Zingiber officinale). J Nat Prod. 1994 May;57(5):658-62.

Erick M. Vitamin B-6 and ginger in morning sickness. J Am Diet Assoc. 1995 Apr;95(4):416.

Ernst E, Pittler MH. Efficacy of ginger for nausea and vomiting: A systematic review of randomized clinical trials. Br J Anaesth. 2000 Mar;84(3):367-71.

Fischer-Rasmussen W, Kjaer SK, Dahl C, Asping U. Ginger treatment of hyperemesis gravidarum. Eur J Obstet Gynecol Reprod Biol. 1991 Jan 4;38(1):19-24.

Grant KL, Lutz RB. Ginger. Am J Health Syst Pharm. 2000 May 15;57(10):945-7.

Grontved A, Brask T, Kambskard J, Hentzer E. Ginger root against seasickness. A controlled trial on the open sea. Acta Otolaryngol. 1988 Jan-Feb;105(1-2):45-9.

Grontved A, Hentzer E. Vertigo-reducing effect of ginger root. A controlled clinical study. ORL J Otorhinolaryngol Relat Spec. 1986;48(5):282-6.

Holtmann S, Clarke AH, Scherer H, Hohn M. The anti-motion sickness mechanism of ginger. A comparative study with placebo and dimenhydrinate. Acta Otolaryngol. 1989 Sep-Oct;108(3-4):168-74.

Janssen PL, Meyboom S, van Staveren WA, de Vegt F, Katan MB. Consumption of ginger (Zingiber officinale roscoe) does not affect ex vivo platelet thromboxane production in humans. Eur J Clin Nutr. 1996 Nov;50(11):772-4.

Jewell D, Young G. Interventions for nausea and vomiting in early pregnancy. Cochrane Database Syst Rev. 2000;(2):CD000145.

Langner E, Greifenberg S, Gruenwald J. Ginger: History and use. Adv Ther. 1998 Jan-Feb;15(1):25-44.

Liu WH. Ginger root, a new antiemetic. Anaesthesia. 1990 Dec;45(12):1085.

Lumb AB. Mechanism of antiemetic effect of ginger. Anaesthesia. 1993 Dec; 48(12):1118.

Lumb AB. Effect of dried ginger on human platelet function. Thromb Haemost. 1994 Jan;71(1):110-1.

Meng HQ. Pharmacological effects of fresh ginger and dried ginger. Chung Hsi I Chieh Ho Tsa Chih. 1990 Oct;10(10):638-40.

Meyer K, Schwartz J, Crater D, Keyes B. Zingiber officinale (ginger) used to prevent 8-Mop associated nausea. Dermatol Nurs. 1995 Aug;7(4):242-4.

Micklefield GH, Redeker Y, Meister V, Jung O, Greving I, May B. Effects of ginger on gastroduodenal motility. Int J Clin Pharmacol Ther. 1999 Jul;37(7):341-6.

Mowrey DB, Clayson DE. Motion sickness, ginger, and psychophysics. Lancet. 1982 Mar 20;1(8273):655-7.

Mustafa T, Srivastava KC. Ginger (Zingiber officinale) in migraine headache. J Ethnopharmacol. 1990 Jul;29(3):267-73.

Phillips S, Hutchinson S, Ruggier R. Zingiber officinale does not affect gastric emptying rate. A randomised, placebo-controlled, crossover trial. Anaesthesia. 1993 May;48(5):393-5.

Phillips S, Ruggier R, Hutchinson SE. Zingiber officinale (ginger)—an antiemetic for day case surgery. Anaesthesia. 1993 Aug;48(8):715-7.

Srivastava KC, Mustafa T. Ginger (Zingiber officinale) in rheumatism and musculoskeletal disorders. Med Hypotheses. 1992 Dec;39(4):342-8.

Stewart JJ, Wood MJ, Wood CD, Mims ME. Effects of ginger on motion sickness susceptibility and gastric function. Pharmacology. 1991;42(2):111-20.

Surh YJ, Lee E, Lee JM. Chemoprotective properties of some pungent ingredients present in red pepper and ginger. Mutat Res. 1998 Jun 18;402(1-2):259-67.

Visalyaputra S, Petchpaisit N, Somcharoen K, Choavaratana R. The efficacy of ginger root in the prevention of postoperative nausea and vomiting after outpatient gynaecological laparoscopy. Anaesthesia. 1998 May;53(5):506-10.

FRUCTOOLIGOSACCHARIDES (FOS)/PREBIOTICS

What Is It?

Fructooligosaccharides (FOS), also called "prebiotics," are a group of nondigestible compounds that stimulate the growth of beneficial microflora (note: this is different than *pro*biotics, or actual beneficial bacteria such as acidophilus and bifidum). In terms of chemistry, a fructooligosaccharide is a glucose molecule bonded to multiple fructose molecules. These bonds cannot be broken down by enzymes in the human small intestine—allowing the FOS to reach the large intestine intact, where it becomes a substrate for colonic bacteria. The effects of short-chain FOS have been studied for nearly two decades. Groups of oligosaccharides can be found in foods such as beans, blueberries, and onions; a liquid supplement is available in Japan, and FOS is available in capsule form in the United States.

Claims

- Lowers serum lipids
- Reduces colon cancer risk
- Increases intestinal calcium absorption
- Reduces the severity of ulcerative colitis
- Alleviates antibiotic-induced diarrhea

Theory

Short-chain FOS is metabolized in the colon (by colonic bacteria) into short-chain fatty acids. These short-chain fatty acids cause a drop in pH, which may inhibit the growth of pathogenic bacteria, facilitate intestinal calcium absorption, and act as a substrate for colonic epithelial cells. By manipulating colonic pH and microflora content, FOS may also play a protective role against colon cancer. Research points to a reduction in liver fatty acid synthesis as a possible mechanism for serum lipid reduction.

Scientific Support

Human studies have shown significant increases in bifidobacteria (beneficial bacteria in the gut) from ingestion of as little as 6 to 8 g of short-chain FOS per day. Research has also shown decreases in pathogenic colonic bacteria following FOS ingestion. There is evidence that short-chain FOS can lower cholesterol and triglycerides, but most of this research has involved animal models. Colon tumors and indicators of cancer have also been reduced in animal models. Although animal studies have given promising results, human studies have failed to show that mineral absorption can be enhanced from FOS ingestion. Overall, the results of human studies on FOS ingestion have been disappointing, but there is clearly a need for more research.

Safety

Since the bonds of FOS are not digestible, bacterial metabolism in the large intestine produces gas and bloating. Flatulence is a common symptom associated with FOS ingestion and can be worse in people who are lactose intolerant (depending on how the FOS is processed). Studies have shown that the severity of symptoms is dose dependent (less FOS means less symptoms). Ingestion of 20 to 30 g per day has been associated with the onset of severe discomfort—but symptoms may be alleviated by starting with a small dose and increasing gradually to the desired amount.

Value

FOS supplements are fairly expensive. At about 20 cents per gram, effective levels of the supplement would cost about $2 per day. FOS is available at most health food stores and natural foods markets. It can be purchased in 100-capsule bottles (usually 750 mg per capsule). Although FOS can also be obtained as part of some acidophilus supplements and only adds about $1 to $2 to the price, it is frequently unclear what dosage of FOS is obtained from these products.

Dosage

Ten g of FOS per day appears to be the optimal dose, since this amount produces a significant increase in bifidobacteria and is fairly well tolerated.

WORKS CONSULTED

Alles MS, Hautvast JG, Nagengast FM, Hartemink R, Van Laere KM, Jansen JB. Fate of fructo-oligosaccharides in the human intestine. Br J Nutr. 1996 Aug;76(2):211-21.

Bouhnik Y, Flourie B, Riottot M, Bisetti N, Gailing MF, Guibert A, Bornet F, Rambaud JC. Effects of fructo-oligosaccharides ingestion on fecal bifidobacteria and selected metabolic indexes of colon carcinogenesis in healthy humans. Nutr Cancer. 1996;26(1):21-9.

Bouhnik Y, Vahedi K, Achour L, Attar A, Salfati J, Pochart P, Marteau P, Flourie B, Bornet F, Rambaud JC. Short-chain fructo-oligosaccharide administration dose-dependently increases fecal bifidobacteria in healthy humans. J Nutr. 1999 Jan;129(1):113-6.

Briet F, Achour L, Flourie B, Beaugerie L, Pellier P, Franchisseur C, Bornet F, Rambaud JC. Symptomatic response to varying levels of fructo-oligosaccharides consumed occasionally or regularly. Eur J Clin Nutr. 1995 Jul;49(7):501-7.

Djouzi Z, Andrieux C. Compared effects of three oligosaccharides on metabolism of intestinal microflora in rats inoculated with a human faecal flora. Br J Nutr. 1997 Aug;78(2):313-24.

Gibson GR. Dietary modulation of the human gut microflora using prebiotics. Br J Nutr. 1998 Oct;80(4):S209-12.

Gmeiner M, Kneifel W, Kulbe KD, Wouters R, De Boever P, Nollet L, Verstraete W. Influence of a synbiotic mixture consisting of Lactobacillus acidophilus 74-2 and a fructooligosaccharide preparation on the microbial ecology sustained in a simulation of the human intestinal microbial ecosystem (SHIME reactor). Appl Microbiol Biotechnol. 2000 Feb;53(2):219-23.

Hartemink R, Van Laere KM, Rombouts FM. Growth of enterobacteria on fructo-oligosaccharides. J Appl Microbiol. 1997 Sep;83(3):367-74.

Jenkins DJ, Kendall CW, Axelsen M, Augustin LS, Vuksan V. Viscous and nonviscous fibres, nonabsorbable and low glycaemic index carbohydrates, blood lipids and coronary heart disease. Curr Opin Lipidol. 2000 Feb;11(1):49-56.

Kaufhold J, Hammon HM, Blum JW. Fructo-oligosaccharide supplementation: Effects on metabolic, endocrine and hematological traits in veal calves. J Vet Med A Physiol Pathol Clin Med. 2000 Feb;47(1):17-29.

Le Blay G, Michel C, Blottiere HM, Cherbut C. Prolonged intake of fructo-oligosaccharides induces a short-term elevation of lactic acid-producing bacteria and a persistent increase in cecal butyrate in rats. J Nutr. 1999 Dec;129(12):2231-5.

May T, Mackie RI, Fahey GC Jr, Cremin JC, Garleb KA. Effect of fiber source on short-chain fatty acid production and on the growth and toxin production by Clostridium difficile. Scand J Gastroenterol. 1994 Oct;29(10):916-22.

Mitsuoka T, Hidaka H, Eida T. Effect of fructo-oligosaccharides on intestinal microflora. Nahrung. 1987;31(5-6):427-36.

Murashova AO, Lisitsin OB, Abramov NA. Bifidogenic factors as drug preparations. Zh Mikrobiol Epidemiol Immunobiol. 1999 Sep-Oct;(5):56-61.

Pierre F, Perrin P, Bassonga E, Bornet F, Meflah K, Menanteau J. T cell status influences colon tumor occurrence in min mice fed short chain fructo-oligosaccharides as a diet supplement. Carcinogenesis. 1999 Oct;20(10):1953-6.

Pierre F, Perrin P, Champ M, Bornet F, Meflah K, Menanteau J. Short-chain fructo-oligosaccharides reduce the occurrence of colon tumors and develop gut-associated lymphoid tissue in Min mice. Cancer Res. 1997 Jan 15;57(2):225-8.

Prosky L. Inulin and oligofructose are part of the dietary fiber complex. J AOAC Int. 1999 Mar-Apr;82(2):223-6.

Rao AV. Dose-response effects of inulin and oligofructose on intestinal bifidogenesis effects. J Nutr. 1999 Jul;129(7 Suppl):1442S-5S.

Roberfroid M. Dietary fiber, inulin, and oligofructose: A review comparing their physiological effects. Crit Rev Food Sci Nutr. 1993;33(2):103-48.

Roberfroid MB. Prebiotics and synbiotics: Concepts and nutritional properties. Br J Nutr. 1998 Oct;80(4):S197-202.

Roberfroid MB, Van Loo JA, Gibson GR. The bifidogenic nature of chicory inulin and its hydrolysis products. J Nutr. 1998 Jan;128(1):11-9.

Sakaguchi E, Sakoda C, Toramaru Y. Caecal fermentation and energy accumulation in the rat fed on indigestible oligosaccharides. Br J Nutr. 1998 Nov;80(5):469-76.

Schaafsma G, Meuling WJ, van Dokkum W, Bouley C. Effects of a milk product, fermented by Lactobacillus acidophilus and with fructo-oligosaccharides added, on blood lipids in male volunteers. Eur J Clin Nutr. 1998 Jun;52(6):436-40.

Sparkes AH, Papasouliotis K, Sunvold G, Werrett G, Clarke C, Jones M, Gruffydd-Jones TJ, Reinhart G. Bacterial flora in the duodenum of healthy cats, and effect of dietary supplementation with fructo-oligosaccharides. Am J Vet Res. 1998 Apr;59(4):431-5.

Sparkes AH, Papasouliotis K, Sunvold G, Werrett G, Gruffydd-Jones EA, Egan K, Gruffydd-Jones TJ, Reinhart G. Effect of dietary supplementation with fructo-oligosaccharides on fecal flora of healthy cats. Am J Vet Res. 1998 Apr;59(4):436-40.

van Dokkum W, Wezendonk B, Srikumar TS, van den Heuvel EG. Effect of nondigestible oligosaccharides on large-bowel functions, blood lipid concentrations and glucose absorption in young healthy male subjects. Eur J Clin Nutr. 1999 Jan;53(1):1-7.

Willard MD, Simpson RB, Delles EK, Cohen ND, Fossum TW, Kolp D, Reinhart G. Effects of dietary supplementation of fructo-oligosaccharides on small intestinal bacterial overgrowth in dogs. Am J Vet Res. 1994 May;55(5):654-9.

PROBIOTICS/ACIDOPHILUS

What Is It?

"Probiotics" refers to a group of beneficial bacteria that help maintain the health and function of the gastrointestinal tract. Acidophilus, or *Lactobacillus acidophilus,* is a popular form of "good" bacteria found in dietary supplements. By displacing other bacteria and yeast, acidophilus (and other beneficial bacteria such as bifidus and bulgaricus) may also play an important role in immune system function and prevention of gastrointestinal problems, including cancer. Each of these three beneficial bacteria can be found in cultured yogurts and in freeze-dried form as dietary supplements.

Claims

- Reduces cholesterol
- Supports immune function
- Maintains healthy digestive system
- Prevents colon cancer

Theory

The digestive system is home to millions of bacteria that help digest, modify, and convert the food we eat. Any alteration in the gastrointestinal environment is likely to influence the activity of these beneficial bacteria— sometimes posing health problems. Maintaining the normal populations of these good bacteria in the intestines, through consuming them as supplements or in cultured yogurt, can help displace (or crowd out) disease-promoting bacteria and yeast that may gain a foothold when the levels of good bacteria drop.

Scientific Support

Acidophilus and other beneficial bacteria are both acid- and bile-resistant, and are, therefore, capable of surviving transit through the gastrointestinal tract after they are ingested. These bacteria are sometimes called "probiotics" because regular consumption is linked to health benefits such as reducing cholesterol, preventing microbial growth, modulation of the immune system, and, possibly, prevention of colon cancer.

Both human and animal studies have shown direct benefits of regular consumption of acidophilus and other beneficial bacteria on immune system function. Overall, consuming probiotic bacteria tends to result in an enhanced ability of the immune system to recognize and destroy invading organisms. Several key components of the immune system, including macrophages, immunoglobulins, and cytokines, are altered by regular intake of beneficial bacteria. Populations of white blood cells are known to increase in number and activity following one to two weeks of consuming beneficial bacteria. Importantly, resistance to viral and bacterial infections is significantly improved following regular intake of probiotics.

Epidemiological studies support the possibility that consumption of beneficial bacteria (from fermented milk and yogurt) may play a role in the prevention of colon cancer. Test-tube studies have shown that acidophilus can decrease the cancer-causing potential (mutagenic activity) of various carcinogens—possibly due to a direct interaction between the carcinogens and the bacteria. Acidophilus consumption has also been shown to reduce levels of cancer-causing enzymes in the digestive tract, supporting the possibility that acidophilus and other beneficial bacteria do indeed play a role in the prevention of colon cancer.

Safety

No safety issues are associated with regular consumption of acidophilus or other probiotic bacteria, although individuals with severe gastrointestinal ailments (Crohn's disease or ulcerative colitis) should consult with their personal physician prior to consuming probiotic supplements.

Value

Dietary supplements providing acidophilus in combination with some of the other beneficial probiotic bacteria are fairly inexpensive. Given the strong evidence for their beneficial effects on immune system function and the possibility that regular consumption may reduce colon cancer risk, these supplements would be a good choice for anybody looking for a general immune system booster. Individuals currently suffering from gastrointestinal ailments, or those who may feel themselves at risk for colon cancer, are strongly advised to consider probiotic supplements (or regular consumption of yogurt with active cultures).

Dosage

Most probiotic products typically list the type of bacteria and the number of live cells on the label or side panel. There are no strict guidelines for dosage intake, but 1 to 8 billion CFUs (colony forming units) is a general rule of thumb. Be sure that you are getting the freshest product possible. The number of live cells decreases relatively quickly with time in most products—so choose one that has a long way to go before it reaches its expiration date.

WORKS CONSULTED

Agerholm-Larsen L, Raben A, Haulrik N, Hansen AS, Manders M, Astrup A. Effect of 8 week intake of probiotic milk products on risk factors for cardiovascular diseases. Eur J Clin Nutr. 2000 Apr;54(4):288-97.

Arunachalam K, Gill HS, Chandra RK. Enhancement of natural immune function by dietary consumption of Bifidobacterium lactis (HN019). Eur J Clin Nutr. 2000 Mar;54(3):263-7.

Barone C, Pettinato R, Avola E, Alberti A, Greco D, Failla P, Romano C. Comparison of three probiotics in the treatment of acute diarrhea in mentally retarded children. Minerva Pediatr. 2000 Mar;52(3):161-5.

Bengmark S. Bacteria for optimal health. Nutrition. 2000 Jul-Aug;16(7-8):611-5.

Bengmark S. Colonic food: Pre- and probiotics. Am J Gastroenterol. 2000 Jan; 95(1 Suppl):S5-7.

Bengmark S. Ecological control of the gastrointestinal tract. The role of probiotic flora. Gut. 1998 Jan;42(1):2-7.

Biancone L, Pallone F. Current treatment modalities in active Crohn's disease. Ital J Gastroenterol Hepatol. 1999 Aug-Sep;31(6):508-14.

Brady LJ, Gallaher DD, Busta FF. The role of probiotic cultures in the prevention of colon cancer. J Nutr. 2000 Feb;130(2S Suppl):410S-4S.

Caplan MS, Jilling T. Neonatal necrotizing enterocolitis: Possible role of probiotic supplementation. J Pediatr Gastroenterol Nutr. 2000;30(Suppl 2):S18-22.

Cerrato PL. Can "healthy" bacteria ward off disease? RN. 2000 Apr;63(4):71-4.

Chin J, Turner B, Barchia I, Mullbacher A. Immune response to orally consumed antigens and probiotic bacteria. Immunol Cell Biol. 2000 Feb;78(1):55-66.

Collins MD, Gibson GR. Probiotics, prebiotics, and synbiotics: Approaches for modulating the microbial ecology of the gut. Am J Clin Nutr. 1999 May;69(5):1052S-7S.

Cunningham-Rundles S, Ahrne S, Bengmark S, Johann-Liang R, Marshall F, Metakis L, Califano C, Dunn AM, Grassey C, Hinds G, Cervia J. Probiotics and immune response. Am J Gastroenterol. 2000 Jan;95(1 Suppl):S22-5.

D'Argenio G, Mazzacca G. Short-chain fatty acid in the human colon. Relation to inflammatory bowel diseases and colon cancer. Adv Exp Med Biol. 1999; 472:149-58.

Davidson GP, Butler RN. Probiotics in pediatric gastrointestinal disorders. Curr Opin Pediatr. 2000 Oct;12(5):477-81.

de Roos NM, Katan MB. Effects of probiotic bacteria on diarrhea, lipid metabolism, and carcinogenesis: A review of papers published between 1988 and 1998. Am J Clin Nutr. 2000 Feb;71(2):405-11.

Dugas B, Mercenier A, Lenoir-Wijnkoop I, Arnaud C, Dugas N, Postaire E. Immunity and probiotics. Immunol Today. 1999 Sep;20(9):387-90.

Dunne C, Murphy L, Flynn S, O'Mahony L, O'Halloran S, Feeney M, Morrissey D, Thornton G, Fitzgerald G, Daly C, Kiely B, Quigley EM, O'Sullivan GC, Shanahan F, Collins JK. Probiotics: From myth to reality. Demonstration of functionality in animal models of disease and in human clinical trials. Antonie Van Leeuwenhoek. 1999 Jul-Nov;76(1-4):279-92.

Dupont C. Bacterial flora in the infant and intestinal immunity: Implication and prospects for infant food with probiotics. Arch Pediatr. 2000 May;7(Suppl 2): 252S-5S.

Erickson KL, Hubbard NE. Probiotic immunomodulation in health and disease. J Nutr. 2000 Feb;130(2S Suppl):403S-9S.

Folwaczny C. Probiotics for prevention of ulcerative colitis recurrence: Alternative medicine added to standard treatment? Z Gastroenterol. 2000 Jun;38(6):547-50.

Friedrich MJ. A bit of culture for children: Probiotics may improve health and fight disease. JAMA. 2000 Sep 20;284(11):1365-6.

Gibson GR, Fuller R. Aspects of in vitro and in vivo research approaches directed toward identifying probiotics and prebiotics for human use. J Nutr. 2000 Feb;130(2S Suppl):391S-5S.

Gibson GR, McCartney AL. Modification of the gut flora by dietary means. Biochem Soc Trans. 1998 May;26(2):222-8.

Gismondo MR, Drago L, Lombardi A. Review of probiotics available to modify gastrointestinal flora. Int J Antimicrob Agents. 1999 Aug;12(4):287-92.

Goldin BR. Health benefits of probiotics. Br J Nutr. 1998 Oct;80(4):S203-7.

Gomez-Gil B, Roque A, Turnbull JF, Inglis V. A review on the use of microorganisms as probiotics. Rev Latinoam Microbiol. 1998 Jul-Dec;40(3-4):166-72.

Gorbach SL. Probiotics and gastrointestinal health. Am J Gastroenterol. 2000 Jan;95(1 Suppl):S2-4.

Guslandi M. The relationship between gut microflora and intestinal inflammation. Can J Gastroenterol. 2000 Jan;14(1):32.

Heyman M. Effect of lactic acid bacteria on diarrheal diseases. J Am Coll Nutr. 2000 Apr;19(2 Suppl):137S-46S.

Hirayama K, Rafter J. The role of probiotic bacteria in cancer prevention. Microbes Infect. 2000 May;2(6):681-6.

Hoerr RA, Bostwick EF. Bioactive proteins and probiotic bacteria: Modulators of nutritional health. Nutrition. 2000 Jul-Aug;16(7-8):711-3.

Holzapfel WH, Haberer P, Snel J, Schillinger U, Huis in't Veld JH. Overview of gut flora and probiotics. Int J Food Microbiol. 1998 May 26;41(2):85-101.

Hove H, Norgaard H, Mortensen PB. Lactic acid bacteria and the human gastrointestinal tract. Eur J Clin Nutr. 1999 May;53(5):339-50.

Hoyos AB. Reduced incidence of necrotizing enterocolitis associated with enteral administration of Lactobacillus acidophilus and Bifidobacterium infantis to neonates in an intensive care unit. Int J Infect Dis. 1999 Summer;3(4):197-202.

Isolauri E. The use of probiotics in paediatrics. Hosp Med. 2000 Jan;61(1):6-7.

Kasper H. Protection against gastrointestinal diseases—present facts and future developments. Int J Food Microbiol. 1998 May 26;41(2):127-31.

Kirjavainen PV, Apostolou E, Salminen SJ, Isolauri E. New aspects of probiotics—a novel approach in the management of food allergy. Allergy. 1999 Sep;54(9):909-15.

Klaenhammer TR. Probiotic bacteria: Today and tomorrow. J Nutr. 2000 Feb;130(2S Suppl):415S-6S.

Kochhar KP. Probiotics and gastrointestinal function in health and disease. Trop Gastroenterol. 2000 Jan-Mar;21(1):8-11.

LaMont JT. The renaissance of probiotics and prebiotics. Gastroenterology. 2000 Aug;119(2):291.

Levy J. Immunonutrition: The pediatric experience. Nutrition. 1998 Jul-Aug; 14(7-8):641-7.

Macfarlane GT, Cummings JH. Probiotics and prebiotics: Can regulating the activities of intestinal bacteria benefit health? BMJ. 1999 Apr 10;318(7189):999-1003.

Matsuzaki T, Chin J. Modulating immune responses with probiotic bacteria. Immunol Cell Biol. 2000 Feb;78(1):67-73.

Orrhage K, Nord CE. Bifidobacteria and lactobacilli in human health. Drugs Exp Clin Res. 2000;26(3):95-111.

Ouwehand AC, Isolauri E, Kirjavainen PV, Tolkko S, Salminen SJ. The mucus binding of Bifidobacterium lactis Bb12 is enhanced in the presence of Lactobacillus GG and Lact. delbrueckii subsp. bulgaricus. Lett Appl Microbiol. 2000 Jan;30(1):10-3.

Reddy BS. Possible mechanisms by which pro- and prebiotics influence colon carcinogenesis and tumor growth. J Nutr. 1999 Jul;129(7 Suppl):1478S-82S.

Reid G. The scientific basis for probiotic strains of Lactobacillus. Appl Environ Microbiol. 1999 Sep;65(9):3763-6.

Roberfroid MB. Prebiotics and probiotics: Are they functional foods? Am J Clin Nutr. 2000 Jun;71(6 Suppl):1682S-7S; discussion 1688S-90S.

Rolfe RD. The role of probiotic cultures in the control of gastrointestinal health. J Nutr. 2000 Feb;130(2S Suppl):396S-402S.

Saavedra JM. Probiotics plus antibiotics: Regulating our bacterial environment. J Pediatr. 1999 Nov;135(5):535-7.

Sanders ME. Considerations for use of probiotic bacteria to modulate human health. J Nutr. 2000 Feb;130(2S Suppl):384S-90S.

Shanahan F. Immunology. Therapeutic manipulation of gut flora. Science. 2000 Aug 25;289(5483):1311-2.

Shanahan F. Probiotics and inflammatory bowel disease: Is there a scientific rationale? Inflamm Bowel Dis. 2000 May;6(2):107-15.

Studd C. Probiotic containing fermented milk supplement may improve the institution of early enteral nutrition. Crit Care Med. 2000 Apr;28(4):1255-6.

Szilagyi A. Prebiotics or probiotics for lactose intolerance: A question of adaptation. Am J Clin Nutr. 1999 Jul;70(1):105-6.

Taylor GR, Williams CM. Effects of probiotics and prebiotics on blood lipids. Br J Nutr. 1998 Oct;80(4):S225-30.

Torrens JK, McWhinney PH. Probiotics and life-threatening infection. J Infect. 1999 Nov;39(3):246.

Vanderhoof JA. Probiotics and intestinal inflammatory disorders in infants and children. J Pediatr Gastroenterol Nutr. 2000;30(Suppl 2):S34-8.

Vanderhoof JA, Whitney DB, Antonson DL, Hanner TL, Lupo JV, Young RJ. Lactobacillus GG in the prevention of antibiotic-associated diarrhea in children. J Pediatr. 1999 Nov;135(5):564-8.

Vanderhoof JA, Young RJ. Use of probiotics in childhood gastrointestinal disorders. J Pediatr Gastroenterol Nutr. 1998 Sep;27(3):323-32.

Vilpponen-Salmela T, Alander M, Satokari R, Bjorkman P, Kontula P, Korpela R, Saxelin M, Mattila-Sandholm T, von Wright A. Probiotic bacteria and intestinal health: New methods of investigation. J Physiol Paris. 2000 Mar-Apr;94(2):157-8.

von Wright A, Salminen S. Probiotics: Established effects and open questions. Eur J Gastroenterol Hepatol. 1999 Nov;11(11):1195-8.

Yasui H, Shida K, Matsuzaki T, Yokokura T. Immunomodulatory function of lactic acid bacteria. Antonie Van Leeuwenhoek. 1999 Jul-Nov;76(1-4):383-9.

Zhou JS, Shu Q, Rutherfurd KJ, Prasad J, Gopal PK, Gill HS. Acute oral toxicity and bacterial translocation studies on potentially probiotic strains of lactic acid bacteria. Food Chem Toxicol. 2000 Feb-Mar;38(2-3):153-61.

SLIPPERY ELM

What Is It?

Slippery elm *(Ulmus rubra, Ulmus fulva)* is a tree that grows in the eastern part of the United States from Canada to Mexico. Its name was derived from the observation that preparations made from the reddish inner bark form a slippery coating over surfaces when they come into contact with liquid. Native Americans traditionally mixed slippery elm with water to form a poultice (dressing or bandage) for injuries, burns, and skin irritations. In the eighteenth and nineteenth centuries, slippery elm became popular in America as a cough and cold remedy. Since it is easily digested, the ground bark was mixed with water or milk to form an oatmeal-like gruel.

Claims

- Soothes mucous membranes irritated by the common cold
- Acts as a digestive remedy for diarrhea, constipation, and Crohn's disease
- Alleviates respiratory dryness associated with coughing and bronchitis
- Forms a skin moisturizer for use in minor irritations, poison ivy, and wounds

Theory

When exposed to liquid, the mucilage of slippery elm gives it the properties for which it is named (mucilage is exactly like what it sounds like—visualize the gooey quality of oatmeal or the "sliminess" of okra). Because slippery elm contains gelatinous mucilage, it is able to coat and soothe irritated mucous membranes, the lining of the throat, and the intestinal lining. By the same theory, it can soothe irritated or wounded skin.

Scientific Support

A search of the scientific literature turned up a grand total of zero studies, with either humans or animals, to provide any scientific basis for the use of slippery elm to treat respiratory, digestive, or dermal ailments (but I found one study on a related species of elm for treating ulcerative colitis). In this case, however, the lack of scientific studies does not seem to be any reason for concern. Unlike the majority of herbal supplements, slippery elm does not have any drug activity associated with it. Therefore, with what is already known about slippery elm, there is not much necessity to study this type of tree bark. In fact, the Food and Drug Administration has acknowledged the soothing properties of slippery elm, and since its actions are not based on intricate molecular mechanisms, the fact that the combination of slippery elm and liquid creates a viscous, soothing, safe substance should speak for itself. Furthermore, the use of slippery elm as a food may have merit—it contains astringent tannins that may help alleviate diarrhea as well as small amounts of nutrients such as calcium and potassium.

Safety

Slippery elm is considered to be safe and effective for use in soothing applications. It is completely nontoxic and has no known drug interactions. Because of a lack of scientific evidence, however, pregnant or lactating women should consult with a doctor or pharmacist before supplementing with slippery elm.

Value

One hundred capsules of ground slippery elm bark generally cost approximately $8 to $10. One serving ranges from two to four capsules (about 800 to 1,500 mg) and may be taken three times daily. Lozenges often contain slippery elm in combination with zinc, vitamin C, and other supplements thought to prevent or battle the common cold to help soothe sore throats and quiet coughs.

Dosage

In capsule form, two or more capsules containing about 400 mg of ground slippery elm bark can be taken three to four times per day, depending on the severity of one's symptoms. As a tea, one to two teaspoonfuls of loose bark make one cup of tea, which can be taken three to four times per day. As a lozenge, follow the instructions on the package, as dosage depends upon whether there are other ingredients in the cough/sore throat drop.

WORKS CONSULTED

Duke, JA. The green pharmacy. Emmaus, PA: Rodale Press, 1997, pp. 170-171.
Ye G, Cao Q, Chen X, Li S, Jia B. Ulmus macrocarpa hance for the treatment of ulcerative colitis—a report of 36 cases. J Tradit Chin Med. 1990 Jun;10(2):97-8.

MASTIC

What Is It?

Mastic *(Pistacia lentiscus)* is a gum (sap) from a tree that grows primarily in Mediterranean and Middle Eastern regions (Italy, Greece, Turkey, Iraq, etc.). The traditional use of mastic in ancient Greece was as a digestive aid to help prevent heartburn, nausea, and ulcers (where it was chewed, or *masticated,* following meals). As a dietary supplement, mastic is composed of oils extracted by distillation of the gum, leaves, and twigs from the tree. Modern use of mastic as a dietary supplement is typically for prevention and treatment of gastric and duodenal ulcers.

Claims

- Prevents and treats gastric (stomach) and duodenal (intestinal) ulcers
- Relieves symptoms of dyspepsia and gastrointestinal discomfort (heartburn)
- Antibacterial effects (against *Helicobacter pylori*—a primary cause of gastric ulcers)
- Reduces bad breath

Theory

The precise mechanism of action for mastic in the treatment of ulcers and dyspepsia is unknown, but the extract appears to reduce stomach secretions (which could balance stomach acid levels) and may have an effect on altering the structural characteristics of *H. pylori* bacteria (which is associated with peptic ulcers).

Scientific Support

A double-blind clinical trial on thirty-eight patients with duodenal ulcers compared 1 g of mastic per day for two weeks to a lactose placebo. A significant reduction in ulcer symptoms was seen in 80 percent of the patients consuming mastic, compared to 50 percent of patients on placebo. Of special note was significant tissue healing (assessed by endoscope—a little camera that was snaked into their gastrointestinal systems to look for damage) in 70 percent of those taking mastic (22 percent of those taking placebo). Mastic was well tolerated and did not produce side effects.

In another study, the effect of mastic on experimentally induced gastric and duodenal ulcers was studied in rats. At oral doses of 500 mg/kg (roughly equivalent to 500 mg per day in a human), mastic reduced gastric secretions, protected cells, and reduced damage to the stomach lining induced by a variety of experimental methods. Mastic also reduced gastric damage following treatment with aspirin (which can cause ulcers), phenylbutazone (an anti-inflammatory), and respirine (a vasodilator)—all of which are medications that should be avoided by patients with peptic ulcers because of their ability to damage the gastric lining. The results of this animal study suggest that mastic may provide mild antiulcer activity, and the findings support human studies on the clinical effectiveness of mastic in the therapy of duodenal ulcers.

In terms of therapy against gastric ulcers, about 1 g of mastic per day for two weeks may be able to speed healing of peptic ulcers. In a test-tube study, mastic has been shown to kill *H. pylori*, possibly by inducing structural changes in the bacteria that make it more susceptible to the body's own immune system.

Safety

No serious side effects are known for mastic when consumed at recommended doses of 1 to 3 g per day.

Value

In the United States, millions of dollars are spent on over-the-counter treatments for ulcers and general stomach irritations such as heartburn. It is estimated that more than 50 percent of individuals over age fifty are infected with the *H. pylori* bacterium and that most cases of duodenal and gastric ulcers are due to *H. pylori* infection. Gastric ulcers can also be induced by frequent use of aspirin and other nonsteroidal anti-inflammatory drugs (NSAIDs). In addition, nonulcer dyspepsia (generalized abdominal discomfort) is widespread in the population (most of us suffer from it from time to time). At least one study has shown that eradication of *H. pylori* can reduce the symptoms of dyspepsia (but another study has shown no benefit). Given this situation and the fact that the conventional treatment for *H. pylori* typically combines both an antisecretory compound (such as omeprazol) along with an antibiotic (such as amoxicillin), the benefits and safety of mastic may represent a very good value (about $30 for a one-month supply) for anybody suffering from ulcers and/or general dyspepsia.

Dosage

Typical dosage recommendations are in the range of 1 to 3 g per day.

WORKS CONSULTED

Al-Habbal MJ, Al-Habbal Z, Huwez FU. A double-blind controlled clinical trial of mastic and placebo in the treatment of duodenal ulcer. Clin Exp Pharmacol Physiol. 1984 Sep-Oct;11(5):541-4.

Al-Said MS, Ageel AM, Parmar NS, Tariq M. Evaluation of mastic, a crude drug obtained from Pistacia lentiscus for gastric and duodenal anti-ulcer activity. J Ethnopharmacol. 1986 Mar;15(3):271-8.

Huwez FU, Al-Habbal MJ. Mastic in treatment of benign gastric ulcers. Gastroenterol Jpn. 1986 Jun;21(3):273-4.

Huwez FU, Thirlwell D, Cockayne A, Ala'Aldeen DA. Mastic gum kills Helicobacter pylori. N Engl J Med. 1998 Dec 24;339(26):1946.

Papageorgiou VP, Bakola-Christianopoulou MN, Apazidou KK, Psarros EE. Gas chromatographic-mass spectroscopic analysis of the acidic triterpenic fraction of mastic gum. J Chromatogr. 1997;769:263-73.

YELLOW DOCK

What Is It?

Yellow dock *(Rumex crispus)* is a relative of the buckwheat family that is native to northern Europe and Asia, but its adaptability has allowed it to spread to many parts of the world. It is also known as curly dock, for the shape of its leaves, and sour dock because of its bitter taste. In ancient times, the Chinese and Romans used yellow dock as a digestive aid and for skin conditions. Today it can be found in many forms and is still used for skin conditions, for liver conditions, and as a mild laxative.

Claims

- Aids with digestive complaints (flatulence, constipation, heartburn)
- Stimulates appetite
- Increases bile flow for better digestion
- Aids with skin conditions such as acne, psoriasis, and eczema (topical application)

Theory

Topically, yellow dock is used as an astringent and an antibacterial, because of its tannin components. Together, these actions could help control skin conditions such as acne that are attributable to bacteria. Furthermore, like other popular herbal laxatives aloe and senna, yellow dock also contains anthraquinone glycosides, explaining the herb's frequent use as a laxative to treat constipation. The tannins in yellow dock also provide a "digestive bitter" quality that could stimulate appetite and bile flow, thereby aiding in the removal of toxic metabolites that could contribute to poor digestion and its unpleasant side effects.

Scientific Support

A number of clinical trials and case reports have documented the beneficial role of yellow dock, either alone or combined with other fibers or herbal laxatives, in alleviating constipation and generalized gastrointestinal complaints—primarily in the elderly and in nursing home residents.

Safety

Aside from a study demonstrating that the anthraquinone glycoside content in yellow dock root is toxic to brine shrimp, yellow dock appears to be quite safe when used as directed for its laxative properties. Caution should be used by anyone with a medical condition or by pregnant or lactating women. Aside from mild diarrhea or nausea, taking yellow dock does not typically produce serious side effects. However, the fresh leaves of yellow dock are high in oxalates. When taken in large doses, oxalates inhibit nutrient absorption and have been known to cause death in grazing sheep. Finally, taking yellow dock for more than sixty days at a time could lead to laxative dependence.

Value

Yellow dock is relatively inexpensive—with a thirty-day supply typically costing less than $10. However, whether it works is not very well substantiated, so you might be better off trying a more reliable therapy.

Dosage

Yellow dock is sold as an entire root and as a root extract in liquid and capsule form. It can be made into a tea by boiling 1 to 2 teaspoons or 5 to 10 g of root in two cups of water for ten minutes. Alternately, 3 to 4 ml of the root extract can be taken three times per day. In capsule form, about 1 g (two 500 mg capsules) can be taken twice daily.

WORKS CONSULTED

Borkje B, Pedersen R, Lund GM, Enehaug JS, Berstad A. Effectiveness and acceptability of three bowel cleansing regimens. Scand J Gastroenterol. 1991 Feb; 26(2):162-6.

Bossi S, Arsenio L, Bodria P, Magnati G, Trovato R, Strata A. Clinical study of a new preparation from plantago seeds and senna pods. Acta Biomed Ateneo Parmense. 1986;57(5-6):179-86.

Brown S, Kerrigan P, Waterston T. A six-year-old suffering from constipation. Practitioner. 2000 Feb;244(1607):63-8.

Maddi VI. Regulation of bowel function by a laxative/stool softener preparation in aged nursing home patients. J Am Geriatr Soc. 1979 Oct;27(10):464-8.

Mueller RS, Bettenay SV, Tideman L. Aero-allergens in canine atopic dermatitis in southeastern Australia based on 1000 intradermal skintests. Aust Vet J. 2000 Jun;78(6):392-9.

Reig R, Sanz P, Blanche C, Fontarnau R, Dominguez A, Corbella J. Fatal poisoning by Rumex crispus (curled dock): pathological findings and application of scanning electronmicroscopy. Vet Hum Toxicol. 1990;32:468-70.

Shen HD, Chang LY, Gong YJ, Chang HN, Han SH. A monoclonal antibody against ragweed pollen cross-reacting with yellow dock pollen. Chung Hua Min. 1985 Nov;18(4):232-9.

van Gorkom BA, Karrenbeld A, van Der Sluis T, Koudstaal J, de Vries EG, Kleibeuker JH. Influence of a highly purified senna extract on colonic epithelium. Digestion. 2000;61(2):113-20.

CAPSICUM/CAYENNE

What Is It?

Capsicum, also known as cayenne, contains capsaicin—the compound that produces the "hot" in hot peppers. Cayenne peppers have been used for centuries as a folk medicine for stimulating circulation, aiding digestion, and relieving pain (topically). Contemporary uses have placed cayenne extracts as thermogenic aids to help increase metabolism.

Claims

- Digestive aid (stimulates gastric secretions)
- Arthritis pain reliever (topical cream)
- Raises metabolic rate
- Reduces allergic symptoms (hay fever-type allergies)
- Prevents migraine headaches

Theory

Anybody who has ever tasted concentrated capsicum or has been unfortunate enough to get it in his or her eyes or other mucous membranes knows of the intense burning sensation that the substance causes. When rubbed on the skin, cayenne can be a very useful analgesic (pain reliever) with benefits in reducing arthritic pain. This effect, called a counterirritant, causes a mild irritation when applied to the skin and "distracts" us from sensing pain from other areas (such as the joint pain common to arthritis). As a digestive aid, cayenne is known to increase secretion of gastric acids in the stomach. Cayenne is often recommended as a thermogenic compound for increasing metabolic rate, which may be related to its ability to dilate blood vessels and cause a local sensation of warming.

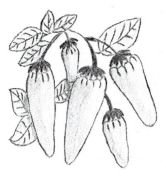

Scientific Support

As indicated, cayenne contains capsaicin, which can relieve pain by interfering with sensory nerve signaling. In addition to the "confusion" that capsaicin induces in sensory nerves, it also results in a temporary depletion of neurotransmitters from sensory nerves, which reduces the ability of the nerve to sense pain in other areas of the body.

Safety

Watch out! Capsaicin creams and supplements can cause not only a mild burning for the first few applications but can also cause severe discomfort if you get it in the wrong place (such as your eyes). Used the right way, however, no serious side effects are expected from capsaicin, either as a topical cream or as an ingested dietary supplement. Caution should be used during pregnancy (to avoid gastrointestinal irritation) and lactation (because capsaicin may pass into breast milk and cause the milk to be unpalatable to the infant).

Value

As a mild digestive aid, cayenne extracts may be somewhat beneficial for individuals with inadequate gastric secretions. For many people, however, gastric secretions are not the primary concern in terms of digestive support (intestinal concerns predominate). As a thermogenic aid to increase metabolism, cayenne may have some modest effects at very high doses (3 g or more), but these effects are small and the risk of gastrointestinal side effects (heartburn) is high.

Dosage

Cayenne/capsaicin products are typically standardized in heat units (HU) and/or percent of capsaicin per capsule. Topical creams often contain 0.02 percent to 0.05 percent capsaicinoids, with dietary supplements providing about 50 to 200 mg per capsule. As a digestive aid, approximately 100 to 500 mg of cayenne extract (0.15 percent to 0.25 percent capsaicin) is recommended two to three times per day with food.

WORKS CONSULTED

Egger G, Cameron-Smith D, Stanton R. The effectiveness of popular, non-prescription weight loss supplements. Med J Aust. 1999 Dec 6-20;171(11-12):604-8.
Guengerich FP. Influence of nutrients and other dietary materials on cytochrome P-450 enzymes. Am J Clin Nutr. 1995 Mar;61(3 Suppl):651S-8S.

Lim K, Yoshioka M, Kikuzato S, Kiyonaga A, Tanaka H, Shindo M, Suzuki M. Dietary red pepper ingestion increases carbohydrate oxidation at rest and during exercise in runners. Med Sci Sports Exerc. 1997 Mar;29(3):355-61.

Lopez-Carrillo L, Hernandez Avila M, Dubrow R. Chili pepper consumption and gastric cancer in Mexico: A case-control study. Am J Epidemiol. 1994 Feb 1;139(3):263-71.

Miller CH, Zhang Z, Hamilton SM, Teel RW. Effects of capsaicin on liver microsomal metabolism of the tobacco-specific nitrosamine NNK. Cancer Lett. 1993 Nov 30;75(1):45-52.

Surh Y. Molecular mechanisms of chemopreventive effects of selected dietary and medicinal phenolic substances. Mutat Res. 1999 Jul 16;428(1-2):305-27.

Yoshioka M, St-Pierre S, Drapeau V, Dionne I, Doucet E, Suzuki M, Tremblay A. Effects of red pepper on appetite and energy intake. Br J Nutr. 1999 Aug;82(2):115-23.

Chapter 14

Supplements for Male Health

INTRODUCTION

The overwhelming market success of the drug Viagra (almost 4 million prescriptions in its first four to five months on the market) underscores the widespread occurrence of male sexual dysfunction. In addition to the 20 to 30 million American men who experience difficulty in achieving and maintaining an erection, millions more suffer from reduced libido and general lack of sexual desire—quite a change from your teenage years when all you could think about was sex.

In addition to problems with sexual function, approximately 50 percent of men will eventually be affected by problems related to their prostate gland—generally benign prostatic hyperplasia (BPH) or prostate cancer. In the case of BPH, the incidence increases with age, so that 90 percent of men over eighty-five years of age are afflicted.

Enough gloomy news. The *good* news is that a number of effective nutritional approaches can help promote sexual function and maintenance of prostate health. The first step, before even exploring any of the many dietary approaches available, is to try to find out the root cause of the sexual dysfunction or prostate trouble. Of utmost importance, particularly in the case of BPH, is an accurate diagnosis to rule out the presence of prostate cancer—which should be aggressively treated by a traditional oncologist (cancer doctor).

ENLARGED PROSTATE

The prostate gland is a tiny little gland near the bladder that can cause some big problems. Its main function is to produce seminal fluid (the stuff that sperm swim around in), but when the prostate gland becomes enlarged, it can obstruct the flow of urine from the bladder through the urethra. The most common prostate-related complaint for most men is a more frequent urge to urinate, often accompanied by difficulty in completely emptying the bladder. Serious complications such as urinary tract infections and kidney damage can result from untreated prostate enlargement.

Benign prostatic hyperplasia is generally caused by increased conversion of the male hormone testosterone into dihydrotestosterone (DHT) in the prostate gland. In the prostate, specialized receptors take up DHT much more readily than testosterone, causing rapid tissue growth and enlargement of the gland. Effective dietary approaches to reducing the uncomfortable side effects of BPH include decreasing alcohol consumption and increasing zinc, selenium, and essential fatty acid (flaxseed) intake. Fish oil supplements and concentrated sources of the essential fatty acids EPA and DHA may promote healthy prostaglandin production and anti-inflammatory effects.

In Europe, herbal remedies account for the vast majority of BPH treatments. Although standardized saw palmetto extracts (at least 85 percent fatty acids and sterols) are among the most popular and effective herbals for BPH, others such as pygeum, urtica (stinging nettle), and various oils are also effective.

Essential oil consumption, possibly due to an anti-inflammatory effect, may be helpful in relieving the symptoms of BPH. One to 2 g per day of flaxseed oil may reduce the frequency of nighttime trips to the bathroom and increase the ability to fully empty urine from the bladder.

In the case of saw palmetto, inhibition of the enzyme (alpha-5-reductase) that converts testosterone to DHT helps to reduce the symptoms associated with BPH. Saw palmetto is at least as effective as the prescription drug Proscar (finasteride), used to treat BPH, and is generally not associated with side effects. Pygeum, on the other hand, appears to inhibit accumulation of fat and cholesterol within the prostate gland and also acts as an anti-inflammatory. Very often, several dietary supplements can be used in conjunction to take advantage of their different mechanisms of action. For example, combinations of standardized extracts of saw palmetto (80 mg), pumpkin seed oil (40 mg), pygeum (10 mg), and urtica (5 mg) may be more effective than any extract alone.

LOW LIBIDO

Switching gears away from prostate-specific conditions, reduced libido or lack of interest in sex is a prevalent concern—particularly considering the hectic pace at which many of us live our lives. A reduced sex drive can be due to a number of factors, including low hormone levels, lack of sleep, emotional issues, and a physical inability to "perform" in terms of a lack of stamina or difficulty achieving or maintaining an erection. Luckily, a number of nutrients and herbal extracts may be effective in boosting energy, normalizing hormonal levels, and putting that spark back in your sex life. Some of them are listed in the next section.

SUPPLEMENTS FOR MALE SEXUAL HEALTH

Ginseng, sometimes called "old man's root" in China, is frequently recommended as an energy-promoting herbal supplement. Occasionally ginseng is promoted as an aphrodisiac for both men and women because of its ability to help stimulate libido. Women may respond better to other herbs such as dong quai.

Sometimes lack of sexual desire is due less to a lack of energy than to an overabundance of stress. In such cases, either kava-kava or valerian may help promote relaxation and allow you to get into the mood.

Ginkgo biloba is most widely known for its memory-boosting effects, resulting from increased blood flow to the brain. It seems, however, that the brain is not the only organ that can benefit from increased blood flow. Ginkgo extracts also appear to increase blood circulation to other parts of the body, including the penis and clitoris, which could help facilitate erection and orgasm. Another herb from Mexico, yohimbe, may also enhance blood flow to the sex organs in both men and women. Yohimbe is not recommended, however, for anybody with high blood pressure or heart disease.

Low zinc levels may reduce testosterone production, and zinc supplements may be effective in returning hormone levels and sex drive to normal. Semen and prostate tissue are particularly rich in zinc, and it has been theorized that inadequate zinc intake may reduce the quality of semen and sperm motility.

Arginine is an amino acid that functions as a precursor to nitric oxide, the principal chemical that relaxes blood vessels and promotes blood circulation in the penis and clitoris. Other amino acids, such as those involved in the production of neurotransmitters such as phenylalanine, tyrosine, and histidine, may be effective in promoting optimal levels of sexual arousal and physical performance during sex. In some cases, a protein-rich diet may be helpful in downregulating the conversion of testosterone to DHT, which may benefit both the prostate and libido.

Chasteberry *(Vitex agnus-castus)* may help normalize hormonal balance (testosterone, estrogen, prolactin) in both men and women, which may lead to increased erectile function and sexual performance.

Vitamin E is often still thought of as a "fertility" or "male potency" nutrient because a deficiency of vitamin E in rats can lead to infertility. Although the same effect is unlikely in humans, many people swallow vitamin E capsules as both an aphrodisiac and a virility booster. Although vitamin E may not directly influence sex drive in humans, it does seem to improve the ability of sperm to fertilize egg cells, possibly by increasing sperm count and sperm motility.

Carnitine, an amino acid with functions in energy production and fat metabolism, has been recommended to maintain normal sperm cell function. Although sperm probably require a lot of energy to support all that "swimming," they actually rely more heavily on carbohydrates (sugar) for energy than they do on fat metabolism (which is what carnitine could potentially help with).

DHEA, a precursor of the hormone testosterone, may be effective in elevating testosterone and boosting libido in those with reduced levels. Another testosterone precursor, androstenedione, is often promoted as a testosterone booster, but evidence for this effect is controversial.

SUMMARY

In many cases, male sexual health, whether affected by prostate issues or other factors related to erections or libido, can be positively influenced by the right combination of proper nutrition, regular exercise, and possibly dietary supplements (see Table 14.1). It must be stressed, however, that both an enlarged prostate gland and/or any difficulty achieving or maintaining an erection need to be fully evaluated by your personal physician to rule out more serious conditions such as prostate cancer or atherosclerosis.

TABLE 14.1. Dietary Supplements for Male Sexual Health

Ingredient	Dose (per day)	Primary claim
Androstenedione	50-200 mg	Increases testosterone levels and sex drive
Arginine	3-6 g	Promotes circulation (treats erectile difficulty)
DHEA	50-100 mg	Increases testosterone levels and sex drive
Ginseng	100-300 mg	Increases energy levels and sex drive
Lycopene	3-6 mg	Reduces prostate cancer risk

Maca	500-900 mg	Boosts libido
Pumpkin seed	Follow label directions	Slows prostate enlargement
Pygeum	50-100 mg	Slows prostate enlargement
Saw palmetto	160-320 mg	Slows prostate enlargement
Selenium	70-200 mcg	Reduces prostate cancer risk
Stinging nettle	300-500 mg	Slows prostate enlargement
Vitamin E	100-400 IU	General "virility" claims
Yohimbe	10-30 mg	Treats erectile difficulty
Zinc	15-30 mg	Sperm production

SAW PALMETTO

What Is It?

Saw palmetto *(Serenoa repens)* is a dwarf palm tree found in the United States from the Carolinas to Texas. For centuries, the crude extracts of saw palmetto have been used to improve sperm production and to increase breast size and sexual vigor, but its most effective and only scientifically based use is to improve the symptoms of benign prostatic hyperplasia (BPH).

Claims

- Aids in the treatment of benign prostatic hyperplasia
- Increases libido
- Increases sperm production
- Increases breast size in women
- Useful as a urinary antiseptic and diuretic
- Prevents hair loss

Theory

The premise for using saw palmetto is that it maintains normal prostate health by decreasing the metabolism and action of male steroids. Saw palmetto has been demonstrated to decrease the activity of 5-alpha reductase, which stimulates the conversion of testosterone to dihydrotestosterone (DHT), its more active form. Since DHT is necessary for excessive growth (hyperplasia) of the prostate and is elevated in men with BPH, inhibition of 5-alpha reductase, and therefore DHT production, may alleviate BPH and the associated compression of the urethra (the tube that runs through the prostate gland to carry urine from the bladder). Additionally, studies have shown that saw palmetto helps to inhibit the production of various inflammatory factors, probably due to an effect of the fatty acids, thus serving to decrease overall prostate inflammation. The prescription medication for treating BPH, finasteride, is available as Proscar for BPH and in a lower potency version called Propecia for treating hair loss in men (because the same conversion of testosterone to DHT is thought to result in thinning and loss of hair).

Scientific Support

In one rather large study using over 1,000 patients over the age of fifty, saw palmetto was found to be as effective as finasteride (Proscar) for the treatment of BPH. In a twelve-week study of 1,334 patients on saw palmetto extract, over 80 percent of patients reported good to excellent results. In another study of forty BPH patients over a sixty-day period, 25 percent of patients had good results and 75 percent had excellent results with respect to BPH severity and symptoms. In a double-blind study of twenty-seven patients, saw palmetto resulted in positive benefits in 43 percent of people receiving the extract versus only 15 percent of subjects in the placebo group. Several recent case reports and small clinical trials have shown a particular combination of saw palmetto and Chinese herbs called "PC-SPES" (chrysanthemum, dyers woad, licorice, reishi, san-qi ginseng, rabdosia, saw palmetto, and baikal skullcap) to be effective in alleviating symptoms of BPH and even in reducing blood levels of prostate-specific antigen (PSA), a marker for prostate cancer. Several other smaller studies have shown significant improvements in symptoms of BPH such as increase in maximum urinary flow rates, reduced number of trips to the bathroom, a greater ability to fully empty the bladder, and an increased quality of life.

Safety

Headaches and gastrointestinal disturbances including diarrhea and nausea have been reported, although these adverse effects are rare. Because saw palmetto has primarily been tested in adult males, it is not recommended for children or for women who are pregnant or lactating. No drug interactions have been reported for saw palmetto. It is important to note that saw palmetto extract may only treat the symptoms of BPH, and therefore those with an enlarged prostate should consult with their physician on a regular basis.

Value

A one-month supply of saw palmetto extract costs approximately $15 to $30. Considering the possible health benefits (similar to the prescription drug Proscar for BPH and Propecia for hair loss) and the fact that saw palmetto appears to be safe and effective in several scientific studies, the value of the herb seems considerable.

Dosage

About 160 mg of the oil-based ("lipophilic") berry extract should be taken twice a day (morning and evening) for at least thirty days (total daily dose approximately 320 mg). Look for a brand that is standardized for fatty acid and sterol content—about 80 to 90 percent total fatty acids and sterols is recommended.

WORKS CONSULTED

Bauer HW, Casarosa C, Cosci M, Fratta M, Blessmann G. Saw palmetto fruit extract for treatment of benign prostatic hyperplasia. Results of a placebo-controlled double-blind study. MMW Fortschr Med. 1999 Jun 24;141(25):62.

Bracher F. Phytotherapy of benign prostatic hyperplasia. Urologe A. 1997 Jan;36(1):10-7.

de la Taille A, Hayek OR, Burchardt M, Burchardt T, Katz AE. Role of herbal compounds (PC-SPES) in hormone-refractory prostate cancer: Two case reports. J Altern Complement Med. 2000 Oct;6(5):449-51.

Dreikorn K, Schonhofer PS. Status of phytotherapeutic drugs in treatment of benign prostatic hyperplasia. Urologe A. 1995 Mar;34(2):119-29.

Ernst E. Herbal medications for common ailments in the elderly. Drugs Aging. 1999 Dec;15(6):423-8.

Gerber GS. Saw palmetto for the treatment of men with lower urinary tract symptoms. J Urol. 2000 May;163(5):1408-12.

Gerber G. What is saw palmetto used for, and does it interact with any medications? Health News. 2000 Jun;6(6):10.

Gerber GS, Zagaja GP, Bales GT, Chodak GW, Contreras BA. Saw palmetto (Serenoa repens) in men with lower urinary tract symptoms: Effects on urodynamic parameters and voiding symptoms. Urology. 1998 Jun;51(6):1003-7.

Glisson J, Crawford R, Street S. The clinical applications of Ginkgo biloba, St. John's wort, saw palmetto, and soy. Nurse Pract. 1999 Jun;24(6):35-6.

Goepel M, Hecker U, Krege S, Rubben H, Michel MC. Saw palmetto extracts potently and noncompetitively inhibit human alpha1-adrenoceptors in vitro. Prostate. 1999 Feb 15;38(3):208-15.

Marks LS, Partin AW, Epstein JI, Tyler VE, Simon I, Macairan ML, Chan TL, Dorey FJ, Garris JB, Veltri RW, Santos PB, Stonebrook KA, deKernion JB. Effects of a saw palmetto herbal blend in men with symptomatic benign prostatic hyperplasia. J Urol. 2000 May;163(5):1451-6.

Marks LS, Tyler VE. Saw palmetto extract: Newest (and oldest) treatment alternative for men with symptomatic benign prostatic hyperplasia. Urology. 1999 Mar;53(3):457-61.

McKinney DE. Saw palmetto for benign prostatic hyperplasia. JAMA. 1999 May 12;281(18):1699.

McPartland JM, Pruitt PL. Benign prostatic hyperplasia treated with saw palmetto: A literature search and an experimental case study. J Am Osteopath Assoc. 2000 Feb;100(2):89-96.

Ondrizek RR, Chan PJ, Patton WC, King A. Inhibition of human sperm motility by specific herbs used in alternative medicine. J Assist Reprod Genet. 1999 Feb;16(2):87-91.

Porterfield H. UsToo PC-SPES surveys: Review of studies and update of previous survey results. Mol Urol. 2000 Fall;4(3):289-92.

Powers JE. That pesky prostate and the saw palmetto. S D J Med. 1997 Dec; 50(12):453-4.

Schilcher H. Is there a rational therapy for symptomatic treatment of benign prostatic hyperplasia with phytogenic drugs? Illustrated with the example of the prostate agent from Serenoa repens. Wien Med Wochenschr. 1999;149(8-10):236-40.

Segars LW. Saw palmetto extracts for benign prostatic hyperplasia. J Fam Pract. 1999 Feb;48(2):88-9.

Shimada H, Tyler VE, McLaughlin JL. Biologically active acylglycerides from the berries of saw-palmetto (Serenoa repens). J Nat Prod. 1997 Apr;60(4):417-8.

Sokeland J. Combined sabal and urtica extract compared with finasteride in men with benign prostatic hyperplasia: Analysis of prostate volume and therapeutic outcome. BJU Int. 2000 Sep;86(4):439-42.

Swoboda H, Kopp B. Serenoa repens—the saw palmetto or dwarf palm. Wien Med Wochenschr. 1999;149(8-10):235.

Wilt TJ, Ishani A, Stark G, MacDonald R, Lau J, Mulrow C. Saw palmetto extracts for treatment of benign prostatic hyperplasia: A systematic review. JAMA. 1998 Nov 11;280(18):1604-9.

PYGEUM

What Is It?

Pygeum *(Pygeum africanum),* also known as African plum, is a large evergreen tree that grows in the high plateaus of southern Africa. The pygeum bark is traditionally powdered and drunk as a tea for genitourinary complaints such as bladder pain and urinary difficulty. As with saw palmetto, pygeum has predominantly been used and tested throughout Europe for the treatment of benign prostatic hyperplasia (BPH).

Claims

Aids in the treatment of mild to moderate cases of BPH by:

- Decreasing frequency of nocturnal urination
- Increasing urine volume (more productive urination)
- Decreasing incidence of incomplete bladder emptying
- Reducing prostate enlargement

Theory

Although the mechanism of action of pygeum is largely unknown, it is theorized to inhibit fibroblast hyperproliferation and prevent bladder contractile dysfunction. As such, pygeum may decrease excessive prostate growth (hyperplasia) and could allow better contraction of the bladder for more productive urination. Both of these actions could improve the quality of life of men with BPH.

Scientific Support

Animal studies indicate that partial bladder obstruction may lead to bladder contractile problems. In a rabbit study, BPH-like symptoms were prevented by pretreatment with pygeum extract. The action of pygeum may be to protect the bladder against lack of oxygen caused by or as a result of injury. In animal studies, 93 percent had an improvement in urine volume, 88 percent had an improvement in maximum bladder capacity, and 38 percent decreased their frequency of urination. In another study, pygeum potently inhibited proliferation of rat prostate cells, although this was not attributed to any effect on 5-alpha reductase, a major enzyme shown to play a role in prostate growth.

In humans, several clinical trials have demonstrated the benefits of pygeum extract in alleviating symptoms of BPH. In one non-placebo-controlled study in Europe, eighty-five men between the ages of fifty and seventy-five with moderate BPH were treated for two months with pygeum (50 mg of extract taken twice daily). In this study, the frequency of nocturnal urination decreased by 32 percent and quality of life improved by 31 percent. In sum, before pygeum treatment, two-thirds of the men were getting up three or more times per night to urinate—but following treatment, they were getting up one or fewer times per night. These improvements persisted for the month of follow-up after the subjects stopped taking pygeum. No changes in prostate volume were reported, and seven men reported an improvement in sexual performance. However, it is important to reiterate that this was not a placebo-controlled study, so bias may have been a factor.

Several placebo-controlled studies have been conducted for pygeum, although effects are not always dramatic. In one placebo-controlled study of 120 subjects, six weeks of pygeum treatment reduced nocturnal urination by 79 percent in those treated, but also by 50 percent in those receiving placebo. In another study of 263 BPH subjects, 50 mg of pygeum twice a day (or placebo) for sixty days reduced nighttime urination by 66 percent in the treated group, compared with 31 percent in the placebo group. However, no symptom scores were taken. In another double-blind study enrolling twenty men, there was no change in subjective or objective improvement.

Safety

Side effects for those taking pygeum are relatively rare (about 5 percent) and mild, and are generally gastrointestinal in nature. No drug interactions have been reported. It is important for any man with an enlarged prostate to consult with his personal physician to determine the cause of prostate enlargement and to rule out prostate cancer. Should you decide to supplement with pygeum, regular physical exams are also recommended.

Value

Sixty capsules (thirty-day supply) of pygeum extract (daily dose of 100 mg per day) costs $15 to $30, depending on the specific formulation and additional support ingredients. For those who cannot swallow capsules, pygeum is also sold as a liquid. Because studies conducted with pygeum have shown some initially positive benefits for men with mild to moderate BPH (and no serious adverse effects), it appears to be a good value.

Dosage

Pygeum africanum bark extract is generally taken twice per day in 50 mg capsules, although taking 100 mg in a single dose has been shown to be just as effective and safe. The extract consists of three groups of active constituents: phytosterols, pentacyclic triterpenoids, and ferulic esters of long-chained fatty alcohols. Thus, this oily extract is typically sold in softgel capsule form.

WORKS CONSULTED

Barlet A, Albrecht J, Aubert A, Fischer M, Grof F, Grothuesmann HG, Masson JC, Mazeman E, Mermon R, Reichelt H, et al. Efficacy of Pygeum africanum extract in the medical therapy of urination disorders due to benign prostatic hyperplasia: Evaluation of objective and subjective parameters. A placebo-controlled double-blind multicenter study. Wien Klin Wochenschr. 1990 Nov 23;102(22):667-73.

Bassi P, Artibani W, De Luca V, Zattoni F, Lembo A. Standardized extract of Pygeum africanum in the treatment of benign prostatic hypertrophy. Controlled clinical study versus placebo. Minerva Urol Nefrol. 1987 Jan-Mar;39(1):45-50.

Breza J, Dzurny O, Borowka A, Hanus T, Petrik R, Blane G, Chadha-Boreham H. Efficacy and acceptability of tadenan (Pygeum africanum extract) in the treatment of benign prostatic hyperplasia (BPH): A multicentre trial in central Europe. Curr Med Res Opin. 1998;14(3):127-39.

Carani C, Salvioli V, Scuteri A, Borelli A, Baldini A, Granata AR, Marrama P. Urological and sexual evaluation of treatment of benign prostatic disease using Pygeum africanum at high doses. Arch Ital Urol Nefrol Androl. 1991 Sep;63(3):341-5.

Chatelain C, Autet W, Brackman F. Comparison of once and twice daily dosage forms of Pygeum africanum extract in patients with benign prostatic hyperplasia: A randomized, double-blind study, with long-term open label extension. Urology. 1999 Sep;54(3):473-8.

Chen MW, Levin RM, Horan P, Buttyan RB. Effects of unilateral ischemia on the contractile response of the bladder: Protective effect of Tadenan (Pygeum africanum extract). Mol Urol. 1999;3(1):5-10.

Choo MS, Bellamy F, Constantinou CE. Functional evaluation of Tadenan on micturition and experimental prostate growth induced with exogenous dihydrotestosterone. Urology. 2000 Feb;55(2):292-8.

Clavert A, Cranz C, Riffaud JP, Marquer C, Lacolle JY, Bollack C. Effects of an extract of the bark of Pygeum africanum (V.1326) on prostatic secretions in the rat and in man. Ann Urol (Paris). 1986;20(5):341-3.

Dagues F, Costa P. Medical treatment of disorders of the bladder sphincter. Rev Prat. 1995 Feb 1;45(3):337-41.

Dufour B, Choquenet C, Revol M, Faure G, Jorest R. Controlled study of the effects of Pygeum africanum extract on the functional symptoms of prostatic adenoma. Ann Urol (Paris). 1984 May;18(3):193-5.

Flamm J, Kiesswetter H, Englisch M. An urodynamic study of patients with benign prostatic hypertrophy treated conservatively with phytotherapy or testosterone. Wien Klin Wochenschr. 1979 Sep 28;91(18):622-7.

Gomes CM, Disanto ME, Horan P, Levin RM, Wein AJ, Chacko S. Improved contractility of obstructed bladders after Tadenan treatment is associated with reversal of altered myosin isoform expression. J Urol. 2000 Jun;163(6):2008-13.

Krzeski T, Kazon M, Borkowski A, Witeska A, Kuczera J. Combined extracts of Urtica dioica and Pygeum africanum in the treatment of benign prostatic hyperplasia: Double-blind comparison of two doses. Clin Ther. 1993 Nov-Dec;15(6):1011-20.

Levin RM, Das AK. A scientific basis for the therapeutic effects of Pygeum africanum and Serenoa repens. Urol Res. 2000 Jun;28(3):201-9.

Longo R, Tira S. Steroidal and other components of Pygeum africanum bark. Farmaco [Prat]. 1983 Jul;38(7):287-92.

Mathe G, Hallard M, Bourut CH, Chenu E. A Pygeum africanum extract with so-called phyto-estrogenic action markedly reduces the volume of true and large prostatic hypertrophy. Biomed Pharmacother. 1995;49(7-8):341-3.

Mathe G, Orbach-Arbouys S, Bizi E, Court B. The so-called phyto-estrogenic action of Pygeum africanum extract. Biomed Pharmacother. 1995;49(7-8):339-40.

Menchini-Fabris GF, Giorgi P, Andreini F, Canale D, Paoli R, Sarteschi ML. New perspectives on the use of Pygeum africanum in prostato-bladder pathology. Arch Ital Urol Nefrol Androl. 1988 Sep;60(3):313-22.

Paubert-Braquet M, Cave A, Hocquemiller R, Delacroix D, Dupont C, Hedef N, Borgeat P. Effect of Pygeum africanum extract on A23187-stimulated production of lipoxygenase metabolites from human polymorphonuclear cells. J Lipid Mediat Cell Signal. 1994 May;9(3):285-90.

Pierini N, Citti F, Di Marzio S, Pozzato C, Quercia V. Identification and determination of N-docosanol in the bark extract of Pygeum africanum and in patent medicines containing it. Boll Chim Farm. 1982 Jan;121(1):27-34.

Solano RM, Garcia-Fernandez MO, Clemente C, Querol M, Bellamy F, Sanchez-Chapado M, Prieto JC, Carmena MJ. Effects of Pygeum africanum extract (Tadenan(R)) on vasoactive intestinal peptide receptors, G proteins, and adenylyl cyclase in rat ventral prostate. Prostate. 2000 Nov 1;45(3):245-52.

Thieblot L, Berthelay S, Berthelay J. Preventive and curative action of a bark extract from an African plant, Pygeum africanum, on experimental prostatic adenoma in rats. Therapie. 1971 May-Jun;26(3):575-80.

Yablonsky F, Nicolas V, Riffaud JP, Bellamy F. Antiproliferative effect of Pygeum africanum extract on rat prostatic fibroblasts. J Urol. 1997 Jun;157(6):2381-7.

YOHIMBE/QUEBRACHO

What Is It?

Yohimbe comes from the bark of an African tree, and the active compound, yohimbine, can also be found in large amounts in the South American herb quebracho *(Aspidosperma quebracho-blanco)*. It has traditionally been used as a stimulant and aphrodisiac in West Africa and South America. In the United States, yohimbe and quebracho are most often promoted in dietary supplements for treating impotence, stimulating male sexual performance (often marketed as "herbal Viagra"), and enhancing athletic performance (as an alternative to anabolic steroids). A purified extract from yohimbe bark yields an alkaloid similar in structure to caffeine and ephedra, called yohimbine, which is regulated as a prescription medication and used for treating erectile dysfunction in males.

Claims

- Enhances sexual performance (aphrodisiac and erectile function)
- Increases muscle mass (boosts testosterone levels)
- Promotes weight loss
- Boosts energy levels
- Relieves depression

Theory

The active compound in yohimbe, an alkaloid called yohimbine, functions as a monoamine oxidase (MAO) inhibitor to increase levels of the neurotransmitter norepinephrine. Yohimbine also acts as a central nervous system stimulator, where it blocks specific receptors (alpha-2 adrenergic receptors) and may increase energy levels and promote fat oxidation. In addition to these effects, yohimbe can also dilate blood vessels, making it a potentially useful treatment for erectile dysfunction and some forms of impotence in men. Because of the MAO inhibition, yohimbe is occasionally recommended as a treatment for mild depression.

Scientific Support

Although yohimbe is frequently promoted as a "natural" way to increase testosterone levels for muscle building, strength enhancement, and fat loss, there is no solid scientific proof that yohimbe is either anabolic or thermogenic.

Results from a few small trials show that yohimbine can increase blood flow to the genitals (which may occur in both men and women). As such, yohimbe may be effective in alleviating some mild forms of both "psychological" and "physical" impotence. In the few studies conducted on the purified form of yohimbine, only about 30 percent of subjects reported beneficial effects in terms of erectile function and sexual performance.

Safety

As the number of yohimbe products on the retail market increases, concerns about their safety are raised because of the reported toxicity of yohimbine (the major alkaloid of the plant). Reported side effects of yohimbe use range from minor complaints such as headaches, anxiety, and tension to more serious adverse events including high blood pressure, elevated heart rate, heart palpitations, and hallucinations. People with high blood pressure and kidney disease should avoid supplements containing yohimbe as should women who are, or who could become, pregnant (due to abortion risk). Also, caution should be used with yohimbe taken in combination with certain foods containing tyramine (red wine, liver, and cheese) as well as with nasal decongestants or diet aids containing ephedrine or phenylpropanolamine (which could lead to dangerous blood pressure fluctuations). Occasionally, yohimbe is combined with serotonergic supplements (such as St. John's wort or 5-HTP) to increase their effectiveness. It is not recommended to combine yohimbe with other antidepressant supplements or medications except under the advice and supervision of a nutritionally oriented physician.

Value

For nearly a century, yohimbe has been used as an aphrodisiac and sexual enhancer—although no effect on human sex drive or performance has been adequately demonstrated. Yohimbine (the drug) has been evaluated in the management of erectile disorder in a few small studies, where it appears to have a modest therapeutic benefit over placebo (especially in "psychological" erectile dysfunction). Laboratory analyses (via chromatogram) of commercial yohimbine extracts, however, indicate that although many products contained measurable quantities of the yohimbine alkaloid, the vast majority are largely devoid of effective levels of the compound. Concentrations of yohimbine in commercial yohimbe products typically range from zero to almost 500 ppm (compared with over 7,000 ppm in authentic yohimbe bark). Because yohimbe bark has been reported to contain up to 6 percent total alkaloids, 10 to 15 percent of which are yohimbine, it is likely that most supplements containing yohimbe also contain undeclared diluents (which you're paying a high price for).

Because there are more effective and safe supplement remedies for increasing circulation to promote erectile function (arginine, cordyceps, and ginkgo biloba), enhancing muscle strength (HMB and creatine), weight loss (green tea, banaba leaf, and gymnema), and relieving mild depression (SAMe, 5-HTP, and St. John's wort), yohimbe is of limited value.

Dosage

Although there are no standard accepted dosage recommendations for yohimbe, it is known that more than 40 mg per day of yohimbine can result in adverse side effects such as dizziness, headaches, loss of coordination, and hallucinations. Typical daily amounts of yohimbine alkaloids found in commercial supplements (label claims) are often in the range of 10 to 30 mg and occasionally standardized to yohimbine or total alkaloid content.

WORKS CONSULTED

Adimoelja A. Phytochemicals and the breakthrough of traditional herbs in the management of sexual dysfunctions. Int J Androl. 2000;23(Suppl 2):82-4.

Betz JM, White KD, der Marderosian AH. Gas chromatographic determination of yohimbine in commercial yohimbe products. J AOAC Int. 1995 Sep-Oct;78(5):1189-94.

De Smet PA, Smeets OS. Potential risks of health food products containing yohimbe extracts. BMJ. 1994 Oct 8;309(6959):958.

Deutsch HF, Evenson MA, Drescher P, Sparwasser C, Madsen PO. Isolation and biological activity of aspidospermine and quebrachamine from an Aspidosperma tree source. J Pharm Biomed Anal. 1994 Oct;12(10):1283-7.

Lyon RL, Fong HH, Farnsworth NR, Svoboda GH. Biological and phytochemical evaluation of plants. XI. Isolation of aspidospermine, quebrachidine, rhazinilam, (–)-pyrifolidine, and akuammidine from Aspidosperma quebracho-blanco (Apocynaceae). J Pharm Sci. 1973 Feb;62(2):218-21.

Riley AJ. Yohimbine in the treatment of erectile disorder. Br J Clin Pract. 1994 May-Jun;48(3):133-6.

Sandler B, Aronson P. Yohimbine-induced cutaneous drug eruption, progressive renal failure, and lupus-like syndrome. Urology. 1993 Apr;41(4):343-5.

Tunmann P, Wolf D. The N(b)-oxide of rhazidigenin, an alkaloid from the bark of Aspidospermia Quebracho blanco Schlecht. Z Naturforsch B. 1969 Dec;24(12):1665-6.

MACA

What Is It?

Maca *(Lepidium meyenii),* also called Peruvian ginseng, is a Peruvian plant (sort of like a radish) used for restoring energy, vitality, and fertility. As folklore has it, when Spanish explorers arrived in Peru in the sixteenth century, their livestock were weak and infertile. Upon the advice of the Incas, the Spaniards fed maca to their horses and other animals. The result was healthy livestock that reproduced normally—and a new "sexual health" was born. In addition to its use for fertility, Inca warriors would supposedly eat maca before battles to promote strength and stamina. Today, maca is still a staple in Peru—the root may be roasted like a potato, or prepared as a jam, pudding, juice, or soup. As an aphrodisiac, maca is typically formulated into a capsule.

Claims

- Boosts libido
- Regulates hormonal secretion
- Increases energy
- Improves memory
- Fights depression

Theory

When the body is well nourished, a person is less likely to be depressed, more likely to have adequate energy levels, and his or her libido will be normal. Because maca is so full of nutrients, it could increase energy, decrease the likelihood of anemia, and affect libido. Sterols found in maca may act on the hormone-producing hypothalamus, pituitary, and adrenal glands, which could all lead to increased energy and libido.

Scientific Support

Although folklore abounds regarding the utility of maca for general health and increased libido, a search of the scientific literature from the past two decades reveals limited information on the worth of maca for sexual function and desire. However, one recent study published as an abstract in the journal *Urology* does give promising results. Male rodents were given maca extract (or a control) and placed with female rodents. Voyeuristic scientists then recorded how many mating events occurred, how many sperm-positive females resulted, and how long it took for male rats to achieve erection. The results revealed that in rodents receiving maca instead of a control, there were more mating events, more sperm-positive females, and fewer rats that consulted their urologists in hopes of obtaining Viagra. The maca-free mice had sex a mere thirteen times in three hours, but the mice who received maca did it sixty-seven times!

The few other scientific studies pertaining to maca relate to its nutritional value. It appears that maca is a good enough source of nutrients that in economically depressed rural areas, consumption of maca can help combat malnutrition. Although scientific studies do not exist that would support the use of maca in improving energy, memory, or fighting depression, it is conceivable that in people who are malnourished in some way, its nutritional value alone could improve mood and mental function.

Safety

Because maca is a food, like oatmeal or sweet potatoes, it is a safe product. It has not been found to cause toxicity or adverse pharmacological effects. However, if you are pregnant, lactating, or have any medical condition, consult your physician before taking maca as a therapeutic.

Value

Maca comes in many forms, but is only widely available in the United States in capsule form (as a maca root extract) or as a liquid. A thirty-day supply of capsules costs approximately $10 to $15.

Dosage

Although it is difficult to assign a dosage to something that is typically eaten as a food, maca capsules generally contain 500 mg of dried maca with dosage recommendations in the range of 3 to 5 g per day (six to ten capsules). As an extract, 900 mg per day is a typical dose (about two capsules per day).

WORKS CONSULTED

Canales M, Aguilar J, Prada A, Marcelo A, Huaman C, Carbajal L. Nutritional evaluation of Lepidium meyenii (MACA) in albino mice and their descendants. Arch Latinoam Nutr. 2000 Jun;50(2):126-33.

Chacon G. La maca (Lepidium peruvianum) Chacon sp. Nov. Y su habitat. Revista Peruana de Biologia. 1990;3:171-272.

Dini A, Migliuolo G, Rastrelli L, Suturnino P, Schettino O. Chemical composition of Lepidium meyenii. Food Chemistry. 1994;49:347-9.

Gomez A. Maca, es alternativa nutricional para el ano 2000. Informe Ojo con su Salud (Lima, Peru). 1997 Aug 15;(58):226-8.

Johns T. The anu and the maca. J Ethnobiol. 1981;1:208-12.

King S. Ancient buried treasure of the Andes. Garden. 1986 Nov/Dec; 16-19.

Leon J. The "maca" (Lepidium Meyenii) a little known food plant of Peru. Econ Bot. 1964;18:122-7.

Quiros C, Epperson A, Hu J, Holle M. Physiological studies and determination of chromosome number in maca, Lepidium meyenii. Economic Botany 1996; 50(2):216-23.

Report of an Ad Hoc Panel of the Advisory Committee on Technical Innovation, Board on Science and Technology for International Development, National Research Council, 1989. Lost Crops of the Incas: Little Known Plants of the Andes with Promise for Worldwide Cultivation. Washington, DC: National Academy Press.

Zheng BL, He K, Kim CH, Rogers LL, Shao L. Effect of a lipidic extract from Lepidium meyenii on sexual behavior in mice and rats. Urology, 2000 (4) 55:598-602.

Chapter 15

Supplements for Female Health

INTRODUCTION

When it comes to female-specific nutrition, the primary concerns are typically menopause, premenstrual syndrome (PMS), breast health, and bone health. Both breast health and bone health are covered in other chapters, so this chapter focuses on nutritional approaches to dealing with menopause and PMS.

MENOPAUSE

In the United States alone, nearly *half* of all women will have experienced menopause within the next fifteen years. Menopause, which most women experience between the ages of forty-five and fifty-five, is simply the cessation of the monthly menstrual cycle. In terms of physical and emotional factors, however, "the pause" represents a significant stage of life and health for all women.

Common side effects associated with the hormonal changes of menopause (reduced estrogen and progesterone levels) include hot flashes, headaches, night sweats, heart palpitations, insomnia, and a variety of anxiety and mood changes. In addition, with the loss of estrogen comes an increased risk of osteoporosis and heart disease. The most common medical approach to this natural time of life is to replace lost hormones through the use of synthetic or derived hormonal medications such as progestin and Premarin. Such hormone replacement therapy (HRT), while beneficial for many women, is not without a significant downside. The most commonly reported side effects of HRT include bloating, breast swelling and tenderness, and nausea—as well as a potentially elevated risk for cancer of the breast and endometrium. Thus it is no wonder that the number of women currently using traditional HRT has been in steep decline for the last decade or so. Luckily, a number of nutritional approaches may be quite helpful in alleviating some of the symptoms associated with menopause.

Stress Relief

For many women, the significant changes that their bodies undergo during menopause can lead to emotional changes such as depression and insomnia, as well as increased levels of stress and anxiety. A wide variety of herbal solutions may be helpful during this important (and remember—*natural*) time of life. St. John's wort may, for many women, be an effective supplement for relieving the mild depression and combating the food cravings and weight gain that often accompany menopause. Calming herbs such as melissa (lemon balm), valerian, and kava-kava may be helpful in relieving anxiety and promoting restful sleep.

Increase Consumption of Soy Foods

Soy-based foods, such as roasted soybeans, isolated soy protein powders, soymilk, tofu, and tempeh are among the richest concentrations of phytoestrogens called isoflavones. In the body, isoflavones act as a weak form of estrogen to provide many of the beneficial effects of estrogen, without the adverse effects associated with high-dose (unopposed) estrogen-replacement therapy. Because isoflavones have a structure similar to the body's natural estrogen, these phytoestrogens are able to bind weakly to estrogen receptors on the surface of cells. This action can block the effects of overproduction of estrogen (when the body produces too much, such as in PMS) while inducing a mild estrogenic effect (when the body fails to produce enough, such as during menopause).

It is well known that in many Asian countries, where the diet contains high levels of soy-based foods (typically 40 to 60 g of soy protein per day), there is also a very low incidence of menopausal symptoms such as hot flashes. In fact, it is widely stated that in Japan, where soy consumption is among the highest in the world, there isn't even a word to describe "hot flash" (because so few women experience the condition). Of special note is the interesting fact that most Asian cultures also enjoy a significantly lower incidence of breast and prostate cancer compared to rates observed in many Western countries, where consumption of soy-based foods is quite low.

Beyond Soy—Supplements for Menopause

In addition to soy-based foods and dietary supplements containing isolated soy isoflavones, there are a number of other herbal sources of phytoestrogens—some of the most popular being black cohosh, dong quai, vitex, red clover, alfalfa, and licorice. Each of these herbs has been shown to have mild to moderate effects in helping to alleviate hot flashes and other menopausal symptoms as well as providing general support in terms of cardiovascular health. Vitamin E, one of the most widely consumed supplements for overall heart health, may also have some mild effects in reducing hot flashes. Wild yam is often recommended as a natural alternative to synthetic progesterone (progesterone balances many of estrogen's effects and also declines during menopause), but the progesterone precursors in wild yam cannot be converted in the body to active progesterone (although this *can* be accomplished in the laboratory). Many menopausal women turn to wild yam creams and progesterone ointments to combat the decreased libido and vaginal dryness that often come with menopause. Although both cardiovascular health and bone health are covered in other chapters, it is important to note that menopause increases the risk of osteoporosis significantly and brings a woman's usually low risk of heart disease almost up to the same level of risk experienced by men of similar age.

PREMENSTRUAL SYNDROME

So if you're not *post*menopausal, then you are *pre*menopausal—meaning that you experience regular (or at least semiregular) monthly menstrual cycles—and that you also have the potential to suffer from premenstrual syndrome. PMS typically strikes toward the end of a regular monthly cycle, just before menstruation begins, and often involves symptoms such as bloating, cramping, breast tenderness, and changes in mood. Although the specific symptoms and their severity can vary significantly from one woman to the next, there are a number of dietary supplements that may be helpful in alleviating some symptoms and preventing others.

Before turning to dietary supplements, however, several aspects of nutrition and lifestyle need to be evaluated. In terms of overall diet, alcohol and caffeine consumption appear to be related, at least moderately, to an increased incidence and severity of PMS symptoms. Some nutritionists suggest avoiding foods containing high levels of sugar and fat (junk food) to help prevent PMS symptoms—but this is generally a prudent approach for anybody looking to feel better through nutrition. In addition, women who exercise regularly tend to report a lower incidence of PMS symptoms (and a reduced severity of any symptoms that do occur) than sedentary women—and lean women have fewer problems than overweight women—so a regular program of physical activity may be as helpful as any approach to combating PMS.

Supplements for PMS

Among dietary supplements, vitamin B_6 is one of the most popular nutrients for treating the symptoms of PMS. Several studies have shown that the overproduction of estrogen commonly thought to be responsible for PMS may be counteracted in some way by 200 to 400 mg of vitamin B_6 per day. It may take two to three months of use before beneficial effects are seen.

Essential fatty acids, such as those provided by fish oil, evening primrose oil, or flaxseed oil, may help resolve some of the fatty acid imbalances that can lead to symptoms of PMS (such as breast tenderness).

Calcium and magnesium, often considered to be supplements only for promoting bone health, also appear to be highly effective in alleviating PMS symptoms. In several recent studies, women consuming the highest levels of calcium suffered fewer episodes of PMS, while other women given calcium supplements (1,000 mg per day) or magnesium supplements (250 mg per day) were found to experience rapid relief from PMS. A number of other vitamins and minerals have been touted as PMS cures, but because most are readily available in a comprehensive multivitamin supplement, a prudent approach is to consume the multi and avoid single-ingredient supplements.

Vitex berry (also called chasteberry) is a popular herbal remedy for some PMS symptoms because of its effects in "balancing" estrogen and progesterone levels throughout the menstrual cycle (perhaps by stimulating progesterone production).

Dong quai, also known as "female ginseng," has been used for centuries as a treatment for various forms of dysmenorrhea (painful menstruation and cramping).

SUMMARY

Many women are looking for alternative approaches to dealing with the common symptoms of menopause and PMS. The growing popularity of dietary supplementation with vitamins, minerals, and herbal extracts has provided women around the world with relief from many of these symptoms and protection from developing related health problems (see Table 15.1). There is little doubt that much more research is needed into the precise mechanisms, long-term effectiveness, and overall safety of popular dietary supplements, but the existing evidence certainly supports the benefits associated with many of the treatments discussed here.

TABLE 15.1. Dietary Supplements for Relief of Menopausal Symptoms and Premenstrual Syndrome

Ingredient	Dose (per day)	Primary claim
Black cohosh	20-40 mg	Menopause
Cranberry	100-500 mg	Urinary tract infections
Damiana	400-800 mg	PMS
Dong quai	250-1,000 mg	PMS
Evening primrose oil	1-4 g	PMS/menopause
Flaxseed oil	10-40 g	PMS/menopause
Gotu kola	60-180 mg	Varicose veins and skin health
Horse chestnut	25-200 mg	Varicose vein therapy
Red clover	20-40 mg	Menopause
Uva ursi	800-2,100 mg	Urinary tract infections
Vitex/chasteberry	150-500 mg	PMS

DAMIANA

What Is It?

Damiana *(Turnera aphrodisiaca)* leaves have been traditionally used as a respiratory, neurological, and sexual medicine by the indigenous cultures of Mexico. This yellow-flowering shrub typically grows in climates that are hot and humid, including Central and South America, and in the state of Texas. Commercially introduced in the United States in 1874, damiana has historically been used as an aphrodisiac and has been claimed to induce euphoria.

Claims

- Acts as an aphrodisiac
- Relieves symptoms of premenstrual syndrome (PMS)
- Relieves anxiety and induces relaxation
- Alleviates depression

Theory

Although there is a clear lack of scientific evidence to support any of the theories for the efficacy attributed to damiana, its seeming ability to induce mild euphoria could support a logical theory that in relatively small quantities, damiana could lead to relaxation and could calm anxiety. Conceivably, those suffering from sexual dysfunction resulting from stress or emotional troubles could benefit from supplementation with this herb.

Scientific Support

It is important to note that only one scientific study exists in the literature that directly examines any physiological functions or effects of damiana. The essential oil from damiana leaves contains several terpene compounds, and a small body of research associates terpenes with pheromones, which are thought to play a role in sexual arousal. Out of four studies mentioning terpenes in relation to sexual behavior, three involve insect mating behavior, while one study found that male white-tailed deer produce terpene-containing pheromones in greater amounts during the breeding season (not exactly compelling "love potion" evidence unless you're a deer or a bug). Furthermore, damiana leaves also contain alkaloids that have been associated with insect pheromones in a variety of studies. Despite this possible link, scientific studies have not been conducted to associate any effect of damiana with pheromone production in humans.

Perhaps the most viable scientific evidence for the age-old use of damiana as an aphrodisiac involves a single recent study demonstrating that damiana extract binds to the progesterone receptor in human breast cancer cells. Despite the fact that oregano extract was found to bind tightly as well, the ability of damiana extract to interact with progesterone receptors may explain claims that damiana supplementation can increase libido. Importantly, many progesterone-binding extracts can have either a neutral or antagonistic effect instead of an agonistic (promoting) effect. However, a variety of scientific studies associate progesterone deficiency, particularly in post-menopausal women, with decreased libido. Thus, if the binding of damiana extract to progesterone receptors indeed mimics the action of progesterone, damiana could theoretically lead to increased libido in women with a progesterone deficiency. Furthermore, because progesterone is one of the major hormones involved in the female reproductive cycle, one may infer that by possibly affecting progesterone detection, damiana extract could ease the cyclical depression and anxiety often associated with the menstrual cycle. However, due to the lack of any controlled clinical trials, all of this is pure speculation.

Safety

Damiana leaves have a mild laxative and stool-softening effect, especially when used at high doses. At high doses, damiana has been reported to cause mild euphoria. Since the scientific community has not rigorously studied damiana, the herb is not recommended for women who are pregnant or lactating, for children, or for anyone with a serious medical condition or who is taking prescription medication.

Value

Both capsule and liquid extract forms of damiana cost approximately $25 to $30 for one month's supply—quite often the herb is combined with other ingredients in a variety of "sexual health" formulas. There are no controlled studies comparing results after taking damiana versus placebo. Additionally, since potential drug interactions and safety have not been investigated, there seems to be little justification for taking damiana when other remedies exist that are much more reliable and well documented.

Dosage

It is generally recommended that 400 to 800 mg of damiana be taken three times daily, but dosage recommendations may vary based on the combination of other ingredients in a particular product.

WORKS CONSULTED

Auterhoff H, Haufel HP. Contents of Damiana drugs. Arch Pharm Ber Dtsch Pharm Ges. 1968 Jul;301(7):537-44.

Lowry TP. Damiana. J Psychoactive Drugs. 1984 Jul-Sep;16(3):267-8.

Zava DT, Dollbaum CM, Blen M. Estrogen and progestin bioactivity of foods, herbs, and spices. Proc Soc Exp Biol Med. 1998 Mar;217(3):369-78.

BLACK COHOSH

What Is It?

Black cohosh *(Cimicifuga racemosa)* is a perennial wildflower native to eastern North America. It has traditionally been used by Native Americans to relieve menstrual cramps and "female complaints" and was used by American colonists to treat amenorrhea (lack of menstruation). Its primary use in modern alternative medicine is for relief of symptoms associated with menopause, including hot flashes and depression.

Claims

Relief of menopausal symptoms such as

- Hot flashes
- Mood swings
- Headache
- Night sweats

Theory

Although the precise chemical makeup and mechanism of action has not been identified for black cohosh, the main active constituents are thought to be the triterpene glycosides, although isoflavones, alkaloids, and phenolic acids may contribute to the overall activity of the plant extract. Some fractions of black cohosh extract are known to bind to estrogen receptors, but it is unclear whether they produce true estrogenic effects in vivo.

Scientific Support

Test-tube studies have shown that black cohosh extracts can inhibit the growth of breast cancer cells, suggesting that black cohosh may block the cancer-promoting effects of estrogen. Animal studies have also suggested a role for black cohosh in bone metabolism due to its inhibition of bone breakdown. Black cohosh extracts have also been shown to bind to serotonin recep-

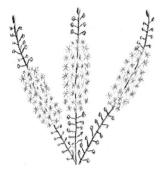

tors, which may explain the traditional use of the plant in treating depressive moods.

A number of clinical studies have been conducted on black cohosh extracts standardized to 1 mg triterpene glycosides per dose. Overall, the studies show a clear reduction in menopausal symptoms (hot flashes, night sweats, headaches) and psychological parameters (depression, sleep disturbances, irritability) following four to eight weeks of treatment. In some cases, subjects have been able to discontinue hormone replacement therapy while taking black cohosh extract.

Safety

Toxicity assessments conducted in rats and cell culture have shown no evidence of toxic or mutagenic effects. Mild to moderate cases of gastrointestinal discomfort have been reported in some subjects. Because of the potential for large doses of black cohosh to induce premature labor, pregnant women should avoid its use.

Value

For women experiencing the physiological changes that accompany menopause, black cohosh may be a natural alternative to estrogen or hormone replacement therapy (ERT/HRT). Many postmenopausal and perimenopausal women elect to discontinue HRT due to the unpleasant side effects associated with the treatment. For these women (as many as 50 percent of American women), black cohosh may provide the symptom relief they are looking for with few side effects.

Dosage

Approximately 20 to 40 mg of black cohosh extract, standardized for triterpene glycoside levels (2.5 percent), should be taken twice per day (total daily dose of 1 to 2 mg triterpene glycosides). A period of four to eight weeks is required for alleviation of menopausal symptoms.

WORKS CONSULTED

Baillie N, Rasmussen P. Black and blue cohosh in labour. N Z Med J. 1997 Jan 24;110(1036):20-1.

Dixon-Shanies D, Shaikh N. Growth inhibition of human breast cancer cells by herbs and phytoestrogens. Oncol Rep. 1999 Nov-Dec;6(6):1383-7.

Duker EM, Kopanski L, Jarry H, Wuttke W. Effects of extracts from Cimicifuga racemosa on gonadotropin release in menopausal women and ovariectomized rats. Planta Med. 1991 Oct;57(5):420-4.

Gunn TR, Wright IM. The use of black and blue cohosh in labour. N Z Med J. 1996 Oct 25;109(1032):410-1.

Hardy ML. Herbs of special interest to women. J Am Pharm Assoc (Wash). 2000 Mar-Apr;40(2):234-42.

Herbal medicine. Black cohosh: The woman's herb? Harv Women's Health Watch. 2000 Apr;7(8):6.

Lieberman S. A review of the effectiveness of Cimicifuga racemosa (black cohosh) for the symptoms of menopause. J Women's Health. 1998 Jun;7(5):525-9.

Liske E. Therapeutic efficacy and safety of Cimicifuga racemosa for gynecologic disorders. Adv Ther. 1998 Jan-Feb;15(1):45-53.

McFarlin BL, Gibson MH, O'Rear J, Harman P. A national survey of herbal preparation use by nurse-midwives for labor stimulation. Review of the literature and recommendations for practice. J Nurse Midwifery. 1999 May-Jun;44(3):205-16.

Pepping J. Black cohosh: Cimicifuga racemosa. Am J Health Syst Pharm. 1999 Jul 15;56(14):1400-2.

Shao Y, Harris A, Wang M, Zhang H, Cordell GA, Bowman M, Lemmo E. Triterpene glycosides from Cimicifuga racemosa. J Nat Prod. 2000 Jul;63(7):905-10.

Wade C, Kronenberg F, Kelly A, Murphy PA. Hormone-modulating herbs: Implications for women's health. J Am Med Women's Assoc. 1999 Fall;54(4):181-3.

DONG QUAI

What Is It?

Dong quai *(Angelica sinensis)* has been used in traditional Chinese medicine (TCM) and Native American medicine for centuries. The plant is related to both parsley and celery and is most commonly used to treat cramps and pain during menstruation as well as to ease some of the symptoms of menopause (hot flashes, night sweats). Dong quai is frequently referred to as "female ginseng" to suggest its "balancing" or adaptogenic effect on the menstrual period.

Claims

- Eases menopausal symptoms (hot flashes, night sweats)
- Reduces symptoms of premenstrual syndrome (PMS)

Theory

The principal active constituents of dong quai roots appear to be a group of coumarin compounds, ferulic acid and ligustilide. Although some popular literature suggests that dong quai acts as a phytoestrogen in the body (similar to isoflavones), there do not appear to be any estrogenic compounds in the plant. Instead, the combined effects of other compounds in areas such as blood flow (coumarins) and muscle relaxation (ferulic acid and ligustilide) are thought to contribute to the overall effects of dong quai.

Phytochemical analyses have found that the natural coumarin derivatives (blood thinners) and additional constituents in dong quai possess antithrombotic and antiarrhythmic properties. In one documented case report, a significant drug interaction between dong quai and an anticoagulant medication (warfarin) resulted in excessive bleeding time.

Scientific Support

Much of the rationale for using dong quai to relieve menopausal symptoms comes from anecdotal and historical reports of traditional use in TCM and other ancient traditions. In Western cultures, hot flashes and related menopausal symptoms are experienced by about 75 percent of perimenopausal and menopausal women. For most women, the experience is a minor annoyance, but for others hot flashes can be an intensely unpleasant sensation. Hot flashes may be triggered by a number of factors including anxiety, stress, high room temperatures, caffeine, and alcohol. Overweight women tend to experience fewer hot flashes than thinner women, probably due to the ability of adipose (fat) tissue to convert circulating precursor hormones such as androstenedione into active forms of estrogen (estrone and estradiol). From a physiological standpoint, hot flashes occur when the body attempts to shed excess heat through vasodilation (opening up blood vessels)—so it is logical that an herbal therapy such as dong quai (which has actions in modulating blood flow and smooth muscle relaxation) may provide some benefits.

Although the blood flow or muscle relaxant mechanism of action has not been subjected to rigorous clinical study, at least one double-blind study has investigated the potential estrogenic activity of dong quai supplements. In the study, seventy-one postmenopausal women received either dong quai or placebo for twenty-four weeks. Measurements included endometrial thickness, vaginal cell maturation, and change in overall menopausal symptoms (including hot flashes). The study found no significant differences between groups in any of the measurements—suggesting that dong quai had no estrogenic effects and was no more helpful than placebo in easing menopausal symptoms.

Safety

Dong quai is generally considered to be quite safe when used as directed. Of potential concern to some individuals, however, is the tendency of dong quai to increase photosensitivity—making those with fair skin even more sensitive to sunlight and increasing the risk of sunburn.

Dong quai is not recommended for use by pregnant or lactating women, and it should not be used in conjunction with other blood-thinning medications or supplements. Because of dong quai's ability to increase bleeding time, use should be discontinued as soon as menstruation begins (if used to control PMS symptoms).

Value

Although dong quai has a long history of use in TCM and Native American medicine, the current level of scientific evidence does not support dong quai as a particularly effective remedy for the uncomfortable symptoms associated with either menopause or PMS. Other dietary supplements such as isoflavone compounds from soybeans and red clover are readily available and have been shown to be effective not only in easing menopausal symptoms but also in providing benefits for heart and bone health.

Dosage

Typical recommendations for using dong quai for the relief of menstrual cramps and menopausal symptoms are in the range of 250 to 1,000 mg per day, taken in two to three divided doses.

WORKS CONSULTED

Fugh-Berman A. Herb-drug interactions. Lancet. 2000 Jan 8;355(9198):134-8.

Hardy ML. Herbs of special interest to women. J Am Pharm Assoc (Wash). 2000 Mar-Apr;40(2):234-42.

Hirata JD, Swiersz LM, Zell B, Small R, Ettinger B. Does dong quai have estrogenic effects in postmenopausal women? A double-blind, placebo-controlled trial. Fertil Steril. 1997 Dec;68(6):981-6.

Page RL 2nd, Lawrence JD. Potentiation of warfarin by dong quai. Pharmacotherapy. 1999 Jul;19(7):870-6.

Shaw CR. The perimenopausal hot flash: Epidemiology, physiology, and treatment. Nurse Pract. 1997 Mar;22(3):55-6, 61-6.

Smolinske SC. Dietary supplement-drug interactions. J Am Med Women's Assoc. 1999 Fall;54(4):191-2, 195.

Yim TK, Wu WK, Pak WF, Mak DH, Liang SM, Ko KM. Myocardial protection against ischaemia-reperfusion injury by a Polygonum multiflorum extract supplemented 'Dang-Gui decoction for enriching blood,' a compound formulation, ex vivo. Phytother Res. 2000 May;14(3):195-9.

Zhu DP. Dong quai. Am J Chin Med. 1987;15(3-4):117-25.

FLAXSEED/LINSEED OIL

What Is It?

Flaxseed is just what it sounds like—the seed of the flax plant. Flaxseed is typically used as a source of the essential fatty acids linolenic acid (LN) and linoleic acid (LA). The oil is about 57 percent LN (an omega-3 acid) and about 17 percent LA (omega-6). LN can be converted into eicosapentaenoic acid (EPA) and docosahexaenoic acid (DHA)—fatty acids that are precursors to anti-inflammatory and antiatherogenic prostaglandins. Another beneficial ingredient found in abundance in flaxseed is lignan, a phytochemical with potential for cancer prevention.

Claims

- Reduces symptoms of PMS and menopause
- Decreases blood pressure
- Reduces risk of stroke and heart attack
- Reduces arthritis pain
- Protects against breast cancer
- Alleviates inflammatory conditions such as multiple sclerosis, eczema, and psoriasis

Theory

Some of the health benefits associated with flaxseed consumption may be due to the presence of compounds known as lignans, which are known to possess various pro- and antiestrogenic properties.

Scientific Support

Studies have shown that large doses (several grams) of flaxseed oil each day can reduce blood clotting by reducing platelet aggregation. Regular flaxseed consumption has also been associated with improvements in the ratio of omega-3 to omega-6 fatty acids in the blood, which may offer protection from atherogenesis and relief from inflammatory conditions. A number of animal studies have shown that flaxseed oil may delay

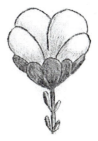

breast cancer progression and protect against colon cancer—sometimes as much as a 50 percent reduction compared to control groups not fed flaxseed. A clear and consistent reduction in proinflammatory markers (tumor necrosis factor and interleukin) has been noted in human subjects supplemented with flaxseed oil.

Safety

Megadoses (more than 100 g) of any type of concentrated oil is likely to induce gastrointestinal distress such as nausea and diarrhea due to a laxative effect. Effective doses of flaxseed or flaxseed oil of 30 to 40 g per day are unlikely to have any adverse side effects. A note of caution is warranted, however, in cases of compromised blood clotting such as hemophilia, due to the tendency of flaxseed to reduce platelet aggregation and prolong bleeding times. A similar cautionary note is advisable for individuals undergoing surgical procedures, which may predispose the patient to excessive bleeding.

Value

Concentrated flaxseed oil is available at health food stores and natural foods markets. Relative to other vegetable oils, it can be quite expensive. A more economical alternative is to use whole flaxseeds (ground or blended), which are often a fraction of the price of the oil, with the added benefits of providing a significant dose of lignans and fiber in addition to the LA and LN essential oils.

Dosage

Beneficial effects have been observed at daily doses of 30 to 40 g (1 to 2 oz) of either concentrated flaxseed oil or whole flaxseeds. Popular uses include salad dressings and spreads for the oil, while the seeds are often used in baked goods or sprinkled on cereal or other foods.

WORKS CONSULTED

Allman MA, Pena MM, Pang D. Supplementation with flaxseed oil versus sunflowerseed oil in healthy young men consuming a low fat diet: Effects on platelet composition and function. Eur J Clin Nutr. 1995 Mar;49(3):169-78.

Beitz J, Mest HJ, Forster W. Influence of linseed oil diet on the pattern of serum phospholipids in man. Acta Biol Med Ger. 1981;40(7-8):K31-5.

Caughey GE, Mantzioris E, Gibson RA, Cleland LG, James MJ. The effect on human tumor necrosis factor alpha and interleukin 1 beta production of diets enriched in n-3 fatty acids from vegetable oil or fish oil. Am J Clin Nutr. 1996 Jan;63(1):116-22.

Goh YK, Jumpsen JA, Ryan EA, Clandinin MT. Effect of omega 3 fatty acid on plasma lipids, cholesterol and lipoprotein fatty acid content in NIDDM patients. Diabetologia. 1997 Jan;40(1):45-52.

Harris WS. n-3 Fatty acids and serum lipoproteins: Human studies. Am J Clin Nutr. 1997 May;65(5 Suppl):1645S-54S.

James MJ, Gibson RA, Cleland LG. Dietary polyunsaturated fatty acids and inflammatory mediator production. Am J Clin Nutr. 2000 Jan;71(1 Suppl):343S-8S.

Kaminskas A, Levaciov M, Lupinovic V, Kuchinskene Z. The effect of linseed oil on the fatty acid composition of blood plasma low- and very low-density lipoproteins and cholesterol in diabetics. Vopr Pitan. 1992 Sep-Dec;(5-6):13-4.

Kelley DS, Nelson GJ, Love JE, Branch LB, Taylor PC, Schmidt PC, Mackey BE, Iacono JM. Dietary alpha-linolenic acid alters tissue fatty acid composition, but not blood lipids, lipoproteins or coagulation status in humans. Lipids. 1993 Jun;28(6):533-7.

Kulakova SN, Gapparova KM, Pogozheva AV, Levachev MM. Evaluation of the effects of fish and vegetable omega-3 PUFA complex on the erythrocyte fatty acid composition in patients with ischemic heart disease and impaired glucose tolerance. Vopr Pitan. 1999;68(5-6):26-9.

Layne KS, Goh YK, Jumpsen JA, Ryan EA, Chow P, Clandinin MT. Normal subjects consuming physiological levels of 18:3(n-3) and 20:5(n-3) from flaxseed or fish oils have characteristic differences in plasma lipid and lipoprotein fatty acid levels. J Nutr. 1996 Sep;126(9):2130-40.

Mantzioris E, James MJ, Gibson RA, Cleland LG. Dietary substitution with an alpha-linolenic acid-rich vegetable oil increases eicosapentaenoic acid concentrations in tissues. Am J Clin Nutr. 1994 Jun;59(6):1304-9.

Mantzioris E, James MJ, Gibson RA, Cleland LG. Differences exist in the relationships between dietary linoleic and alpha-linolenic acids and their respective long-chain metabolites. Am J Clin Nutr. 1995 Feb;61(2):320-4.

McManus RM, Jumpson J, Finegood DT, Clandinin MT, Ryan EA. A comparison of the effects of n-3 fatty acids from linseed oil and fish oil in well-controlled type II diabetes. Diabetes Care. 1996 May;19(5):463-7.

Mest HJ, Beitz J, Heinroth I, Block HU, Forster W. The influence of linseed oil diet on fatty acid pattern in phospholipids and thromboxane formation in platelets in man. Klin Wochenschr. 1983 Feb 15;61(4):187-91.

Morton MS, Wilcox G, Wahlqvist ML, Griffiths K. Determination of lignans and isoflavonoids in human female plasma following dietary supplementation. J Endocrinol. 1994 Aug;142(2):251-9.

Pang D, Allman-Farinelli MA, Wong T, Barnes R, Kingham KM. Replacement of linoleic acid with alpha-linolenic acid does not alter blood lipids in normolipidaemic men. Br J Nutr. 1998 Aug;80(2):163-7.

Sanders TA, Younger KM. The effect of dietary supplements of omega 3 polyunsaturated fatty acids on the fatty acid composition of platelets and plasma choline phosphoglycerides. Br J Nutr. 1981 May;45(3):613-6.

Singer P, Wirth M, Berger I. A possible contribution of decrease in free fatty acids to low serum triglyceride levels after diets supplemented with n-6 and n-3 polyunsaturated fatty acids. Atherosclerosis. 1990 Aug;83(2-3):167-75.

EVENING PRIMROSE OIL

What Is It?

Evening primrose oil (EPO) is made from the seeds of the herb *Oenothera biennis*, which grows wild in arid environments such as sand dunes. True to its name, evening primrose flowers open in the evening and fade in bright sunlight. First documented medicinally in England, evening primrose oil is most commonly used for relieving premenstrual syndrome, fibrocystic breasts, and menopausal symptoms such as hot flashes.

Claims

- Relieves PMS and breast pain associated with the menstrual cycle
- Alleviates hot flashes resulting from menopause
- Reduces risk of heart disease
- Improves eczema and dermatitis
- Improves rheumatoid arthritis
- Aids in weight loss

Theory

Sixty to 80 percent of evening primrose oil is the essential (not produced by the body) fatty acid, linoleic acid. Gamma linoleic acid (GLA) is synthesized by the body from linoleic acid and makes up 8 to 14 percent of the oil. GLA is a precursor of prostaglandin E_1 (PGE_1)—the deficiency of which has been documented in some women with PMS and cyclical breast pain. Since decreased levels of PGE_1 can increase the pain-inducing effects of the hormone prolactin on breast tissue, it is thought that low PGE_1 levels may be a primary cause of many of the symptoms associated with PMS.

In addition to its applications for specific detrimental effects of the menstrual cycle, theories for non–gender-related uses for evening primrose oil are prevalent. PGE_1 has beneficial anti-inflammatory, blood-thinning, and vasodilating properties. Also, since GLA increases PGE_1 levels, supplementation with evening primrose oil could provide benefits in rheumatoid arthritis and coronary artery disease. Because essential fatty acids are claimed to have positive effects on certain skin dis-

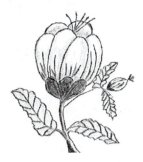

eases, supplementation with evening primrose oil, composed mostly of essential fatty acids, could also alleviate eczema and dermatitis. Finally, people with GLA deficiencies are thought to produce more fat in their bodies—so claims abound for evening primrose oil supplements to promote fat loss.

Scientific Support

Most scientific literature related to evening primrose oil supplementation involves its use for promoting well-being during the menstrual cycle. Among nine studies of the effects of evening primrose oil on PMS, including the symptoms of irritability, depression, bloating, and breast pain, only four were properly controlled. Since PMS symptoms are highly subjective, there is known to be a high incidence of the placebo effect (25 to 80 percent). Thus, placebo control is crucial for a well-controlled, reliable study.

In two controlled studies, subjects received 4 to 6 g of evening primrose oil or placebo for three to four months—but neither trial was able to demonstrate a significant benefit of the supplements. It is worth noting, however, that one other placebo-controlled study *did* show significant benefits of supplementation with evening primrose oil, but only after six months of treatment. In the treatment of cyclic breast pain, evening primrose oil has been found to be more effective than placebo (44 percent versus 19 percent, respectively). When compared to treatment with the prescription drugs bromocriptine and danazol, evening primrose oil was as effective as bromocriptine but less effective than danazol in alleviating breast pain. In one well-controlled study to evaluate the use of evening primrose oil for the relief of hot flashes associated with menopause, fifty-six women were treated for six months with either 4 g of evening primrose oil or placebo. In this study, no significant benefits were attributed to taking evening primrose oil.

Perhaps the most convincing evidence for supplementing with evening primrose oil involves its use in those with coronary artery disease. A study in ten patients with high cholesterol levels showed that 3.6 g of evening primrose oil taken daily for eight weeks significantly decreased LDL ("bad") cholesterol by 9 percent. However, for patients with high triglyceride and cholesterol levels, no such reductions occurred. In a double-blind crossover study in men taking either fish oil alone or fish oil plus evening primrose oil, the combination led to a significant 12 percent decrease in atherogenic markers, whereas fish oil alone led to a nonsignificant 6 percent decrease in the same markers. Finally, evening primrose oil has been demonstrated to decrease platelet aggregation and atherosclerotic plaques in rabbits (one of the most common animal models for coronary artery disease).

There are many other claims for the use of evening primrose oil, although the scientific findings are rather disappointing. In a six-week, double-blind, placebo-controlled study of fifty-eight children who required treatment with topical skin steroids for atopic dermatitis (twenty-two of which also had asthma), no significant difference was found between the placebo and the evening primrose oil group. Likewise, no effect on asthma symptoms was seen. In a twenty-four week, double-blind, placebo-controlled study of thirty-nine patients with chronic hand dermatitis, no therapeutic value was shown following 600 mg of daily GLA supplements (compared to placebo). No scientific evidence is available to support any benefit of evening primrose oil in alleviating rheumatoid arthritis or in aiding weight loss.

Safety

Evening primrose oil appears to be quite safe. Potential adverse effects include gastrointestinal upset and headache. Additionally, seizure has been reported in three subjects taking evening primrose oil, but all were in patients with documented cases of schizophrenia. Because evening primrose oil hinders platelet aggregation, this supplement may increase the anticoagulant effect of drugs such as warfarin. Therefore, anyone taking anticoagulants should consult with his or her personal physician before taking evening primrose oil.

Value

Evening primrose oil concentration varies quite a bit among different brands and delivery forms (capsule or liquid), but a thirty-day supply generally costs around $10 to $20. It appears that evening primrose oil may be a useful alternative to prescription medication for symptoms of PMS, especially breast pain associated with the menstrual cycle. Perhaps the most promising use for evening primrose oil is its cardioprotective effect.

Dosage

The most common dose of evening primrose oil is 1 to 4 g per day with approximately 10 percent GLA.

WORKS CONSULTED

al-Shabanah OA. Effect of evening primrose oil on gastric ulceration and secretion induced by various ulcerogenic and necrotizing agents in rats. Food Chem Toxicol. 1997 Aug;35(8):769-75.

Bordoni A, Biagi PL, Turchetto E, Serroni P, De Jaco AP, Orlandi C. Treatment of premenstrual syndrome with essential fatty acids. G Clin Med. 1987 Jan;68(1):23-8.

Budeiri D, Li Wan Po A, Dornan JC. Is evening primrose oil of value in the treatment of premenstrual syndrome? Control Clin Trials. 1996 Feb;17(1):60-8.

Cerin A, Collins A, Landgren BM, Eneroth P. Hormonal and biochemical profiles of premenstrual syndrome. Treatment with essential fatty acids. Acta Obstet Gynecol Scand. 1993 Jul;72(5):337-43.

Chenoy R, Hussain S, Tayob Y, O'Brien PM, Moss MY, Morse PF. Effect of oral gamolenic acid from evening primrose oil on menopausal flushing. BMJ. 1994 Feb 19;308(6927):501-3.

Cheung KL. Management of cyclical mastalgia in oriental women: Pioneer experience of using gamolenic acid (Efamast) in Asia. Aust N Z J Surg. 1999 Jul;69(7):492-4.

Collins A, Cerin A, Coleman G, Landgren BM. Essential fatty acids in the treatment of premenstrual syndrome. Obstet Gynecol. 1993 Jan;81(1):93-8.

de Vries JE. Painful breasts. Ned Tijdschr Geneeskd. 1998 May 30;142(22):1291.

Dirks J, van Aswegen CH, du Plessis DJ. Cytokine levels affected by gamma-linolenic acid. Prostaglandins Leukot Essent Fatty Acids. 1998 Oct;59(4):273-7.

Dove D, Johnson P. Oral evening primrose oil: Its effect on length of pregnancy and selected intrapartum outcomes in low-risk nulliparous women. J Nurse Midwifery. 1999 May-Jun;44(3):320-4.

Gateley CA, Maddox PR, Pritchard GA, Sheridan W, Harrison BJ, Pye JK, Webster DJ, Hughes LE, Mansel RE. Plasma fatty acid profiles in benign breast disorders. Br J Surg. 1992 May;79(5):407-9.

Gateley CA, Miers M, Mansel RE, Hughes LE. Drug treatments for mastalgia: 17 years experience in the Cardiff Mastalgia Clinic. J R Soc Med. 1992 Jan;85(1):12-5.

Goldfien A. Premenstrual syndrome. Curr Ther Endocrinol Metab. 1994;5:219-22.

Grajeta H, Biernat J. Effect of high-fat cholesterol enriched diets on hypolipemic action of Oenothera paradoxa oil in rats. Part 2. Blood serum and liver fatty acids. Nahrung. 1997 Feb;41(1):50-2.

Haslett C, Douglas JG, Chalmers SR, Weighhill A, Munro JF. A double-blind evaluation of evening primrose oil as an antiobesity agent. Int J Obes. 1983; 7(6):549-53.

Horrobin DF. The role of essential fatty acids and prostaglandins in the premenstrual syndrome. J Reprod Med. 1983 Jul;28(7):465-8.

Horrobin DF. Evening primrose oil and premenstrual syndrome. Med J Aust. 1990 Nov 19;153(10):630-1.

Horrobin DF. The effects of gamma-linolenic acid on breast pain and diabetic neuropathy: Possible non-eicosanoid mechanisms. Prostaglandins Leukot Essent Fatty Acids. 1993 Jan;48(1):101-4.

Horrobin DF, Ells KM, Morse-Fisher N, Manku MS. The effects of evening primrose oil, safflower oil and paraffin on plasma fatty acid levels in humans: Choice of an appropriate placebo for clinical studies on primrose oil. Prostaglandins Leukot Essent Fatty Acids. 1991 Apr;42(4):245-9.

Joe LA, Hart LL. Evening primrose oil in rheumatoid arthritis. Ann Pharmacother. 1993 Dec;27(12):1475-7.

Johnson SR. Premenstrual syndrome therapy. Clin Obstet Gynecol. 1998 Jun; 41(2):405-21.

Khoo SK, Munro C, Battistutta D. Evening primrose oil and treatment of premenstrual syndrome. Med J Aust. 1990 Aug 20;153(4):189-92.

Kleijnen J. Evening primrose oil. BMJ. 1994 Oct 1;309(6958):824-5.

Martens-Lobenhoffer J, Meyer FP. Pharmacokinetic data of gamma-linolenic acid in healthy volunteers after the administration of evening primrose oil (Epogam). Int J Clin Pharmacol Ther. 1998 Jul;36(7):363-6.

McFayden IJ, Forrest AP, Chetty U, Raab G. Cyclical breast pain—some observations and the difficulties in treatment. Br J Clin Pract. 1992 Autumn;46(3):161-4.

Munoz SE, Piegari M, Guzman CA, Eynard AR. Differential effects of dietary Oenothera, Zizyphus mistol, and corn oils, and essential fatty acid deficiency on the progression of a murine mammary gland adenocarcinoma. Nutrition. 1999 Mar;15(3):208-12.

Rahbeeni F, Hendrikse AS, Smuts CM, Gelderblom WC, Abel S, Blekkenhorst GH. The effect of evening primrose oil on the radiation response and blood flow of mouse normal and tumour tissue. Int J Radiat Biol. 2000 Jun;76(6):871-7.

Reilly JD, Hopegood L, Gould L, Devismes L. Effect of a supplementary dietary evening primrose oil mixture on hoof growth, hoof growth rate and hoof lipid fractions in horses: A controlled and blinded trial. Equine Vet J Suppl. 1998 Sep;(26):58-65.

Veale DJ, Torley HI, Richards IM, O'Dowd A, Fitzsimons C, Belch JJ, Sturrock RD. A double-blind placebo controlled trial of Efamol Marine on skin and joint symptoms of psoriatic arthritis. Br J Rheumatol. 1994 Oct;33(10):954-8.

Viikari J, Lehtonen A. Effect of primrose oil on serum lipids and blood pressure in hyperlipidemic subjects. Int J Clin Pharmacol Ther Toxicol. 1986 Dec;24(12):668-70.

Warren G, McKendrick M, Peet M. The role of essential fatty acids in chronic fatigue syndrome. A case-controlled study of red-cell membrane essential fatty acids (EFA) and a placebo-controlled treatment study with high dose of EFA. Acta Neurol Scand. 1999 Feb;99(2):112-6.

Yoshimoto-Furuie K, Yoshimoto K, Tanaka T, Saima S, Kikuchi Y, Shay J, Horrobin DF, Echizen H. Effects of oral supplementation with evening primrose oil for six weeks on plasma essential fatty acids and uremic skin symptoms in hemodialysis patients. Nephron. 1999 Feb;81(2):151-9.

RED CLOVER

What Is It?

Red clover *(Trifolium pratense)* is a member of the legume family—the same class of plants in which we find chickpeas and soybeans. Red clover extracts are used as dietary supplements for their high content of isoflavone compounds, which possess weak estrogenic activity and have been associated with a variety of health benefits during menopause (reduction of hot flashes, promotion of heart health, and maintenance of bone density).

Claims

- Elevates/balances moods
- Improves sleeping patterns
- Reduces hot flashes
- Improves libido
- Supports cardiovascular health
- Promotes maintenance of bone mass

Theory

As a source of plant estrogens, red clover extract can help reduce some of the side effects associated with a decline in estrogen levels in midlife (menopause). Plant estrogens, most commonly found in soy products, are substances present in plants that are able to mimic the effects of estrogens because of similarities in chemical structure. By interacting with estrogen receptors on cellular surfaces, isoflavone compounds are thought to deliver some of the beneficial effects of estrogen (fewer hot flashes, better bone preservation, and cardiovascular health) without the potential adverse estrogen side effects (increased risk of breast and endometrial cancer).

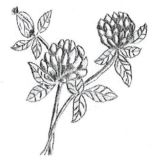

Scientific Support

Red clover supplements standardized to contain 40 mg of isoflavones per tablet (290 mg of the red clover extract) have been examined in several clinical studies.

The unique point of difference between isoflavones derived from red clover and those extracted from soybeans is that red clover extracts contain four different isoflavones (genistein, daidzein, biochanin, formononetin), while soybeans contain only two (genistein and daidzein). No comparative studies have been done to examine whether any differences in effectiveness exist between isoflavones from red clover or soybeans. Studies on soy and red clover isoflavones have shown beneficial effects on reducing menopausal symptoms (hot flashes, night sweats, reduced libido, vaginal dryness), improving cardiovascular risk factors (cholesterol levels, arterial compliance), and maintaining bone density (by reducing bone loss).

Safety

No serious adverse side effects are expected with regular use of red clover extract. Levels of as much as 160 mg per day have been evaluated as safe.

Value

The amount of red clover isoflavones typically recommended (40 mg per day) is equivalent to a glass of soymilk plus 4 cups of chickpeas. Prices are in the $20 to $30 range for a thirty-day supply—not a high price for a product that can deliver some real quality-of-life benefits.

Dosage

Typical dosage recommendations call for 40 mg of isoflavones per day for at least four to six weeks.

WORKS CONSULTED

Cassady JM, Zennie TM, Chae YH, Ferin MA, Portuondo NE, Baird WM. Use of a mammalian cell culture benzo(a)pyrene metabolism assay for the detection of potential anticarcinogens from natural products: Inhibition of metabolism by biochanin A, an isoflavone from Trifolium pratense L. Cancer Res. 1988 Nov 15;48(22):6257-61.

Glencross RG, Festenstein GN, King HG. Separation and determination of isoflavones in the protein concentrate from red clover leaves. J Sci Food Agric. 1972 Mar;23(3):371-6.

Grunert E, Woelke G. Isoflavones in some white and red clover varieties and their oestrogenic effect in juvenile mice. Dtsch Tierarztl Wochenschr. 1967 Sep 1;74(17):431-4.

Howes JB, Sullivan D, Lai N, Nestel P, Pomeroy S, West L, Eden JA, Howes LG. The effects of dietary supplementation with isoflavones from red clover on the lipoprotein profiles of post menopausal women with mild to moderate hyper-cholesterolaemia. Atherosclerosis. 2000 Sep;152(1):143-7.

Kallela K, Heinonen K, Saloniemi H. Plant oestrogens; the cause of decreased fertility in cows. A case report. Nord Vet Med. 1984 Mar-Apr;36(3-4):124-9.

Leont'eva TP, Kazakov AL, Ryzhenkov VE. Effect of the total flavonoids from red clover and chick-pea on the lipid content in the blood and liver of rats. Vopr Med Khim. 1979 Jul-Aug;25(4):444-7.

Lindner HR. Occurrence of anabolic agents in plants and their importance. Environ Qual Saf Suppl. 1976;(5):151-8.

Lundh T. Metabolism of estrogenic isoflavones in domestic animals. Proc Soc Exp Biol Med. 1995 Jan;208(1):33-9.

Nestel PJ, Pomeroy S, Kay S, Komesaroff P, Behrsing J, Cameron JD, West L. Isoflavones from red clover improve systemic arterial compliance but not plasma lipids in menopausal women. J Clin Endocrinol Metab. 1999 Mar;84(3):895-8.

Saloniemi H, Wahala K, Nykanen-Kurki P, Kallela K, Saastamoinen I. Phyto-estrogen content and estrogenic effect of legume fodder. Proc Soc Exp Biol Med. 1995 Jan;208(1):13-7.

Schultz G. Estrogen-effective isoflavones in Trifolium pratense (red clover). Distri-bution in superterranean parts of plants and occurrence as "bound" isoflavones. Dtsch Tierarztl Wochenschr. 1965 Jun 1;72(11):246-51.

van der Schouw YT, de Kleijn MJ, Peeters PH, Grobbee DE. Phyto-oestrogens and cardiovascular disease risk. Nutr Metab Cardiovasc Dis. 2000 Jun;10(3):154-67.

Widyarini S, Spinks N, Reeve VE. Protective effect of isoflavone derivative against photocarcinogenesis in a mouse model. Redox Rep. 2000;5(2-3):156-8.

VITEX/CHASTEBERRY

What Is It?

Vitex agnus-castus is a shrub native to the Mediterranean and Central Asia, but can also be found growing from Maryland to Florida and west to Texas. It bears small, reddish-black fruits that look, smell, and taste like black peppercorns. Vitex has been used since the fourth century B.C., when Hippocrates suggested it for expelling the placenta after birth, among other uses. Because at one point vitex was thought to cause a loss of libido, it earned the nickname "chaste tree." More recently, vitex has been used for everything from increasing lactation to "purifying" the brain and the liver. Today, vitex is generally marketed for symptoms associated with the menstrual cycle and with female hormonal imbalances.

Claims

- Alleviates premenstrual syndrome (PMS)
- Stabilizes menstrual abnormalities
- Eases menopausal symptoms
- Helps restore fertility in women
- Serves as an acne treatment

Theory

The main active compounds in vitex are found in its ripe dried fruit, and its main constituents are the flavonoids, which include casticin (the predominant flavonoid), isovitexin, and orientin. Vitex also contains terpenes and plant steroids, although it is not clear how these compounds act to perform the effects for which vitex is known. Because vitex appears to effect changes in key hormones that regulate the menstrual cycle, it is thought that taking vitex can help normalize the ratio of hormones required for menstrual function and fertility. Normal hormonal balance is also essential for fertility, so vitex is sometimes recommended after discontinuing use of birth control pills to restore normal ovulation. It is theorized that vitex helps to restore normal hormone pulsatility during the luteal phase of the menstrual cycle and may help

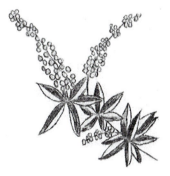

alleviate PMS symptoms. Before you guys run out and buy vitex for your girlfriend, wife, sister, mother, or daughter, however, keep in mind that the mechanism behind PMS is still not understood and that the causes of PMS may differ from one woman to the next.

Scientific Support

Several studies have evaluated the claims for using vitex. In a well-controlled study of fifty-two women with hyperprolactinemia (too much prolactin), 20 mg per day of vitex for three months normalized most menstrual hormone levels and caused a significant reduction in PMS symptoms. In an open study (no controls), eighteen infertile women with abnormal progesterone levels were given vitex for three months. Progesterone levels were restored to normal in eleven women, and two women became pregnant by the end of the study. Because of results such as this, vitex is often used as an initial fertility treatment if other causes of sterility have been ruled out.

In a well-controlled study to evaluate the effect of vitex on premenstrual tension syndrome (PMTS), 105 women were given either 4 mg of vitex or 100 mg of pyridoxine (vitamin B_6). After three months of treatment, vitex was considered 77 percent effective, while pyridoxine was considered 61 percent effective.

In addition to its uses for fertility and menstrual symptoms, vitex has been used as a treatment for acne. In a study of 118 subjects treated with vitex, the treatment group was found to heal more quickly than subjects who received conventional acne therapy.

Safety

Side effects of taking vitex include headache, nausea, gastrointestinal and abdominal discomfort, and a reversible skin rash. No serious adverse effects have been documented as a result of taking vitex. Because the mechanism by which this supplement works is not entirely clear, it is very important to consult a physician before taking vitex if you have any medical condition, are taking any medication, or are pregnant or lactating.

Value

Vitex is not only considered a safe supplement, it is also relatively inexpensive. A variety of studies support its usefulness, and a month's supply costs as little as $5.

Dosage

No established dosage is documented for Vitex, but most capsules, tablets, and liquids contain 150 to 500 mg per dose, with one morning dose recommended per day. Clinical studies have demonstrated efficacy with as little as 4 mg per day.

WORKS CONSULTED

Amann W. Premenstrual water retention. Favorable effect of Agnus castus (Agnolyt) on premenstrual water retention. ZFA (Stuttgart). 1979 Jan 10;55(1):48-51.

Amann W. Amenorrhea. Favorable effect of Agnus castus (Agnolyt) on amenorrhea. ZFA (Stuttgart). 1982 Feb 10;58(4):228-31.

Burdina LM. Benign breast diseases: Diagnosis and treatment. Ter Arkh. 1998; 70(10):37-41.

Dixon-Shanies D, Shaikh N. Growth inhibition of human breast cancer cells by herbs and phytoestrogens. Oncol Rep. 1999 Nov-Dec;6(6):1383-7.

Fikentscher H. Aetiology, diagnosis and therapy of mastopathy and mastodynia. Experiences of treatment with mastodynon. Med Klin. 1977 Aug 26;72(34):1327-30.

Gerhard I, Patek A, Monga B, Blank A, Gorkow C. Mastodynon(R) bei weiblicher Sterilitat. Forsch Komplementarmed. 1998;5(6):272-8.

Halaska M, Raus K, Beles P, Martan A, Paithner KG. Treatment of cyclical mastodynia using an extract of Vitex agnus castus: Results of a double-blind comparison with a placebo. Ceska Gynekol. 1998 Oct;63(5):388-92.

Hernandez MM, Heraso C, Villarreal ML, Vargas-Arispuro I, Aranda E. Biological activities of crude plant extracts from Vitex trifolia L. (Verbenaceae). J Ethnopharmacol. 1999 Oct;67(1):37-44.

Hillebrand H. The treatment of premenstrual aphthous ulcerative stomatitis with Agnolyt. Z Allgemeinmed. 1964 Dec 31;40(36):1577.

Hirobe C, Qiao ZS, Takeya K, Itokawa H. Cytotoxic flavonoids from Vitex agnuscastus. Phytochemistry. 1997 Oct;46(3):521-4.

Kubista E, Muller G, Spona J. Conservative therapy of mastopathy. Zentralbl Gynakol. 1983;105(18):1153-62.

Kubista E, Muller G, Spona J. Treatment of mastopathy with cyclic mastodynia: Clinical results and hormone profile. Gynakol Rundsch. 1986;26(2):65-79.

Kubista E, Muller G, Spona J. Treatment of mastopathies with cyclic mastodynia. Clinical results and hormonal profiles. Rev Fr Gynecol Obstet. 1987 Apr;82(4):221-7.

Loch EG, Selle H, Boblitz N. Treatment of premenstrual syndrome with a phytopharmaceutical formulation containing Vitex agnus castus. J Women's Health Gend Based Med. 2000 Apr;9(3):315-20.

Madjar H, Vetter M, Prompeler H, Breckwoldt M, Pfleiderer A. Doppler measurement of breast vascularity in women under pharmacologic treatment of benign breast disease. J Reprod Med. 1993 Dec;38(12):935-40.

Milewicz A, Gejdel E, Sworen H, Sienkiewicz K, Jedrzejak J, Teucher T, Schmitz H. Vitex agnus castus extract in the treatment of luteal phase defects due to latent hyperprolactinemia. Results of a randomized placebo-controlled double-blind study. Arzneimittelforschung. 1993 Jul;43(7):752-6.

Opitz G, Liebl A. Conservative treatment of mastopathy with Mastodynon. Ther Ggw. 1980 Jul;119(7):804-9.

Roeder D. Treatment of mastodynia and mastopathy using Mastodynon. Med Welt. 1976 Mar 19;27(12):591-2.

Roeder D. Experiences with mastodynon in the treatment of the premenstrual syndrome. Fortschr Med. 1977 May 5;95(17):1175-8.

Schwalbe E. Treatment of mastodynia. ZFA (Stuttgart). 1979 Aug 10;55(22):1239-42.

Sliutz G, Speiser P, Schultz AM, Spona J, Zeillinger R. Agnus castus extracts inhibit prolactin secretion of rat pituitary cells. Horm Metab Res. 1993 May; 25(5):253-5.

Tschudin S, Huber R. Treatment of cyclical mastalgia with a solution containing a Vitex agnus castus extract: Results of a placebo-controlled double-blind study. Breast 1999;8:175-81. Forsch Komplementarmed Klass Naturheilkd. 2000 Jun; 7(3):162-4.

UVA URSI/BEARBERRY

What Is It?

Uva ursi *(Arctostaphylos uva-ursi)* is a woody plant also known as bearberry. It may also be referred to scientifically as *Arbutus uva-ursi*. The first mention of its use in European medicine dates from the thirteenth century. Currently, German extracts of uva ursi leaves are licensed for use in medicinal teas to treat mild urinary tract infections. The leaves, but not the berries, contain at least seven active ingredients including arbutin, which has antibacterial activity. Uva ursi is used in herbal medicinal teas to help prevent and treat urinary tract infections. It may also act as a mild diuretic and can be found in diet teas.

Claims

- Urinary antiseptic (antibacterial effect in the urine)
- Diuretic (increases urine output)
- Treatment of cystitis (inflammation of the bladder, typically following a urinary tract infection)
- Treatment of pyelonephritis (inflammation of the kidney)
- Used for mild urinary tract infections

Theory

Bearberry leaves (uva ursi) contain compounds that have antibacterial and diuretic properties. These compounds are absorbed via the gastrointestinal tract, transported to the kidneys via the blood, and excreted from the body via the urine. When the urine is alkaline (pH 8), the compounds in uva ursi can perform antibacterial functions. It is theorized that these compounds also act as mild diuretics and result in an increase in urine output.

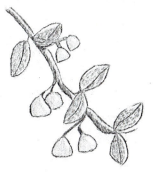

Scientific Support

The active ingredient in bearberry extract is considered to be arbutin. Arbutin is split into glucose (a sugar) and hydroquinone. Hydroquinone combines with glucuronic acid, and this compound is excreted in the urine. If the urine is alkaline (pH 8), hydroquinone is unbound and released in the urinary tract where it exhibits a bacteria-killing effect. If the urine is not alkaline, hydroquinone remains bound and is inactive. Although arbutin and its metabolite hydroquinone are considered the most important active ingredients, there are other compounds extracted from bearberry leaves that are thought to have antibacterial properties. The peak antibacterial action takes place within three to four hours of ingestion.

No scientific studies in humans have examined the effectiveness of uva ursi in curing urinary tract infections. Some studies have been conducted in laboratory rats. A long history of use speaks to its safety, and many individuals claim effectiveness—but that is not the same as having scientific studies that document its safety and effectiveness.

Controversy surrounds the claim that uva ursi is a mild diuretic. Several sources question whether uva ursi has any diuretic effect at all, while other sources suggest a mild diuretic effect of nonarbutin fractions of bearberry leaf extracts.

Safety

Uva ursi is not recommended during pregnancy or lactation or if you have kidney disease. Except for those conditions, uva ursi is thought to be safe, although it may irritate the stomach due to its high tannin content. Treatment should not continue for more than seven days.

Value

The addition of uva ursi to a diet tea (a common modern use) appears to have little or no value. At best, it may contribute a small diuretic effect. Even so, losing body water is generally not the goal of those seeking weight loss. There is no evidence, scientific or anecdotal, that uva ursi helps reduce body fat.

Perhaps the best use of uva ursi is for self-treatment of a urinary tract infection with a seven-day course of a medicinal tea or dietary supplement containing the leaf extract. Some nutritionally oriented physicians will treat mild urinary tract infections with uva ursi first, followed by prescription antibiotics if the infection persists.

Dosage

Medicinal teas can be made by steeping 3 g of dried leaf in 150 ml (5 fluid oz) of boiling water for up to 15 minutes (repeat up to four times per day for as long as one week). Dietary supplements are generally standardized for total arbutin content, which should approximate 400 to 700 mg per dose to be taken two to four times daily.

WORKS CONSULTED

Beaux D, Fleurentin J, Mortier F. Effect of extracts of Orthosiphon stamineus Benth, Hieracium pilosella L., Sambucus nigra L. and Arctostaphylos uva-ursi (L.) Spreng. in rats. Phytother Res. 1999 May;13(3):222-5.

Bradley PR, ed. Uva ursi. British Herbal Compendium, Vol.1. Dorset, England: British Herbal Medicine Association; 1992;211-3.

Brinker, FJ. Arctostaphylos Spp. Eclectic Dispensatory of Botanical Therapeutics, Vol. 2. Sandy, OR: Eclectic Medical Publications; 1995;19-23.

Dombrowicz E, Zadernowski R, Swiatek L. Phenolic acids in leaves of Arctostaphylos uva ursi L., Vaccinium vitis idaea L. and Vaccinium myrtillus L. Pharmazie. 1991 Sep;46(9):680-1.

Duke JA. Arctostaphylos uva-ursi (L.) Spreng. (Ericaceae)—bearberry. CRC Handbook of Medicinal Herbs. Boca Raton, FL: CRC Press, Inc.;1985;55-6.

Floresne Vari H, Verzarne Petri G, Kutasi M. Microbiological testing of uva ursi species. Acta Pharm Hung. 1984 Jul;54(4):170-5.

Foster S, Tyler, VE. Uva ursi. Tyler's Honest Herbal: A Sensible Guide to the Use of Herbs and Related Remedies. Binghamton, NY: Haworth; 1999;375-6.

Frohne D. The urinary disinfectant effect of extract from leaves uva ursi. Planta Med. 1970 Jan;18(1):1-25.

Grases F, Melero G, Costa-Bauza A, Prieto R, March JG. Urolithiasis and phytotherapy. Int Urol Nephrol. 1994;26(5):507-11.

Grieve, M. Bearberry. A Modern Herbal. New York: Dover Publications; 1931;89-90.

Jahodar L, Jilek P, Paktova M, Dvorakova V. Antimicrobial effect of arbutin and an extract of the leaves of Arctostaphylos uva-ursi in vitro. Cesk Farm. 1985 Jun;34(5):174-8.

Jahodar L, Leifertova I, Lisa M. Investigation of iridoid substances in Arctostaphylos uva-ursi. Pharmazie. 1978 Aug;33(8):536-7.

Leifertova I, Kudrnacova I, Prokes J, Melicharova E. Evaluation of phenolic substances in Arctostaphylos uva ursi L. III. Hydroquinone determination in leaves during the vegetation period. Cesk Farm. 1975 Jun;24(4-5):197-200.

Matsuda H, Nakamura S, Tanaka T, Kubo M. Pharmacological studies on leaf of Arctostaphylos uva-ursi (L.) Spreng. V. Effect of water extract from Arctostaphylos uva-ursi (L.) Spreng. (bearberry leaf) on the antiallergic and antiinflammatory activities of dexamethasone ointment. Yakugaku Zasshi. 1992 Sep;112(9):673-7.

Matsuo K, Kobayashi M, Takuno Y, Kuwajima H, Ito H, Yoshida T. Antityrosinase activity constituents of Arctostaphylos uva-ursi. Yakugaku Zasshi. 1997 Dec;117(12):1028-32.

Mykytyn MS, Demianchuk A. Inhibiting effect of the aqueous extract of Arctostaphylos uva-ursi on myrosinase activity from Brassica napus seeds. WMJ. 1998 Jul-Aug;70(4):122-6.

Shipochliev T. Uterotonic action of extracts from a group of medicinal plants. Vet Med Nauki. 1981;18(4):94-8.

Swanston-Flatt SK, Day C, Bailey CJ, Flatt PR. Evaluation of traditional plant treatments for diabetes: Studies in streptozotocin diabetic mice. Acta Diabetol Lat. 1989 Jan-Mar;26(1):51-5.

Wahner C, Schonert J, Friedrich H. Knowledge of the tannin contained in leaves of the bearberry (Arctostaphylos uva-ursi L). Pharmazie. 1974 Sep;29(9):616-7.

Weiss RF. Cystitis and pyelonephritis. Herbal Medicine. Portland, OR: Medicina biologica. 1991;244-5.

HORSE CHESTNUT

What Is It?

You've probably seen horse chestnut trees at your local park or lining streets in your town. The trees were once found only in Asia but are now widely distributed across most parts of the world. In dietary supplements, extracts of the seeds of the chestnut are also known as *Aesculus hippocastanum*, escin, or aescin and sometimes by the German name, Rosskastanie. Horse chestnut seeds have been used traditionally to treat both hemorrhoids and varicose veins. It seems that horse chestnut extracts may strengthen the veins to prevent leakage of fluid out of the vessels and into the tissue space, which leads to edema (swelling).

Claims

- Reduces swelling in the legs
- Prevents/treats varicose veins
- Strengthens veins
- Treatment for minor injuries (sprains/strains)

Theory

Veins that are either weak or under chronic stress (or both) are more likely to fail and are therefore more likely to allow leakage of fluid from the vessels into the tissue space, leading to swelling. Fluid accumulation is more common in the legs and far more likely in individuals who stand for extended periods of time. Prolonged standing and obesity can increase pressure within leg veins, causing weak veins to swell, leak, and deteriorate into varicose veins. The active compound in horse chestnut, aescin, performs an antioxidant function and has a general vasoprotective role by protecting collagen and elastin (the two chief proteins that form the structure of veins). By protecting these key vessel proteins, veins and capillaries are able to stay strong and maintain their structural integrity when exposed to stress.

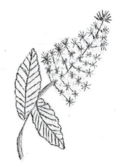

Scientific Support

The first-line therapy for varicose veins is often the use of compression stockings as an external mechanical aid to combat swelling and venous insufficiency. The problem, however, is that most people either forget or refuse to wear them—and even when they are used, they only seem to slow down progression of varicose veins without either stopping or repairing vessel damage. When compression therapy fails, surgery to remove damaged veins is necessary.

Faced with these undesirable options, an effective dietary supplement, in the form of horse chestnut seed, is a welcome remedy. The aescin in horse chestnut can provide vasoprotection through its role as an antioxidant and an inhibitor of enzymes such as collagenase and elastase (which can break down venous structures). Aescin also seems to function as an anti-inflammatory, which can help reduce swelling and fluid accumulation.

At least a dozen clinical studies have been conducted on the effects of horse chestnut seed extract on various measures of venous insufficiency. Overall, these studies show a reduction in lower-leg volume and leg circumference at the calf and ankle, indicating that swelling and fluid accumulation can be controlled with the supplement. Improved integrity of veins and capillaries is accompanied by a reduction in fluid leakage (by about 20 percent) and is roughly equivalent to the effectiveness of compression therapy. In addition, common symptoms that accompany lower-leg swelling, such as leg pain, heaviness, and fatigue, are typically reduced in individuals taking horse chestnut seed extract.

Safety

When used as directed—as a dietary supplement to relieve lower-leg swelling and fluid accumulation—horse chestnut appears to be safe and effective in reducing symptoms. In rare cases, large doses of aescin may be associated with kidney or liver damage, so individuals with diseases of these organs should avoid horse chestnut (as should pregnant or lactating women).

Value

Because approximately half of middle-aged Americans suffer from varicose veins, horse chestnut seed could provide benefits to millions of people. Individuals who could benefit most are those at highest risk for developing varicose veins, which includes women (especially after pregnancy), people who are overweight, and older individuals.

Dosage

Doses of horse chestnut providing 50 to 200 mg of aescin per day for two weeks have been shown to deliver beneficial effects in cases of venous insufficiency (lower-leg swelling, fluid accumulation, leg pain, and heaviness). Smaller maintenance doses of 25 to 100 mg per day may be effective once symptoms improve. It is recommended to select a horse chestnut supplement that has been standardized for 15 to 20 percent aescin content.

WORKS CONSULTED

Antoniuk VO. Isolation of lectin from horse chestnut (Aesculus hippocastanum L.) seeds and study of its interaction with carbohydrates and glycoproteins. WMJ. 1992 Sep-Oct;64(5):47-52.

Balansard P, Joanny P, Bouyard P. Comparison of the vein tonus effect of dried horse chestnut extract and a combination of essential phospholipids and dried horse chestnut extract. Therapie. 1975 Nov-Dec;30(6):907-17.

Beck M. Horse chestnut seed extract. Lancet. 1990 Jun 16;335(8703):1467.

Berti F, Omini C, Longiave D. The mode of action of aescin and the release of prostaglandins. Prostaglandins. 1977 Aug;14(2):241-9.

Bielanski TE, Piotrowski ZH. Horse-chestnut seed extract for chronic venous insufficiency. J Fam Pract. 1999 Mar;48(3):171-2.

Bisler H, Pfeifer R, Kluken N, Pauschinger P. Effects of horse-chestnut seed extract on transcapillary filtration in chronic venous insufficiency. Dtsch Med Wochenschr. 1986 Aug 29;111(35):1321-9.

Bogs U, Bremer D. Horse chestnut seeds and their prepared extracts. Pharmazie. 1971 Jul;26(7):410-8.

Diehm C, Trampisch HJ, Lange S, Schmidt C. Comparison of leg compression stocking and oral horse-chestnut seed extract therapy in patients with chronic venous insufficiency. Lancet. 1996 Feb 3;347(8997):292-4.

Diehm C, Vollbrecht D, Amendt K, Comberg HU. Medical edema protection—clinical benefit in patients with chronic deep vein incompetence. A placebo controlled double blind study. Vasa. 1992;21(2):188-92.

Dworschak E, Antal M, Biro L, Regoly-Merei A, Nagy K, Szepvolgyi J, Gaal O, Biro G. Medical activities of Aesculus hippocastaneum (horse-chestnut) saponins. Adv Exp Med Biol. 1996;404:471-4.

Greeske K, Pohlmann BK. Horse chestnut seed extract—an effective therapy principle in general practice. Drug therapy of chronic venous insufficiency. Fortschr Med. 1996 May 30;114(15):196-200.

Guillaume M, Padioleau F. Veinotonic effect, vascular protection, antiinflammatory and free radical scavenging properties of horse chestnut extract. Arzneimittelforschung. 1994 Jan;44(1):25-35.

Horacek J. Experience with horse chestnut containing medium in the treatment of varicose leg ulcers. Z Haut Geschlechtskr. 1969 Sep 15;44(18):743-6.

Li Y, Matsuda H, Wen S, Yamahara J, Yoshikawa M. Structure-related enhancing activity of escins Ia, Ib, IIa and IIb on magnesium absorption in mice. Bioorg Med Chem Lett. 1999 Sep 6;9(17):2473-8.

Lochs H, Baumgartner H, Konzett H. Effect of horse chestnut extracts on venous tone. Arzneimittelforschung. 1974 Sep;24(9):1347-50.

Matsuda H, Li Y, Murakami T, Ninomiya K, Yamahara J, Yoshikawa M. Effects of escins Ia, Ib, IIa, and IIb from horse chestnut, the seeds of Aesculus hippocastanum L., on acute inflammation in animals. Biol Pharm Bull. 1997 Oct;20(10):1092-5.

Nehring U. On the demonstration of efficacy of horse chestnut extract on venous tonus following its oral administration. Med Welt. 1966 Aug 6;32:1662-5.

Neiss A, Bohm C. Demonstration of the effectiveness of the horse-chestnut-seed extract in the varicose syndrome complex. MMW Munch Med Wochenschr. 1976 Feb 13;118(7):213-6.

Nill HJ, Fischer H. Comparative investigations concerning the effect of extract of horse chestnut upon the pressure-volume-diagramm of patients with venous disorders. Arztl Forsch. 1970 May 10;24(5):141-3.

Obolentseva GV, Khadzhai II. On the effect of aescin and flavonoid complex from horse chestnut on inflammatory edema. Farmakol Toksikol. 1969 Mar-Apr;32(2):174-7.

Pittler MH, Ernst E. Horse-chestnut seed extract for chronic venous insufficiency. A criteria-based systematic review. Arch Dermatol. 1998 Nov;134(11):1356-60.

Rehn D, Unkauf M, Klein P, Jost V, Lucker PW. Comparative clinical efficacy and tolerability of oxerutins and horse chestnut extract in patients with chronic venous insufficiency. Arzneimittelforschung. 1996 May;46(5):483-7.

Rotblatt MD. Cranberry, feverfew, horse chestnut, and kava. West J Med. 1999 Sep;171(3):195-8.

Rothkopf M, Vogel G. New findings on the efficacy and mode of action of the horse chestnut saponin escin. Arzneimittelforschung. 1976 Feb;26(2):225-35.

Schrader E, Schwankl W, Sieder C, Christoffel V. Comparison of the bioavailability of beta-aescin after single oral administration of two different drug formulations containing an extract of horse-chestnut seeds. Pharmazie. 1995 Sep;50(9):623-7.

Schrodter A, Loew D, Schwankl W, Rietbrock N. The validity of radioimmunologic determination of bioavailability of beta-escin in horse chestnut extracts. Arzneimittelforschung. 1998 Sep;48(9):905-10.

Senatore F, Mscisz A, Mrugasiewicz K, Gorecki P. Steroidal constituents and anti-inflammatory activity of the horse chestnut (Aesculus hippocastanum L.) bark. Boll Soc Ital Biol Sper. 1989 Feb;65(2):137-41.

Simini B. Horse-chestnut seed extract for chronic venous insufficiency. Lancet. 1996 Apr 27;347(9009):1182-3.

Steiner M. Conservative therapy of chronic venous insufficiency. The extent of the edema-preventive effect of horse chestnut seed extract. Vasa Suppl. 1991;33:217.

Vayssairat M, Debure C, Maurel A, Gaitz JP. Horse-chestnut seed extract for chronic venous insufficiency. Lancet. 1996 Apr 27;347(9009):1182; discussion 1183.

Vogel G, Marek ML, Oertner R. Studies on the mechanism of the therapeutic and toxic action of the horse chestnut saponin aescin. Arzneimittelforschung. 1970 May;20(5):699-703.

Yoshikawa M, Murakami T, Matsuda H, Yamahara J, Murakami N, Kitagawa I. Bioactive saponins and glycosides. III. Horse chestnut. (1): The structures, inhibitory effects on ethanol absorption, and hypoglycemic activity of escins Ia, Ib, IIa, IIb, and IIIa from the seeds of Aesculus hippocastanum L. Chem Pharm Bull (Tokyo). 1996 Aug;44(8):1454-64.

Yoshikawa M, Murakami T, Otuki K, Yamahara J, Matsuda H. Bioactive saponins and glycosides. XIII. Horse chestnut. (3): Quantitative analysis of escins Ia, Ib, IIa, and IIb by means of high performance liquid chromatography. Yakugaku Zasshi. 1999 Jan;119(1):81-7.

Yoshikawa M, Murakami T, Yamahara J, Matsuda H. Bioactive saponins and glycosides. XII. Horse chestnut. (2): Structures of escins IIIb, IV, V, and VI and isoescins Ia, Ib, and V, acylated polyhydroxyoleanene triterpene oligoglycosides, from the seeds of horse chestnut tree (Aesculus hippocastanum L., Hippocastanaceae). Chem Pharm Bull (Tokyo). 1998 Nov;46(11):1764-9.

CRANBERRY

What Is It?

Cranberry *(Vaccinium macrocarpon)* consumption was first documented in North America in 1621 (at the Pilgrim Thanksgiving dinner). In the mid-1800s, German chemists discovered that the urine of those who ate cranberries contained a bacteriostatic (antibacterial) compound. Today, cranberry juice is a common home remedy used to prevent bacterial urinary tract infections (UTI).

Claims

- Maintains a healthy urinary tract
- Prevents/treats urinary tract infections

Theory

The most likely mechanism of action for cranberry is its ability to inhibit bacterial adhesion to the urinary tract lining (*Escherichia coli* is the most common culprit in causing UTIs). Cranberries contain several organic acids and fatty acids that prevent bacteria from adhering to urinary tract cells. Cranberry ingestion also lowers the pH of urine, thereby making conditions for bacterial growth less favorable. In addition, another constituent of cranberry, parasorbic acid, has been found to give plants some protection from fungal attack.

Scientific Support

Studies conducted to test the therapeutic utility of supplementing with cranberry have been quite favorable. In one controlled study, 153 elderly women were given a daily dose of either 300 ml (about 9 oz) of low-calorie cranberry juice or placebo for six months. Not only did in vitro (test-tube) tests show that the juice prevented adhesion of *E. coli* to urinary tract cells, only 15 percent of urine samples from supplemented subjects contained *E. coli*, while over 28 percent of urine samples from placebo subjects showed the pres-

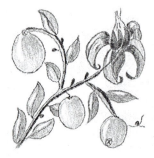

ence of the bacteria. In a study of sexually active women with UTI symptoms, antibiotic therapy for ten days along with 400 mg of cranberry was significantly better than antibiotic therapy alone. Other scientific studies have demonstrated similar findings—cranberry supplementation prevents and limits the severity of UTI. In elderly subjects, cranberry has also been found to decrease urine odor, and to reduce the incidence of constipation and incontinence.

Safety

Cranberry is an incredibly safe supplement, as there are no documented side effects resulting from its use. With very large quantities, however (three to four liters per day), cranberry juice can cause diarrhea and other gastrointestinal symptoms, but very few people would ever attempt to drink this much. For those prone to kidney stones, it is important to note that cranberries contain oxalates, the compounds that form the stones. However, limiting intake to one liter of cranberry juice per day minimizes the risk of forming stones. No contraindications have been reported for pregnant or lactating women.

Value

Cranberry is available in a wide variety of forms (berries, juice, etc.) and can generally be purchased in standardized dietary supplement forms for $10 to $20 for a one-month supply. As a supplement for preventing and treating urinary tract infections and promoting the antibacterial effects of antibiotics, cranberry represents a great value.

Dosage

As a treatment for UTIs, 12 to 32 oz of cranberry juice is recommended. Capsules are also marketed in cranberry extract and in powder form, and these should be standardized to at least 30 percent total organic acid content. Typical daily doses of cranberry for UTI prevention:

- 100 to 500 mg of a standardized cranberry extract (30 percent organic acids)
- ½ cup of fresh cranberries or ¼ cup of dried cranberries
- 3 oz of a 30 percent pure cranberry juice cocktail (taken four times per day)

WORKS CONSULTED

Fleet JC. New support for a folk remedy: Cranberry juice reduces bacteriuria and pyuria in elderly women. Nutr Rev. 1994 May;52(5):168-70.

Jackson B, Hicks LE. Effect of cranberry juice on urinary pH in older adults. Home Health Nurse. 1997 Mar;15(3):198-202.

Kerr KG. Cranberry juice and prevention of recurrent urinary tract infection. Lancet. 1999 Feb 20;353(9153):673.

Kolmos HJ. Cranberry juice: An effective agent against urinary tract infection. Ugeskr Laeger. 1995 Feb 6;157(6):753-4.

Kuzminski LN. Cranberry juice and urinary tract infections: Is there a beneficial relationship? Nutr Rev. 1996 Nov;54(11 Pt 2):S87-90.

Nazarko L. Infection control. The therapeutic uses of cranberry juice. Nurs Stand. 1995 May 17-23;9(34):33-5.

Reid G. Potential preventive strategies and therapies in urinary tract infection. World J Urol. 1999 Dec;17(6):359-63.

Schlager TA, Anderson S, Trudell J, Hendley JO. Effect of cranberry juice on bacteriuria in children with neurogenic bladder receiving intermittent catheterization. J Pediatr. 1999 Dec;135(6):698-702.

Walker EB, Barney DP, Mickelsen JN, Walton RJ, Mickelsen RA Jr. Cranberry concentrate: UTI prophylaxis. J Fam Pract. 1997 Aug;45(2):167-8.

Wilson T, Porcari JP, Harbin D. Cranberry extract inhibits low density lipoprotein oxidation. Life Sci. 1998;62(24):PL381-6.

GOTU KOLA

What Is It?

Gotu kola *(Centella asiatica)* is a vinelike plant native to India and Southeast Asia. In India and Indonesia, gotu kola has a long history of use to promote wound healing and treat skin diseases. In Europe, extracts of *Centella asiatica* are used as drugs for the treatment of wound healing defects. Gotu kola should not be confused with kola nut, which is completely unrelated and is often used in dietary supplements as a natural source of caffeine.

Claims

- Helps prevent varicose veins and hemorrhoids
- Helps heal scars/burns/wounds
- Reduces skin inflammation and skin wrinkles (smoother skin)
- Cellulite reduction
- Increases energy levels
- Improves memory and circulation
- Reduces anxiety and promotes restful sleep

Theory

Gotu kola contains a blend of compounds including at least three triterpenes (asiatic acid, madecassic acid, and asiaticoside) that appear to have antioxidant benefits and an ability to stimulate collagen synthesis for tissue regeneration.

Scientific Support

Perhaps the best feature of gotu kola is its ability to improve symptoms of varicose veins, particularly overall discomfort, tiredness, and swelling. In human studies, gotu kola extract (30 to 180 mg per day for four weeks) leads to improvements in various measurements of vein function (foot swelling, ankle edema, and fluid leakage from the veins) compared to placebo. Gotu kola appears to have a generally beneficial effect on connective tissues,

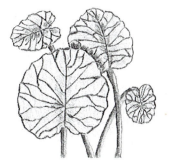

where it may improve the structure and function of the connective tissue in the body, keeping veins stronger and also possibly reducing the symptoms of other connective-tissue diseases. In one animal study, asiatic acid and asiaticoside were the most active of the three triterpenes, but all three were effective in stimulating collagen synthesis and glycosaminoglycan synthesis. Radiation injury to the skin of laboratory rats can be reduced by treatment with madecassol (one of the triterpene compounds in gotu kola)—suggesting a skin regeneration and anti-inflammatory activity.

The activity of asiaticoside has been studied in normal as well as delayed wound healing. In one animal study, topical applications of asiaticoside (0.2 percent solution) produced a 56 percent increase in hydroxyproline, a 57 percent increase in tensile strength, and elevated collagen content. In streptozotocin diabetic rats, where healing is delayed, topical application of 0.4 percent solution of asiaticoside over wounds increased tissue hydroxyproline and collagen content and tensile strength, which facilitated healing. In each of these studies, asiaticoside was also shown to be active by the oral route (at 1 mg/kg dose), suggesting that gotu kola may work by stimulating synthesis of collagen and increasing connective tissue strength.

Other studies have indicated an antioxidant effect of asiaticoside. When applied topically (0.2 percent solution) twice daily for seven days to skin wounds in rats, results showed an increase in both enzymatic and nonenzymatic antioxidants, such as superoxide dismutase (35 percent), catalase (67 percent), glutathione peroxidase (49 percent), vitamin E (77 percent), and ascorbic acid (36 percent) in newly formed tissues. It also resulted in a severalfold *decrease* in free radical damage and lipid peroxide levels (69 percent). This enhancement of antioxidant levels at the initial stage of healing may be an important contributing factor in the healing properties of gotu kola.

There is no credible evidence supporting the claims of gotu kola to benefit energy levels, memory enhancement, cellulite reduction, or restful sleep, but at least two reports indicate a mild antianxiety activity of gotu kola.

Safety

Orally, gotu kola appears to be nontoxic, and it seldom causes any side effects other than the occasional allergic skin rash. There are some concerns that gotu kola may be carcinogenic if applied topically to the skin—although this has not appeared as a major concern in animal models of wound healing. There is some anecdotal evidence that gotu kola use may result in elevated blood sugar levels, which could be of concern to individuals with diabetes.

Value

The primary benefits of gotu kola appear to be an enhancement of wound healing and an improvement in overall vein function (especially for varicose veins and hemorrhoids). Selling for anywhere between $15 and $30 for a one-month supply, gotu kola represents a good value for people who suffer from varicose veins or swollen ankles as well as for anybody recovering from a connective tissue injury such as a muscle or tendon strain, ligament sprain, or skin abrasion.

Dosage

Typical dosage recommendations are in the range of 60 to 180 mg per day, usually consumed in divided doses of 20 to 60 mg three times daily for at least four weeks. It is important to look for an extract standardized to contain triterpene compounds—typically 30 to 40 percent and including asiaticoside, asiatic acid, madecassic acid, and madecassoside (these compounds typically occur at only 1 to 4 percent in the whole herb).

WORKS CONSULTED

Belcaro GV, Grimaldi R, Guidi G. Improvement of capillary permeability in patients with venous hypertension after treatment with TTFCA. Angiology. 1990 Jul;41(7):533-40.

Cesarone MR, Laurora G, De Sanctis MT, Incandela L, Grimaldi R, Marelli C, Belcaro G. The microcirculatory activity of Centella asiatica in venous insufficiency. A double-blind study. Minerva Cardioangiol. 1994 Jun;42(6):299-304.

Chen YJ, Dai YS, Chen BF, Chang A, Chen HC, Lin YC, Chang KH, Lai YL, Chung CH, Lai YJ. The effect of tetrandrine and extracts of Centella asiatica on acute radiation dermatitis in rats. Biol Pharm Bull. 1999 Jul;22(7):703-6.

Gonzalo Garijo MA, Revenga Arranz F, Bobadilla Gonzalez P. Allergic contact dermatitis due to Centella asiatica: A new case. Allergol Immunopathol (Madr). 1996 May-Jun;24(3):132-4.

Hausen BM. Centella asiatica (Indian pennywort), an effective therapeutic but a weak sensitizer. Contact Dermatitis. 1993 Oct;29(4):175-9.

Maquart FX, Chastang F, Simeon A, Birembaut P, Gillery P, Wegrowski Y. Triterpenes from Centella asiatica stimulate extracellular matrix accumulation in rat experimental wounds. Eur J Dermatol. 1999 Jun;9(4):289-96.

Shukla A, Rasik AM, Dhawan BN. Asiaticoside-induced elevation of antioxidant levels in healing wounds. Phytother Res. 1999 Feb;13(1):50-4.

Shukla A, Rasik AM, Jain GK, Shankar R, Kulshrestha DK, Dhawan BN. In vitro and in vivo wound healing activity of asiaticoside isolated from Centella asiatica. J Ethnopharmacol. 1999 Apr;65(1):1-11.

Suguna L, Sivakumar P, Chandrakasan G. Effects of Centella asiatica extract on dermal wound healing in rats. Indian J Exp Biol. 1996 Dec;34(12):1208-11.

Tenni R, Zanaboni G, De Agostini MP, Rossi A, Bendotti C, Cetta G. Effect of the triterpenoid fraction of Centella asiatica on macromolecules of the connective matrix in human skin fibroblast cultures. Ital J Biochem. 1988 Mar-Apr;37(2):69-77.

Widgerow AD, Chait LA, Stals R, Stals PJ. New innovations in scar management. Aesthetic Plast Surg. 2000 May-Jun;24(3):227-34.

Young GL, Jewell D. Creams for preventing stretch marks in pregnancy. Cochrane Database Syst Rev. 2000;(2):CD000066.

Chapter 16

Supplements for Support During Cancer

INTRODUCTION

In the year 2000, more than 1.2 million new cases of cancer were detected, and almost 600,000 Americans died from the disease—almost evenly split between men and women. For women, breast cancer is the obvious main concern (175,000 women deal with this disease each year), while for men, prostate cancer is the second most prevalent form (180,000 cases and 37,000 deaths last year) following lung cancer. Because a recent study in the journal *Cancer* (2000:88:615-19) suggested that as many as one-third of cancer patients supplement their conventional medical treatment with alternative therapies such as dietary supplements, it is important for both physicians and patients to understand how dietary supplements may help or hinder conventional oncology treatments.

WHAT IS CANCER?

Cancer, aside from being one of the most dreaded words in any language, can be defined as the uncontrolled growth of abnormal cells derived from normal tissues. The aspect of cancer that can make it so deadly is that it can spread from the site of origin to other locations within the body and cause organ failure. There are approximately 200 different types of cancer—and this chapter will do little more than scratch the tip of this deadly iceberg. For example, cancers can arise from the epithelial cells that line body cavities (carcinomas) or from the mesenchymal cells that make up connective tissues, blood, and the lymphatic system (sarcomas). Perhaps the simplest way to describe cancer is as a cellular malignancy that leads to unregulated growth, lack of differentiation, and ability to invade and spread to surrounding tissues (metastasize).

What Causes Cancer?

Perhaps the next question after learning about what cancer *is* typically concerns what *causes* cell growth to go awry in the first place. The short answer is that lots of things promote cancer development and, aside from smoking and poor diet, it is difficult to point out any single lifestyle factor as a dominant contributor (see Table 16.1). Instead, it is often instructive to understand a bit about the epidemiology of cancer to help outline the "who, what, and why" of cancer risk. Here are a few statistics to consider.

Age has the most significant impact on the incidence of and mortality from cancer. For those who live in the United States, the incidence of cancer doubles every five years after the age of twenty-five, with almost 70 percent of all cancer deaths occurring after the age of sixty-five. In particular, cancers of the prostate, stomach, and colon appear to be the most age-specific, with the highest rates between the ages of sixty and eighty. In contrast, children age ten or under tend to suffer a greater incidence of blood cell cancers such as leukemia (acute lymphoblastic leukemia).

Cancer risk follows a *geographic pattern,* with certain parts of the country and the world exhibiting greater rates of specific cancers. For example, the risk of breast cancer in Japan is quite low, while the average American woman has a one-in-eight chance of contracting breast cancer in her lifetime. Almost exclusively due to cigarette smoking, worldwide rates of lung cancer have increased steadily over the past seven decades, so that now nearly *half* of all premature deaths in the Western world are tobacco related. Scary, isn't it? Across the United States, the mortality from cancer appears to be higher in the New England and Mid-Atlantic states, while being somewhat lower in the West and Southwest. Overall, the American Cancer Society pegs the annual cancer death rate in the United States at 174 deaths per 100,000 people.

TABLE 16.1. Causes of Cancer Deaths (United States)

Type of cancer	Cause	Percentage of Total
Lung, bladder, kidney, pancreas, cervix	Tobacco	30-35
Colon, breast, prostate, ovary, endometrium, liver	Diet-related	30-35
Skin	Sunlight, tanning beds	2

Gender plays an obvious role in the development of certain cancers—after all, men do not have breasts and women do not have prostate glands. For men, prostate cancer is the major concern, occurring in about one out of every eight men over a lifetime. For women, breast cancer also occurs at a rate of about one in eight over a lifetime. Both of these cancers are particularly insidious in that they can strike a man or woman in the prime of their lives. Lung cancer, however, is an "equal opportunity" killer and is the most common cause of cancer death in both sexes (although colon cancer is the runner-up to lung cancer in terms of both incidence and mortality across the genders).

It is also quite true that *family history* can play a role in the development of certain cancers. The problem is that even with the ongoing development of powerful gene-screening tools, there is nothing that we can do about our individual risk of developing an inherited cancer (or other inherited disease). Short of choosing our parents wisely, we all need to rely on the same general lifestyle choices (diet, exercise, supplements) that are presented here.

Controllable Risk Factors

It makes sense that since 30 to 35 percent of cancers are diet-related and tobacco-related cancers are another 30 to 35 percent of all cancers, these two controllable risk factors are the place to start. First and foremost on your cancer prevention "to do" list is simple—*stop smoking* (and stop exposing yourself and others to secondhand smoke). Next, get yourself up and out the door for some *exercise*. A sedentary lifestyle is associated with a higher risk of many cancers, and the simple act of walking a few miles several times each week can help reduce cancer risk for the colon, breast, prostate, and lung.

The nutritionally linked cancers include cancer of the esophagus, stomach, liver, colon, rectum, breast, prostate, endometrium, and ovary. The *dietary aspects* most commonly associated with these cancers are pickled foods, salted foods, alcohol, nitrates/nitrosamines, mycotoxins, fried foods, and hydroxyl radicals (caused by barbecuing). This does not mean that you have to memorize each of these classes of chemicals and then religiously avoid them. This laundry list is presented simply as a means to help you realize that the simple incorporation of a higher proportion of *fruits and vegetables* (and the associated *phytonutrients* and *fiber*) can go a long way toward reducing cancer risk and helping your body fight any cancers that you may already be battling.

In many cases, when people learn of their heightened risk for cancer, or they or a loved one are diagnosed with the disease, it spurs them to radically change their approach to eating. Some of the more popular diets, including Mediterranean, Asian, vegetarianism, macrobiotic, and high protein/low carbohydrate, are outlined in the next section. Several types of low-fat, primarily vegetarian-based diets have very strong evidence for cancer protection due to a reduced exposure to carcinogens (fewer processed foods) and an increased intake of anticarcinogenic phytonutrients.

SPECIALIZED DIETS

Mediterranean and *Asian* diets both tend to rely on a "semivegetarian" combination of foods—lots of fruits and vegetables, small amounts of protein (mostly fish), and little (if any) eggs or dairy products. The key difference between the two diets is that the Mediterranean diet also includes a relatively high intake of olive and flax oils (which supply omega-3 fatty acids), while the Asian diet has a higher consumption of soy-based foods (which supplies isoflavones). Even though the Mediterranean diet is not particularly low in fat (at about 40 percent of total calories), breast cancer rates in Greece and Italy are much lower than might be expected. Asian diets, on the other hand, are quite low in total fat content and have also been associated with reduced rates of breast cancer—possibly due to the anti-cancer effects of isoflavones and other compounds found in tofu, fish, garlic, and green tea.

Vegetarianism is the practice of living on a diet that includes foods derived exclusively, or almost exclusively, from plants. Vegetarians do not eat meat, although many of the less strict vegetarians may include small amounts of dairy products or eggs ("lacto-ovo" vegetarians). Strict vegetarians, called vegans, eat no meat, fish, poultry, eggs, or dairy products. Because their diets are devoid of the richest sources of protein and vitamin B_{12}, vegans need to be especially careful about combining plant sources of protein (such as rice and beans) in adequate amounts to meet daily protein requirements.

In most cases, a vegetarian diet is healthier than the way most Americans normally eat (largely because it incorporates a large amount of fruits and vegetables). Leading health organizations have encouraged a reduction of animal fats and an increase in fruits and vegetables in the American diet for decades. It is well known that excessive saturated fat intake contributes to an increased risk for many cancers (as well as heart disease). Most health professionals recognize that diets which rely on whole grains and fresh fruits and vegetables can result in better overall health. It is also well supported that vegetarian diets can help reduce obesity and constipation, and there is growing evidence that such diets may be effective in reducing the risk of cancers of the lung, colon, breast, and prostate as well.

Macrobiotic diets became popular in the early 1960s as more of a spiritual movement than a healthy lifestyle. Today, macrobiotic diets still incorporate a high degree of spirituality by combining diet, consciousness, and social philosophy to promote healing and healthful living. Macrobiotic diets are generally based on one of several Eastern philosophies (Chinese and Indian are common) and may incorporate the concept of "balancing" various universal factors. For example, the Chinese/Japanese principle of "yin and yang" assigns opposite values to every component of life and nature (such as hot/cold, male/female, light/dark), with the overall concept that to achieve health and happiness, one must first achieve balance in yin and yang. The macrobiotic diet is intended to be yin-yang balanced and, therefore, healthy.

The macrobiotic concept includes more than just a diet or simple food selection. It requires special methods of food preparation as well as the assessment of yin-yang values in each geographic location. In other words, it is a *major* effort for most people and a paradigm shift away from the typical American diet and lifestyle. Macrobiotic philosophy dictates that only pots, pans, and utensils made of certain materials may be used; however, most wood, glass, ceramic, stainless steel, and enamel cookware pieces are allowed, while copper and aluminum are excluded. From a practical standpoint, this diet and philosophical approach can take a lot of planning and may cost more in time and dollars than other dietary approaches.

The typical macrobiotic diet (if there is such a thing) is generally composed of about 50 percent to 60 percent whole grains because they are thought to be neutral in the yin-yang continuum. Vegetables make up another 25 to 30 percent of the diet, with the remainder being various beans, seaweed, and soups (miso soup is quite popular). Dairy, eggs, sugar, meats, and processed foods are generally not part of most macrobiotic diets. Like vegetarian diets, a macrobiotic diet may help reduce cholesterol, body weight, and heart disease as well as certain cancers—most notably colon, prostate, and breast cancers.

High protein/low carbohydrate (HPLC) diets have been popular for decades—these fad diets come and go with the changing of the seasons. You may recognize this type of diet by its more popular names such as The Atkins Diet, Protein Power, Carbohydrate Addicts, Sugar Busters, and many others. The primary reason that most people follow one of these diets is for the rapid and effortless weight loss that is promised. Although there are no direct cancer-reducing benefits of such diets (aside from an indirect benefit of any weight loss), there may be a very real *cancer-promoting* side effect of HPLC diets due to their promotion of high fat intakes.

In most cases, HPLC diets are extremely low (or devoid) of carbohydrates (less than 20 percent of total calories) such as breads, rice, pasta, cereals, almost all fruits, and certain types of vegetables. This leaves protein and fat, from which dieters are encouraged to consume the bulk of their daily calorie needs. Although most of the popular diet books recommend that the majority of fat intake come from unsaturated varieties (poly- and monounsaturated oils), this message is lost on the vast majority of dieters, who feel that the diets are a license to eat all the fat, of whatever type, that they want (think bacon and mayonnaise sandwiches). The chief problem with a high dietary intake of saturated fat (and low intake of fiber) is an increased risk of heart disease and cancer because certain fatty acids can turn on oncogenes and increase the risk for breast, colon, and prostate cancer.

Although an HPLC diet may be quite effective for achieving short-term weight loss in some people, much of the loss in body weight will come from body water and glycogen losses, and the restrictions on carbohydrates, fruits, and vegetables are very difficult to adhere to for any prolonged period of time.

What to Look for in a Diet

- Never follow a diet that eliminates whole food groups. Eliminating whole food groups can increase the chances of a vitamin or mineral deficiency.
- Always eat a diet that is varied and not monotonous. Eating a wide variety of foods virtually ensures a consistent intake of many vitamins, minerals, and other health-promoting agents.
- Avoid eating fast foods. Avoiding fast foods and fried foods is an easy way to keep your fat and caloric intake under control.
- Try to eat food that has a low sugar content. This means avoid foods that have a high level of simple sugars.
- Take a multivitamin/mineral supplement daily. In addition, always inform your health care provider of the type of diet that you follow and any and all dietary supplements that you may take.

DIETARY SUPPLEMENTS

Let's start off with a *very* important point: *Dietary supplements cannot prevent or cure cancer on their own.* Although some of the supplements outlined in this chapter may be beneficial when added to a healthy diet and regular excise program, *none* of them present any sort of "miracle" in terms of cancer prevention or treatment (despite what the breathless marketing materials might lead you to believe). A large number of clinical trials are under way with selected vitamins, minerals, phytonutrients, and other supplement ingredients to determine their relative anticancer properties (or lack thereof). Thus far, this research appears to be quite promising for selenium, green tea, and some other vitamins, but the research to date has largely been conducted in test tubes and lab animals—and it is *far* from being conclusive regarding any beneficial effects in humans.

The bottom line, in terms of nutrition, for preventing cancer is to eat a diet that is high in fruits, vegetables, and whole grains while also being low in saturated fat and processed meats. That said, the following supplement recommendations are cautiously presented with the recommendation that any cancer patient should work with his or her oncologist to optimize a specific treatment regimen—whether it includes dietary supplements or not.

PC-SPES is a combination of eight different herbs that appear to have mild antihormone activity and positive effects during prostate cancer treatment. Recent case reports point to an improvement in quality of life measurements, reduction in metastatic pain, and a reduction in levels of prostate-specific antigen (PSA). PC-SPES has also been found to have a tumor-shrinking effect in an animal model. PC-SPES is sold over the counter, but great caution should be taken when using or incorporating PC-SPES into your treatment plan. No one should use PC-SPES without his or her oncologist approving it or at least being aware of it.

Antioxidant nutrients, whether vitamins (C and E), minerals (selenium and zinc), or phytonutrients (catechins and flavonoids), have shown terrific promise in the prevention of skin cancer (which affects as many as one in four people). Although most cases of skin cancer are highly treatable if caught early enough, prevention of the disease in the first place is the better choice. The most serious form of skin cancer, melanoma, was once quite rare in the United States, but rates are increasing faster than those of any other form of cancer. Melanoma is expected to affect approximately one in every 100 people and account for 9,000 to 10,000 deaths in 2002 alone. Because the greatest risk factor for developing skin cancer is sun exposure (and a fair complexion), the best preventive measure is to avoid excessive exposure by using sunscreens, sunglasses, and clothing. Several studies have suggested a beneficial role of antioxidants used both internally as supplements and externally as topical cosmetics, with combinations of vitamins A, C, E, selenium, and beta-carotene actually resulting in an increase in the skin's own ability to resist sun damage (sort of like an internal sunscreen). The Skin Cancer Foundation recommends that skin cancer risk can be reduced by minimizing your sun exposure between 10 a.m. and 3 p.m. and using a sunscreen with SPF-15 or higher (apply to all exposed areas and reapply every two hours).

Vitamin C, the primary water-soluble antioxidant nutrient in the diet, is known to be depleted in people afflicted with various cancers. Although studies of vitamin C supplements have shown conflicting results with regard to cancer prevention, its role in "regenerating" the antioxidant effects of vitamin E provides support for including vitamin C in any antioxidant supplement regimen. It may be that vitamin C, like beta-carotene, is but one dietary substance needed for overall chemoprotection and that mixed sources (from foods) are your best protection against cancer. Several studies have found a strong association between high vitamin C intake from foods and a reduced incidence of cancers of the stomach, bladder, throat, colon, and breast—perhaps by suppressing the formation of carcinogenic nitrosamines in the gastrointestinal tract.

Niacin (vitamin B_3) is known to increase levels of NAD in various tissues, which may lead to an enhanced capacity to repair cellular damage that could lead to cancer.

Milk thistle (silymarin) is a popular herbal supplement for "liver detoxification," but it also possesses powerful effects as an antioxidant. A number of animal studies (in rodents) have shown a reduced occurrence of several cancers, perhaps due to a modulation of liver enzyme pathways.

Grape seed extract and green tea extract are both rich sources of polyphenol compounds such as proanthocyanidins (in grape seed) and catechins (in green tea). Polyphenols are potent antioxidants that deliver powerful antitumor properties in rodent models of cancer. Grapes also contain several phytonutrient compounds, such as resveratrol and quercetin, that have additional antiestrogen and anti-inflammatory properties.

Sulforaphane and indoles are compounds found in broccoli, cabbage, cauliflower, and related cruciferous vegetables that are thought to possess anticancer properties by enhancing the liver's ability to detoxify certain carcinogens more effectively.

Isoflavones, such as daidzein and genistein (from either soy or red clover), possess both antioxidant and weak estrogenic activity. The antiestrogen effect of small doses of isoflavones may be beneficial in certain forms of hormone-sensitive cancer, such as breast, uterine, and prostate, but very high doses could theoretically *increase* cancer cell proliferation and promote tumor growth. For this reason, it may be prudent to consume isoflavone supplements at levels that are achievable from a high-soy diet (probably no more than 50 to 100 mg per day). We know from animal studies that soy-based diets are associated with reduced cancer risk, so it may be speculated that a similar effect *may* be observed in humans.

Vitamin E, as the major fat-soluble antioxidant in the body, can be quite effective in protecting delicate structures in the skin and eyes from the damaging effects of sun-induced oxidative stress. Several animal studies have shown vitamin E's ability to reduce skin cancer whether used orally or topically, and human population studies suggest a beneficial role of vitamin E in preventing prostate cancer (400 to 800 IU per day). In one human study, 50 mg of synthetic vitamin E reduced the incidence of prostate cancer by more than 30 percent and the death rate from prostate cancer by more than 40 percent, while colon cancer was reduced by 16 percent. In other studies, colon cancer risk has been cut by 30 to 70 percent depending on the dose and duration of vitamin E supplementation (usually around 200 IU per day), and positive benefits have been noted for vitamin E supplements (400 to 800 IU per day) in cancers of the liver, mouth, and stomach. For some reason, vitamin E does not appear to be particularly effective against lung cancer.

Selenium deficiency has been associated with an increased risk of several forms of cancer, and supplements (200 mcg per day) are thought to protect against cancers of the prostate, colon, and lung (but probably not against skin cancer). In one of the best studies, subjects received either 200 mcg per day of selenium or a placebo. Those receiving the selenium supplements showed dramatic reductions in cancer of the prostate (66 percent), colon (50 percent), and lung (40 percent) as well as an overall 50 percent reduction in cancer deaths. The best supplemental sources of selenium should supply 100 to 200 mcg per day in a bioavailable form such as selenomethionine, selenium-rich yeast, or high-selenium garlic (instead of an inorganic form such as sodium selenite). Caution is urged in using higher doses of selenium, however, which can lead to toxic effects at doses above 900 mcg to 1 mg per day (gastrointestinal distress, loss of hair or fingernails, forgetfulness, etc.).

Garlic may be helpful in reducing the risk of colon cancer by as much as 30 percent—possibly via either its antioxidant properties (garlic is high in selenium) or through its ability to influence certain detoxification enzyme pathways in the liver. Several population studies conducted in China, Europe, and the United States have shown that people with the highest dietary consumption of garlic have a significantly reduced risk of developing colon cancer.

Beta-carotene, although possessing powerful antioxidant properties, may *not* be the ideal supplement for cancer prevention. In fact, there is some fairly strong evidence that although mixed carotenoids from fruits and vegetables may provide a cancer-preventive effect, high-dose supplements of purified beta-carotene may actually *promote* certain forms of cancer in specific populations, such as lung cancer in lifelong heavy smokers. We know from population studies that lung cancer risk is reduced by almost 75 percent by consuming a diet rich in fruits and vegetables (particularly cruciferous veggies such as broccoli and cauliflower). However, at least two very large intervention studies conducted in the mid-1990s, the Alpha-Tocopherol, Beta-Carotene (ATBC) study and the Beta-Carotene and Retinol Efficacy Trial (CARET), showed a clear 18 to 46 percent *increase* in lung cancer occurrence among smokers and those exposed to asbestos. The ATBC study used 20 mg doses of beta-carotene daily for five to eight years. A related population study, the Physicians' Health Study, found no adverse effects of 25 mg per day of beta-carotene (nor any beneficial effects), but only about 10 percent of the participants were smokers.

Lycopene is another carotenoid (found in tomatoes, pink grapefruit, and watermelon) that has powerful antioxidant activity (about twice as good as beta-carotene). Like selenium, lycopene may be especially effective in the prevention of prostate cancer. Several studies show a strong association between dietary intake of tomatoes and tomato products (pizza sauce, tomato sauce, and ketchup) and a reduced rate of cancers of the prostate, breast, stomach, lung, and colon.

Green tea extract has been shown in a wide variety of studies to provide cancer-preventive benefits. Rodent studies show a clear benefit of green tea consumption on rates of skin cancer, while test-tube and population studies suggest beneficial effects of green tea on cancers of the stomach, colon, prostate, breast, lung, and liver. The human studies suggest that consumption of eight to ten cups of either green or black tea daily can reduce cancer incidence by 30 to 40 percent. Like vitamin C, the polyphenol/catechin compounds are thought to reduce the formation of carcinogenic nitrosamines in the body and may have the additional benefit of providing a direct antitumor effect by blocking the activity of certain cancer-specific enzymes. General dosage recommendations for green tea supplements are in the range of 300 to 600 mg per day (three divided doses of 100 to 200 mg each)—or about the amount that you might find in three to six cups of brewed green or black tea.

Folic acid deficiency is known to increase the risk of cancers of the colon, breast, and lung, but it is not known whether dietary supplements may help reduce cancer risk. Because of the other well-known health benefits of folic acids supplements (400 mcg per day), such as cardiovascular health (reduced serum homocysteine levels) and reproductive health (reduced risk of neural tube birth defects), this vitamin should be part of almost everybody's daily supplement regimen (as part of a balanced multivitamin that includes B_{12} and B_6).

Flaxseed supplements (the whole seed, *not* flaxseed oil) contain isoflavone-like compounds known as lignans that are associated with a reduced risk of certain cancers (flaxseed *oil* is a good source of omega-3 fatty acids, which have cardioprotective benefits). Like isoflavones from soy or red clover, flaxseed lignans may prevent estrogen from attaching to cells and promoting hormone-sensitive cancers (breast, uterine, and prostate).

Shark cartilage is widely touted (mostly on the Internet) as a "miracle" cure for cancer. While it is quite true that shark cartilage (as well as other sources of cartilage such as chicken, beef, and pork) contains various anti-angiogenesis compounds that inhibit blood vessel growth (which could theoretically choke off tumor growth), test-tube studies have yet to be completed in human trials. For a summary of supplements see Table 16.2.

Supplement Use During Chemotherapy and Radiation Therapy

A controversy in the dietary supplement industry right now is that, while we have some evidence that certain dietary supplements may be beneficial in terms of reducing the risk of developing certain forms of cancer *(prevention)*, we are not absolutely sure whether dietary supplements should be recommended *during* treatment of existing cancer. There are certainly very logical arguments on both sides of the issue, but neither side has the necessary scientific data to "prove" their point of view.

Arguing in favor of using dietary supplements during chemotherapy and radiation treatment is the knowledge that antioxidant supplements can help protect healthy cells from the damaging effects of cancer treatment. In many cases, this may result in a better tolerance of the highly toxic cancer treat-

TABLE 16.2. Dietary Supplements for Cancer Prevention and Support During Treatment

Ingredient	Dose (per day)	Primary claim
Green tea	125-500 mg	General antioxidant benefits ("cell protection")
Lycopene	10-40 mg	General antioxidant, prostate cancer protection
Milk thistle	175-350 mg	Liver health and "detoxification"
Schisandra	200-800 mg	Liver health and "detoxification"
Shark cartilage	250-1,000 mg	Slows tumor growth (anti-angiogenesis)
Spirulina	2-3 g	General antioxidant

ments and an ultimately more positive health outcome of therapy. Arguing against using dietary supplements during cancer treatment is the theory that cancer cells may also be able to use the protective qualities of some supplements to actually reduce the effectiveness of treatments designed to kill tumors. There is some evidence that tumor cells are able to take up and accumulate high levels of vitamin C—resulting in tumors that become highly resistant to radiation treatment. Although this may indicate that high-dose vitamin C supplements are ill advised during cancer treatment, there is simply a lack of scientific evidence for most other supplements.

In other studies, primarily in animals and test tubes, there is evidence that some nutritional supplements may actually help chemotherapy work better. Some of the drugs used during chemotherapy are known to interfere with vitamin and mineral metabolism. For example, *methotrexate* interferes with folic acid metabolism—so cancer patients taking methotrexate should be careful to consume about 400 mcg of folate, but no more without the guidance of their oncologist (high-dose supplements can reduce the effectiveness of the drug). Another chemotherapy drug, *Adriamycin,* can lead to heart damage that appears to be reduced by higher dietary levels of antioxidants, B-complex vitamins, and coenzyme Q10. In some cases, vitamin E may enhance the ability of Adriamycin to slow tumor growth (suggested by test-tube studies). *Cisplatin,* one of the most potent chemotherapy drugs, can deplete the body of magnesium and other nutrients—yet some of the toxic side effects may be counteracted by supplements designed to promote glutathione synthesis (such as alpha-lipoic acid, selenium, and cysteine).

WORKS CONSULTED

Alaejos MS, Diaz Romero FJ, Diaz Romero C. Selenium and cancer: Some nutritional aspects. Nutrition. 2000 May;16(5):376-83.

Andlauer W, Stehle P, Furst P. Chemoprevention—a novel approach in dietetics. Curr Opin Clin Nutr Metab Care. 1998 Nov;1(6):539-47.

Berkow R, Fletcher AJ, Beers MH. The Merck Manual of Diagnosis and Therapy. Sixteenth edition. Rahway, NJ: Merck and Co., Inc., 1992.

Cravo ML, Pinto AG, Chaves P, Cruz JA, Lage P, Nobre Leitao C, Costa Mira F. Effect of folate supplementation on DNA methylation of rectal mucosa in patients with colonic adenomas: Correlation with nutrient intake. Clin Nutr. 1998 Apr;17(2):45-9.

Halliwell B. Can oxidative DNA damage be used as a biomarker of cancer risk in humans? Problems, resolutions and preliminary results from nutritional supplementation studies. Free Radic Res. 1998 Dec;29(6):469-86.

Hercberg S, Preziosi P, Galan P, Faure H, Arnaud J, Duport N, Malvy D, Roussel AM, Briancon S, Favier A. "The SU.VI.MAX Study": A primary prevention trial using nutritional doses of antioxidant vitamins and minerals in cardiovascular diseases and cancers. SUpplementation on VItamines et Mineraux Antio-Xydants. Food Chem Toxicol. 1999 Sep-Oct;37(9-10):925-30.

John EM, Schwartz GG, Dreon DM, Koo J. Vitamin D and breast cancer risk: The NHANES I Epidemiologic follow-up study, 1971-1975 to 1992. National Health and Nutrition Examination Survey. Cancer Epidemiol Biomarkers Prev. 1999 May;8(5):399-406.

Kampman E, Slattery ML, Caan B, Potter JD. Calcium, vitamin D, sunshine exposure, dairy products and colon cancer risk. Cancer Causes Control. 2000 May; 11(5):459-66.

Lamson DW, Brignall MS. Antioxidants in cancer therapy; their actions and interactions with oncologic therapies. Alt Med Rev. 1999;4:304-27.

McCarthy D, Weihofen D. The effect of nutritional supplements on food intake in patients undergoing radiotherapy. Oncol Nurs Forum. 1999 Jun;26(5):897-900.

Murphy GP, Lawrence W, Lenhard RE. American Cancer Society Textbook of Clinical Oncology. Second edition. Atlanta, Georgia: American Cancer Society, 1995.

Navarro-Alarcon M, Lopez-Martinez MC. Essentiality of selenium in the human body: Relationship with different diseases. Sci Total Environ. 2000 Apr 17; 249(1-3):347-71.

Nitenberg G, Raynard B. Nutritional support of the cancer patient: Issues and dilemmas. Crit Rev Oncol Hematol. 2000 Jun;34(3):137-68.

Novaes MR, Lima LA. Effects of dietetic supplementation with L-arginine in cancer patients. A review of the literature. Arch Latinoam Nutr. 1999 Dec;49(4):301-8.

Pfeifer BL, Pirani JF, Hamann SR, Klippel KF. PC-SPES, a dietary supplement for the treatment of hormone refractory prostate cancer. Brit J Urology Int. 2000;85(4):481-5.

Rock CL, Michael CW, Reynolds RK, Ruffin MT. Prevention of cervix cancer. Crit Rev Oncol Hematol. 2000 Mar;33(3):169-85.

Rosenblatt KA, Thomas DB, Jimenez LM, Fish B, McTiernan A, Stalsberg H, Stemhagen A, Thompson WD, Curnen MG, Satariano W, Austin DF, Greenberg RS, Key C, Kolonel LN, West DW. The relationship between diet and breast cancer in men. Cancer Causes Control. 1999 Apr;10(2):107-13.

Slattery ML, Edwards SL, Boucher KM, Anderson K, Caan BJ. Lifestyle and colon cancer: An assessment of factors associated with risk. Am J Epidemiol. 1999 Oct 15;150(8):869-77.

Terry P, Lagergren J, Ye W, Nyren O, Wolk A. Antioxidants and cancers of the esophagus and gastric cardia. Int J Cancer. 2000 Sep 1;87(5):750-4.

Tiwari RK, Geliebter J, Garikapaty VP, Yedavelli SP, Chen S, Mittelman A. Antitumor effects of PC-SPES, an herbal formulation in prostate cancer. Int J Oncol. 1999;14(4):713-9.

Yun TK. Update from Asia. Asian studies on cancer chemoprevention. Ann N Y Acad Sci. 1999;889:157-92.

GREEN TEA

What Is It?

Green tea *(Camellia sinensis)* is the second-most-consumed beverage in the world (water is the first) and has been used medicinally for centuries in India and China. A number of beneficial health effects are attributed to regular consumption of green tea, and dried or powdered extracts of green tea are available as dietary supplements. Green tea is prepared by picking, lightly steaming the leaves, and allowing them to dry. Black tea, the most popular type of tea in the United States, is made by allowing the leaves to ferment before drying. Due to differences in the fermentation process, a portion of the active compounds are destroyed in black tea, but remain in green tea. The active constituents in green tea are a family of polyphenols (catechins) with potent antioxidant activity. Tannins, large polyphenol molecules, form the bulk of the active compounds in green tea, with catechins making up nearly 90 percent. Several catechins are present in significant quantities: epicatechin (EC), epigallocatechin (EGC), epicatechin gallate (ECG), and epigallocatechin gallate (EGCG). EGCG makes up about 10 to 50 percent of the total catechin content and appears to be the most powerful of the catechins—with antioxidant activity about 25 to 100 times more potent than vitamins C and E. A cup of green tea may provide 10 to 40 mg of polyphenols and has antioxidant activity greater than a serving of broccoli, spinach, carrots, or strawberries. A number of commercial green tea extracts are standardized to total polyphenol content and/or EGCG content.

Claims

- Anticancer
- General antioxidant
- Antiatherogenic/reduces cholesterol and triglycerides
- Reduces blood clotting
- Enhances immune function
- Enhances weight loss

Theory

Because the active compounds, the catechins, found in green tea are known to possess potent antioxidant activity, they may provide beneficial health effects by protecting the body from oxidative damage from free radicals. A number of chronic disease states have been associated with free radical–induced oxidative damage, including cancer, heart disease, suppressed immune function, and accelerated aging.

Scientific Support

Although numerous laboratory investigations have shown the powerful antioxidant activity of green tea and green tea extracts, prospective clinical studies in humans are few. From the laboratory findings, it is clear that green tea is an effective antioxidant, that it provides protection from experimentally induced DNA damage, and that it can slow or halt the initiation and progression of cancerous tumor growth. There is also evidence from some studies that green tea provides significant immunoprotective qualities, particularly in the case of cancer patients undergoing radiation or chemotherapy. White blood cell count appears to be maintained more effectively in cancer patients consuming green tea than in nonsupplemented patients.

Several epidemiological studies show an association between consumption of total flavonoids in the diet and the risk for cancer and heart disease. Men with the highest consumption of flavonoids (from fruits and vegetables) have approximately *half* the risk of heart disease and cancer compared to those with the lowest intake. The primary catechin in green tea, EGCG, appears to inhibit the growth of cancer cells as well as to play a role in stimulating apoptosis (programmed cell death), both of which are crucial aspects of cancer prevention.

In terms of heart disease protection, the potent antioxidant properties of polyphenols would be expected to reduce free radical damage to cells and prevent the oxidation of LDL cholesterol—both of which would be expected to inhibit the formation of atherosclerotic plaques.

Aside from the clear benefits of green tea as an antioxidant, recent studies have suggested a role for catechins in promoting weight loss. In one animal study, the antiobesity effect of green tea was evaluated by feeding different levels of green tea (1 to 4 percent in their diets) to female mice for four months. The study found that the mice receiving the green tea in their diets had a significant suppression of food intake, body weight gain, and fat tissue accumulation. In addition, levels of cholesterol and triglycerides were lower in mice receiving the green tea diet. Perhaps the most interesting finding from this study was that leptin levels in serum showed a decrease with green tea treatments, indicating that green tea may have a direct effect on the regulation of body weight (downward).

In some studies, green tea is associated with a mild increase in thermogenesis (increased caloric expenditure), which is generally attributed to its caffeine content. However, a handful of studies have shown that green tea extract stimulates thermogenesis to an extent much greater than can be attributed directly to its caffeine content alone—meaning that the thermogenic properties of green tea may be due to an interaction between caffeine and its high content of catechin-polyphenols. A probable theory for the thermogenic effect of green tea is an increase in levels of norepinephrine—because catechin-polyphenols are known to inhibit catechol-O-methyltransferase (the enzyme that degrades norepinephrine). One study examined this theory, and the effect of green tea extract on twenty-four-hour energy expenditure, in ten healthy men, who each consumed three treatments of green tea extract (50 mg caffeine and 90 mg epigallocatechin gallate), caffeine (50 mg), and placebo (at breakfast, lunch, and dinner). The results of the study showed that, relative to placebo, the green tea extract resulted in a significant (4 percent) increase in twenty-four-hour energy expenditure (approximately 800 calories per day) and a significant increase in the body's use of fat as an energy source (twenty-four-hour respiratory quotient). In addition, twenty-four-hour urinary norepinephrine excretion was 40 percent higher during treatment with the green tea extract than with the placebo. It is interesting to note that treatment with caffeine in amounts equivalent to those found in the green tea extract (50 mg) had no effect on energy expenditure or fat oxidation, suggesting that the thermogenic properties of green tea are due to compounds other than its caffeine content alone.

Safety

Green tea consumption of as much as twenty cups per day has not been associated with any significant side effects. In high doses, however, teas that contain caffeine may lead to restlessness, insomnia, heart palpitations, and tachycardia (rapid heartbeat). Decaffeinated versions of green tea and green tea extracts are available, but due to differences in caffeine extraction methods, the amounts of phenolic/catechin compounds can vary between extracts. Be sure to choose an extract that is decaffeinated as well as standardized for total polyphenol content and/or catechin concentrations. In addition, individuals taking aspirin or other anticoagulant agents (including vitamin E and ginkgo biloba) on a daily basis should be aware of the possible inhibition of platelet aggregation (blood clotting) associated with green tea (in some cases, green tea may prolong bleeding times).

Value

Green tea may be especially beneficial for individuals at high risk for cancer (e.g., family history) or for those undergoing or recovering from chemotherapy or radiation treatment. It is also beneficial as a general protective measure and dietary "insurance" of adequate polyphenol intake. Recent data provides strong evidence that green tea may be effective in stimulating thermogenesis, increasing caloric expenditure, promoting fat oxidation, and controlling body weight.

Dosage

Typical dosage recommendations are for 125 to 500 mg per day—preferably of an extract standardized to at least 60 percent polyphenols and/or EGCG as a marker compound (this should be equivalent to four to ten cups of brewed green tea).

WORKS CONSULTED

Anderson JW, Diwadkar VA, Bridges SR. Selective effects of different antioxidants on oxidation of lipoproteins from rats. Proc Soc Exp Biol Med. 1998 Sep;218(4):376-81.

Benzie IF, Szeto YT, Strain JJ, Tomlinson B. Consumption of green tea causes rapid increase in plasma antioxidant power in humans. Nutr Cancer. 1999;34(1):83-7.

Dulloo AG, Duret C, Rohrer D, Girardier L, Mensi N, Fathi M, Chantre P, Vandermander J. Efficacy of a green tea extract rich in catechin polyphenols and caffeine in increasing 24-h energy expenditure and fat oxidation in humans. Am J Clin Nutr. 1999 Dec;70(6):1040-5.

Dulloo AG, Seydoux J, Girardier L, Chantre P, Vandermander J. Green tea and thermogenesis: Interactions between catechin-polyphenols, caffeine and sympathetic activity. Int J Obes Relat Metab Disord. 2000 Feb;24(2):252-8.

Graham HN. Green tea composition, consumption, and polyphenol chemistry. Prev Med. 1992 May;21(3):334-50.

Gupta S, Ahmad N, Mohan RR, Husain MM, Mukhtar H. Prostate cancer chemoprevention by green tea: In vitro and in vivo inhibition of testosterone-mediated induction of ornithine decarboxylase. Cancer Res. 1999 May 1;59(9):2115-20.

Hasegawa R, Chujo T, Sai-Kato K, Umemura T, Tanimura A, Kurokawa Y. Preventive effects of green tea against liver oxidative DNA damage and hepatotoxicity in rats treated with 2-nitropropane. Food Chem Toxicol. 1995 Nov; 33(11):961-70.

Hirose M, Hoshiya T, Akagi K, Futakuchi M, Ito N. Inhibition of mammary gland carcinogenesis by green tea catechins and other naturally occurring antioxidants in female Sprague-Dawley rats pretreated with 7,12-dimethylbenz [alpha] anthracene. Cancer Lett. 1994 Aug 15;83(1-2):149-56.

Kao YH, Hiipakka RA, Liao S. Modulation of endocrine systems and food intake by green tea epigallocatechin gallate. Endocrinology. 2000 Mar;141(3):980-7.

Lin JK, Liang YC, Lin-Shiau SY. Cancer chemoprevention by tea polyphenols through mitotic signal transduction blockade. Biochem Pharmacol. 1999 Sep 15;58(6):911-5.

Muramatsu K, Fukuyo M, Hara Y. Effect of green tea catechins on plasma cholesterol level in cholesterol-fed rats. J Nutr Sci Vitaminol (Tokyo). 1986 Dec;32(6):613-22.

Sato D. Inhibition of urinary bladder tumors induced by N-butyl-N-(4-hydroxybutyl)-nitrosamine in rats by green tea. Int J Urol. 1999 Feb;6(2):93-9.

Satoh K, Sakagami H. Ascorbyl radical scavenging activity of polyphenols. Anticancer Res. 1996 Sep-Oct;16(5A):2885-90.

Sayama K, Lin S, Zheng G, Oguni I. Effects of green tea on growth, food utilization and lipid metabolism in mice. In Vivo. 2000 Jul-Aug;14(4):481-4.

Schubert SY, Lansky EP, Neeman I. Antioxidant and eicosanoid enzyme inhibition properties of pomegranate seed oil and fermented juice flavonoids. J Ethnopharmacol. 1999 Jul;66(1):11-7.

Tanaka H, Hirose M, Kawabe M, Sano M, Takesada Y, Hagiwara A, Shirai T. Post-initiation inhibitory effects of green tea catechins on 7,12-dimethylbenz[a]anthracene-induced mammary gland carcinogenesis in female Sprague-Dawley rats. Cancer Lett. 1997 Jun 3;116(1):47-52.

Wang ZY, Huang MT, Ho CT, Chang R, Ma W, Ferraro T, Reuhl KR, Yang CS, Conney AH. Inhibitory effect of green tea on the growth of established skin papillomas in mice. Cancer Res. 1992 Dec 1;52(23):6657-65.

Weisburger JH, Rivenson A, Aliaga C, Reinhardt J, Kelloff GJ, Boone CW, Steele VE, Balentine DA, Pittman B, Zang E. Effect of tea extracts, polyphenols, and epigallocatechin gallate on azoxymethane-induced colon cancer. Proc Soc Exp Biol Med. 1998 Jan;217(1):104-8.

Xu Y, Ho CT, Amin SG, Han C, Chung FL. Inhibition of tobacco-specific nitrosamine-induced lung tumorigenesis in A/J mice by green tea and its major polyphenol as antioxidants. Cancer Res. 1992 Jul 15;52(14):3875-9.

Yang TT, Koo MW. Hypocholesterolemic effects of Chinese tea. Pharmacol Res. 1997 Jun;35(6):505-12.

Yang TT, Koo MW. Chinese green tea lowers cholesterol level through an increase in fecal lipid excretion. Life Sci. 2000;66(5):411-23.

Zhu M, Gong Y, Ge G. Effects of green tea on growth inhibition and immune regulation of Lewis lung cancer in mice. Chung Hua Yu Fang I Hsueh Tsa Chih. 1997 Nov;31(6):325-9.

MILK THISTLE

What Is It?

Milk thistle *(Silybum marianum)* is an edible plant, the leaves of which can be eaten like artichokes and the seeds of which can be roasted and brewed like coffee. *Silybum marianum* has been used for over 2,000 years as a traditional medicine specifically for liver ailments. Milk thistle is rumored to have received its name because of its ability to stimulate milk production in lactating women.

Claims

- Protects/regenerates liver tissue
- Alleviates inflammation
- General antioxidant

Theory

Milk thistle contains a compound called silymarin, an antioxidant that scavenges damaging free radicals. Silymarin, as well as an isolated flavono-lignan compound called silybin, have a particular effect in the liver where they can prevent or counteract damage caused by toxins such as alcohol and acetaminophen (Tylenol), as well as environmental and bacterial toxins, and even some poisons such as those found in the lethal death cap mushroom.

Scientific Support

A very large and impressive body of scientific evidence supports the therapeutic utility of milk thistle for various indications related to liver health. The name silymarin is a general term for the active chemicals, known as flavonolignans, which are found only in the seeds of the milk thistle plant. Heavy metals and many drugs and poisons cause liver toxicity through the production of free radicals and, more specifically, lipid peroxidation. Silymarin has been shown to combat lipid peroxidation in the liver of rats. Likewise, it has been demonstrated that silymarin may hasten the restoration

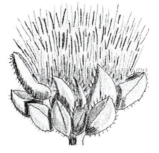

of liver cells in damaged liver tissue. Excessive alcohol consumption is known to cause liver damage by depleting levels of glutathione, the body's most important antioxidant. Silymarin and silybin can actually elevate liver glutathione levels in rats given alcohol. Furthermore, in rabbits with liver damage, those given silymarin had increased survival times relative to those that did not receive the extract. The results of animal studies have been repeated in large, well-controlled human trials. Subjects with liver damage caused by chronic alcoholism, cirrhosis, hepatitis, or other toxicities were significantly benefited by treatment with silymarin. However, silymarin appears to have its most profound effect in those with less severe liver damage.

Safety

Milk thistle is quite safe as a supplement. Neither toxicity nor drug interactions have been reported following high doses of milk thistle or its components. The only common side effect that has been reported following supplementation with milk thistle is a mild laxative effect. Because long-term studies have not been conducted with milk thistle or its derivatives, pregnant women should not take this supplement, and lactating women who may take milk thistle to promote milk production should first consult with their physicians.

Value

Because of its well-documented effect on liver health, combined with its strong safety profile, milk thistle seems to be an excellent supplement for preventing liver damage. Standardized extracts generally sell for $12 to $20 for a one-month supply.

Dosage

Milk thistle is typically marketed as a standardized extract of the milk thistle seed. The preferred formulation of the extract contains 80 percent silymarin flavonoids (silybin, silydianin, and silychristin). Typical dosage recommendations are for 175 mg of 80 percent silymarin extract, taken one to three times per day.

WORKS CONSULTED

Beckmann-Knopp S, Rietbrock S, Weyhenmeyer R, Bocker RH, Beckurts KT, Lang W, Hunz M, Fuhr U. Inhibitory effects of silibinin on cytochrome P-450 enzymes in human liver microsomes. Pharmacol Toxicol. 2000 Jun;86(6):250-6.

Berkson BM. A conservative triple antioxidant approach to the treatment of hepatitis C. Combination of alpha lipoic acid (thioctic acid), silymarin, and selenium: Three case histories. Med Klin. 1999 Oct 15;94(Suppl 3):84-9.

De Martiis M, Fontana M, Assogna G, D'Ottavi R, D'Ottavi O. Milk thistle (Silybum marianum) derivatives in the therapy of chronic hepatopathies. Clin Ter. 1980 Aug 15;94(3):283-315.

De Martiis M, Fontana M, Sebastiani F, Parenzi A. Silymarin, a membranotropic drug: Clinical and experimental observations. Clin Ter. 1977 May 31;81(4):333-62.

Deak G, Muzes G, Lang I, Niederland V, Nekam K, Gonzalez-Cabello R, Gergely P, Feher J. Immunomodulator effect of silymarin therapy in chronic alcoholic liver diseases. Orv Hetil. 1990 Jun 17;131(24):1291-2, 1295-6.

Flora K, Hahn M, Rosen H, Benner K. Milk thistle (Silybum marianum) for the therapy of liver disease. Am J Gastroenterol. 1998 Feb;93(2):139-43.

Fromming KH, Saller R, Wachter W. Silymarin-containing phytopharmaceuticals—biopharmacy as an essential therapeutic quality criterion. Z Arztl Fortbild Qualitatssich. 1999 Jun;93(4):VI-XI.

Gil'miiarov EM, Radomskaia VM, Kretova IG, Vinogradova LN, Babichev AV, Ponomareva LA, Samykina LN, Sheshunov IV, Gil'miiarov EM. Biologically active additive from milk thistle in the solution of public health problems. Vopr Pitan. 1998;(3):33-5.

Kiesewetter E, Leodolter I, Thaler H. Results of two double-blind studies on the effect of silymarine in chronic hepatitis. Leber Magen Darm. 1977 Oct;7(5):318-23.

Luper S. A review of plants used in the treatment of liver disease: Part 1. Altern Med Rev. 1998 Dec;3(6):410-21.

Maitrejean M, Comte G, Barron D, El Kirat K, Conseil G, Di Pietro A. The flavanolignan silybin and its hemisynthetic derivatives, a novel series of potential modulators of P-glycoprotein. Bioorg Med Chem Lett. 2000 Jan 17;10(2):157-60.

Margaroli P, Rossi M, Arcabasso GD, Cosini I, Malacrida C. Evaluation of the therapeutic effects of silymarin. Clin Ter. 1980 Dec 31;95(6):663-72.

Morelli I. Constituents of Silybum marianum and their therapeutic use. Boll Chim Farm. 1978 May;117(5):258-67.

Par A, Roth E, Rumi G Jr, Kovacs Z, Nemes J, Mozsik G. Oxidative stress and antioxidant defense in alcoholic liver disease and chronic hepatitis C. Orv Hetil. 2000 Jul 23;141(30):1655-9.

Pepping J. Milk thistle: Silybum marianum. Am J Health Syst Pharm. 1999 Jun 15;56(12):1195-7.

Quaglia MG, Bossu E, Donati E, Mazzanti G, Brandt A. Determination of silymarine in the extract from the dried silybum marianum fruits by high performance liquid chromatography and capillary electrophoresis. J Pharm Biomed Anal. 1999 Mar;19(3-4):435-42.

Realini S, Gonvers JJ, Hofstetter JR. Clinical investigation of silymarin in chronic liver diseases. Schweiz Rundsch Med Prax. 1975 May 13;64(19):595-8.

Reutter FW, Haase W. Clinical experience with silymarin in the treatment of chronic liver disease. Schweiz Rundsch Med Prax. 1975 Sep 9;64(36):1145-51.

Rumiantseva ZN. The pharmacodynamics of hepatic protectors from the lady's-thistle. Vrach Delo. 1991 May;(5):15-9.

Saliou C, Rihn B, Cillard J, Okamoto T, Packer L. Selective inhibition of NF-kappaB activation by the flavonoid hepatoprotector silymarin in HepG2. Evidence for different activating pathways. FEBS Lett. 1998 Nov 27;440(1-2):8-12.

Sawaryn T, Szymonski K, Machalska M. Sylimarine in the treatment of chronic hepatitis. Przegl Epidemiol. 1977;31(4):445-50.

Silybum marianum (milk thistle). Altern Med Rev. 1999 Aug;4(4):272-4.

Sonnenbichler J, Scalera F, Sonnenbichler I, Weyhenmeyer R. Stimulatory effects of silibinin and silicristin from the milk thistle Silybum marianum on kidney cells. J Pharmacol Exp Ther. 1999 Sep;290(3):1375-83.

Stickel F, Egerer G, Seitz HK. Hepatotoxicity of botanicals. Public Health Nutr. 2000 Jun;3(2):113-24.

Zhao J, Sharma Y, Agarwal R. Significant inhibition by the flavonoid antioxidant silymarin against 12-O-tetradecanoylphorbol 13-acetate-caused modulation of antioxidant and inflammatory enzymes, and cyclooxygenase 2 and interleukin-1alpha expression in SENCAR mouse epidermis: Implications in the prevention of stage I tumor promotion. Mol Carcinog. 1999 Dec;26(4):321-33.

SCHISANDRA/SCHIZANDRA

What Is It?

Schisandra *(Schisandra chinensis)*, also known as wu-wei-wi and sometimes spelled with a "z" (schizandra), has a long history of use in traditional Chinese medicine as an herb capable of promoting general well-being and enhancing vitality. Schisandra and its products originate from the red berries that grow on a vine belonging to the magnolia family (sometimes the leaves are used as well). Approximately twenty-five species of schisandra exist, and all are indigenous to Asia except for a rare form of the vine that grows in wooded areas in North Carolina and surrounding states. In their dried form, schisandra berries are referred to as wu-wei-zi. In addition to its traditional uses for promoting energy and alleviating exhaustion caused by stress, schisandra has historically been taken to strengthen the sex organs, promote mental function, beautify the skin, and treat night sweats, asthma, cough, and insomnia.

Claims

- Improves the body's response to stress and boosts mood
- Promotes liver and kidney health
- Enhances aerobic capacity and energy levels
- Improves mental function

Theory

Schisandra is touted as a member of the adaptogen family, along with ginseng and related herbs, because of the presence of compounds thought to balance bodily functions related to stress. Lignans are a main constituent of schisandra; these compounds, which are a concentrated component of the seeds of the schisandra berry, may stimulate the immune system, protect the liver, increase the body's ability to cope with stress, and cause a calming or mild sedative effect. The more prominent lignans found in schisandra are schizandrin, wuweizisu C, and gomisin A. Schisandra extract also contains essential oils and acids, as well as vitamins and minerals that together could produce the claimed effects by increasing cellular efficiency in processing wastes, delivering more oxygen, and creating and using energy.

Scientific Support

A few scientific studies have been conducted to test specific effects of schisandra supplementation. In a very well controlled study performed in 1988, twenty-six patients with a specific heart malady (dilated cardiomyopathy) were given a combination of *Panax ginseng, Radix ophiopogonis,* and schisandra seed extract. Subject improvement was measured via an echocardiogram as well as a treadmill tolerance test. Subjects served as their own controls by taking the concoction or a placebo for twenty days, taking nothing for ten days, and then taking either the placebo or the mixture for twenty more days. After taking the herbs, left ventricular function improved significantly, and exercise tolerance increased from an average of 7.2 minutes to 10.7 minutes. Despite these positive results, it is not clear which of the ingredients are responsible, or whether the combination is necessary to produce beneficial results.

In a Japanese study using rats with liver injury, wuweizisu C was found to reduce measures of liver damage such as cell death and inflammatory cell infiltration. The authors of the study concluded that wuweizisu C may be useful in protecting the liver in human hepatitis as well as other liver ailments. A study testing the endurance of mice in running on a treadmill and swimming showed that treatment with schisandra extract resulted in a significant increase in work capacity.

Safety

Schisandra is generally considered to be safe and nontoxic when used as directed. Reported side effects of schisandra ingestion include mild indigestion and skin rash. Because schisandra may induce uterine muscle contractions, pregnant women should not take this herb.

Value

Schisandra is sold in liquid and capsule form as well as in the natural dried berry form. It is also found in combination with other herbs, vitamins, and minerals for immune enhancement, stress reduction, and for energy and sexual stamina. Schisandra supplements generally sell for $10 to $15 for a one-month supply.

Dosage

Typical dosage recommendations for liver health and energy are in the range of 200 to 800 mg per day.

WORKS CONSULTED

Hsieh MT, Tsai ML, Peng WH, Wu CR. Effects of Fructus schizandrae on cyclo-heximide-induced amnesia in rats. Phytother Res. 1999 May;13(3):256-7.

Ko KM, Ip SP, Poon MK, Wu SS, Che CT, Ng KH, Kong YC. Effect of a lignan-enriched fructus schisandrae extract on hepatic glutathione status in rats: Protection against carbon tetrachloride toxicity. Planta Med. 1995 Apr;61(2):134-7.

Li PC, Poon KT, Ko KM. Schisandra chinensis-dependent myocardial protective action of sheng-mai-san in rats. Am J Chin Med. 1996;24(3-4):255-62.

Liu GT. Advances in research of the action of components isolated from Fructus schizandrae chinensis on animal livers. Chung Hsi I Chieh Ho Tsa Chih. 1983 May;3(3):182-5.

Liu KT, Lesca P. Pharmacological properties of Dibenzo[a,c]cyclooctene derivatives isolated from Fructus Schizandrae Chinensis III. Inhibitory effects on carbon tetrachloride-induced lipid peroxidation, metabolism and covalent binding of carbon tetrachloride to lipids. Chem Biol Interact. 1982 Jul 15;41(1):39-47.

Liu KT, Lesca P. Pharmacological properties of dibenzo[a,c]cyclooctene derivatives isolated from Fructus Schizandrae chinensis. I. Interaction with rat liver cytochrome P-450 and inhibition of xenobiotic metabolism and mutagenicity. Chem Biol Interact. 1982 Apr;39(3):301-14.

Yan-yong C, Zeng-bao S, Lian-niang L. Studies of Fructus schizandrae. IV. Isolation and determination of the active compounds (in lowering high SGPT levels) of Schizandra chinensis Baill. Sci Sin. 1976 Mar-Apr;19(2):276-90.

LYCOPENE

What Is It?

Lycopene is a carotenoid (like beta-carotene) that is responsible for giving tomatoes their red color. Although there are about 600 carotenoids, lycopene is the most abundant form found in the U.S. diet (beta-carotene is number two). More than 80 percent of the lycopene consumed in the United States comes from tomato sauce, pizza sauce, and ketchup. The lycopene content of tomatoes can be influenced dramatically during the ripening process, and large differences are noted between various types of tomatoes (e.g., red varieties have more lycopene than yellow). The bioavailability of lycopene is increased following cooking—so processed tomato products such as ketchup, tomato juice, and pizza sauce have more bioavailable lycopene than do fresh tomatoes.

Claims

- Protects against cancer
- General antioxidant
- Protects against cardiovascular disease

Theory

In 1999, the H.J. Heinz Company (the tomato ketchup people) launched a consumer awareness campaign about lycopene. The ads were accompanied by the headline "Lycopene may help reduce the risk of prostate and cervical cancer"—not bad for a bottle of ketchup. Because lycopene is a potent antioxidant and seems to inhibit growth of cancer cells, it is logical that a higher intake of this carotenoid may indeed be associated with reduced incidence of cancer. In addition, lycopene may also help prevent heart disease through the same antioxidant mechanism via an inhibition of LDL cholesterol oxidation. Finally, lycopene is known to play a role, along with beta-carotene, in protecting the skin from the damaging effects of ultraviolet light radiation.

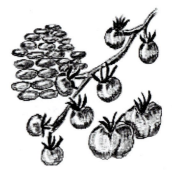

Scientific Support

The theory behind lycopene's cancer preventive benefits is logical. Indeed, plasma lycopene levels are clearly reduced, by about 40 to 50 percent, in smokers whose lungs are exposed to a high degree of oxidative damage, and several epidemiological studies have shown that consumption of foods high in lycopene (tomatoes, pizza sauce, and tomato juice) is associated with lower rates of prostate cancer. Dietary supplements containing 10 to 40 mg of lycopene have been shown to reduce DNA damage in white blood cells—probably due to the reduction in oxidative damage to DNA and lipoproteins. However, it is important to remember the recent history of lycopene's carotenoid cousin, beta-carotene, which was associated with reduced disease incidence when consumed in *foods,* but appeared less effective, and in some cases *detrimental,* when consumed as isolated high-dose dietary supplements.

In a study of patients suffering from prostate cancer, lycopene supplements have been shown to slow tumor growth. In subjects consuming the lycopene supplement, prostate tumors shrank and produced lower levels of prostate-specific antigen (PSA), a marker compound produced by active prostate cancer cells. An interesting note with this study was that the supplement used was not a purified lycopene supplement, but a high-lycopene tomato concentrate, suggesting that other tomato compounds in addition to lycopene may contribute to the protective effect. Another study concluded that regular consumption of a variety of processed tomato products—such as ketchup, tomato juice, and tomato sauce—significantly raises blood levels of lycopene.

Safety

No significant adverse side effects are associated with regular consumption of supplemental levels of lycopene, but owing to the controversy surrounding high doses of supplemental beta-carotene (which appears to increase lung cancer risk), doses of lycopene should remain in the range of levels attainable from a diet high in tomato-based products (10 to 40 mg per day).

Value

Until recently, virtually all lycopene supplements were extremely expensive, and many still are. Recently, however, supplement manufacturers have introduced a synthetic lycopene that should cut the cost of lycopene-containing supplements about five times. Although the new synthetic lycopene appears to match the natural food form in terms of chemical configuration (predominantly all-*trans*), the question still remains whether purified lycopene supplements or the more expensive tomato extracts are more effective.

As an antioxidant, lycopene is twice as effective as beta-carotene in protecting white blood cells from membrane damage due to free radicals. For individuals undergoing pharmaceutical treatment of high cholesterol or triglycerides, it is important to be aware that common treatments such as cholestyramine and probucol have been shown to reduce plasma lycopene levels by 30 to 40 percent.

Dosage

The most compelling cancer prevention data suggests that ten servings of tomato products per week can reduce the risk of prostate cancer by approximately 35 percent. Depending on the specific food sources consumed, lycopene intake may fall in the 20 to 100 mg range. Regular consumption of tomato products is recommended as your primary lycopene source, with 10 to 40 mg of supplemental lycopene for added antioxidant support.

WORKS CONSULTED

Agarwal S, Rao AV. Tomato lycopene and its role in human health and chronic diseases. CMAJ. 2000 Sep 19;163(6):739-44.

Amir H, Karas M, Giat J, Danilenko M, Levy R, Yermiahu T, Levy J, Sharoni Y. Lycopene and 1,25-dihydroxyvitamin D3 cooperate in the inhibition of cell cycle progression and induction of differentiation in HL-60 leukemic cells. Nutr Cancer. 1999;33(1):105-12.

Arab L, Steck S. Lycopene and cardiovascular disease. Am J Clin Nutr. 2000 Jun;71(6 Suppl):1691S-5S; discussion 1696S-7S.

Bohm V, Bitsch R. Intestinal absorption of lycopene from different matrices and interactions to other carotenoids, the lipid status, and the antioxidant capacity of human plasma. Eur J Nutr. 1999 Jun;38(3):118-25.

Bramley PM. Is lycopene beneficial to human health? Phytochemistry. 2000 Jun;54(3):233-6.

Casso D, White E, Patterson RE, Agurs-Collins T, Kooperberg C, Haines PS. Correlates of serum lycopene in older women. Nutr Cancer. 2000;36(2):163-9.

Davies J. Tomatoes and health. J R Soc Health. 2000 Jun;120(2):81-2.

De Stefani E, Oreggia F, Boffetta P, Deneo-Pellegrini H, Ronco A, Mendilaharsu M. Tomatoes, tomato-rich foods, lycopene and cancer of the upper aerodigestive tract: A case-control in Uruguay. Oral Oncol. 2000 Jan;36(1):47-53.

Gann PH, Ma J, Giovannucci E, Willett W, Sacks FM, Hennekens CH, Stampfer MJ. Lower prostate cancer risk in men with elevated plasma lycopene levels: Results of a prospective analysis. Cancer Res. 1999 Mar 15;59(6):1225-30.

Giovannucci E. Tomatoes, tomato-based products, lycopene, and cancer: Review of the epidemiologic literature. J Natl Cancer Inst. 1999 Feb 17;91(4):317-31.

Grant WB. Calcium, lycopene, vitamin D and prostate cancer. Prostate. 2000 Feb 15;42(3):243.

Heber D. Colorful cancer prevention: Alpha-carotene, lycopene, and lung cancer. Am J Clin Nutr. 2000 Oct;72(4):901-2.

Hughes DA, Wright AJ, Finglas PM, Polley AC, Bailey AL, Astley SB, Southon S. Effects of lycopene and lutein supplementation on the expression of functionally associated surface molecules on blood monocytes from healthy male nonsmokers. J Infect Dis. 2000 Sep;182(Suppl 1):S11-5.

Karas M, Amir H, Fishman D, Danilenko M, Segal S, Nahum A, Koifmann A, Giat Y, Levy J, Sharoni Y. Lycopene interferes with cell cycle progression and insulin-like growth factor I signaling in mammary cancer cells. Nutr Cancer. 2000;36(1):101-11.

Kelloff GJ, Lieberman R, Steele VE, Boone CW, Lubet RA, Kopelovitch L, Malone WA, Crowell JA, Sigman CC. Chemoprevention of prostate cancer: Concepts and strategies. Eur Urol. 1999;35(5-6):342-50.

Lowe GM, Booth LA, Young AJ, Bilton RF. Lycopene and beta-carotene protect against oxidative damage in HT29 cells at low concentrations but rapidly lose this capacity at higher doses. Free Radic Res. 1999 Feb;30(2):141-51.

Mayne ST, Cartmel B, Silva F, Kim CS, Fallon BG, Briskin K, Zheng T, Baum M, Shor-Posner G, Goodwin WJ Jr. Plasma lycopene concentrations in humans are determined by lycopene intake, plasma cholesterol concentrations and selected demographic factors. J Nutr. 1999 Apr;129(4):849-54.

Michaud DS, Feskanich D, Rimm EB, Colditz GA, Speizer FE, Willett WC, Giovannucci E. Intake of specific carotenoids and risk of lung cancer in 2 prospective US cohorts. Am J Clin Nutr. 2000 Oct;72(4):990-7.

Norrish AE, Jackson RT, Sharpe SJ, Skeaff CM. Prostate cancer and dietary carotenoids. Am J Epidemiol. 2000 Jan 15;151(2):119-23.

Paetau I, Rao D, Wiley ER, Brown ED, Clevidence BA. Carotenoids in human buccal mucosa cells after 4 wk of supplementation with tomato juice or lycopene supplements. Am J Clin Nutr. 1999 Oct;70(4):490-4.

Pellegrini N, Riso P, Porrini M. Tomato consumption does not affect the total antioxidant capacity of plasma. Nutrition. 2000 Apr;16(4):268-71.

Porrini M, Riso P. Lymphocyte lycopene concentration and DNA protection from oxidative damage is increased in women after a short period of tomato consumption. J Nutr. 2000 Feb;130(2):189-92.

Rao AV, Agarwal S. Role of antioxidant lycopene in cancer and heart disease. J Am Coll Nutr. 2000 Oct;19(5):563-9.

Rao AV, Fleshner N, Agarwal S. Serum and tissue lycopene and biomarkers of oxidation in prostate cancer patients: A case-control study. Nutr Cancer. 1999;33(2):159-64.

Riso P, Pinder A, Santangelo A, Porrini M. Does tomato consumption effectively increase the resistance of lymphocyte DNA to oxidative damage? Am J Clin Nutr. 1999 Apr;69(4):712-8.

Sengupta A, Das S. The anti-carcinogenic role of lycopene, abundantly present in tomato. Eur J Cancer Prev. 1999 Aug;8(4):325-30.

Shi J, Le Maguer M. Lycopene in tomatoes: Chemical and physical properties affected by food processing. Crit Rev Food Sci Nutr. 2000 Jan;40(1):1-42.

Siems WG, Sommerburg O, van Kuijk FJ. Lycopene and beta-carotene decompose more rapidly than lutein and zeaxanthin upon exposure to various pro-oxidants in vitro. Biofactors. 1999;10(2-3):105-13.

Slattery ML, Benson J, Curtin K, Ma KN, Schaeffer D, Potter JD. Carotenoids and colon cancer. Am J Clin Nutr. 2000 Feb;71(2):575-82.

Sutherland WH, Walker RJ, De Jong SA, Upritchard JE. Supplementation with tomato juice increases plasma lycopene but does not alter susceptibility to oxidation of low-density lipoproteins from renal transplant recipients. Clin Nephrol. 1999 Jul;52(1):30-6.

Wright AJ, Hughes DA, Bailey AL, Southon S. Beta-carotene and lycopene, but not lutein, supplementation changes the plasma fatty acid profile of healthy male non-smokers. J Lab Clin Med. 1999 Dec;134(6):592-8.

SHARK CARTILAGE/BOVINE TRACHEAL CARTILAGE

What Is It?

Cartilage extracts are just what you think they are—from sharks, the fins are typically used, while cartilage from the trachea (windpipe) of cows is used in bovine cartilage supplements. The cartilage is then pulverized, powdered, and packed into capsules.

Claims

- Cures/prevents cancer
- Promotes wound healing
- Relieves arthritis pain and stiffness

Theory

Cartilage has been linked to healing of connective tissue injuries since the middle part of the century (much as HCP/gelatin, glucosamine, and chondroitin are today). In the early 1980s, cartilage extracts became a popular alternative treatment for reducing the pain and stiffness associated with arthritis (although gelatin, SAMe, and glucosamine all appear to be more effective in this regard). Today, the most common use of cartilage supplements is as a cancer treatment. As the theory goes, cartilage supplements inhibit tumor growth by inhibiting angiogenesis (growth of new blood vessels) and choking off the blood supply that the tumor needs to survive and grow. This popular, but unproven, theory generated a wave of media attention in the 1980s following publication of a popular pseudoscientific book titled *Sharks Don't Get Cancer* (but they actually *do*).

Scientific Support

Although there is certainly no shortage of testimonials for "miracle" cartilage products that "cure" cancer, the scientific evidence for such effects is lacking. Despite the promotion of shark and bovine cartilage supplements as cancer cures, careful scientific study in people with advanced tumors has shown these claims to be wildly optimistic at best and completely bogus in many cases. It is estimated that more than 100,000 U.S. cancer victims have tried shark cartilage, either alone or in conjunction with standard chemotherapy. Unfortunately, the majority of studies that have tested shark cartilage on cancer patients have found little or no effect in slowing the disease or improving quality of life. In one recent study, sixty patients with various cancers saw no improvements in tumor size or disease stage.

An interesting 1983 report in the prestigious journal *Science,* however, indicates that shark cartilage does indeed contain compounds that can inhibit tumor angiogenesis. This means that *something* in cartilage prevents the growth of new blood vessels toward tumors, thereby restricting tumor growth. The inhibitor is probably not a typical protein, but may be a heat-stable form of proteoglycans (long chains of sugars and amino acids). Whatever this factor happens to be, it turns out that there is quite a lot of it in shark cartilage compared to cartilage from mammalian sources (such as cows). A major problem with the shark cartilage theory of tumor prevention, however, has always been the lack of clinical proof that this antiangiogenesis factor could even get into the body when consumed as a dietary supplement.

However, studies reported over the last two to three years suggest that oral administration of liquid cartilage extract delivers an antiangiogenic effect in humans similar to that previously observed in lab animals and test-tube studies. In one study, subjects (twenty-nine healthy males) received either a placebo or a liquid shark cartilage extract (7 to 21 ml) each day for three to four weeks. Midway through the supplementation period (day twelve), a special sponge was inserted subcutaneously (under the skin of each subject's arm) that was removed on day twenty-three. Researchers then counted the number of cells that had grown into the sponge as an indirect measurement of angiogenesis. Results from the study showed that cell density was significantly lower in subjects who had received the liquid cartilage extract than in subjects who had received the placebo. These results are the first to show that the antiangiogenic component of cartilage extracts is bioavailable in humans by oral administration and that oral intake of such extracts can actually reduce blood vessel growth in the body. The next step will be to conduct controlled clinical trials in cancer patients to see whether cartilage extracts can indeed choke off cancerous tumors and live up to the claims made for many of the supplements currently on the market.

One of the largest manufacturers of shark cartilage supplements has funded several small studies of their supplements in treating cancer—unfortunately, results have been mixed. The National Cancer Institute has recently announced its intention to fund a phase III clinical trial of shark cartilage for treatment of cancer—with a portion of the money for the study coming from a legal judgment against shark cartilage companies for making false claims about the ability of these products to cure cancer.

Safety

Although no specific safety studies have been conducted on cartilage extracts, the doses commonly suggested are not expected to cause any significant side effects (or benefits). In some isolated cases, bovine tracheal cartilage has been associated with contamination by thyroid tissue (the trachea is located adjacent to the thyroid gland), which could potentially lead to thyroid hormone toxicity.

Value

At this time, cartilage extracts do not appear to provide significant value as a dietary supplement. As research into this area progresses, perhaps new findings will provide evidence that cartilage extracts prevent angiogenesis in cancer patients. Until then, consider other supplements with proven benefits in joint health and wound healing (HCP/gelatin, SAMe, glucosamine, and chondroitin) and cancer prevention (green tea and soy isoflavones).

Dosage

If you *do* choose to supplement with cartilage extracts, typical dosage recommendations are likely to be in the range of 250 to 1,000 mg per day, although significant differences may exist between products.

WORKS CONSULTED

Ashar B, Vargo E. Shark cartilage-induced hepatitis. Ann Intern Med. 1996 Nov 1;125(9):780-1.

Berbari P, Thibodeau A, Germain L, Saint-Cyr M, Gaudreau P, Elkhouri S, Dupont E, Garrel DR, El-Khouri S. Antiangiogenic effects of the oral administration of liquid cartilage extract in humans. J Surg Res. 1999 Nov;87(1):108-13.

Blackadar CB. Skeptics of oral administration of shark cartilage. J Natl Cancer Inst. 1993 Dec 1;85(23):1961-2.

Chen JS, Chang CM, Wu JC, Wang SM. Shark cartilage extract interferes with cell adhesion and induces reorganization of focal adhesions in cultured endothelial cells. J Cell Biochem. 2000 Jun 6;78(3):417-28.

Couzin J. Beefed-up NIH center probes unconventional therapies. Science. 1998 Dec 18;282(5397):2175-6.

Davis PF, He Y, Furneaux RH, Johnston PS, Ruger BM, Slim GC. Inhibition of angiogenesis by oral ingestion of powdered shark cartilage in a rat model. Microvasc Res. 1997 Sep;54(2):178-82.

Dupont E, Savard PE, Jourdain C, Juneau C, Thibodeau A, Ross N, Marenus K, Maes DH, Pelletier G, Sauder DN. Antiangiogenic properties of a novel shark cartilage extract: Potential role in the treatment of psoriasis. J Cutan Med Surg. 1998 Jan;2(3):146-52.

Ernst E. Shark cartilage for cancer? Lancet. 1998 Jan 24;351(9098):298.

Ernst E, Cassileth BR. How useful are unconventional cancer treatments? Eur J Cancer. 1999 Oct;35(11):1608-13.

Felzenszwalb I, Pelielo de Mattos JC, Bernardo-Filho M, Caldeira-de-Araujo A. Shark cartilage-containing preparation: Protection against reactive oxygen species. Food Chem Toxicol. 1998 Dec;36(12):1079-84.

Fontenele JB, Araujo GB, de Alencar JW, Viana GS. The analgesic and anti-inflammatory effects of shark cartilage are due to a peptide molecule and are nitric oxide (NO) system dependent. Biol Pharm Bull. 1997 Nov;20(11):1151-4.

Fontenele JB, Viana GS, Xavier-Filho J, de-Alencar JW. Anti-inflammatory and analgesic activity of a water-soluble fraction from shark cartilage. Braz J Med Biol Res. 1996 May;29(5):643-6.

Gomes EM, Souto PR, Felzenszwalb I. Shark-cartilage containing preparation protects cells against hydrogen peroxide induced damage and mutagenesis. Mutat Res. 1996 Apr 6;367(4):204-8.

Gotay CC, Dumitriu D. Health food store recommendations for breast cancer patients. Arch Fam Med. 2000 Aug;9(8):692-9.

Horsman MR, Alsner J, Overgaard J. The effect of shark cartilage extracts on the growth and metastatic spread of the SCCVII carcinoma. Acta Oncol. 1998; 37(5):441-5.

Hunt TJ, Connelly JF. Shark cartilage for cancer treatment. Am J Health Syst Pharm. 1995 Aug 15;52(16):1756, 1760.

Lane IW and Comac L. Sharks Don't Get Cancer. Garden City, NY: Avery Publishing, 1992.

Lee A, Langer R. Shark cartilage contains inhibitors of tumor angiogenesis. Science. 1983 Sep 16;221(4616):1185-7.

Liang JH, Wong KP. The characterization of angiogenesis inhibitor from shark cartilage. Adv Exp Med Biol. 2000;476:209-23.

Markman M. Shark cartilage: The Laetrile of the 1990s. Cleve Clin J Med. 1996 May-Jun;63(3):179-80.

Mathews J. Media feeds frenzy over shark cartilage as cancer treatment. J Natl Cancer Inst. 1993 Aug 4;85(15):1190-1.

McGuire TR, Kazakoff PW, Hoie EB, Fienhold MA. Antiproliferative activity of shark cartilage with and without tumor necrosis factor-alpha in human umbilical vein endothelium. Pharmacotherapy. 1996 Mar-Apr;16(2):237-44.

Miller DR, Anderson GT, Stark JJ, Granick JL, Richardson D. Phase I/II trial of the safety and efficacy of shark cartilage in the treatment of advanced cancer. J Clin Oncol. 1998 Nov;16(11):3649-55.

Morris GM, Coderre JA, Micca PL, Lombardo DT, Hopewell JW. Boron neutron capture therapy of the rat 9L gliosarcoma: Evaluation of the effects of shark cartilage. Br J Radiol. 2000 Apr;73(868):429-34.

Newman V, Rock CL, Faerber S, Flatt SW, Wright FA, Pierce JP. Dietary supplement use by women at risk for breast cancer recurrence. The Women's Healthy Eating and Living Study Group. J Am Diet Assoc. 1998 Mar;98(3):285-92.

Oikawa T, Ashino-Fuse H, Shimamura M, Koide U, Iwaguchi T. A novel angiogenic inhibitor derived from Japanese shark cartilage (I). Extraction and estimation of inhibitory activities toward tumor and embryonic angiogenesis. Cancer Lett. 1990 Jun 15;51(3):181-6.

Oneschuk D, Fennell L, Hanson J, Bruera E. The use of complementary medications by cancer patients attending an outpatient pain and symptom clinic. J Palliat Care. 1998 Winter;14(4):21-6.

Sheu JR, Fu CC, Tsai ML, Chung WJ. Effect of U-995, a potent shark cartilage-derived angiogenesis inhibitor, on anti-angiogenesis and anti-tumor activities. Anticancer Res. 1998 Nov-Dec;18(6A):4435-41.

Simone CB, Simone NL, Simone CB 2nd. Shark cartilage for cancer. Lancet. 1998 May 9;351(9113):1440.

Steurer J. Shark cartilage on the Internet. Schweiz Med Wochenschr. 1999 Dec 28;129(51-52):1996-7.

SPIRULINA/BLUE-GREEN ALGAE

What Is It?

The term "spirulina" includes various species of primitive unicellular blue-green algae, most commonly *Spirulina maxima* and *Spirulina platensis*. These microscopic plants grow naturally in lakes rich in salt, particularly in Central and South America, Australia, and Africa. The bulk of these microscopic aquatic plants used in supplements are grown and harvested in outdoor tanks in California, Hawaii, and Asia. Since ancient times, natives of Mexico and Africa have eaten spirulina for its nutritive value. More recently, however, scientific studies have supported its roles as an antiviral, antimutagenic, and cholesterol-lowering agent—primarily due to the presence of carotenoids and other nutrients and antioxidants in the tiny plants.

Claims

- Prevents and inhibits cancerous oral lesions
- Stimulates immune defenses and inhibits replication of certain viruses
- Prevents heart disease (lowers cholesterol)
- Provides antioxidants and other nutrients
- Improves weight loss

Theory

Because spirulina is a whole organism, it contains many important nutrients, including all of the essential amino acids (those which the human body cannot produce), vitamins, minerals, and essential fatty acids. It also contains chlorophyll and carotenoids, both of which have antioxidant properties. Because spirulina contains high levels of protein and low levels of fat, powder made from this alga is often mixed with juice as a supplement to low-calorie diets. Spirulina is also a rich source of gamma-linoleic acid (GLA), an essential fatty acid found in foods as well as in dietary supplements such as evening primrose oil. Because people with GLA deficiencies are thought to produce more fat in their bodies, it is hypothesized that supplementing with GLA could promote loss of body fat. Spirulina also contains a novel polysaccharide called calcium spirulan (Ca-SP) that may have antiviral and antithrombic (clot-busting) activity. Because it is a rich source of antioxidants and other nutrients, spirulina may have modest cancer-fighting activities as well.

Scientific Support

Support for the use of spirulina in preventing and treating oral cancer is quite encouraging. In a study performed in India, supplementation with 1 g per day of spirulina for twelve months led to complete regression of oral cancerous lesions in twenty of forty-four subjects (45 percent), all of whom were tobacco chewers. A year after discontinuation of spirulina supplementation, nine out of twenty of the responders (45 percent) redeveloped lesions. These results were also duplicated using animal models of oral cancer, but whether the positive results from these studies are due simply to spirulina's high beta-carotene content remains to be studied.

To investigate its antiviral properties, using human immune cell lines (a test-tube study), scientists found that an extract from *Spirulina platensis* was effective in inhibiting HIV-1 replication and infectivity by up to 50 percent, and Ca-SP isolated from spirulina may inhibit the replication of other viruses.

No scientific studies were found to support the role of spirulina as a weight loss agent in humans. However, the theory behind its potential use may have a kernel of truth or merit. Since spirulina is a rich source of nutrients with only 5 percent fat (mostly composed of essential fatty acids), supplementation with spirulina could be viewed as a general, if somewhat nonspecific, method of increasing phytonutrient intake. Furthermore, it is thought that people with low dietary intakes of GLA may also have a more difficult time losing body fat. Normalizing GLA levels by supplementing with spirulina (or evening primrose oil) could help one lose excess body fat. Unfortunately, scientific support does not exist to bolster either of these claims.

Safety

Studies in animals fed large quantities of spirulina have shown no toxic effects. However, in rare cases, people have experienced allergic reactions to spirulina. Studies in pregnant rats have shown that even at very high levels, dietary ingestion of spirulina was not associated with any fetal toxicity or birth defects. The most important safety concern with regard to spirulina supplementation has to do with the environment in which the spirulina is grown. Spirulina that is grown in water contaminated with toxic metals such as lead, mercury, and cadmium can result in contaminated supplements. Therefore, it is very important to carefully select a well-respected manufacturer that performs regular screening to rule out heavy metal contamination. Finally, although spirulina is often advocated as a safe source of the micronutrient vitamin B_{12}, studies have shown that the B_{12} contained in spirulina is not readily absorbed. Therefore, spirulina should not be taken for the explicit purpose of combating B_{12} deficiency. Finally, because spirulina may have mild anticlotting actions, anybody who is taking blood-thinning medications should not take spirulina unless otherwise advised by a physician.

Value

Spirulina is available in tablet, capsule, or powder form at an average cost of approximately $10 to $30 per month. For people with oral cancer, spirulina may be a relatively inexpensive and safe supplement to try.

Dosage

Typical dosage recommendations are in the range of 2 to 3 g (2,000 to 3,000 mg) of spirulina per day. Most tablets and capsules provide 400 to 500 mg and need to be taken several times per day. Spirulina is also sold in flake or powder form and may be added to juice or sprinkled onto food or into soups.

WORKS CONSULTED

Chamorro G, Salazar M. Teratogenic study of Spirulina in mice. Arch Latinoam Nutr. 1990 Mar;40(1):86-94.

Chamorro G, Salazar M, Salazar S. Teratogenic study of Spirulina in rats. Arch Latinoam Nutr. 1989 Dec;39(4):641-9.

Delpeuch F, Joseph A, Cavelier C. Consumption and nutritional contribution of the blue algae (Oscillatoria platensis) among some populations of Kanem. Ann Nutr Aliment. 1975;29(6):497-516.

Gonzalez de Rivera C, Miranda-Zamora R, Diaz-Zagoya JC, Juarez-Oropeza MA. Preventive effect of Spirulina maxima on the fatty liver induced by a fructose-rich diet in the rat, a preliminary report. Life Sci. 1993;53(1):57-61.

Hayashi O, Hirahashi T, Katoh T, Miyajima H, Hirano T, Okuwaki Y. Class specific influence of dietary Spirulina platensis on antibody production in mice. J Nutr Sci Vitaminol (Tokyo). 1998 Dec;44(6):841-51.

Hayashi O, Katoh T, Okuwaki Y. Enhancement of antibody production in mice by dietary Spirulina platensis. J Nutr Sci Vitaminol (Tokyo). 1994 Oct;40(5):431-41.

Iwata K, Inayama T, Kato T. Effects of Spirulina platensis on plasma lipoprotein lipase activity in fructose-induced hyperlipidemic rats. J Nutr Sci Vitaminol (Tokyo). 1990 Apr;36(2):165-71.

Kapoor R, Mehta U. Effect of supplementation of blue green alga (Spirulina) on outcome of pregnancy in rats. Plant Foods Hum Nutr. 1993 Jan;43(1):29-35.

Kapoor R, Mehta U. Supplementary effect of spirulina on hematological status of rats during pregnancy and lactation. Plant Foods Hum Nutr. 1998;52(4):315-24.

Kay RA. Microalgae as food and supplement. Crit Rev Food Sci Nutr. 1991;30(6):555-73.

Maranesi M, Barzanti V, Carenini G, Gentili P. Nutritional studies on Spirulina maxima. Acta Vitaminol Enzymol. 1984;6(4):295-304.

Mitchell GV, Grundel E, Jenkins M, Blakely SR. Effects of graded dietary levels of Spirulina maxima on vitamins A and E in male rats. J Nutr. 1990 Oct;120(10):1235-40.

Paredes-Carbajal MC, Torres-Duran PV, Diaz-Zagoya JC, Mascher D, Juarez-Oropeza MA. Effects of dietary Spirulina maxima on endothelium dependent vasomotor responses of rat aortic rings. Life Sci. 1997;61(15):PL 211-9.

Ross E, Dominy W. The nutritional value of dehydrated, blue-green algae (Spirulina platensis) for poultry. Poult Sci. 1990 May;69(5):794-800.

Salazar M, Chamorro GA, Salazar S, Steele CE. Effect of Spirulina maxima consumption on reproduction and peri- and postnatal development in rats. Food Chem Toxicol. 1996 Apr;34(4):353-9.

Salazar M, Martinez E, Madrigal E, Ruiz LE, Chamorro GA. Subchronic toxicity study in mice fed Spirulina maxima. J Ethnopharmacol. 1998 Oct;62(3):235-41.

Torres-Duran PV, Miranda-Zamora R, Paredes-Carbajal MC, Mascher D, Ble-Castillo J, Diaz-Zagoya JC, Juarez-Oropeza MA. Studies on the preventive effect of Spirulina maxima on fatty liver development induced by carbon tetrachloride, in the rat. J Ethnopharmacol. 1999 Feb;64(2):141-7.

Torres-Duran PV, Miranda-Zamora R, Paredes-Carbajal MC, Mascher D, Diaz-Zagoya JC, Juarez-Oropeza MA. Spirulina maxima prevents induction of fatty liver by carbon tetrachloride in the rat. Biochem Mol Biol Int. 1998 Apr;44(4):787-93.

Venkataraman LV, Somasekaran T, Becker EW. Replacement value of blue-green alga (Spirulina platensis) for fishmeal and a vitamin-mineral premix for broiler chicks. Br Poult Sci. 1994 Jul;35(3):373-81.

Chapter 17

Supplements for Support During Diabetes

INTRODUCTION

Nearly 16 million people in the United States have diabetes, and another 14 million have impaired fasting glucose or the "prediabetes" that is a precursor to development of the metabolic syndrome. Every day, over 2,000 people are newly diagnosed with the condition, while many millions more are completely unaware that they too may be affected. In the long term, diabetes typically leads to complications, such as blindness (retinopathy and cataract), heart disease, stroke, kidney failure, amputations, and painful nerve damage.

The two major types of diabetes are known as type 1 and type 2 diabetes. Type 1 diabetes (also known as insulin-dependent diabetes mellitus, IDDM, or juvenile diabetes) accounts for only about 5 to 10 percent of diabetes cases. It is considered an autoimmune disease because the immune system attacks the insulin-producing beta cells in the pancreas, resulting in the production of little or no insulin.

Over 90 percent of people with diabetes have type 2 diabetes (also known as non–insulin-dependent diabetes mellitus or NIDDM). Type 2 diabetes most often affects adults over age forty, especially when overweight. In type 2 diabetes, the pancreas usually produces insulin, but the body does not use the insulin effectively. In other words, the body's cells and tissues are more or less insulin-resistant or insulin-insensitive. Ultimately, blood sugar increases, since the body can't use it. The symptoms of type 2 diabetes develop gradually and include fatigue, frequent urination, thirst, blurred vision, slow healing of sores, and frequent infections.

The condition known as "impaired fasting glucose" is the silent (often undiagnosed) precursor of type 2 diabetes. It is important to detect impaired fasting glucose early, because at this stage, the condition responds well to lifestyle changes (diet, exercise, and supplements), which may prevent or delay the progression into full-blown type 2 diabetes.

Good management of diabetes, i.e., keeping blood glucose near normal, can significantly lower the risk and progression of eye, kidney, nerve, and cardiovascular complications and improve quality of life. Effective diabetes management usually includes drug therapy together with lifestyle changes, such as regular physical activity, balanced diet, and prudent dietary supplementation.

SUPPLEMENTS THAT MAY HELP

People with diabetes can benefit greatly from a number of the dietary supplements outlined in this chapter. When combined with a proper diet and exercise regimen, these supplements can provide one or more of the following three major health benefits:

1. Addressing the specific nutrient deficiencies common in people with diabetes
2. Improving blood sugar levels and insulin function
3. Reducing the development and/or severity of diabetes complications, such as diabetic neuropathy (nerve damage), retinopathy (eye retina damage), cataract, microangiopathy (blood vessel damage), and kidney disease

A few words of caution though, before reading on: First, don't view supplements as drugs. Although some nutrients or herbs may be able to lower blood sugar levels and improve insulin function, they are not intended to replace drug therapy. However, as you will see, many nutritional and herbal supplements can lower blood sugar levels. Diabetic people who start a nutritional supplementation program may need to reduce the dosage of insulin or oral hypoglycemic medications. If you don't watch your blood sugar levels closely and adjust medications accordingly, you may experience hypoglycemia. Finally, supplements work best when you also make other lifestyle changes, such as maintaining a normal body weight, regular exercise, and eating a healthy diet.

Chromium is a trace mineral that's essential for normal insulin function. Dietary studies indicate that most people in the United States and other industrialized countries don't get enough chromium, and deficiencies appear to be even more common in diabetic people. Many clinical studies support the benefits and safety of chromium supplementation in diabetic people. Supplemental chromium can lower blood insulin levels, improve glucose tolerance, and decrease hemoglobin glycosylation in people with type 2 diabetes. Chromium also helps maintain healthy blood levels of triglycerides and HDL cholesterol. Experts from the U.S. Dept. of Agriculture recommend chromium supplementation in daily amounts of 200 to 1,000 mcg. Clinical studies show that the inorganic forms of chromium, such as chromium chloride, are not as effective as the organic or chelated forms, such as chromium polynicotinate, picolinate, glycine-niacin chelate, GTF chromium, and chromium yeast. However, recent laboratory studies questioned the safety of chromium picolinate and in particular of picolinic acid at very high concentrations. Since people with diabetes may wish to supplement with chromium long-term at high levels, e.g., up to 1,000 mcg per day, they may be well advised to avoid chromium picolinate for the time being.

Vanadium is another trace element involved in promoting normal insulin function. Safe and adequate dietary intakes range from approximately 10 to 100 mcg of vanadium per day. Some studies have shown that megadoses of vanadium as vanadyl sulfate can improve glucose tolerance in type 2 diabetics. However, the vanadium doses used in these studies are 200 to 1,000 times above safe dietary intakes, and the long-term safety of these pharmacological doses has not been established. High-dose vanadyl sulfate (i.e., above 100 mcg per day) should only be taken under the supervision of your physician. Supplementation with up to 100 mcg per day is safe and will cover the body's nutritional vanadium needs, including the proposed functions of vanadium in insulin and glucose metabolism.

Magnesium is an essential mineral for nerve function, heart rhythm, energy metabolism, and bone structure. Most of us don't get enough magnesium from our diets, and people with diabetes are at even higher risk of magnesium deficiency. Experts recommend magnesium supplementation for people with diabetes. Daily magnesium intakes of 150 to 400 mg are safe and effective, provided that the magnesium is in a form that is bioavailable. The most widely available form is magnesium oxide, but it has very poor bioavailability. Much better absorption is typically seen with magnesium forms such as aspartate, amino acid chelate, and glycinate.

Zinc deficiency is also quite common in people with diabetes. Zinc is an essential trace mineral for immune function, antioxidant protection, and reproduction. Three out of four of us do not meet the recommended intakes for zinc. Zinc supplementation is especially important for diabetics because it also promotes normal insulin function. However, to avoid unwanted nutrient interactions, zinc should not be supplemented in high doses (e.g., above 30 mg daily) and is best taken in balance with other trace elements.

Antioxidant supplements can play an important role for people with diabetes, because diabetics have much higher levels of free radical damage than nondiabetics do. Dozens of clinical studies show that dietary supplementation with antioxidant nutrients can help slow down the development and progression of secondary diabetes complications such as cataract, retinopathy, nerve damage (neuropathy), kidney disease, and microvascular disease. The most important antioxidant nutrients to consider as supplements for diabetics are alpha-lipoic acid, vitamin E, and vitamin C. These antioxidant nutrients are best supplemented in combination rather than as megadose single-nutrient products, because the body's antioxidant defense system consists of many interacting and synergistic components that depend on a variety of dietary antioxidants.

Alpha-lipoic acid has been established by many European and U.S. studies as an important antioxidant for diabetics. Alpha-lipoic acid has been named "the universal antioxidant" because it reacts with many different free radicals. In people with diabetes, alpha-lipoic acid supplementation enhances insulin action and can reduce or reverse peripheral neuropathy (nerve damage). The most effective daily dose in these studies is 600 mg. Higher doses (1,200 to 1,800 mg per day) are not significantly more useful than 600 mg per day, and can cause some tolerance problems. People with diabetic neuropathy may try 600 mg per day for two to three months, and then go down to about 100 mg per day for maintenance. A dose of 100 mg per day is also appropriate for more general antioxidant support and nerve protection in diabetics without neuropathy.

Vitamin E nutrition is generally very poor in the U.S. population and in people with diabetes. Vitamin E supplementation enhances antioxidant protection of the nervous system and protects body proteins in diabetics. Vitamin E at 100 IU daily can reduce protein glycosylation (hemoglobin) and platelet aggregation in people with diabetes. The common practice of high-dose supplementation with only the alpha-tocopherol form of vitamin E has been criticized because it disturbs the body's balance of other important forms of vitamin E, especially gamma-tocopherol. Thus, it seems prudent to recommend daily supplementation with moderate doses, such as 100 to 200 IU of vitamin E, preferably from mixed natural tocopherols.

Vitamin C transport into cells may be impaired in many diabetics due to high levels of a sugar derivative called sorbitol—potentially resulting in a cellular vitamin C deficiency. Many studies show that blood levels of vitamin C are low in people with diabetes. Supplemental vitamin C helps normalize sorbitol metabolism, protects various proteins from free radical and glucose-induced damage, and may also promote normal blood lipid levels in diabetic people. Supplementing with moderately high doses of vitamin C (600 to 1,000 mg daily) is generally quite safe and well tolerated. People who are sensitive to acidic foods may wish to consider buffered forms of vitamin C, such as calcium ascorbate or Ester-C.

Glutathione is probably the body's most important antioxidant, especially for the eyes, including lens and retina. In diabetics and older non-diabetics, levels of glutathione in the lens of the eye rapidly decline—a factor that is linked to the development of cataracts. Cataracts are due to oxidized lens proteins, which have become cloudy enough to impair vision. Experts suggest that it is crucial to promote normal glutathione levels in the eyes. Dietary glutathione supplements, however, are ineffective, because glutathione is not efficiently absorbed by the intestinal tract. The best strategy to support the body's own glutathione synthesis is to supplement the diet with alpha-lipoic acid along with vitamins C and E, which recycle and/or spare the body's glutathione. A number of human studies support long-term supplementation with vitamins C and E to maintain normal eye health. Supplementation with N-acetylcysteine (NAC) also increases the body's glutathione production, because NAC is the most important building block of glutathione. NAC supplementation, however, is most beneficial in fairly large amounts (1 to 5 g daily) to augment the body's glutathione levels.

Among the B vitamins, folic acid (folate), B_{12}, and B_6 are important for cardiovascular health, primarily because they help reduce blood levels of a potentially dangerous amino acid called homocysteine. High blood levels of homocysteine are now considered to be a major risk factor for cardiovascular disease. Several clinical studies have shown that people with diabetes often have high homocysteine levels. Considering that most of us do not meet the Recommended Dietary Allowances (RDAs) for folic acid, B_{12}, and B_6, daily supplementation at RDA levels or higher can be recommended. Multivitamin supplements that deliver all B vitamins at such levels are usually adequate for this purpose.

Niacin is another B vitamin of special importance to diabetics, because 100 mg per day of niacin has been shown to improve glucose tolerance and fasting blood sugar in diabetics when cosupplemented with chromium. Although megadose niacin (1.5 to 3 g daily) may preserve pancreas function and lower blood sugar, the evidence is controversial, and many people experience skin flushing as well as a higher risk of liver damage. Megadose niacin should only be taken under the supervision of a physician.

Essential fatty acids may provide unique benefits in terms of nerve function to people with diabetes. Supplements containing evening primrose oil or fish oil are a convenient way for many people to add these essential fatty acids to their diets. Double-blind clinical studies show that daily supplementation with 6 g of evening primrose oil can improve nerve function in people with diabetic neuropathy. Evening primrose oil is generally well tolerated and safe, and is widely available in soft gel capsules of 500 to 1,000 mg. Supplementation with large amounts (10 to 30 g daily) of fish oil (rich in omega-3 fatty acids) can lower blood viscosity (platelet aggregation) and serum triglyceride levels and therefore address some of the cardiovascular concerns of diabetic people. Fish oil may also improve kidney function. However, some clinical studies also found a worsening of blood sugar control in diabetics, which may be overcome by simultaneous vitamin E supplementation. When supplementing with high-dose fish oil, diabetic patients should carefully monitor their blood sugar levels and take additional vitamin E (e.g., 5 IU for each gram of fish oil).

Gymnema sylvestre is a woody vine used in traditional Ayurvedic medicine in India. In Hindi, it is referred to as *gurmar,* which means "sugar destroyer." *Gymnema sylvestre*'s active compounds are poorly understood; however, saponins known as gymnemic acids and a protein compound called gurmarin appear to play a role. The standardization level for gymnemic acids is not fully known, and other constituents in the crude extract have been reported to inhibit nutrient absorption. A *Gymnema sylvestre* extract called GS4 was developed that supposedly has these absorption inhibitors removed. It's not entirely understood how GS4 lowers blood sugar, but it seems to inhibit glucose absorption in the intestine. Two open-label clinical studies showed that GS4 lowered blood sugar in people with type 1 and type 2 diabetes at doses of 200 to 400 mg daily. No side effects were reported, but in one of these studies some subjects with type 2 diabetes needed to adjust their insulin doses to avoid hypoglycemia.

Banaba leaf extract is a newcomer among standardized diabetes herbs and is currently sold under the trade name Glucosol. The active marker compound in Glucosol, corosolic acid, has been shown to promote the transport of blood sugar into cells. Glucosol is standardized to provide a minimum of 1 percent corosolic acid. The extract has been shown to be well tolerated and safe in humans and in animal studies. Compared to other herbal extracts used by people with diabetes, Glucosol offers the advantage that it can lower blood sugar in diabetic people without causing hypoglycemia and can do so at a low dose of 16 to 48 mg daily. A series of recent and still unpublished clinical studies showed significant benefits of Glucosol when taken daily for thirty days at 32 to 48 mg per day. One of these studies was a randomized, double-blind crossover study with twelve diabetic subjects taking 48 mg of the extract. Glucosol lowered fasting blood sugar in people with type 2 diabetes, and the effect was sustained for several weeks even after discontinuation of the supplement.

Bitter melon *(Momordica charantia)* fruit has been used traditionally in Asia and South America as a folk remedy for diabetes and other ailments. Small, poorly designed studies of various bitter melon juices and powders indicate that it may lower blood sugar in diabetic people, but the overall evidence is inconclusive. High doses taken for long periods of time may cause liver toxicity. Based on current findings, bitter melon cannot be recommended for people with diabetes.

Panax (Asian) *ginseng* has been used for over 1,000 years as a folk remedy in China and Korea. Various animal studies show that Asian ginseng can lower blood sugar, improve glucose utilization, and increase insulin production. A placebo-controlled clinical study showed that 100 to 200 mg of an Asian ginseng extract reduced hemoglobin glycosylation and improved glucose tolerance in type 2 diabetic patients without side effects. The standard dose is 100 to 200 mg daily of extracts standardized to 4 to 7 percent ginsenosides. However, the antidiabetic activity appears to be due to compounds other than the ginsenosides, and this lack of standardization can result in variable activity of commercially available Asian ginseng extracts. High doses may result in hypertension in susceptible people and are not recommended during pregnancy and for people who have elevated blood pressure.

Fenugreek is a well-known spice that has been used in Asia and Africa to treat various ailments including diabetes. The active, blood sugar–lowering principles of fenugreek have not been entirely elucidated, but dietary fiber and saponins may contribute. The available clinical studies used defatted fenugreek seeds, and the trials were small and not well designed. The major drawback of fenugreek is that it takes a lot (15 to 100 g daily) of fenugreek seeds to obtain an effect. Mild gastrointestinal upset is the most common side effect.

SUMMARY

There are a number of well-documented nutritional and herbal ingredients that can be very useful in the management of type 1 and type 2 diabetes as well as metabolic syndrome X and prediabetes. A good supplement for people with diabetes should address potential nutrient deficiencies, antioxidant support, nerve protection, and blood sugar/insulin function. The recommended ingredients are listed in Table 17.1. All of these nutrients or herbs should be taken with meals for maximum benefit and tolerance. Pregnant and lactating women and people with diabetes should seek the advice of a qualified health care professional before starting to use these and other dietary supplements.

TABLE 17.1. Dietary Supplements for Support During Diabetes

Ingredient	Dose (per day)	Primary claims and notes
Alpha-lipoic acid	100-600 mg/day	Antioxidant; protects from nerve damage. Higher doses not necessarily better.
Banaba leaf extract	32-48 mg/day of Glucosol extract	Promotes normal blood sugar and glucose tolerance. Look for extracts standardized to min. 1 percent corosolic acid.
Chromium	200-1,000 mcg/day	Corrects deficiency; needed for insulin action. Best from organically bound sources.
Evening primrose oil	3-6 g/day	Improves nerve function.
Fish oil	10-30 g/day	Improves blood lipids and blood viscosity. Look for at least 5 IU vitamin E/g.
Folic acid (folate)	400-1,000 mcg/day	Lowers homocysteine. Best from multivitamin.
Gymnema sylvestre	200-400 mg/day of GS4 extract	Promotes normal blood sugar. Look for extracts standardized to min. 25 percent gymnemic acids.
Magnesium	150-400 mg/day	Corrects deficiency; nerve and heart function. Best from organic acid salts and chelates.
Vanadium	10-100 mcg/day	Needed for insulin action. Megadoses (over 100 mcg) may not be safe.
Vitamin B_{12}	Min. 6 mcg/day	Lowers homocysteine. Best from multivitamin.
Vitamin B_6	2-50 mg/day	Lowers homocysteine. Best from multivitamin.
Vitamin C	600-1,000 mg/day	Antioxidant; helps normalize sorbitol levels. Best tolerated as calcium ascorbate.
Vitamin E	100-200 IU/day	Antioxidant; protects proteins and has cardiovascular benefits. Preferably from natural mixed tocopherols.
Zinc	7.5-30 mg/day	Corrects deficiency; needed for insulin action. Best taken as part of a multivitamin.

CHROMIUM

What Is It?

Chromium is an essential trace mineral that aids in glucose metabolism, regulation of insulin levels, and maintenance of healthy blood levels of cholesterol and other lipids. Chromium forms part of a compound in the body known as glucose tolerance factor (GTF), which is involved in regulating the actions of insulin in maintaining blood sugar levels and, possibly, in helping to control appetite. Food sources include brewer's yeast, whole grain cereals, broccoli, prunes, mushrooms, and beer. The most widely available supplements are chromium salts such as chromium polynicotinate, chromium picolinate, and chromium chloride.

Claims

- Lowers blood sugar
- Increases insulin sensitivity
- Reduces body fat
- Controls hunger/suppresses appetite
- Reduces cholesterol and triglyceride levels
- Increases lean body mass/muscle mass

Theory

Chromium deficiency is known to lead to glucose intolerance and insulin resistance—symptoms commonly encountered in people with diabetes. Since chromium helps regulate the actions of insulin (as a constituent of glucose tolerance factor), chromium supplements may help support the many functions of insulin in the body, such as maintaining blood sugar and cholesterol levels and controlling appetite (particularly sweet cravings). Chromium is notorious for its poor absorption by the body, so many supplements are combined with another, more efficiently absorbed compound such as a vitamin (such as niacin in chromium polynicotinate) or an amino acid derivative (such as picolinic acid, a derivative of tryptophan, in chromium picolinate).

Scientific Support

Chromium supplementation rapidly gained popularity in the mid and late 1980s when studies suggested chromium supplements (200 mcg per day) were associated with anabolic effects (increased muscle mass and reduced body fat). In diabetic and overweight individuals, chromium supplements have been shown to reduce triglyceride levels by almost 20 percent, improve glucose tolerance, and normalize insulin levels. Supplements of 400 mcg have helped overweight women lose about 50 percent more fat in three months than a placebo group. Subsequent studies, however, have been equivocal on the effect of chromium on muscle and fat mass—with nearly a 50/50 split between studies showing a beneficial effect of the supplements and those showing no effect. Some of the "positive" studies have been criticized for using inaccurate or imprecise measures of body composition to arrive at their conclusions that chromium is beneficial for weight loss.

What we *do* know about chromium, however, is that deficiency of the mineral results in insulin resistance that can be easily corrected by supplements. Chromium deficiency is not unknown in the United States and is thought to contribute to insulin resistance in many people. It is estimated that 90 percent of Americans consume less than the recommended amount of chromium each day. Also, the urinary excretion of chromium is known to increase in people who exercise, suggesting that active people and athletes may have higher dietary requirements for chromium.

Safety

Although the vast majority of studies of chromium supplementation reveal no side effects except mild gastrointestinal upset, they tend to be of short duration (a few weeks to a few months). Recent anecdotal reports, however, have suggested a variety of adverse side effects such as anemia, memory loss, and DNA damage—in most cases for a particular form of chromium known as chromium picolinate.

A handful of laboratory (test-tube) studies have shown that chromium in the picolinate form (chromium III) causes DNA breakage in isolated cells. Such DNA effects are thought to lead to genetic mutations and cancer, but it is important to note that these cell studies in the test tube are far removed from the case of a human ingesting an essential trace mineral. In one of the most publicized studies, Dartmouth researchers demonstrated that chromium picolinate is absorbed into cells intact (at least in the test tube), where it causes breaks in chromosomal DNA in hamster ovary cells (a common test model for cancer researchers). The upshot of the study was that other chromium salts, such as nicotinate and chloride, were not taken up into the cells as efficiently as the picolinate version.

There have been a few case reports of adverse effects following high-dose chromium supplementation. In one, a twenty-four-year-old female bodybuilder developed rhabdomyolysis, a serious condition causing muscle and kidney toxicity, after ingesting 1,200 mcg of chromium picolinate over forty-eight hours. This is six to twenty-four times the daily recommended allowance of 50 to 200 mcg. Another case of toxicity following chromium picolinate ingestion (1,200 to 2,400 mcg for four to five months) involved a thirty-three-year-old woman who was taking it to enhance weight loss. The supplement increased blood chromium levels to two to three times normal and caused anemia, blood abnormalities, liver dysfunction, and renal failure.

Both case reports demonstrate the fact that intakes of chromium picolinate at levels above the recommended dosage should be avoided. In an animal study conducted by the USDA, rats fed a diet rich in chromium picolinate for twenty-four weeks showed no adverse side effects. No clinical studies show harmful effects in humans from supplements containing chromium picolinate. It would seem prudent, however, to avoid excessive intake of supplements containing chromium picolinate and, where possible, to select supplements that use alternate forms of chromium such as nicotinate, chloride, or other amino acid chelates.

Value

A few years ago, the Federal Trade Commission cracked down on several chromium companies for making unsubstantiated claims about the ability of chromium to "magically" melt away body fat without diets or exercise. The majority of claims now are couched in the "maintain and promote" terminology permitted by the Dietary Supplement Health and Education Act. However, because more than 90 percent of American diets fail to provide the recommended amount of chromium, and chromium supplements have been shown to be effective in maintaining insulin function and in helping some dieters lose body fat, chromium supplements may be an effective supplement for individuals seeking better control of blood sugar and appetite (sweet cravings).

Dosage

The most widely available supplements are chromium salts such as chromium polynicotinate, chromium picolinate, and various chromium/amino acid chelates, which help increase the absorption and availability compared to isolated chromium salts such as chromium chloride (which has an extremely low gastrointestinal absorption rate).

No RDA has been established for chromium, but the ESADDI (estimated safe and adequate daily dietary intake) is 50 to 200 mcg. Natural forms of supplemental chromium, such as chromium-rich yeast, may be absorbed somewhat more efficiently than inorganic forms of chromium, such as chloride, which are found in some supplements. One ounce of brewer's yeast provides approximately 100 to 200 mcg of chromium.

WORKS CONSULTED

Anderson RA. Effects of chromium on body composition and weight loss. Nutr Rev. 1998 Sep;56(9):266-70.

Bahadori B, Wallner S, Schneider H, Wascher TC, Toplak H. Effect of chromium yeast and chromium picolinate on body composition of obese, non-diabetic patients during and after a formula diet. Acta Med Austriaca. 1997;24(5):185-7.

Cerulli J, Grabe DW, Gauthier I, Malone M, McGoldrick MD. Chromium picolinate toxicity. Ann Pharmacother. 1998 Apr;32(4):428-31.

Flatt PR, Juntti-Berggren L, Berggren PO, Gould BJ, Swanston-Flatt SK. Failure of glucose tolerance factor-containing Brewer's yeast to ameliorate spontaneous diabetes in C57BL/KsJ DB/DB mice. Diabetes Res. 1989 Mar;10(3):147-51.

Grant KE, Chandler RM, Castle AL, Ivy JL. Chromium and exercise training: Effect on obese women. Med Sci Sports Exerc. 1997 Aug;29(8):992-8.

McCarty MF. Chromium and other insulin sensitizers may enhance glucagon secretion: Implications for hypoglycemia and weight control. Med Hypotheses. 1996 Feb;46(2):77-80.

Reading SA. Chromium picolinate. J Fla Med Assoc. 1996 Jan;83(1):29-31.

Trent LK, Thieding-Cancel D. Effects of chromium picolinate on body composition. J Sports Med Phys Fitness. 1995 Dec;35(4):273-80.

Uusitupa MI, Mykkanen L, Siitonen O, Laakso M, Sarlund H, Kolehmainen P, Rasanen T, Kumpulainen J, Pyorala K. Chromium supplementation in impaired glucose tolerance of elderly: Effects on blood glucose, plasma insulin, C-peptide and lipid levels. Br J Nutr. 1992 Jul;68(1):209-16.

Walker LS, Bemben MG, Bemben DA, Knehans AW. Chromium picolinate effects on body composition and muscular performance in wrestlers. Med Sci Sports Exerc. 1998 Dec;30(12):1730-7.

VANADIUM

What Is It?

Vanadium is an essential trace mineral that has only recently been identified as being truly essential in humans. A normal diet typically provides about 10 to 30 mcg of vanadium per day. Although no RDA is currently established, this amount appears to be adequate for most healthy adults. Supplemental vanadium is usually in the vanadyl or vanadate forms. Vanadium is thought to play a role in metabolism of carbohydrates and may have functions in cholesterol and blood lipid metabolism. In diabetics, vanadium supplements may have a positive effect in regulating blood glucose levels. Food sources of vanadium include seafood, mushrooms, some cereals, and soybeans.

Claims

- Mimics insulin action
- Lowers blood sugar
- Increases muscle mass
- Increases muscle vascularity and blood flow ("pumped feeling")
- Increases glycogen synthesis and storage

Theory

Vanadium, or the most common supplemental form, vanadyl sulfate, is thought to mimic the physiological effects of insulin by a mechanism that remains unclear. Through this insulin-mimetic effect, vanadium is thought to promote glycogen synthesis, maintain blood glucose levels, and stimulate protein synthesis for muscle growth.

Scientific Support

Vanadyl sulfate supplements have been shown to normalize blood glucose levels and reduce glycosylated hemoglobin levels in patients with non–insulin-dependent diabetes mellitus (NIDDM). Also in NIDDM patients, vanadium sulfate (100 mg per day—a *huge* dose) can reduce fasting glucose levels by about 20 percent and decrease hepatic insulin resistance. Normal (nondiabetic) subjects typically do not exhibit a significant change in glucose uptake or lipolysis, but vanadyl sulfate may acutely stimulate amino acid transport into skeletal muscle. Studies of vanadyl sulfate for

weight loss and exercise performance have been variable, with most showing only modest (if any) effects on body composition. Although vanadium
has become a popular dietary supplement among bodybuilders, there is limited data to support claims of increased muscle mass and strength.

Safety

Limited information is available about vanadium toxicity. Traditionally,
vanadium is considered quite safe in humans (because of its poor absorption). Some studies have suggested, however, that patients with bipolar
disorder have elevated blood and tissue levels of vanadium. In one safety
study, 100 mg of vanadyl sulfate (close to 10,000 times higher than dietary
needs) was given to NIDDM subjects for four weeks (50 mg twice per day).
Gastrointestinal side effects were experienced by 75 percent of the subjects
during the first week, but the supplements were well tolerated after that. The
authors of the study concluded that vanadyl sulfate resulted in modest reductions of fasting plasma glucose, but they cautioned that the safety of
large doses of vanadium supplements for long periods remained uncertain.
It is thought that prolonged exposure to excessive vanadium could cause
muscle cramps, emotional depression, and damage to the nervous system
and other organs. Some animal studies have suggested the possibility of hematological and biochemical changes, reproductive and developmental toxicity, and pro-oxidative effects on glutathione, ascorbic acid, and lipids following prolonged vanadium supplementation.

Value

Vanadium is an essential trace mineral that is not contained in many multi-
vitamin/mineral supplements. It is thought, however, that we obtain enough
vanadium from our diets. For individuals concerned with maintaining blood
glucose levels, such as diabetics or people with hypoglycemia (low blood
sugar), a vanadium supplement may be beneficial. Some bodybuilding and
diabetic dietary supplements contain vanadium at *milligram* levels—when
dietary needs are likely to be only in *microgram* amounts (1,000 times lower).
Prolonged consumption of high-dose vanadium supplements is not recommended.

Dosage

There is no Daily Value or Recommended Dietary Allowance for vanadium. Vanadium is now considered an essential trace mineral, and 10 mcg

per day is thought to satisfy the body's basic needs (our diets probably contain about 10 to 30 mcg of vanadium per day).

WORKS CONSULTED

Clarkson PM, Rawson ES. Nutritional supplements to increase muscle mass. Crit Rev Food Sci Nutr. 1999 Jul;39(4):317-28.

Cohen N, Halberstam M, Shlimovich P, Chang CJ, Shamoon H, Rossetti L. Oral vanadyl sulfate improves hepatic and peripheral insulin sensitivity in patients with non-insulin-dependent diabetes mellitus. J Clin Invest. 1995 Jun;95(6):2501-9.

Dehghani GA, Ahmadi S, Omrani GR. Effects of vanadyl sulphate on glucose homeostasis in severe diabetes induced by streptozotocin in rats. Indian J Med Res. 1997 Nov;106:481-5.

Goldfine AB, Patti ME, Zuberi L, Goldstein BJ, LeBlanc R, Landaker EJ, Jiang ZY, Willsky GR, Kahn CR. Metabolic effects of vanadyl sulfate in humans with non-insulin-dependent diabetes mellitus: In vivo and in vitro studies. Metabolism. 2000 Mar;49(3):400-10.

Halberstam M, Cohen N, Shlimovich P, Rossetti L, Shamoon H. Oral vanadyl sulfate improves insulin sensitivity in NIDDM but not in obese nondiabetic subjects. Diabetes. 1996 May;45(5):659-66.

Hoeger WW, Harris C, Long EM, Hopkins DR. Four-week supplementation with a natural dietary compound produces favorable changes in body composition. Adv Ther. 1998 Sep-Oct;15(5):305-14.

Jandhyala BS, Hom GJ. Minireview: Physiological and pharmacological properties of vanadium. Life Sci. 1983 Oct 3;33(14):1325-40.

Kreider RB. Dietary supplements and the promotion of muscle growth with resistance exercise. Sports Med. 1999 Feb;27(2):97-110.

McCarty MF. Complementary measures for promoting insulin sensitivity in skeletal muscle. Med Hypotheses. 1998 Dec;51(6):451-64.

Nechay BR. Mechanisms of action of vanadium. Annu Rev Pharmacol Toxicol. 1984;24:501-24.

Preuss HG, Jarrell ST, Scheckenbach R, Lieberman S, Anderson RA. Comparative effects of chromium, vanadium and Gymnema sylvestre on sugar-induced blood pressure elevations in SHR. J Am Coll Nutr. 1998 Apr;17(2):116-23.

Zorbas YG, Federenko YF, Naexu KA. Urinary excretion of microelements in endurance-trained volunteers during restriction of muscular activity and chronic rehydration. Biol Trace Elem Res. 1994 Mar;40(3):189-202.

BANABA LEAF/COROSOLIC ACID

What Is It?

Banaba *(Lagerstroemia speciosa)* is a medicinal plant that grows in India, Southeast Asia, and the Philippines. Traditional uses include brewing tea from the leaves as a treatment for diabetes and hyperglycemia (elevated blood sugar). The hypoglycemic (blood sugar-lowering) effect of banaba leaf extract is similar to that of insulin, which induces glucose transport from the blood into body cells.

Claims

- Balances blood sugar
- Promotes healthy insulin levels
- Controls appetite and food craving (especially carbohydrate cravings)
- May promote weight loss

Theory

Banaba leaf extract contains a triterpenoid compound known as corosolic acid, which has actions in stimulating glucose transport into cells. As such, banaba plays a role in regulating levels of blood sugar and insulin in the blood. For some people, fluctuations in blood sugar and insulin are related to appetite, hunger, and various food cravings—particularly craving for carbohydrates such as bread and sweets. By keeping blood sugar and insulin levels in check, banaba may be an effective supplement for promoting weight loss in certain individuals.

Scientific Support

The blood sugar-regulating properties of banaba have been demonstrated in cell culture, animal, and human studies. In isolated cells, the active ingredient in banaba extract, corosolic acid, is known to stimulate glucose uptake. In diabetic mice, rats, and rabbits, banaba feeding reduces elevated blood sugar and insulin levels to normal. In humans with type II diabetes, banaba extract, at a dose of 16 to 48 mg per day for four to eight weeks, has been shown to be effective in reducing blood sugar levels (5 to 30 percent reduction) and maintaining tighter control of blood sugar fluctuations. An interesting side effect of tighter control of blood sugar and insulin levels is a significant tendency of banaba to promote weight loss (an average of 2 to

4 lb per month)—without significant dietary alterations. It is likely that modulation of glucose and insulin levels reduces total caloric intake somewhat and encourages moderate weight loss.

Safety

At suggested doses, 16 to 48 mg per day, no adverse side effects are expected from banaba extract. Higher doses should be avoided, however, to prevent possible hypoglycemic effects (headache, dizziness, fatigue) commonly associated with extremely low blood glucose levels.

Value

As a dietary supplement to help reduce elevated levels of sugar and insulin in the blood, banaba extract has been shown to be safe and effective. As a weight loss aid, a handful of small studies in humans have suggested that tighter control of blood glucose and insulin can help promote moderate weight loss.

Dosage

Doses of banaba extract in the range of 16 to 48 mg per day, consumed in divided doses with meals, are effective in reducing or modulating blood glucose and insulin levels. Higher doses should be avoided due to the potential for hypoglycemia (low blood sugar).

WORKS CONSULTED

Kakuda T, Sakane I, Takihara T, Ozaki Y, Takeuchi H, Kuroyanagi M. Hypoglycemic effect of extracts from Lagerstroemia speciosa L. leaves in genetically diabetic KK-AY mice. Biosci Biotechnol Biochem. 1996 Feb;60(2):204-8.

Murakami C, Myoga K, Kasai R, Ohtani K, Kurokawa T, Ishibashi S, Dayrit F, Padolina WG, Yamasaki K. Screening of plant constituents for effect on glucose transport activity in Ehrlich ascites tumour cells. Chem Pharm Bull (Tokyo). 1993 Dec;41(12):2129-31.

Suzuki Y, Unno T, Ushitani M, Hayashi K, Kakuda T. Antiobesity activity of extracts from Lagerstroemia speciosa L. leaves on female KK-AY mice. J Nutr Sci Vitaminol (Tokyo). 1999 Dec;45(6):791-5.

FENUGREEK

What Is It?

Fenugreek seeds *(Trigonella foenum-graecum)* are used as a traditional spice in Asia and Europe. They have a slight maple taste and are often used in the production of imitation maple flavorings. Fenugreek seeds contain a high proportion (40 percent) of a soluble fiber known as mucilage. This fiber forms a gelatinous structure (similar to guar gum), which may have effects on slowing the digestion and absorption of food from the intestine.

Claims

- Reduces blood sugar (controls diabetes)
- Lowers cholesterol levels
- Suppresses appetite and promotes weight loss

Theory

There is certainly a large body of evidence that dietary intake of soluble fiber can slow down the digestion and absorption of food and may result in a slower rise in blood sugar in some individuals. Other compounds identified through chemical analysis of the seeds, such as the saponins, may have a beneficial role in lowering cholesterol production in the liver.

Scientific Support

At least a few studies have shown a beneficial effect of fenugreek in reducing blood glucose levels and improving glucose tolerance in patients with diabetes. In terms of weight control, the soluble fiber in fenugreek seeds can reduce dietary fat absorption by binding to fatty acids as well as creating a sensation of fullness to reduce appetite. Finally, because fenugreek seeds contain estrogen-like saponins, blood levels of total cholesterol, LDL, and triglycerides can be reduced (with no change in HDL)— providing an important heart benefit.

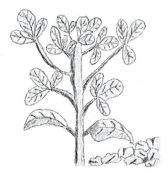

In one study, 15 g of powdered fenugreek seeds soaked in water significantly reduced postprandial glucose and insulin levels following a meal in non–insulin-dependent diabetics. Another study showed that an amino acid extracted from fenugreek seeds (4-hydroxy-isoleucine) may stimulate insulin secretion via a direct stimulation of beta cells and help control blood sugar levels in rats and dogs. In a group of insulin-dependent diabetic patients, defatted fenugreek seed powder (100 g given in two doses of 50 g each at lunch and dinner) significantly reduced fasting blood sugar and improved glucose tolerance over a ten-day period. There was also a 54 percent reduction in urinary glucose excretion and a significant reduction in blood levels of total cholesterol, LDL, VLDL, and triglycerides with no change in HDL levels.

Safety

The soluble fiber in fenugreek seeds has the potential to reduce the absorption of fats as well as many vitamins and minerals when consumed in large amounts, so caution is warranted to ensure proper dietary intake. Pregnant women should avoid consuming fenugreek due to reports that it may stimulate uterine contractions.

Value

The levels of fenugreek seed that have been associated with lower blood sugar and cholesterol values are quite high at 15 to 20 g per day. Few, if any, commercial preparations supply anywhere near this level of fenugreek, so check the labels.

Dosage

Defatted fenugreek seed powder is available as raw powder to be added to other foods or liquids and in capsule or tablet form. Consumption of 15 to 20 g per day is effective in controlling blood sugar, while higher levels (up to 100 g) may be needed to effectively suppress appetite for weight loss purposes.

WORKS CONSULTED

Bhardwaj PK, Dasgupta DJ, Prashar BS, Kaushal SS. Control of hyperglycaemia and hyperlipidaemia by plant product. J Assoc Physicians India. 1994 Jan;42(1):33-5.
Bordia A, Verma SK, Srivastava KC. Effect of ginger (Zingiber officinale Rosc.) and fenugreek (Trigonella foenumgraecum L.) on blood lipids, blood sugar and

platelet aggregation in patients with coronary artery disease. Prostaglandins Leukot Essent Fatty Acids. 1997 May;56(5):379-84.

Broca C, Gross R, Petit P, Sauvaire Y, Manteghetti M, Tournier M, Masiello P, Gomis R, Ribes G. 4-Hydroxyisoleucine: Experimental evidence of its insulino-tropic and antidiabetic properties. Am J Physiol. 1999 Oct;277(4 Pt 1):E617-23.

Genet S, Kale RK, Baquer NZ. Effects of vanadate, insulin and fenugreek (Trigonella foenum graecum) on creatine kinase levels in tissues of diabetic rat. Indian J Exp Biol. 1999 Feb;37(2):200-2.

Gupta D, Raju J, Baquer NZ. Modulation of some gluconeogenic enzyme activities in diabetic rat liver and kidney: Effect of antidiabetic compounds. Indian J Exp Biol. 1999 Feb;37(2):196-9.

Khosla P, Gupta DD, Nagpal RK. Effect of Trigonella foenum graecum (Fenu-greek) on blood glucose in normal and diabetic rats. Indian J Physiol Pharmacol. 1995 Apr;39(2):173-4.

Madar Z, Abel R, Samish S, Arad J. Glucose-lowering effect of fenugreek in non-insulin dependent diabetics. Eur J Clin Nutr. 1988 Jan;42(1):51-4.

Pavithran K. Fenugreek in diabetes mellitus. J Assoc Physicians India. 1994 Jul;42(7):584.

Puri D. Therapeutic potentials of fenugreek. Indian J Physiol Pharmacol. 1998 Jul;42(3):423-4.

Raju J, Gupta D, Rao AR, Baquer NZ. Effect of antidiabetic compounds on glyoxalase I activity in experimental diabetic rat liver. Indian J Exp Biol. 1999 Feb;37(2):193-5.

Ravikumar P, Anuradha CV. Effect of fenugreek seeds on blood lipid peroxidation and antioxidants in diabetic rats. Phytother Res. 1999 May;13(3):197-201.

Riyad MA, Abdul-Salam SA, Mohammad SS. Effect of fenugreek and lupine seeds on the development of experimental diabetes in rats. Planta Med. 1988 Aug;54(4):286-90.

Sauvaire Y, Ribes G, Baccou JC, Loubatieeres-Mariani MM. Implication of steroid saponins and sapogenins in the hypocholesterolemic effect of fenugreek. Lipids. 1991 Mar;26(3):191-7.

Sharma RD, Raghuram TC, Rao NS. Effect of fenugreek seeds on blood glucose and serum lipids in type I diabetes. Eur J Clin Nutr. 1990 Apr;44(4):301-6.

Swanston-Flatt SK, Day C, Flatt PR, Gould BJ, Bailey CJ. Glycaemic effects of traditional European plant treatments for diabetes. Studies in normal and streptozotocin diabetic mice. Diabetes Res. 1989 Feb;10(2):69-73.

GYMNEMA/GURMAR

What Is It?

Gymnema sylvestre is a plant used medicinally in India and Southeast Asia for treatment of "sweet urine," or what we refer to in the West as diabetes or hyperglycemia. Gymnema leaves, whether extracted or infused into a tea, suppress glucose absorption and reduce the sensation of sweetness in foods—effects that may deliver important health benefits for individuals who want to reduce blood sugar levels or body weight.

Claims

- Reduces blood sugar levels
- Lowers blood cholesterol levels
- Balances insulin levels
- Promotes weight loss
- Reduces sugar cravings

Theory

Gymnema sylvestre leaves contain gymnemic acids, which are known to suppress transport of glucose from the intestine into the bloodstream, and a small protein, gurmarin, that can interact with receptors on the tongue to decrease the sensation of sweetness in many foods. This dual action has been shown to reduce blood sugar and cholesterol levels in diabetic animals and humans and may provide some benefits in terms of regulating appetite control and food cravings.

Scientific Support

The hypoglycemic (blood sugar-lowering) effect of gymnema has been known for centuries. Modern scientific methods have isolated at least nine different fractions of gymnemic acids that possess hypoglycemic activity. The effect of gymnema extract on lowering blood levels of glucose, cholesterol, and triglycerides is fairly gradual—typically taking a few days to several weeks. Very high doses of the dried gymnema leaves may even help to repair the cellular damage that causes diabetes by helping to regenerate the insulin-producing beta cells in the pancreas.

Several human studies conducted on gymnema for treatment of diabetes have shown significant reduction in blood glucose, glycosylated hemoglobin (an index of blood sugar control), and insulin requirements (so insulin therapy could be reduced). Gymnema appears to increase the effectiveness of insulin rather than causing the body to produce more—although the precise mechanism by which this occurs remains unknown. As with other natural ingredients for control of blood sugar and insulin levels, such as banaba leaf, a common side effect is weight loss, probably due to a combination of appetite suppression and control of food cravings (especially for carbohydrates and sweets).

Safety

At typical recommended doses (see Dosage), dietary supplements containing gymnema are not associated with significant adverse side effects. Mild gastrointestinal upset may occur if gymnema is taken on an empty stomach, so consumption with meals is recommended. Caution is urged, however, with extremely high doses, which may have the potential to induce hypoglycemia (abnormally low blood sugar) in susceptible individuals. In those with active diabetes, it is recommended to consult your personal physician before and during use of gymnema, as alterations to your dosage of insulin or other antidiabetic medications may be warranted. Certain medications, including antidepressants (St. John's wort) and salicylates (white willow and aspirin) can enhance the blood sugar-lowering effects of gymnema, whereas certain stimulants such as ephedra (ma huang) may reduce its effectiveness.

Value

As a dietary supplement to enhance control of blood glucose and insulin, *Gymnema sylvestre* appears to be effective—particularly in the case of individuals with diabetes or hyperglycemia (elevated blood sugar). As an agent to promote weight loss, gymnema may help control appetite and carbohydrate cravings, which may be helpful in some individuals attempting weight loss.

Dosage

Most human studies have been conducted in diabetic patients and have used 400 mg of gymnema extract per day in conjunction with conventional oral antidiabetic medications to lower blood glucose and reduce insulin requirements. In nondiabetics, smaller doses may be effective in helping to control blood sugar and insulin fluctuations—and the associated swings in appetite and food cravings. Because it acts gradually, gymnema extract should be consumed regularly with meals for several days or weeks and can be taken for months or years with no significant side effects.

WORKS CONSULTED

Baskaran K, Kizar Ahamath B, Radha Shanmugasundaram K, Shanmugasundaram ER. Antidiabetic effect of a leaf extract from Gymnema sylvestre in non-insulin-dependent diabetes mellitus patients. J Ethnopharmacol. 1990 Oct;30(3):295-300.

Chattopadhyay RR. Possible mechanism of antihyperglycemic effect of Gymnema sylvestre leaf extract. Gen Pharmacol. 1998 Sep;31(3):495-6.

Fushiki T, Kojima A, Imoto T, Inoue K, Sugimoto E. An extract of Gymnema sylvestre leaves and purified gymnemic acid inhibits glucose-stimulated gastric inhibitory peptide secretion in rats. J Nutr. 1992 Dec;122(12):2367-73.

Khare AK, Tondon RN, Tewari JP. Hypoglycaemic activity of an indigenous drug (Gymnema sylvestre, 'Gurmar') in normal and diabetic persons. Indian J Physiol Pharmacol. 1983 Jul-Sep;27(3):257-8.

Miyasaka A, Imoto T. Electrophysiological characterization of the inhibitory effect of a novel peptide gurmarin on the sweet taste response in rats. Brain Res. 1995 Apr 3;676(1):63-8.

Murakami N, Murakami T, Kadoya M, Matsuda H, Yamahara J, Yoshikawa M. New hypoglycemic constituents in "gymnemic acid" from Gymnema sylvestre. Chem Pharm Bull (Tokyo). 1996 Feb;44(2):469-71.

Okabayashi Y, Tani S, Fujisawa T, Koide M, Hasegawa H, Nakamura T, Fujii M, Otsuki M. Effect of Gymnema sylvestre, R.Br. on glucose homeostasis in rats. Diabetes Res Clin Pract. 1990 May-Jun;9(2):143-8.

Ota M, Shimizu Y, Tonosaki K, Ariyoshi Y. Role of hydrophobic amino acids in gurmarin, a sweetness-suppressing polypeptide. Biopolymers. 1998 Mar;45(3):231-8.

Ota M, Shimizu Y, Tonosaki K, Ariyoshi Y. Synthesis, characterization, and sweetness-suppressing activities of gurmarin analogues missing one disulfide bond. Biopolymers. 1998 Aug;46(2):65-73.

Shanmugasundaram ER, Gopinath KL, Radha Shanmugasundaram K, Rajendran VM. Possible regeneration of the islets of Langerhans in streptozotocin-diabetic rats given Gymnema sylvestre leaf extracts. J Ethnopharmacol. 1990 Oct;30(3):265-79.

Shanmugasundaram ER, Rajeswari G, Baskaran K, Rajesh Kumar BR, Radha Shanmugasundaram K, Kizar Ahmath B. Use of Gymnema sylvestre leaf extract in the control of blood glucose in insulin-dependent diabetes mellitus. J Ethnopharmacol. 1990 Oct;30(3):281-94.

Shanmugasundaram KR, Panneerselvam C, Samudram P, Shanmugasundaram ER. The insulinotropic activity of Gymnema sylvestre, R. Br. An Indian medical herb used in controlling diabetes mellitus. Pharmacol Res Commun. 1981 May;13(5):475-86.

Shimizu K, Abe T, Nakajyo S, Urakawa N, Atsuchi M, Yamashita C. Inhibitory effects of glucose utilization by gymnema acids in the guinea-pig ileal longitudinal muscle. J Smooth Muscle Res. 1996 Oct;32(5):219-28.

Shimizu K, Iino A, Nakajima J, Tanaka K, Nakajyo S, Urakawa N, Atsuchi M, Wada T, Yamashita C. Suppression of glucose absorption by some fractions extracted from Gymnema sylvestre leaves. J Vet Med Sci. 1997 Apr;59(4):245-51.

Shimizu K, Ozeki M, Tanaka K, Itoh K, Nakajyo S, Urakawa N, Atsuchi M. Suppression of glucose absorption by extracts from the leaves of Gymnema inodorum. J Vet Med Sci. 1997 Sep;59(9):753-7.

Srivastava Y, Nigam SK, Bhatt HV, Verma Y, Prem AS. Hypoglycemic and life-prolonging properties of Gymnema sylvestre leaf extract in diabetic rats. Isr J Med Sci. 1985 Jun;21(6):540-2.

Suttisri R, Lee IS, Kinghorn AD. Plant-derived triterpenoid sweetness inhibitors. J Ethnopharmacol. 1995 Jun 23;47(1):9-26.

Yoshikawa M, Murakami T, Kadoya M, Li Y, Murakami N, Yamahara J, Matsuda H. Medicinal foodstuffs. IX. The inhibitors of glucose absorption from the leaves of Gymnema sylvestre R. Br. (Asclepiadaceae): Structures of gymnemosides a and b. Chem Pharm Bull (Tokyo). 1997 Oct;45(10):1671-6.

Yoshikawa M, Murakami T, Matsuda H. Medicinal foodstuffs. X. Structures of new triterpene glycosides, gymnemosides-c, -d, -e, and -f, from the leaves of Gymnema sylvestre R. Br.: Influence of gymnema glycosides on glucose uptake in rat small intestinal fragments. Chem Pharm Bull (Tokyo). 1997 Dec;45(12):2034-8.

DIETARY SUPPLEMENT MASTER CHART

Supplement Ingredient	Weight	Sports	Energy	Bone	Joint	Brain	Heart	Immune	Eye	GI	Male	Female	Cancer	Diabetes
5-Hydroxytryptophan (5-HTP)	S					P								
Alfalfa							P							
Aloe vera										P				S
Alpha-lipoic acid									P					
Amino acids		P												
Androstenedione		P									S			
Antioxidants		S							P					
Arginine		S					P							
Astragalus								P						
Banaba														P
B-complex vitamins	S	S	P											
Bee Pollen		S	P											
Beta-carotene									P					
Beta-glucans								P						
Bilberry									P					
Black cohosh												P		
Bladderwrack	P											S		
Boron				P	S						S			
Boswellia		S			P						S			
Branched-chain amino acids		P				S								
Brewer's yeast		S	P											
Caffeine	S		P									S		
Calcium				P										

P = Primary indication
S = Secondary usage

Supplement Ingredient	Weight	Sports	Energy	Bone	Joint	Brain	Heart	Immune	Eye	GI	Male	Female	Cancer	Diabetes
Capsicum/cayenne	S									P				
Carnitine	P	S					S							
Carnosine		P												
Cat's claw								P						
Chitosan	P													
Choline						P								
Chondroitin					P									
Chromium	S	S												P
Citrus aurantium (synephrine)	P	S	S											
Coenzyme Q10		S	S				P	P						
Colostrum		S						S						
Conjugated linoleic acid (CLA)	P	P											S	
Cordyceps		P	S											
Cranberry												P		
Creatine		P												
Damiana											S	P		
Devil's claw					P									
DHEA		P									S	P		
Dong quai												P		
Echinacea								P						
Essential fatty acids					S	S	P							
Evening primrose oil							S					P		
Fenugreek	S													P
Feverfew						P								

P = Primary indication
S = Secondary usage

Supplement Ingredient	Weight	Sports	Energy	Bone	Joint	Brain	Heart	Immune	Eye	GI	Male	Female	Cancer	Diabetes
Fiber							S		S	P				
Flaxseed/linseed							P					S		
Folic acid							P					S		
GABA		P				S								
Gamma-Oryzanol		P												
Garlic							P							
Ginger										P				
Ginkgo biloba						P	S							
Ginseng		S	P											
Glucomannan	P													
Glucosamine					P									
Glutamine		S						P						
Glycerol		P												
Goldenseal								P						
Gotu kola												P		
Grape seed/pine bark		S						S	P				S	
Green-lipped mussel					P									
Green tea	S						S						P	
Guarana	P		S											
Gymnema	S													P
Hawthorn							P							
HMB		P												
Horse Chestnut							S					P		
Huperzine A						P								

P = Primary indication
S = Secondary usage

Supplement Ingredient	Weight	Sports	Energy	Bone	Joint	Brain	Heart	Immune	Eye	GI	Male	Female	Cancer	Diabetes
Hydrolyzed collagen protein		S			P									
Hydroxycitric acid (HCA)	P													
Inosine		S	P											
Iodine	P													
Kava kava						P								
Lutein/zeaxanthin									P					
Lycopene							S				P		S	
Ma Huang	P		S											
Maca											P			
Magnesium				P			S							
Mastic										P				
Medium chain triglycerides		P												
Melatonin						P								
Methylsulfonylmethane (MSM)		S			P									
Milk Thistle									S				P	
N-acetylcysteine (NAC)		S						S	P				S	
NADH		S	P											
Niacin							P							
Omega-3 fatty acids/Fish oil					S	S	P							
Ornithine alpha-ketoglutarate		P												
Perilla seed oil							S	P						
Phenylalanine (DLPA)		S				P								
Polyphenols							S	S	P				S	
Prebiotics/FOS										P				

P = Primary indication
S = Secondary usage

Supplement Ingredient	Weight	Sports	Energy	Bone	Joint	Brain	Heart	Immune	Eye	GI	Male	Female	Cancer	Diabetes
Probiotics (acidophilus)										P				
Protein	S	P												
Proteolytic enzymes		P			S									
Pygeum											P			
Pyruvate	P	S												
Quercetin	S								P					
Red clover				S			S					P		
Red yeast rice				S			P							
Rhodiola		S	P											
Ribose		P												
Royal Jelly		S	P											
S-adenosylmethionine					S	P								
Saw palmetto											P			
Schisandra			S										P	
Sea buckthorn			P											
Sea cucumber					P									
Selenium		S							S				P	
Shark/bovine cartilage					S								P	
Slippery elm										P				
Sodium bicarbonate		P		S										
Soy				S			P					S		
Spirulina			S											
St. John's wort	S					P							P	
Tribulus		P									S			

P = Primary indication
S = Secondary usage

Supplement Ingredient	Weight	Sports	Energy	Bone	Joint	Brain	Heart	Immune	Eye	GI	Male	Female	Cancer	Diabetes
Uva ursi/Bearberry														
Valerian						P						P		
Vanadium	S	S												P
Vinpocetine						P								
Vitamin A								P						
Vitamin B$_1$		S	P											
Vitamin B$_{12}$						S	P							
Vitamin B$_2$		S	P											
Vitamin B$_6$							P	S						
Vitamin C		S			S		P	S			S	S		
Vitamin D				P	S									
Vitamin E		S				S		P	S				S	
Vitamin K				P										
Vitex/chasteberry												P		
Whey protein		P												
White willow bark	P				S									
Yellow dock										P				
Yohimbe/quebracho		S									P			
Zinc		S		S	S			P			S			

P = Primary indication
S = Secondary usage

673

Index